FOUNDATIONS OF MORPHODYNAMICS IN OSTEOPATHY

An integrative approach to cranium, nervous system, and emotions

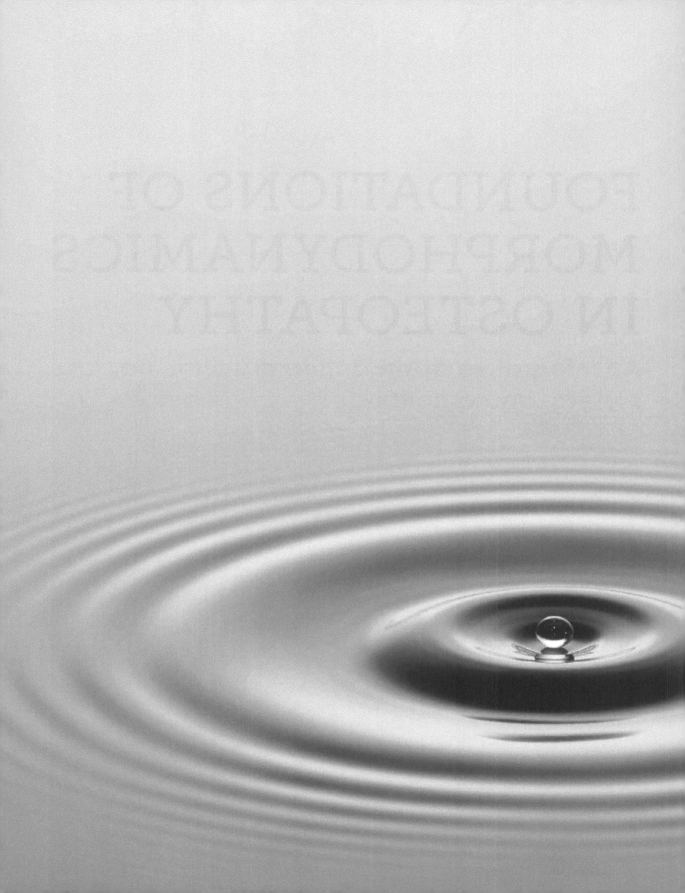

FOUNDATIONS OF MORPHODYNAMICS IN OSTEOPATHY

An integrative approach to cranium, nervous system, and emotions

Editors

Torsten LIEM and Patrick van den HEEDE

Forewords by
John Glover and Jean-Pierre Barral

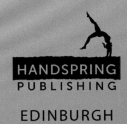

HANDSPRING PUBLISHING

EDINBURGH

HANDSPRING PUBLISHING LIMITED
The Old Manse, Fountainhall,
Pencaitland, East Lothian
EH34 5EY, Scotland
Tel: +44 1875 341 859
Website: www.handspringpublishing.com

First published 2017 in the United Kingdom by Handspring Publishing. This book is a much expanded
and revised translation of *Morphodynamik in der Osteopathie*, second edition (2013), published by Haug
Verlag, part of the Thieme Publishing Group.

2

ISBN (print version) 978-1-909141-24-7
ISBN (electronic version) 978-1-909141-63-6

British Library Cataloguing in Publication Data
A catalogue record for this book is available from the British Library

Library of Congress Cataloguing in Publication Data
A catalog record for this book is available from the Library of Congress

Notice
Neither the Publisher nor the Author assumes any responsibility for any loss or injury and/or damage to
persons or property arising out of or relating to any use of the material contained in this book. It is the
responsibility of the treating practitioner, relying on independent expertise and knowledge of the patient, to
determine the best treatment and method of application for the patient.

All reasonable efforts have been made to obtain copyright clearance for illustrations in the book for which the authors or publishers do not own the rights. If you believe that one of your illustrations has been used without such
clearance please contact the publishers and we will ensure that appropriate credit is given in the next reprint.

Commissioning Editor Andrew Stevenson
Copy Editor Joannah Duncan
Designer Bruce Hogarth, KinesisCreative
Indexer Aptara
Typesetter DiTech
Printer Ashford Colour Ltd

The authorised representative in the EEA is Hachette Ireland,
8 Castlecourt Centre, Dublin 15, D15 XTP3, Ireland (email: info@hbgi.ie)

Contents

Foreword

When Torsten Liem asked me to write a foreword to this book, I did not hesitate. I agreed to do it as I have now known Torsten and held him in the highest regard for a good 25 years.

These years have been defined by a vigorous exchange of ideas that has continued to develop and thus allowed our friendship to mature. From the beginning, I found myself delighted by Torsten's therapeutic curiosity and his constant pursuit of depth in osteopathic teaching. Both of these characteristics are reflected in this book.

A good textbook is built around current teaching methodology. It should also pose questions and deliver answers in line with documented research, yet at the same time reflect the plurality of scientific opinions. Most importantly, it should invite its readers to enter into a dialogue.

This completely revised and extended edition of Torsten's successful osteopathic guide *Morphodynamics in Osteopathy* reviews the state of the art, courageously breaking new ground and presenting both trainee and practising osteopaths with further perspectives and new approaches.

After Still's publications, *Foundations of Morphodynamics in Osteopathy* is one of the most inspiring of its kind in modern-day osteopathy. Therefore I am honored to have recognized some of my own approaches on reading it.

Jean-Pierre Barral DO

Former Chairman, International College of Osteopathy, St Etienne, France; former Chief, Department of Visceral Manipulation, Faculty of Medicine, Université de Paris Nord, France

Le Cailar, France, 2016

Foundations of Morphodynamics in Osteopathy is written in a way that challenges traditional osteopathic thinking and asks the reader to expand the osteopathic concept into new dimensions. The influences of dynamic morphology are portrayed in a very distinctive manner and are integrated into an osteopathic way of thinking and treatment: rhythmic, physical, biologic, developmental dynamics, emotional, and mental, as well as spiritual aspects. Philosophic concepts in the context of osteopathic procedures are discussed.

The reader is led step by step to understand that it is not enough to postulate the unity of 'body, mind, spirit'. We have to integrate the fine differentiations and dialectic dynamics of these subjective, intersubjective, and objective levels of reality into our daily actions.

The contributors, all experts in their field, build on the work, expanding on various aspects. The implications of the book for osteopathic thinking and approaches to the patient are numerous and may only be fully understood in the future.

Osteopathic Energetics is an important milestone in osteopathic literature!

John Glover DO, FAAO

Professor and Chairman, Department of Osteopathic Manipulative Medicine, Touro University College of Osteopathic Medicine, California

Vallejo, California, 2016

Preface to the English edition

This book is an expanded version of the originally published book by Torsten Liem *Morphodynamik in der Osteopathie* (2006). Each chapter of the earlier book has been completely revised and many new chapters added. This process took more than two years. Finally, a completely new book has emerged, with, as in the earlier book, a strong focus on the practical application of the osteopathic visions presented. Whilst the content of the work is rooted in the traditions of osteopathic philosophy, principles, models, approaches and techniques, in fact it reaches far beyond these foundations.

The central focus of this book lies on the *interplay between body and mind*, based on biological, neurophysiological and psychological interactions, as well as developmental and genetic influences on the human organism and how the knowledge of these factors can be embedded into the osteopathic treatment.

Based on evolutionary and ontogenetic evidence, one should consider *body-mind interaction* and *mind-body interaction* as two successive episodes of ontogenetic differentiation. They appear as two faces of the same medal. The concept of 'body' or 'embodiment' is an adaptive process that integrates information into matter and exposes this integrated information to an evolutionary wave pattern of adaptability to an ever changing and integrative essay of refinement of these elements.

The specificity of mind seems related to a specific transformation, when the mind starts to be 'personalized' by relating to a particular form of matter. The acuteness of appearance of certain types of disease could depend on time-related information that starts to interfere with the integrity of certain types of body-mind organization, which may be sensible at that moment for that specific information. It is clear that when energy and matter interfere, they create an evolutionary pattern of space-time relation that is specific for that particular form. Mind can be conceived as an

interactive expression between these two components, which, depending on its evolutionary level, creates an increasing probability of awareness and finally, consciousness.

The concept of *inner consciousness* is explored in more detail in several chapters of this book. Whilst mind is considered as requiring a foundation (body matter) first in order to be explicit and expressive, it then starts to inform and transform the body across changing space-time units of consciousness and awareness inside the 'most subtle and refined components of its constituents'. The ontology of mind is a story of mind building and maturation within a genetic and epigenetic landscape of body ontogenesis (ontogeny), whilst the phenomenology of mind is a story of condensation of space and time into the finest fractions of body awareness. *Body* matter potentiates mind maturation; later on, *mind* matter reorganizes body matter. *In fact, there is no separation between the two.*

The content of this book is organized by first approaching the frameworks of approximations to health, disease and healing. Then, body systems of regulation are discussed, followed by detailed descriptions of ontogenetic patterns of body and mind – always focused on the practical implications. Finally, diagnostic and treatment principles and the specific osteopathic approaches to cranium, nervous system, and emotions are outlined.

To a certain extent we can only perceive and palpate what we allow ourselves to perceive. This will depend on our expectations. For that, the chapters 'Paradigms of healing', 'The osteopathic object – reloaded', 'What is health? What is disease?' and 'Thoughts on the significance of systems theory for osteopathic diagnosis and therapy' are of significant importance. In these chapters, the development of healing systems and perspectives on health, disease and healing in relation to osteopathic approaches are discussed, allowing experiential space structures and horizons to develop and aid our palpatory perception. But questions are also raised and in attempting to formulate answers, an inner reflection and maturation process is set in motion, albeit with open ending.

The chapters 'Biological rhythms', 'Physical principles', 'Neurobiological principles', and 'The effect of formative and regulatory forces on living organisms' exploit basic organizational levels that may be considered as part of a holistic treatment. Hence, these chapters also include practical considerations. In chapters 7 to 11, ontogenetic dynamics are illustrated based on objective and subjective viewpoints, and are made accessible to the osteopath. These are important prerequisites to understanding and treating patients in their dynamics and development. They not only provide essential knowledge for the palpatory approach but also sensitize us to being empathic towards the earliest developmental stages of ontogeny. The chapters 'Evolution of the mind-body-spirit unit', 'Touch as therapeutic intervention', and 'The practitioner and therapeutic interaction' raise awareness of the many different aspects of the body-mind-spirit unit in the interaction between practitioner and patient.

The osteopathic specific concept of 'Somatic dysfunction and compensation' is presented and explored from different angles. This chapter is essential for understanding and implementing an osteopathic diagnostic assessment and diagnosis formation. Here, viewpoints of osteopathic philosophy, osteopathic principles and various osteopathic models are reflected and elaborated on.

The 'Experience of fulcrums' and 'The emergence of stillness' are key concepts within osteopathy, with phenomenological perspectives illustrated that provide possible approaches for clinical practice.

The chapters 'Principles of diagnosis' and 'Treatment principles' are the centerpiece of the book. The many threads that have been developed in previous chapters combine and merge here. Yet, at best they only represent practical suggestions for diagnosis and treatment. Every practitioner should seek to modify and add to them, according to their personal experiences, opinions and beliefs as well as the needs of the individual patient.

In the following chapters, specific osteopathic approaches are introduced, such as total rhythmic balanced interchange after Becker, and various approaches to midline structures. Energy bodies, including the chakra system, and the fluid body are illustrated in further chapters from developmental dynamic aspects, and conclusions for different therapeutic principles are provided.

Osteopathic approaches and principles are applied and implemented to structures of the head region in the chapters 27 to 36. Developmental dynamics of the bones of the skull, brain structures and cranial nerves and their approximation are made accessible to the osteopath by detailed descriptions of specific techniques. Here, some completely new approaches are presented. For example, in the chapter 'Developmental patterns and influence upon body organization', the palpation of cranial stages of flexion is described.

It is clear that these are not techniques in the strict sense, but rather therapeutic approximations towards dynamic interactions of structural and functional relationships. In fact, from our point of view, we would prefer not to speak of techniques, but instead 'deductions through possibilities', which generally arise during interaction of individual practitioners with the tissue structures of individual patients. In this sense, the palpatory approximations rather represent resonance phenomena of different density levels of tissue and time/space units, which are influenced by the mental images of the practitioner and their perceptions in the therapeutic context, and the process of dialogue between patient and practitioner.

Finally, chapter 37 discusses practical implications of the polyvagal theory, and chapter 38 presents an osteopathic approach to the treatment of trauma and emotional integration.

In summary, the purpose of this book is to outline and discuss the potential importance of these illustrated therapeutic models and phenomena for osteopathic practice as well as giving detailed descriptions of possible treatment approaches that address these factors. However, as with all knowledge that is passed on, questions will arise in the minds of those who consume this knowledge. We welcome all such questions in the hope and expectation that they will lead to fruitful discussions and new solutions.

Torsten Liem DO
Hamburg, October 2016

Patrick van den Heede DO
Orroir, October 2016

Preface to the first German edition

'Our wholeness, that part of it which is tangible, is the body, together with everything and every process within it. We inhabit this, as if living in an eerily enchanted castle—as oppressive as some fantastical vision conjured up by Kafka or Kubin. Masters we may be, but where is our dominance? Here we sit in the turret of our consciousness. Through its windows we see the world outside; through its doorway float the sounds of the castle's interior. We issue our orders, the service is delivered— but often enough strange faces bring the delivery, and in strange and confusing ways. They bring what we have not ordered, and what we did want often does not arrive—or, when it does, it is late or comes at an inconvenient time. The house is under a malign spell; we cannot find our way around its labyrinth. The servant hall seems often in league against us, or perhaps its denizens have flown or are engaged in festivities of their own. We can never be sure that there will not be insurrection; surely the place is haunted? Noises the other side of the wall, maybe poltergeists? Guests that we have not invited? Could it be the mob of servants whispering and arguing? What kind of life are these people living, and how many of them are there?

Heinrich Zimmer

When I began my search for an appropriate title to this book, I discussed this with Jim Jealous. At that time we thought 'Dynamics of Primary Respiration' would be a suitable title. After much further discussion and consideration, I arrived at 'Morphodynamics in Osteopathy' as best reflecting the content of the present book. One of the central questions that the book addresses concerns the influences, interactions and governing principles that determine the morphological dynamics and their application in osteopathic practice.

Human beings are more than the sum of soma and psyche; they are an indivisible psychosomatic unity. The tissue, the external element, is present throughout, extending up to the highest inner element, the highest consciousness. The increasing complexity of material form that emerges in the course of evolution goes hand in hand with an increasing sophistication of energies and inner consciousness; the more complex the basic material forms, the more subtle the accompanying energy patterns and fields. The material element (including the energy fields associated with it) is constantly present in this dynamic, which is both phylogenetic and ontogenetic. This external, objective element, the external form, permeates through to the highest inner, subjective level, the highest possible consciousness. The subjective reality of inner consciousness is the opposite number of the objective reality of the tissue structures and their associated energies. It is embedded in interobjective realities (the person's sociobiological environment) and intersubjective ones (culture and family).

However, it would be a mistake to suppose that inner experiences can be reduced to the energetic or physical level. If we are to treat the 'wholeness' of the person adequately, it is not enough to treat just the corresponding aspect of the tissue or the energy. We also need the capacity to discover the inner component of the consciousness that is being evidenced, and to take it into consideration.

Osteopaths' ability to perceive patterns of tissue-energy-consciousness in their patients will be determined by the extent of their own consciousness or awareness of their own inner selves with their sensorimotor, vital, emotional, mental and spiritual components, and that of their patients. This ability enables them to see the association between tissue and energy patterns and the inner dimensions, and to take account of them. The more they can do this, the more likely it is that treatment will not evoke further dissociative patterns.

When seeking solid methods for the treatment of tissue dysfunction complexes and the associated subjective patterns of consciousness, it helps to distinguish the various osteopathic approaches and their particular appropriateness, and to consider the developing interrelationships of structure and function.

This is the central theme of the present book. The methods presented should be seen as options; on no account should they be seen as dogmatically prescriptive. Each osteopath is invited to develop them further, to reconsider them in context, to differentiate or to integrate the suggestions.

The present-day demands placed on osteopathic treatment cannot be met either by a purely objective, scientific approach, or by visionary approaches with perhaps religious overtones.

Treatment methods do not exist in a vacuum; they develop in the particular context of their own historical, cultural and social environment. This formative environment, however, is generally taken so much for granted that the underlying belief patterns are not seen. If osteopathy is seen as a kind of visionary approach, this risks denying the cultural, social and scientific conditions of the time in which osteopathy developed (or in which osteopathic concepts such as 'somatic dysfunction' took shape). That closes off access to the potential of evolutionary developments. To arrive at a mature understanding of osteopathic methods of diagnosis and treatment, we need to realize how paradigms in the art of healing and our understanding of the body have changed over time. This book offers a detailed discussion of the ways in which these may have influenced osteopathy. It also discusses the differentiation between integrative approaches, and looks at their application in the therapeutic interaction. We can also draw on areas such as phenomenology and systems theory to find ideas that help osteopaths extend their diagnostic and therapeutic perspectives.

Although, from the point of view of phylogenetics, humanity has already achieved significant advances as compared to other living creatures, the situation is different when seen ontologically. Here, each individual human starts as it were from square one. As an individual, each has to pass through all the various levels as they encounter them in the course of their development. However, this also brings the risk that something may go wrong at any of these levels of development. The individual may fail to achieve the necessary differentiation and fail to transcend; or the process may remain incomplete. Osteopathy can help here. It can release

restrictions that are the result of conditioning, and can promote the development toward a more profound sense of balance.

Therefore healing need not necessarily mean restoring a previous state of health. Healing acquires a quite different and more far-reaching meaning when we recognize that there is a process of development taking place, one that began (ontologically speaking) at conception, but which is by no means complete by the time the individual reaches adulthood. Once this is realized, practitioners are freed from the limitations of a rigid treatment structure whose narrow focus simply seeks to restore a lost, past state of health. It is by understanding the inherent relationship between health and the developing higher-order integration in the person that we expand the potential of the therapeutic interaction.

As we gain insights into the biological rhythms and developmental dynamics, this deepens our understanding of homeostasis and the state of health. That leads on to more adequate and specific treatment of the patient.

A major part of the present book deals with the detailed presentation of objective and subjective factors of developmental dynamics and the physical, biological, emotional, mental and spiritual levels in the therapeutic interaction.

Presentation of these factors shows clearly just how many dynamics and levels of reality are involved in the treatment. If we take just one of the levels and try to generalize on that basis in the therapeutic interaction, we inevitably limit the therapeutic potential. If on the other hand we take the various levels into consideration, we are able to provide a more "holistic" osteopathic treatment.

A word of caution: The therapeutic interaction can only be learnt step by step. The essential prerequisites are a sound knowledge of every tissue, the structural-functional unit to which each belongs and the many interactions of tissue and organ systems; also, of the palpatory approach needed for the particular tissue and how to approach the entirety of the tissue dynamics. These stages of learning cannot be bypassed.

If we try to make our approach intuitively without these fundamentals, all we can achieve is a prerational kind of touch that fails to differentiate. Attempting to achieve intuitive insight into the organization that exists in the patient's body without being able to identify a given dysfunction—in the lesser omentum, for example, or the palmaris muscle—or to see the connections between, say, a dysfunctional vascular supply to the cecum and the rest of the organization, is not osteopathy.

This book does not offer slick recipes for treatment, magic formulae or techniques. Its aim, in line with the philosophy of Still, is to give osteopaths a sense of certain ways of seeing and invite them to take a journey of discovery, one that:

- expands their understanding of themselves, their patients, and the therapeutic interaction
- deepens the process of seeing, thinking, knowing fingers
- and, last but not least, enriches treatment.

Torsten Liem
Hamburg, February 2006

Acknowledgments

Above all we should like to express our very great thanks to all our co-authors. Thank you too for the lively and inspiring correspondence and exchange of ideas. This book could never have come about without the outstanding contributions of the following: Prof. Dr Lev E. Beloussov, Dr Bruno Chikly DO, Terence Dowling, Marie-Odile Fessenmeyer DO, Dr med. Lorenz Fischer, Dr Matthias Flatscher, Jochen Frühwein DO, Prof. Dr Brian Freeman, Dr med. Rüdiger Goldenstein DO, Michael Habecker, Dr Anne Jäkel, Dr med. Ludwig Janus, Tsafi Lederman and Prof. Dr.Eyal Lederman DO, Prof. Dr Maximilian Moser, James McGovern, PhD, Rene McGovern, PhD, Michael M. Patterson, PhD, Stephen Paulus, DO, Prof. Stephen W. Porges PhD, Peter Sommerfeld, DO, Dr med. G.H. van der Bie and Dr.med. Jaap van der Wal. Special thanks to David Hohenschurz-Schmidt for all his help.

Our sincere thanks also go to Elaine Richards, David Beattie, Renate FitzRoy, Roy Macdonald, Karolin Krell, Jörg Wentzel, and Isabelle Lang for translation, as well as Christian Fossum DO, Sibylle Heck, Prof. Dr Paul Klein DO, Prof. Dr Karl W. Kratky, Rüdiger Krause DO, Christoph Newiger, Sotorius Pappas, Jenny Parkinson, and Prof. Dr med. Johannes W. Rohen for their help in dealing with matters of editing, resolving numerous queries and for the stimulating discussions in the course of producing the book.

We would also like to thank for the following graphic artists: Chryssa Dardamissis, Heike Hübner, Piotr and Malgorzata Gusta, Jörg Pekarsky, Stefanie Lenk, Jan Porthun and Christina Sieg.

We are also grateful to my friend and valued colleague Cristian Ciranna Raab DO, BSc for his help in the work on this book. Time and again he provided a listening ear when I felt in my practice that my journey was taking me away from familiar shores while the new was not yet in sight, and in those times when my 'knowing fingers' seemed to me more and more unknowing and powerless.

Torsten Liem would also like to thank Marina Horbatsch of Hippokrates Verlag, my first publisher, for all her support in the production and publication of the book from its inception. Her patience through the multitude of corrections has been truly superhuman.

We are very grateful for Andrew Stevenson and Handspring Publishers for their patience and support for the current edition.

Lev Beloussov, PhD Emeritus Professor of Developmental Embryology, Faculty of Biology, Moscow State University, Moscow

Guus van der Bie MD Formerly Lecturer in Anatomy and Embryology, Utrecht State University, Netherlands

Bruno Chikly MD, DO Registered Osteopath; Brain Curriculum Developer and Instructor; Lymph International Seminar Leader; Founder of the Chikly Health Institute Scottsdale, Arizona; Past Adjunct Professor at the Union Institute and University Graduate College (University of Ohio)

Terence Dowling MA, PhD Psychotherapist; Lecturer, German School of Osteopathy

Marie-Odile Fessenmeyer Osteopath, member of the Association for Multidisciplinary Research into Cephalic and Cervical Anomalies, France

Lorenz Fischer, Dr. med. Professor, Head of Department of Neural Therapy, Co-Director IKOM, University of Bern, Switzerland

Matthias Flatscher PhD Lecturer, Institute of Philosophy, University of Vienna; Lecturer, Hagen Open University, Austria

Brian Freeman PhD Honorary Associate Professor, School of Medical Sciences, The University of New South Wales, Sydney, Australia

Jochen Frühwein BSc Ost. Osteopath; Lecturer, German Osteopathic School, Germany

Rüdiger Goldenstein MSC paed. Ost., DO (DAAO), DPO Orthopedist; Lecturer in Osteopathy, Germany

Michael Habecker Writer and Musician; Author (with Thomas Feichtinger) of *Innen Leben - eine Entdeckungsreise*

Patrick van den Heede, DO, MSc Osteopath; Co-Founder, Integrative Institute of Morphology, Belgium

Anne Jäkel BSc (Hons) Ost, DPhil Head of Research, European School of Osteopathy, Maidstone UK

Ludwig Janus, Dr. med. Psychoanalyst and Psychotherapist; Past-President, International Society for the Study of Prenatal and Perinatal Psychology and Medicine, Germany

Eyal Lederman DO, PhD Osteopath, Honorary Senior Lecturer University College London, researcher and author in manual and physical therapies; director of CPDO Ltd

Tsafi Lederman MA UKCP psychotherapist, supervisor (manual therapy & psychotherapy), trainer group facilitator and director of CPDO Ltd, London, UK

Torsten Liem, MSc Ost., MSc paed. Ost., DO, DPO Joint Principal, German School of Osteopathy, Germany

James McGovern, MS, PhD Past-President, A T Still University, Kirksville, Missouri

Rene McGovern MA, MS, PhD, ABPP (Clinical Health Psychology) Professor, Clinical Psychology, Arizona School of Professional Psychology, Phoenix, Arizona; Associate Professor of Psychiatry, Case Western Reserve University; President, Arizona Psychological Association

Max Moser PhD Professor in Physiology, Medical University Graz and Human Research Institute, Weiz, Austria; Head of the Human Research Institute and Professor at the Institute for Physiology, Medical University, Graz, Austria

Michael M. Patterson, PhD, DO (Hon) Emeritus Professor of Osteopathic Medicine, Associate Editor for International Affairs of the Journal of the American Osteopathic Association, USA

Stephen Paulus, DO, MS Board certified in Osteopathic Manipulative Medicine and Family Practice. Practising osteopathic physician; teacher of osteopathic medicine and philosophy, USA

Stephen Porges, PhD Distinguished University Scientist, Kinsey Institute, Indiana University Bloomington; Research Professor, Department of Psychiatry, University of North Carolina at Chapel Hill.

Peter Sommerfeld, DO, MSc, Lecturer, German School of Osteopathy, Germany

Jaap van der Wal MD PhD Formerly, Associate Professor, Anatomy & Embryology, University of Maastricht. Freelance teacher of phenomenological embryology (Embryo in Motion) under auspices of Dynamension (www.embryo.nl), Netherlands

Paradigms of healing

Torsten Liem

Evil cannot altogether arrest the course of life on the highway and rob it of its possessions. For the evil has to pass on, it has to grow into good, it cannot stand and give battle to the All. If the least evil could stop anywhere indefinitely, it would sink deep and cut into the very roots of existence.

…and knowledge is nothing but the continually burning up of error to set free the light of truth.

R. Tagore[1]

Introduction

Healing methods do not exist or develop in a vacuum. They arise within a defined, historical framework of a culture and society. This framework is often taken for granted, and the underlying beliefs often remain in the unconscious.

Those who see osteopathy as nothing short of a revelation are in danger of ignoring the cultural, social, and epistemological factors that helped it into existence, and are therefore denying it any potential for further evolution.

In order fully to appreciate the diagnostic and therapeutic methods of osteopathy, it is important to acquire an awareness of the changes, and an understanding of the healing processes that the body underwent at the time. Familiarity with these paradigms will enable the reader to arrive at a more balanced view of the beliefs and dynamic developments involved in osteopathy. Reductionist elements that may hamper the potential for healing through osteopathy may thus be recognized. A deeper understanding of the beliefs and social context in which osteopathy is embedded will enable osteopaths to play an active and enlightened role in developing the discipline further, e.g., by identifying postmodern therapeutic elements and, by a differentiated approach, implementing integral methods in therapeutic interaction. It is not a matter of rejecting traditional views, but one of resisting claims of an absolute truth that reflects a limited perspective. Instead, these limited perspectives should be brought together to create a bigger picture. The objective is to unfold the best possible healing potential in a patient using osteopathic diagnostic and therapeutic methods.

Looking at the history of science, Kuhn was able to identify certain repeated processes.[2] Once established, paradigms in science tend to perpetuate themselves. Accepted ideas determine what route research will take in order to underpin and legitimize the current paradigm. Divergence, anomalies, or studies and hypotheses that do not fit in with the paradigm of the day are largely met with obstruction and then ignored. Further along the road, attempts are made to reconcile inconsistencies and get rid of anomalies. However, with increasing anomalies, the paradigm must give in and adapt in order to accommodate new insights, until a point is reached where the existing paradigm can no longer do so and breaks down under the weight of unresolved contradictions. At this point of crisis, chaos reigns and, from this state of instability, a revolution or transformation arises that results in a new perspective. A new paradigm is born. Again, this new paradigm will persist until new anomalies arise that will bring about another revolutionary change. This pattern, also known as dialectics, not only applies to the art of healing, but also to all other kinds of holons (see below).

Evolving paradigms in the art of healing

- Archaic: symbolic actions (pre-rational symbolic view) where human, spiritual, and external reality/environment are perceived as one.

- Magical (largely pre-rational, magic-related perspective): vague idea of self as mind and body, and the natural and spiritual world interwoven with each other and firmly grounded in the here and now. In the early days of humankind, diseases that could not be explained by obvious causes were seen as the work of demons.[3] Healing could be achieved through magic, such as incantations, voodoo, ecstatic dances, and fetishes as well as exorcism. By practicing one of these forms of magic, a practitioner induces healing. In the age of magic, personal belongings have a life of their own, and nature acts on behalf of humans (anthropocentrism). Images and symbols arising in the mind are projected onto the outside world, resulting in a sensation of human omnipotence that is detached from reality. The transition phase from magical to mythical is characterized by the use of magic rituals in order to make spirits or gods intervene to heal a patient.

- Mythical (analogous, mythical, mythic-rational perspective): a context is created on the basis of analogies. Physical similarities are interpreted as hints towards specific actions (e.g., the shape of a walnut is reminiscent of the brain; therefore, walnuts are good for the brain). Knowledge of diseases and their cure is intermingled with religious ideas on the influence of godheads. While in the magical paradigm the power of working miracles was thought to be in the hands of individuals such as magicians, the mythical paradigm attributes these powers to gods or other supernatural forces. Accordingly, in slave-owning societies, disease was viewed as punishment by a just god for sins committed. Priests acted as mediators between the offended godhead and affected sinners, trying to achieve mitigation through prayers, offerings, and other forms of atonement.[3] The following is an example from ancient Greece. When the god Apollo brought the plague upon Greek warriors, they responded by making offerings as well as using home remedies. The spiritual and the natural world are experienced as two profoundly different things. The divine becomes essential. The transition phase from the mythical to the rational is characterized by the rationalization of traditionally mythical topics. Mythology undergoes scrutiny from a rational perspective.

- Rational: modern era (rational, logical perspective, cause and effect). The modern era began about 500 years ago with Copernicus and continued with Kepler, Galileo and Descartes (and we are just witnessing the change to the postmodern era). The world is seen as a given, with no personal attributes that can be measured through objective means. This paradigm enabled humans not only to understand nature through their senses and technological extensions, but also to manipulate it. However, it largely ruled out other intuitive ways of acquiring knowledge. The enlightenment of the eighteenth century, championing autonomy of thought, is a continuation of the principles laid down by Francis Bacon (1561–1626) in *The Advancement of Learning*.[4] It is characterized by empiricism and rationalism, an objective perspective, systematic observation and experimentation, mechanistic, animistic, and vitalistic concepts, and the strict separation of the clerical and medical professions, i.e., religion and medicine.

Hoffmann (1660–1742), in continuation of Descartes' ideas, takes an iatromechanical point of view: life processes are dependent on a mechanism created by God and kept in motion by the forces of the cosmic ether. Form and size, movement and interaction among parts of an organism determine whether processes run smoothly or are disrupted in a mechanical way.

Stahl (1659–1742) takes an animistic or psychodynamic approach. In contrast to the mechanistic perspective: the human body is not viewed as a Cartesian machine, but as an animated organism full of vital force. Its components are brought into life by a sentient soul that recognizes them and controls them by its willpower. This view makes space for the effect of emotions (joy, grief, anger, hope, or love) on the functioning of organs and tissue. Disease and organic dysfunction are seen as caused by the psyche. Hence, the healing power lies with the psyche.

The characteristics of osteopathic principles are recognizable in both Hoffmann's iatromechanistic (model of somatic dysfunction) and Stahl's animistic perspectives (e.g., self-healing potential of the body), although the psychogenic etiology was less influential on the diagnostic and therapeutic methods of osteopathy. Although Still may not have included psychological aspects sufficiently in his theory, he was aware that osteopathic treatment must develop an understanding of these aspects.[5]

Under the influence of changes brought about by the Industrial Revolution, the medical science of the Enlightenment evolves into the modern science-based medicine of the nineteenth century in the West, which is characterized by the application of physical, chemical, and biological approaches (cell pathology) in medicine. The diagnostic methods evolve into physical examinations, while patients are increasingly given medication.

- Postmodern era: system-based approaches (systemic rational perspective), complementary medicine, diversity of paradigms, and wide choice of available treatments. The osteopathic diagnostic and therapeutic approach can be seen as a process of communication, thus illustrating the relationship between osteopath and patient in a systems theoretical context (see Chapter 16). What is usually missing, however, is the inclusion of the "inner context" of the individual (i.e., psychological etiology).

The transition stage towards the transpersonal (integral/multiperspective, holonic, partially post-rational view) involves the recognition and inclusion of consciousness as an integral part of the healing process and is a key element of postmodern medicine – the acceptance of ascending as well as descending causality between the material world and the consciousness.

Postmodern treatment is based on the differentiation among and integration of physical, biological, and mental levels – in other words, of body and mind. Crucially, however, this differs from pre-rational concepts of the unity of body and mind in its post-rational integration of body and mind found in poststructuralism. Osteopathy has always claimed the need for such unity, albeit not always in a very differentiated form. Osteopathic treatment approaches have multiple ways of affecting patients' behavior and development favorably. One example could be the resolution of dysfunctional conditioning – a kind of regression therapy under osteopathic auspices. However, osteopathic concepts have focused especially on verifiable interaction between tissue and function. This left little room for inner subjective experiences of patients. Neither was it possible to account for psychological concepts of mental levels and their inter-

action with somatic levels. Such interactions would enhance the holistic approach of osteopathic treatment in a concrete situation.

- Mystic aspects: the immediate experience of a fulcrum (as part of treatment) gives our existence a transpersonal canvas. It is essential that the practitioner as well as the patient develop abilities to observe and become a witness. With these growing abilities, the space that opens up to let in this light will grow even further.

The mystic stage of development is characterized by the convergence of two perspectives – one worldly and one other-worldly. In the psyche, the physical, biological, and mental levels meet and are unified, transcending the dualism of subject and object for the first time (sacred medicine).

With regard to palpation, the mystic paradigm means that it is not a separate self that touches another because there is no self that can be distinguished from the overall being and the process of touching (a unity that is not expressed as antirational regression and an indistinct, preconscious twilight, but an awareness beyond one-dimensional, positivist rationality).

If the self does not exist, the other person does not exist either. This aspect of physical contact can be traced back to a fulcrum where emptiness is form and form is emptiness, overcoming dualism as well as monism. There is neither an entity that acts as opposed to an entity that is being touched, thus relating to each other, nor is there a shared physical contact.

Some mystic aspects exist in osteopathy, e.g., the wider idea of primary respiration and the postconceptual consciousness of immediate experience through therapeutic interaction. However, it is necessary to differentiate further the interrelation between tissue and function in emotional, mental, and spiritual contexts. In the mystic paradigm, healing requires not only a rational/pre-rational understanding of objective (condition of tissue, environmental factors, etc.) and subjective/intersubjective contexts (world of the patient's experience), but also intuitive awareness in both the practitioner and the patient. In this paradigm, actual healing is closely linked to an increased awareness in the patient. Healing thus comes about as the coherent, super-conscious experience of the inner world and its outer context. It seems to me that these are things that have not been clearly pointed out in osteopathic methodology and in most treatment settings. In order to foster a development that takes care of these aspects, reductionist popular physics, iatromechanical models of treatment, embryo-centered healing doctrines, nature mysticism, as well as pre-rational magic, and mythical fundamentalist approaches must be looked at without prejudice and distinguished on their merits. This will not be easy, by any means, and will lead to conflict, as all these perspectives and attitudes are usually associated with dogmatic and elitist rationalization, as well as irrational and authoritarian defense mechanisms on the side of their followers. What might mitigate conflict is the view that everything these perspectives have to offer will be preserved. The only thing that will be given up is the idea of absolute truth and elitist, narrow dogmatism in order to be transcended into an overriding postpersonal and mystic perspective.

Changes in the perception of the body

The way the human body was perceived and interpreted from the Middle Ages through early modernism (seventeenth century) and the late modern era (late twentieth century) or even early postmodernism, underwent fundamental changes.[6] These changes played an important role in the development of healing paradigms (Table 1.1). Based on these paradigms, Levin and Solomon distinguish seven perceptions of the body[6] (Table 1.2).

The origins of osteopathy

A. T. Still may have experienced the birth of osteopathy as a sort of personal revelation, but there is clear evidence that historico-cultural circumstances and medical ideas of his time may have influenced osteopathic philosophy, even if he made no reference to this (with few exceptions) in his writings.

Confronted with personal tragedy as well as the frequent and strong adverse effects caused by the medical practice of this day that he saw working as a medical doctor[55], A.T. Still was motivated to search for a better method of healing.

"I have observed for thirty years the workings of long-protected systems of stupendous, unpardonable ignorance, criminal ignorance, called allopathy, homeopathy, eclecticism, all of them using drugs without exception".

Still had exposed himself to the three main medical disciplines. Even if the latter two made use of less aggressive medication, they were still not effective in his opinion. He replaced the administration of drugs with a fundamentally different system of treatment.

First clues of this development can already be found in Still's childhood. He was raised in the tradition of the Methodist church, whose founder John Wesley advocated a strict abstinence from alcohol (even if the original medical practice of Wesley and other Methodist preachers was quite similar to heroic medicine), which might well have sensitized Still against the administration of drugs of any kind, especially as alcohol was then also used as a medical remedy. Also his close relationship with nature, which can be found in all his publications, has been an evident part of his life from early childhood.

The most important influences were the changing perceptions of the body that were concomitant with the industrial revolution and the laws of Newton, the developing upsurge of anatomy, the spiritual impact of the Methodist faith, American Transcendentalism with its branches spiritism and Swedenborgianism, as well as the emerging concepts of evolution.

Still's original act was the synthesis of healing facilitated by magnetism and bone setting[56,57], which he combined with an anatomical conceptual framework and the aforementioned influences. Still's creative contribution consists largely in the development of a theory, which describes how the flow of life is interrupted and how this could be transferred into diagnostic and therapeutic action. This is the theory of the lesion.

In the process he put the focus on the adjustment and the alignment of the musculoskeletal system, whilst taking into account new ideas of his time from the areas of neuroscience and fluid circulation.

It appears conceivable that his formative experiences made earlier in life as well as the heroic medicine he was confronted with as a young doctor caused him to take a stand against any implementation of pharmacology into the curriculum-even at a later stage, when a shift in medicine in America had occurred[58].

Parameter	Middle ages	Early modern	Late modern	Early postmodern
From the abstract to the concrete	Abstract concept and idealized projection of speculative reasoning; the actual body was hardly looked at	Empirical examination of the actual body	Breakdown of the mechanistic paradigm, wider concept of a living body	The body as a meaningful experience
From the outer to the inner	Humors and dispositions	The body as a complex, solid, and opaque machine that could be inspected by dissection	The idea of separate inner and outer body realities begins to disappear and is replaced by the concept of interaction between the two	Paradigms on the basis of psycho-neuroimmunological research
From qualities to causalities	The body as an amalgamation of qualities, substance of timeless different stages and conditions	Causes of disease are found in anatomic pathology, such as in virology and bacteriology (modern age)	Host environment, communicative systems, interactive fields, local economy, the body as a unity of time and space	Multifactorial causality, web
From states to processes	Application of Aristotelian logic of qualities to understand the functioning of the body	Structural differentiation of the body	Functional complexity of the body	Recognition of conditions and systemic processes, even beyond mechanistic concepts
From analysis to holism	The body as an organic entity within a pre-established system of categories	Concrete, empirical, analytical, mechanistic concept of the body consisting of separately functioning parts	The body interacts with its cultural environment, system-theoretical concept of the body as an organic entity, based on analysis	Process holism in a systemic context
From mechanical isolation to systemic integration	The body as a sacred entity	Empirical knowledge of a profane body mechanism, separate from the surrounding world	Self-regulated body depending on continuous (e.g., psychological) interaction with social, cultural, historical, and biological environments; disease as meaningful epidemiological processes	Systemic integration of the body in all its dimensions and interactions

TABLE 1.1: Chronology of body interpretations (according to Levin and Solomon)[6]

Body	Period	Body perceived as
Rational body	Middle Ages	Abstract concept and idealized projection of speculative reasoning; sacred and universal body that reflects a greater cosmos
Anatomic body	Early modernism	Structure; the body of organs reflecting to some extent the concept of humors
Physiological body	Modernism	Complex machine whose parts worked together in a functional system, based on knowledge gained from dissections
Biochemical body (cell, molecules)	Modernism	Complex system of tissue, cells, molecular and bio-chemical interactions and processes; based on technology giving insight into the invisible side of the physical presence ("the flesh")
Psychosomatic body	Late modernism	Unity of body and spirit – an approach that was not consistently applied throughout the medical field, but only to certain pathologies
Psychoneuroimmunological body	Early postmodernism	System of organized processes with mutual interaction within a multi-factorial web of cause and effect; the body is no longer restricted to its substance; disease is no longer perceived as an entirely biological process, but within an interactive social, cultural, and historical environment
Experienced meaning of the body	Postmodernism	Differentiated correlation between the body as a phenomenological concept of experienced meaning and conditions in the medical body, as well as between illness/healing and experienced meaning; depending on the subjective experience of the patient (and the therapist) and medical knowledge

TABLE 1.2: Seven perceptions of the body (according to Levin and Solomon)[6]

Conventional and complementary medicine

Classical model of orthodox medicine (Tables 1.3 and 1.4)

Over the past 100–150 years, orthodox medicine was largely shaped by the following paradigms:

- Fragmentism: everything can be traced back to particles, molecules, cells, and viruses that interact with each other. These interactions constitute over-arching entities, and it is often a question of practicability rather than the underlying reality[7] as to whether treatment starts at the part or the entity. Any treatment methodology has to resort to some

Orthodox medicine	Complementary medicine
Academically taught medicine	Alternative medicine
Conventional medicine	Unconventional medicine
Taught medicine	Experience-based healing
Medicine based on natural sciences	Naturopathy
Experimental medicine	Empirical medicine
Technocratic medicine	Biological medicine
Hi-tech medicine	Gentle medicine
Medicine treating organs	Regulatory medicine

TABLE 1.3: Key terms that characterize conventional and complementary medicine (according to Stacher)[8]

reduction. Therefore, reductionism is not a concept that contradicts holism. The holon concept shown below resolves the dichotomy often found in discussions on conventional models of medicine versus complementary medicine (see page 13f.).

- *Causa efficiens*: this approach is usually restricted to an Aristotelian notion of cause and effect. Thus, the preferred approach is etiological–analytical, following closely causality chains. To a large extent, linear, monocausal explanation patterns are used (see p. 67) without referring to other Aristotelian concepts of cause. Orthodox medicine relies predominantly on the laws of chemistry, on Newton's classical linear physics (i.e., cause and effect must be proportional), and on Virchow's cellular pathology. This approach is mainly successful in treating life-threatening situations and infections. It seems to be less successful in the treatment of chronic disease.

- Darwinism: chance and selection determine who will have an evolutionary advantage. Changes that occur are not directed.

- Statistical Reductionism: scientific knowledge in medicine is predominantly based on large comparative case studies, thus denying the importance of individual cases. Placebo effects are either not accepted or excluded by the setup of trials, but certainly not accounted for.

- Separation of body, mind, and psyche.

Model of complementary medicine/ biological medicine

Complementary or "biological" medicine, by contrast, has developed on the basis of holistic concepts (as laid out for the first time in 1927 by Smuts[8a] in his book *Holism and Evolution*). In holism, all life phenomena are viewed in the context of a self-organizing entity. Thus, complementary medicine is characterized by taking the following into account:[9]

- Multiparticularity: biological processes involve not just one particle, but always dozens or hundreds of different molecules.

- Multirelationality: interactions between cells and molecules in biological processes. The effect of a molecule or a cell on a biological process may be modified by the presence of another cell or molecule. Biological processes are complex because they involve a multitude of

Orthodox medicine	Complementary medicine
General	Individual
Objective	Subjective
Reproducible (statistics)	Unique
Finding	Feeling
Neglecting pointers (hard facts)	Over-interpretation (superstition)
False hopelessness	False hope
Coincidence and placebo effects must be ruled out	Coincidence and placebo effects may be helpful
Underlying cause	Symptom, syndrome, disharmony patterns
Causal, sequential (effective compound)	Analogue, parallel
Disease	Sick person
Focus on the outside ("enemy")	Focus on the inside (immune system)
Responsibility of the doctor	Responsibility of the patient
Doctor as active agent	Self-healing, self-regulation
Action	Waiting for healing to happen
Rapid progress, new methods	Methods largely unchanged
Solidary and cellular pathology	Humoral pathology
Matter	Energy

TABLE 1.4: Criteria for the distinction of medical schools according to Kratky[10]

interacting molecules and cells. Tensegrity models in living organisms point in the same direction.

- Pleiotropy, pluripotency, and multifunctionality: cells or molecules (e.g., cytokines) are characterized by a large variability in their impact on many different specific cells or biological processes.

- Redundancy: diverse cells and molecules can have identical effects on cells or biological processes.

- Context-dependency of effects: the effects of molecules or cells on other cells or molecules depend on the context. The same molecule or cell may have an opposite effect in a different context. Due to such complex interactions, it makes no sense to look at parts in isolation only. The entire organism must be taken into account. Thus, osteopathic diagnosis progresses from the general to the specific (i.e., deductive principle) and not vice versa. Symptoms are only part of the whole spectrum of information an osteopath will look at. During treatment as well, the osteopath's attention will focus not only on therapeutic palpation, but to some extent also on the entire patient, thus attempting to keep an eye on the interaction between parts and the whole entity during treatment, and not just from one treatment to the next.

- No strict separation between the subjective and the objective: both are closely interrelated and interwoven.

- "Biological medicine" mainly applies principles of modern, nonlinear physics (quantum physics, chaos theory, and the thermodynamics of energetically open systems) to biological systems as well as following the ground regulations system developed by Pischinger and Heine.[10a,b] They focus more on the extracellular space that is upstream of organ parenchymal cells. Usually, disturbances of information and regulation caused by various sources (interference fields, heavy metals) precede the disease of an organ parenchymal cell. "Ce n'est pas le microbe, c'est le terrain" (Béchamp). An effort is therefore made to reduce or resolve the stress on the ground system. Fischer gives the following explanation of this approach:[11]

For a reaction to take place in an interconnected organism, the stored information and the energetic state in a patient must be "nudged" by an adequate individual application of therapeutic stimuli. Such a stimulus usually not only elicits a local, but also a global/general reaction in the organism. The smallest possible targeted stimulus seems to be most effective. Thus, a response to an osteopathic manipulation may take place far from the manipulation site and even outside any segmental limits. Nonlinear effects of positive feedback can lead to extraordinary transformations.

- Principles of self-organization. One of the basic laws of self-organization is the correspondence between structure and function (one of the main fields in osteopathy). The self-organization of open nonlinear systems is characterized by the following processes and principles:

- Structural determination: no exact prediction can be made of how living systems react to external stimuli or how they organize themselves in response. The processes set in motion within the system depend on the system's own determinants and effective forces.

Osteopathic treatment encourages reorganization by providing therapeutic stimuli or information or by breaking up pathologic stress patterns. How the system reacts or how it reorganizes itself cannot be predicted. Hence, treatment is always individual and accommodates subjective as well as objective findings. Palpation has an eminent role to play here, although it goes without saying that other findings are not neglected.

- Cyclical, nonlinear processes: functional chains within living systems take not only a linear route, but also form loops relating back to the original state (hypercycle), i.e., a causes b, b causes c, and c has an effect on a. When an external stimulus initiates a possible transformation from one state to another, this usually involves all parts of a system. Changes in partial states affect the whole cycle, which reflects on the partial states and their potential to bring about constructive change and growth (i.e., development of new partial systems).

In this closed cycle of transformation or catalytic processes, the structure renews itself by exchanging parts of the system, while the organization of the entity remains in place. In biological systems, cause and effect are not proportional. This, as well as the development of loops, creates a rather complex pattern of self-organization. Hence, the treatment principle "strong healing stimulus – strong healing effect" rarely applies, if at all, and then only as a way of suppressing life-threatening illness.

- Autopoiesis: an autopoietic unit – a self-renewing system – is characterized by a certain autonomy regarding its environment. It has the ability to recreate itself, determining its shape, size, boundaries, and even its own environment, independent

Orthodox approach	Approach of "biological medicine"
Treatment by tackling/suppressing symptoms	Treatment by cooperation with nature to free the body from disease
Disease as separate, independent units – the causes of disease are mostly unknown	Taking into account pathophysiology and etiology – disease as various grades of adaptation, e.g., persistent sympathicotonus
Specialization into disciplines	A condition is never looked at in isolation
Acute and chronic diseases are considered to be separate and independent	Acute illness is seen as an attempt to recreate homeostasis
Treatment of the disruption in order to achieve adaptation (stimulation in order to achieve control)	Addresses psychoneuroendocrine imbalances
Attempting to regulate internal homeostasis externally (through medication)	Inclusion of environmental factors that led to the imbalance in the treatment
Technically oriented	Following principles
Short-term treatment results (e.g., by palliative strategies such as ever stronger medication) that maintain the sympathicotonus (potentially resulting in a shift of symptoms or chronification)	Long-term healing without suppression of body reactions, retrograde symptom development is intended and considered indispensable for the healing process
Treatment of disease by tackling/suppressing symptoms, as the symptom is considered to be the disease (see also, e.g., symptom-oriented tissue manipulation)	Chronic disease is taken back to its acute form. "Acute" conditions undergo a supported healing process
Eclectic, i.e., no overall philosophical concept of disease	The holistic approach leads to a constitutional psychoneuroendocrinological diagnosis, taking in the whole picture
"Osteopathic lesion" is a joint with limited movement in a changed position (somatic dysfunction)	Osteopathic lesion is a sympathetic dysfunction (i.e. the degree to which the adaptive status is maintained)

TABLE 1.5: Treatment in orthodox medicine and biological medicine*

*According to Beardmore, modified (conference presentation at the Institute for Classical Osteopathy, Maidstone, October 2005.)

from surrounding nutritional resources. Adapting to internal (organ systems) and external conditions, a living system can create a new state of order, comprising innumerable intricately interwoven and interfering material regulatory cycles, e.g., neuroendocrine immunological processes, organ functions, circulatory, and respiratory volumes, as well as the body's own electromagnetic or morphogenetic fields, which, in turn, are not independent of internal material regulatory cycles and external fields.

Similar to other biological treatment approaches, osteopathy has an interest in stimulating self-healing powers in the sense of autopoiesis. What it definitely does not do is push toward partial reactions in a patient by interfering in cyclical processes.

Just as in orthodox medicine, much of the training is spent diagnosing certain diseases and assigning treatments to them; so in the technocratic approach to osteopathy, diagnosis and treatment will focus on somatic and visceral dysfunction. The dysfunction may be localized in a place different from where the symptoms show. Thus, even a technocratic osteopathic approach is more individualistic and less reductionist than disease-focused medical treatment. In fact, no two patients with the same symptoms will receive the same treatment in osteopathy, as their treatment will be based on osteopathic findings (e.g., palpation of somatic dysfunction, primary dysfunction complexes, etc.).

- Structural coupling: self-organizing systems are tied to suitable environmental conditions. Thus, humans are also tied to physical, biological, emotional, cultural, and biosocial environmental conditions from birth to death. Self-organization takes place under the tension of the relative autonomy of the autopoietic unit on the one hand and the relative dependency on suitable environmental conditions on the other.

It is therefore a priority in osteopathy to perceive the patient from the angle of this tension and treat accordingly. This can mean that we must raise the patient's awareness of some aspects of their lives that are particularly damaging, such as malnutrition, stress, not enough sleep or exercise, too much noise, alcohol/caffeine/tobacco, interference fields, work, over-stimulation, etc. Like any living organism, humans have ways of cleansing and healing themselves when they are no longer poisoned and stressed. Table 1.5 lists the differences between orthodox and biological-medical treatment.

Biopsychosocial model

Human beings are not only autopoietic, they are also cognitive entities, which is acknowledged by the biopsychosocial model. This model was first introduced by G.L. Engel in 1977.[12] Engel stated that orthodox medicine took a reductionist approach by looking

- Solid matter
- Physiological/biochemical regulation (acid/base balance, redox potentials, bioelectric regulation, etc.)
- Comprehensive regulatory systems – nervous system, hormonal regulation, immune system, ground regulation of the connective tissue system, etc.
- Bioenergetic level – electromagnetic fields biophotons
- "Bioinformation" level of subtle energies (potentials, scalar waves, etc.)
- Transpersonal level of the "implicit order" and the "united field or vacuum"

TABLE 1.6: Differentiation according to Bischof[20]

for the causes of disease in biological/somatic pathology, neglecting psychological and sociological factors (i.e., biomedical model). According to Engel, the historical reasons for this lie in the Cartesian dualism of body and mind, harking back to the influence of the Orthodox Church. Engel favored an approach that maintained the advantages of a biomedical model, but put its absolute claim into perspective by integrating biosocial factors. Engel's approach was founded on general, system-theoretical concepts, emphasizing how each of the systems included was whole in itself as well as being part of an overarching whole. He was thus able to take account of psychosocial factors in the treatment of patients.

It has been argued that the biopsychosocial approach is not really a theory, but a response to reductionist tendencies in orthodox medicine, and that its general outline on the integration of psychological and sociological factors remains incomplete. Besides, it cannot be considered to be a proper model on the basis of which its ideas can be taken further.[13] The approach also failed to discuss subjective and inter-subjective factors in therapeutic interaction.

Phenomenological approach

From a phenomenological point of view, a human being cannot be understood on the basis of biology only, as is predominantly done in the objective approach of biological medicine. Phenomenology raises an important point: we only reach consciousness through inner perception.

- Subjective/intersubjective knowledge: health and disease are seen in the context of the meaning of general phenomena, such as dimensions of time and space, the physiological aspect of existing, sharing a world with other beings, the general mood, memory and history, being mortal, and the open-endedness of being. To give room to all these aspects of being is to develop toward the freedom of human existence.[14]

- Interconnection: these characteristics of human existence are all interconnected, and if one of them suffers it will affect all the other characteristics. The aspects named above are, according to Boss, experienced by both body and soul; in stark contrast to Descartes'[15] separation of body and soul.

Husserl, founder of the discipline of phenomenology, suggested the term "somatology" for the description of methodological studies of subjective experiences of the body using objective science. Referring to the phenomenological method, Hannah defined "somatics" as an area of study covering physical sensation and the perception of the body from a first-person perspective, as opposed to the biomedical method that takes a third-person perspective.[16] In order to clarify his approach, Husserl emphasizes that consciousness is the subject as well as the object of a stream of awareness, which is self-contented and not externally determined (i.e., intentional synthesis of consciousness).[17]

Phenomenological pathology sees individuals with a disease as individuals for whom an existence has been previously outlined, which is then restricted in its possibilities by pathological events.[18] However, translating human and inter-human phenomena into exclusively anatomical and physiological processes – as is often done in current osteopathy – may bear the risk of looking at a person in those reduced terms. Thus, structural–physiological dynamics may be a necessary but not a sufficient condition for human phenomena.

Energy medicine model of the organism (body as a whole)

The term was coined in the mid-eighties for methods using energy fields in diagnosis and treatment. The energy-medical model is hierarchically organized and comprises complex regulation levels of biological functions. Energy medicine comprises all energetic and informal interactions that arise from self-regulation or other energetic connections between mind and body.[19] However, the term 'energy medicine' is not very precise, as it is not always energy that is involved, but partially (solid) matter as well as energy and information (i.e., bioinformation level).[7]

Different perspectives or looking at the world from a Huna perspective

Four perceptions of reality in complementary medicine may be clarified using Hawaiian thinking and healing traditions (Table 1.7). These can also be applied to osteopathic treatment:

- Logical–systematic approach: effective causes lead to somatic dysfunction, which, in turn, may elicit compensatory changes in the organism. The osteopath tries to understand the causal chain, supporting the resolution or integration of somatic dysfunction.

- Dynamic–systemic perspective: the organism is a chaotic open system. Highly individual osteopathic treatment targets the storage of information and the balance of energy in the patient. Ever so slight, targeted stimulation triggers not only local, but global (systemic) responses that enable transformation into different states.

- Constructivist–symbolic perspective: this perspective gives an insight into the significance and interpretation of symptoms and dysfunction complexes. The practitioner tries to understand the particular meaning of a symptom in the life of a patient. It is the diseased individual, not the symptom that is treated. The presence of a symptom indicates the absence of something else. What the patient lacks, according to this approach, is a consciousness of certain aspects of life. Symptoms and symptomatic dysfunction are not a nuisance that must be overcome and removed, but provide a pathway for the patient to become a more healthy and whole person. The symptoms are intimately connected to the person showing them. The symptom becomes a symbol, an instrument that enables the individual to develop into a more conscious being.

- Holistic–symbiotic perspective: this is, in a sense, the beginning of a post-rational, transpersonal level

	1	2	3	4
Symbol	→●→●→	(cycle symbol)	=	●
Occurrence	Classical natural sciences	Chaos studies, social sciences	Human sciences	Spirituality
Characteristics	Logical/systematic	Dynamic/systemic	Constructivist/symbolic	Holistic/symbiotic
	Everything has spatial and temporal limitations	Everything is linked to everything else and follows cycles	Everything is symbolic, standing for something else	Everything is one, part of oneness
	Either – or If – then	One as well as the other	On the one hand – on the other TWO sides of a coin	Two sides of ONE coin
	Objectivity Hierarchy Reproducibility Predictability	Subjectivity Reference to itself Exchange Complexity	Analogy Rituals Metaphors Hermeneutics Mirror effect Placebo	Identification Mystical experience of unity Mass panic Ecstasy

TABLE 1.7: Perspectives of the Huna according to Kratky[21]

of experience where therapeutic interaction is based on the mystic experience of the interconnection that exists between all forms of life and an underlying common ground.

Depending on the case, one or the other perspective may appear more appropriate. However, all four perspectives are found in the healing tradition of Huna, opening up different treatment pathways, some of which may be followed up simultaneously. If dysfunction is due, for example, to an accident in the past, a logical–systematic approach may be helpful to establish causal relationships in order to treat key components in the dysfunction complex. As a consequence of the accident, several compensatory changes may already have occurred at various levels. These could include fascial, postural, psychoneuroendocrine, immunological changes, and it would therefore be sensible to apply a

dynamic–systemic approach to all diagnostics in further treatment. The effect of a therapeutic stimulus is never quite predictable in such a patient. A symbolic interpretation may be appropriate in a patient who is accident-prone, to explain the meaning of such strings of accidents.

Holon concept and the AQAL model according to Wilber[22]

Wilber tries to reconcile objective and subjective approaches by combining the four-quadrant model with the holon concept. Wilber thus integrates orthodox medical approaches (i.e., biomedical model, objective science, and empiricism), complementary medicine, the biopsychosocial model, system theory, phenomenology, hermeneutics, and structuralism. His model has far-reaching consequences regarding the holistic or integral character of osteopathic approaches. It develops perspectives for

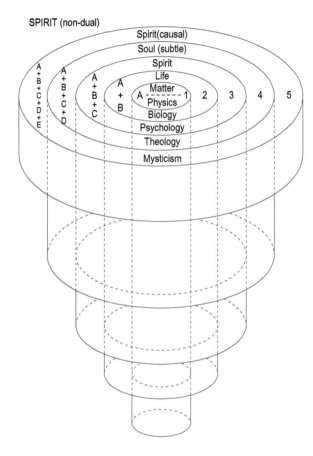

SPIRIT (non-dual)

Spirit(causal)
Soul (subtle)
Spirit
Life
Matter
Physics
Biology
Psychology
Theology
Mysticism

holistic or integral osteopathic treatment of humans, as well as showing its limitations.[23]

The holon concept according to Koestler and Wilber

According to the holon concept, originally thought out by Koestler and then further developed by Wilber, reality is neither a whole nor does it consist of parts, but it is composed of wholes/parts that are called holons.

All phenomena are thus whole as well as part of something else. Every whole exists as part of another whole. This concept applies to things as well as processes. It applies to atoms, molecules, cells, tissue, and organisms, and hence to humans. It applies to somatic dysfunction as well as to the idea of health. A whole in itself does not exist, but only the wholes/parts that integrate into a higher as well as a lower level on the scale.

There are certain uniform phenomena in the evolutionary process, universal patterns of evolution, but there is also discontinuity. Wilber, as well as Jantsch et al., point out that the continuous process of self-transcendence engenders discontinuity. Mental activities cannot be put down to biology, and biological processes cannot be put down to matter and physics only.

Wilber's model of the Cosmos (as opposed to the physical Cosmos or universe) describes structures and processes in all dimensions of existence. It comprises the physiosphere (material level), the biosphere (biological level, including inherent autopoiesis), the noosphere (level of the mind, world soul), and the theosphere (divine sphere). There are some striking resemblances (in spite of some incongruences and diverging interpretations by osteopaths*) between Still's perspective and Wilber's cosmology (see Tables 1.8 and 1.9).

Wilber made the following fundamental statements to characterize holons:

1 The reality or the Cosmos consists neither of things nor processes, but of holons, i.e., of wholes/parts – of entities that are at the same time part of other entities while also having a certain autonomy as parts. According to this concept, disease and somatic dysfunction are not independent entities, but temporary phenomena that interrelate with their environment, i.e., other wholes/parts.

---

*Pöttner sees in Still's triune (tri-unus – three united as one) concept a reflection of the Christian trinity idea, albeit a very distant one. According to Pöttner, the mind is not part of the soul for Still, but intellect that manifests in logical reasoning. The intellect, just like the spiritual being, has God-like characteristics, and both have a long tradition in the over 2000-year-old history of Christianity.

	Interpretation according to Dippon	Interpretation according to Stark	Equivalent in Spencer's matter/motion/force according to Townbridge
Material body	Body as inanimate matter	Body as inanimate matter	Matter
Spiritual body	Soul inseparably linked to the body, bringing life to the body through movement and action and sensual perception	Vitalist or physiological perspective. Principle of action, excitability, sensitivity, accessibility, arteries, veins, nerves, lymph, etc. as carriers of vitality; biochemical or genetic secrets of the body	Motion
Being of mind	Mind as the entity above the vital forces of the body–soul entity that coordinates chaotic movement and sensual impressions in a meaningful way	Soul in the sense of an entity mediating between the body and a spiritual being that exists as something divine, independent of the body	Force
Comment: Dippon thinks that Stark's representation of Still's triune concept is a rather spiritual interpretation. Pöttner[29] disagrees. See further comment*			

TABLE 1.8: Interpretations of Still's Triune Concept[24–28]

*Pöttner agrees with Stark's interpretation of Still's triune concept, seeing the three times subdivided unity as a step further from the rigid opposition of the physical and the spiritual. The triune concept permits a gradual transition from one to the other. According to Pöttner, this interpretation is borne out by Still's background in American transcendentalism, which had a strong influence on his ideas on osteopathy. Although Spence is also aware of this tradition and uses similar terminology, he does not adopt the triune model from transcendentalism, as Still did.

2 Holons have four fundamental capacities:

a Horizontal capacity:

i Agency/self-preservation: this describes a tendency towards self-preservation, self-assertion, and assimilation and is an expression of wholeness. Wholeness, autonomy, and identity of a holon, and its agency must be preserved. If its autonomy is under threat, this will affect its existence. A holon, therefore, strives to keep its wholeness in the face of environmental constraints. This is true at all levels, whether atoms, molecules, cells, tissues, organisms, or mental entities.

ii Communion/self-adaptation: these refer to a tendency to enter relationships and fit in as a way of expressing its partness aspect. Being always part of something else, a holon must adapt to its environment. If it can no longer be part of its environment and another entity, this can also be a threat to its existence. Agency and communion characterize the horizontal capacity of a holon.

Elements	Properties	Manifestations	Approaches	Kosmos according to Wilber
Material body or physical being or matter	Matter, physical functioning parts of the body (bones and muscle origins)	Matter	Mechanical	Physiosphere
Spiritual side of a vitalist or physiological perspective	Action principle, excitability, sensitivity, accessibility. Arteries, veins, lymph, nerves, etc. which are the main carriers of vitality. Biochemical or genetic mysteries of the body	Action	Vitalist	Biosphere
Spirit or spiritual existence within a religious concept	Principle that governs the body and provides it with purposeful action. Vital force	Movement	Spiritual	Noosphere
Soul, the "inner self", the human spirit from a spiritualist perspective. The truth of life until after death. Spiritual substance spiritualist				Theosphere

TABLE 1.9: Still's view of a human being. Elements, properties, manifestations, and approaches (according to Stark). Last column augmented by Liem[30]*

*This concept clearly diverges from Wilber's classification. For Wilber, the noosphere is a spiritual level that has transcended the body sphere, for instance in the sense that the mind has some control over the body and its desires (sensomotoric consciousness). The noosphere, according to Wilber, is not linked to a spiritual approach (although the spiritual touches other levels), and neither can it be attributed to the vital force, which would be part of the biosphere.

b Vertical Capacity

i Self-immanence: a healthy descending drive where the higher embraces the lower, e.g., a molecule embraces its atoms. Its dysfunctional form is self-dissolution. If neither agency nor communion can be maintained, regression occurs. The higher dissolves into the lower – in other words the holon dissolves into its subholons. Thus, a molecule may disintegrate into atoms. The process of holon dissolution reverses the process of holon building.

ii Self-transcendence: Jantsch calls the evolution "self-realization through self-transcendence," describing an evolutionary drive towards a higher level. In this transcendence process, from which new holons emerge, what exists is transcended. Preceding holons are embraced by new holons.

A holon is exposed to these four forces and carries them within.

In osteopathy, the unity of the body/organism and its intimate interaction with physical, mental, emotional, and spiritual factors[31] within the unity is emphasized. Individuals are integrated, regulated, and coordinated by the independent functions of many different associated anatomical, physiological, and psychosocial systems. Even the "partial aspect" of humans in limbo between self-preservation and self-adaptation as well as between self-dissolution and self-transformation is taken into account in osteopathy, although not always very clearly. Osteopathic diagnosis and treatment includes questions such as: is the person deficient in his/her ability to maintain wholeness and/or to define boundaries? How does the patient adapt to his/her cultural, social, and biosocial environments? Where can balance be found as opposed to the current imbalance? Are the patient's symptoms an outlet for processes veering towards self-dissolution or self-transcendence? Or what are the opportunities/challenges/resources for a patient in self-transcendence (i.e., converting an imbalance into a balance of a higher order)? What are the dangers of self-dissolution?

The same applies to the patient's subholons, e.g., organs or tissues. An organ must define its boundaries in its environment and maintain relative autonomy, while also being able to adapt to its surroundings and function as part of the wholeness of a human being.

1 Holons emerge: evolution can be partially understood as a process of self-transcendence that leads beyond what exists. During the emergence of holons, new units are created from fragments – a creative process. According to Wilber, the Cosmos unfolds in quantum leaps of such creative emergence. It is important to emphasize that a level/holon cannot be reduced to its components. Thus, the analysis of the components of a holon will give insight into its parts, but not regarding its wholeness. Wilber and Jantsch point out that the continuous process of self-transcendence results in discontinuity, e.g., the transformation of biological existence leads to mental existence, whereas mental activity cannot be reduced to its biology. Biological life, in turn, cannot be reduced to matter (physics). The challenge for osteopathy lies in the development of more adequate methods of differentiation, e.g., in order to integrate the mental level into the treatment context.

Wilber equals the principle of self-transcending creativeness to the mind. According to him, calculations show that the dynamics of evolution are not simply driven by chance. Creative evolution is characterized by an effort to overcome chance. The Cosmos gives rise to form in its drive toward organizing shape in increasingly coherent holons. This drive comes out of the Buddhist principle of emptiness.

2 Holons emerge holarchically: there is a natural hierarchy of increasing wholeness (e.g., particles→atoms→cells →tissue→human being or physiosphere→biosphere→noosphere, etc.). According to Koestler, reality is built out of holons: he coined the term "holarchy" to describe a state where on a higher/lower organizational level, the whole is more than the sum of its parts (subholons).

In an osteopathic context, disease could thus be understood as a dysfunctional disproportion or imbalance of wholeness and partness. Within the human holon, the wholeness may have shifted in relation to its partialness or vice versa. Such shifts are perceived in osteopathy as specific dysfunction patterns or complexes. The practitioner must identify them.

3 Each emerging holon transcends and incorporates its predecessors: an emerging holon retains its preceding entities (subholons) by keeping its basic functions and structures intact, while overcoming their separateness and isolation by incorporating them in a more comprehensive identity. This improves their potential for communion. Thus, a cell transcends the molecules of which it consists while at the same time including them. The molecules, in turn, transcend and embrace atoms, etc. A molecule possesses characteristics beyond those of atoms, however numerous they may be. The same applies to the cell in relation to the molecule – it has new properties, as has the biosphere beyond what could be explained by purely material laws. Similarly, the emergence of the spiritual goes beyond the purely biological. Thus, the higher level always includes the properties of the lower, while the higher is not completely contained in the lower. Everything lower is contained in the higher, but not everything higher is contained in the lower level. Thus, the higher levels cannot be reduced to the lower levels. Hence, the human organism cannot be entirely reduced to its biological, biochemical dynamics, and quantum physical laws (e.g., as attempted in conventional medicine), or its vitalistic and biomechanical dynamics (as in osteopathy), or its psychodynamics (as sometimes in psychology). A holon at a certain level provides an outer shell for lower systems (subholons) as well as an inner world for higher level systems.

Morphogenetic fields are organized hierarchically.[32] Morphogenetic fields of a higher order define and structure their components without violating the patterns and laws pertaining to the components. Physicochemical processes within the molecular components of cell organelles are regulated by the relevant cell organelles, while the processes involving cell organelles are subject to higher-ranking fields within the cells, which, in turn, are subject to the fields of tissues, which belong to organ fields, and finally the field of the entire organism. On each of these levels, the superior level has an effect on the lower by structuring processes/dynamics that would otherwise be unstructured and uncoordinated. Lower levels are not destroyed, but embraced, as the higher level represents a kind of probability structure that stabilizes the lower levels by supporting certain processes and making others less likely.

4 The lower sets the possibilities of the higher; the higher sets the probabilities of the lower. The lower sets a framework for the higher. These are certain conditions that do not restrict the higher. Thus, the higher cannot be defined by the lower or reduced by the lower, e.g., biological properties cannot be reduced to physical or quantum physical laws, and the spiritual level cannot be reduced to the biosphere. The transcendence of the lower and the integration into higher holons goes beyond the subholon setting without violating or ignoring subholon rules and basic patterns. This means that, even where the biological goes beyond pure physics, it is still subject to physical laws. Likewise, the spiritual is always subject to biological laws while at the same time going beyond the biosphere. Freud, for example, mainly worked on the psychological level, but always strived to understand the connection between psyche and soma, which, he emphasized, were closely interconnected and interacted with each other, but were subject to different laws.[33]

Still, on the other hand, apparently looked at somatic levels in his publications. According to Stark, Still regarded the body as an amalgamation of matter, movement, and mind, penetrating each other as in transcendentalism. He apparently dealt with the mechanics, and what he did not spell out had to be read between the lines.[34]

Although from a holon perspective, Still did not sufficiently integrate the mental and physical levels in his writings and was not very elaborate on the interactions and mutual impacts of the mental and somatic levels and their holarchic ties (see point 7) – given his local, regional, and general social and cultural environment when he initiated osteopathy – he emphasized the need for the osteopath to gain an understanding of the mental aspects of a patient's personality.[5] According to many experts on the history of osteopathy, such as Stark and Paulus, he had deep insight into the spiritual world. Dippon claims that he was deeply rooted in the Christian Methodist view of the world. However, it can only be guessed how deep his knowledge of the spiritual world really was, as it can usually only be read between the lines.** The mind (sometimes used by Still as synonymous with the soul) lives in the subject he is writing about on the day. In his autobiography, he talks of "the material house in which the spirit of life dwells" (autobiography 1897, p. 99). Conversely, he states on p. 104 of his *Philosophy of Osteopathy*[51] that "The eye is an organized effect, the lymphatics the cause; in them the spirit of life more abundantly dwells." These quotes show that you cannot just pick one sentence that may permit a certain interpretation and neglect the rest. When writing, he had to start writing somewhere, and the fact that he describes things one after the other does not mean that they form a linear sequence.[34]

According to Hulett, Still's osteopathic principles aimed at establishing a normal/healthy relationship between the individual and the environment which could apply beyond the body itself, e.g., to the adjustment of bodily relationships, intellectual and moral relationships, as well as to conditions in the environment. For Hulett, this amounts to the realization of the harmony principle.[35]

** Still's interest in spirituality was not necessarily shared or tolerated by his surroundings, and notably his wife, who went as far as tearing out pages of a book Still was reading, with the title *Religious Denominations of the World* (Miller V.I., updated by Brown J.N. in 1973). Still left the following annotation in his copy: "my good wife is an honest Methodist woman and has torn out pages 47, 48, 49, and 50 as she was (satisfied?) they were a bill of slanderous lies on a good people. She is right" (from Still's family library). Only recently, it emerged that Still was probably a Freemason.[36] To what extent Freemasonry has shaped his writing can only be surmised.

Characteristics of a holon at any level:
a Qualitative emergence
b Asymmetry or breaks in symmetry
c Inclusive principle (the higher includes the lower, but not vice versa)
d A developmental logic (the higher safeguards the lower, but overcomes its separateness)
e Chronological indicator: the higher follows the lower chronologically, although not everything that came later is necessarily higher.

5 The number of levels that a hierarchy comprises determines whether it is "shallow" or "deep": a small number is described as shallow, while a large number is considered deep. The larger the vertical extension of a holon, the larger its depth. The number of holons at one level is shown on a horizontal scale (i.e., quantity: wide–narrow): the more holons there are at the same level, the larger the span.

6 Each successive level of evolution produces greater depth and less span (compared to its previous level): in a holarchy, a high (i.e., deep) holon has a narrower span, compared to a lower holon, and more depth. It is not the number of its parts at one level that make a holon higher – on the contrary – the number of entities is always smaller than that of its parts (more atoms than molecules, more molecules than cells, more cells than tissues, etc.). It follows that the deeper a holon, the more it depends on internal holons. Wilber stipulates that the higher the depth of a holon, the higher the degree of consciousness. A molecule has less consciousness than a cell, a cell less consciousness than a plant, a plant less consciousness than an animal, etc.

True spirituality would thus be a measure of depth. According to Wilber, the negation of God through reasoning requires more spirituality than affirmation of God's existence through myths, simply because negation is the expression of a higher depth.[37]

Changes at the horizontal level are called translations, whereas vertical changes are referred to as transformations. Agency and communion affect the horizontal, while self-transcendence and self-dissolution act on the vertical. The agency/self-preservation of a holon acts according to the organizational level/codex of the relevant holon, i.e., a holon does not simply recognize a given external world, but only perceives it selectively, depending on the coherence with its codex or disposition. This is important for the understanding of holons. External stimuli that do not fit the organizational pattern of a holon are simply ignored, they are not taken in. They do not exist as far as the holon is concerned. Thus, according to Varela,[33] holons are relatively autonomous entities that follow a "logic of coherence," and a subatomic particle is unable to respond to biological forces such as hunger, nor is it capable of understanding a painting by Klee or the meaning of somatic dysfunction. The deeper a holon (deep structure), the wider the range of worlds it responds to. Transformation leads to the emergence of a completely new organizational structure of the agency. A newly emerged holon can thus access completely new aspects of a pre-existing world. Every transformation comprises all pre-existing lower levels, but at the same time, something totally new emerges, i.e., it embraces and transcends all previous subholons, thus conveying to the emerging holon a deeper understanding and perception of the world. Wilber calls this a gradual internalization of the external. "Translation is change of the surface structure, transformation is change in the deep structure (vertical). Translation is the shifting about of parts; transformation creates a whole."

Even if seen from the phylogenetic point of view, man in contrast to other species has reached already a great depth or deepness or profoundness, every single human being as an individual or as an individual person starts from an ontogenetic point of view as if from point zero, going though all developmental stages. This means that at each developmental level, something may go wrong and differentiation and transcendence remain incomplete or do not happen at all. Here, osteopathy, like many other methods, can support differentiation and transformation processes by dissolving limiting conditions and promoting orientation towards a deeper state of balance.

7 Destroy any type of holon, and you will destroy all of the holons above it and none of the holons below it. Accordingly, dissolving a holon means regression to

the next lower holon level. Wilber has thus described an extremely useful tool to decide which holon is higher or lower in evolutionary terms. We simply must ask ourselves which holons would be destroyed if a certain type of holon were to be dissolved. Everything that is destroyed with it is higher, while everything that remains intact is lower. For example, if the prefrontal cortex is damaged, the lower areas of the brain that control basic biological functions in a patient remain intact. Damasio gives a lively description of patients who have lapses in consciousness in the course of persistent vegetative state. Although they retain normal basic body functions, their mind is totally inert, with no sense of self and no awareness of their closest relations.[38] The less depth a holon has (i.e., the shallower it is), the more fundamental it is for the Cosmos. By contrast, the more deep structure a holon has, the more significant it is for the universe because it integrates more Cosmos in its wholeness. Thus, living matter is more significant than nonliving matter. Emotions are more significant than the biological level, and the mental level, in turn, more significant than the emotional level, and the spiritual level more significant than the mental level. The emergence undergoes individual variation and is evolutionarily directed and must be taken into account when looking at health and illness in a patient. Fundamental holons have an impact on all following holons, creating an ascending chain of causality. Thus, for example, nutrition and the biological status of a person may affect emotional, mental, and spiritual levels. Genetic defects may equally affect higher levels or even prevent higher developmental levels from forming. It can generally be said that the earlier (in development) a major trauma appears, the more fundamental its potential effects on the organism. Here is another example: if all molecules in the universe were to be destroyed, biological life would be impossible, although atoms and subatomic particles would not be affected. There can also be causal chains operating in the descending direction. We can, for example, "think ourselves" into a state of illness.

If possible emotional trauma – either in the sense of evolutionary emergence or as the synchronous objective and subjective expression of dysfunction –

is neither recognized nor taken into account in the process of resolving the somatic dysfunction, treatment can only result in translational compensation. This may sometimes be necessary in order to prevent physical collapse or temporarily halt self-dissolving tendencies. However, genuine transformative processes can also thus be prevented, at least until the onset of the next period of instability, disorder, or the development of symptoms. On the other hand, it is possible that a patient may use the energy gained in the symptom-free period to sustain genuine transformative processes.

Here is a functional/physiological example – Porges[39] distinguishes between three stress responses. A person who feels relatively safe may respond to stress by involving the autonomic system, which is also, phylogenetically, the most recent system and includes the myelinated vagus and its associated cranial nerves (V, VII, IX, X, and XI). In other words, the response involves facial expression, vocalization, and listening. At the same time, the lower brain stem structures (including the sympathetic trunk and the non-myelinated vagus) are inhibited. If the threat becomes stronger or the former strategy proved unsuccessful, older structures are disinhibited. First, the sympathetic trunk kicks in, exhibiting fight and flight mechanisms. If that proves unsuccessful, the non-myelinated vagus (immobilization) takes over. This has been described as the theory of dissolution (according to Jackson[39a]). Again, this shows that if one holon level does not function (although not irreversibly here!), the lower level offers a fallback position. It is important in osteopathy to remember that if a higher or more significant integration level has stopped operating, for whatever reason (e.g., past trauma), dysfunctional transfer to lower levels may occur (e.g., sympathetic response or even immobility). Such dysfunctional conditioning, in turn, may cause further physiological disruption.

8 Holarchies co-evolve: no holon exists on its own, but all holons exist in field in fields in fields... The basic unit is "holon plus environment." Both are inseparable and mutually influence their evolution (according to Jantsch,[39b] micro- and macro-evolution). Here is an example from biology: there is mutual interaction

between a cell and its surroundings, e.g., via ground regulation according to Pischinger,[39c] via integrins and architecture of the cytoskeleton in the tensegrity model, via structural coupling and autopoiesis, or via morphogenetic effects in embryonic development.

9 Micro and macro interact and exchange at all levels: at each level, holons exist and maintain themselves through interaction with other holons at the same holarchic level (exchange at the same level). Wilber gives the example of the three main levels in a human: matter (physiosphere), life (biosphere), and mind (noosphere). In the physiosphere, humans are in exchange with other physical levels (e.g., gravity, material forces, light, or water). In the biosphere, there is exchange with other biological systems and ecosystems, while in the noosphere, there is exchange with cultural and symbolic contexts.

10 Evolution has directionality: directionality exists not only in the biosphere but in all domains of evolution and is characterized by differentiation, polymorphism, complexity, and organization.

a Increasing complexity: in the evolutionary process, macro- and microcosm developed intricate interdependent structures, resulting in interlacing functional and structural differentiation and integration processes.

b Increasing differentiation/integration: differentiation leads to the development of parts where new shapes emerge. Integration is the way from polymorphism to unity. The inherent force of evolution, gradually increasing differentiation and integration, enhances coherent heterogeneity and thus the formation of holarchically organized holons (whole/parts). This is a continuous, never-ending process: one holon leading to another and another ad infinitum.

These differentiations and integrations are explained extensively in this book in respect of the physiosphere (Chapter 4) and for the biosphere (Chapter 5). The noosphere is explained to a certain extent (Chapters 11 and 12). In the noosphere, this process can be observed as aggression (drive towards differentiation) or Eros (drive towards integration). Osteopathic treatment generally strengthens the processes of increasing differentiation and

integration in the organism (focusing mainly on the biological level, but potentially able to integrate other levels as well (Chapter 20).

c Increasing organization/structuring: in evolution, there is an inherent drive toward the formation of ever more complex or higher organizational levels. Teilhard de Chardin[40] took the view that matter unfolds spirally through all evolutionary stages and, with increasing complexity, consciousness becomes more self-centered. He uses the analogy of a lamp with several veils, between the light source and the outside, which dampen the light. While minerals have a thick veil that lets hardly any light penetrate, the lamp in plants is shaded by a slightly thinner veil, allowing more light to penetrate. With the phylogenetic development from fish to mammals and the ongoing development of the brain, the veil becomes ever thinner. The thinnest veil in evolution is that found in humans. Once the veil has been completely lifted, we can see the pure spirit. The same light shines behind the various veils, whether coarse or delicate, and, accordingly, the light of pure consciousness appears behind all forms of life and can be perceived as completely unveiled consciousness in some saints. According to Jantsch, evolution occurs in breaks in symmetry, i.e., the increasing complexity of holons induces a hypercycle that elevates holons to a higher level of organizational structure (formation of a super holon). Each new organizational level represents a simplification of system functions and structures. At the same time, however, structural and organizational complexity increases. (In relation to his quadrant model, Wilber explains that the higher the complexity of material form – upper right quadrant – the higher the internalized consciousness level – upper left quadrant – that can develop within such forms (Figure. 1.2).)

d Increase in relative autonomy: for Wilber, this means an increase in self-preservation ability (agency) under changing environmental conditions – not to be confused with hardiness and durability. Indeed, stones can be much more durable than, for example, biological holons. The latter, however, are able to exist as a self-renewing system,

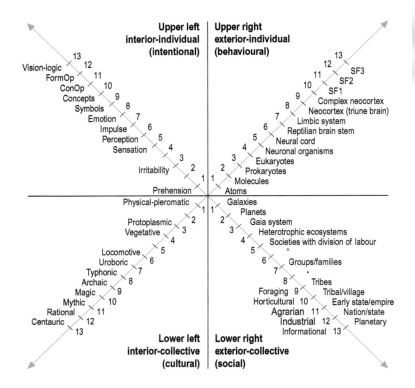

Figure 1.2
Four Quadrants according to Wilber.[45]

in the absence of thermodynamic equilibrium (Chapter 6). Relative autonomy increases, as in the course of evolution, and external forces affecting holons become internal forces through transformation. Relative autonomy can go too far in humans, leading to a pathological dissociation of the mind from the biological level (e.g. anorexia) or the environment (e.g. environmental destruction) – an indicator of the relativity of autonomy. A holon may be a whole, but it is also part of a wider context/environment.

Dissociations can show as subjective or objective changes. The resulting tension can be picked up by the osteopath and not only through palpation, although palpation will be the main avenue for treatment.

e Increasing telos: the defined telos of a holon exists as a relative whole, while in its property as a part (of another holon) it is influenced by a telos out-

side itself. The deep structure, the morphogenetic field, as well as the end point of the system, act as attractors for the system in question. Attractors provide quasi-patterns of higher probability or a kind of attraction that acts as an engine, driving the development of a holon in a certain direction. Certain defining contexts of a holon can thus not be resolved within the holon itself. The holon exists in its entirety, separated from the world outside and within its own, limited, perspective; over time, its internal inconsistencies will increase, initiating transformation/transcendency. Deeper holons (the outside) exert an attraction on the defining context of an existing holon, until the outside transcends to an inside. The type of attractor can be identified by looking at a series of system states. Static attractors govern evolution when system states are relatively at rest; periodic attractors govern those systems that go through

Mind	Pure consciousness, spirit, consciousness of God, emptiness (Brahman in Hinduism)
Matter	The entirety of phenomena in the world (Maya in Hinduism)
Motion	Maya evolving towards increasing complexity, differentiation and internalization (Wilber's holon concept)

TABLE 1.10: Vedanta interpretation of Still's "matter, motion, mind"*

*Omega point: complex unit in which the organized sum of the reflected elements of the world becomes irreversible in embrace of a transcendent super-ego.

recognizable periodic repetitions of the same cycle. If, however, the sequences are irregular, this may hint at a chaotic attractor. Chaotic attractors may seem chaotic on the surface, but there are some patterns of order hidden in their complex structure, which give direction and structure to seemingly accidental system activities.

During the evolution of transformative processes, it has been established that increasing fluctuations in a system imply that interactive dynamics can no longer be stabilized by static or periodic attractors in the current state. This is where chaotic attractors come in, creating a critical threshold state with chaotic manifestations. This critical state can result in a symmetry break and lead to a transformation of the system at a higher organizational level. New static and periodical attractors replace the chaotic attractors to ensure the dynamic stability of the new holon (Chapter 4).

A telos has been described not only for the biosphere (e.g. the development of a plant out of a seed or of an animal out of a fertilized egg), but also for the physiosphere and the noosphere. As far as the noosphere is concerned, Freud's and Piaget's approaches are based on the presence of a telos, toward which the psyche develops. The end points of these developments vary, depending on the author, which is understandable considering the variation in context and environmental factors on which the authors based their considerations. From a holon concept perspective, the question arises as to whether a final telos can be defined. Certainly not in the world of phenomena, which

seems to consist of an endless pattern of holons – holons in holons in holons, etc. – or endless dynamics towards ever-deeper holons.

It would, however, be conceivable that there is an extreme, all-pervading telos, emptiness: the primary foundation of all holarchies and of all being. This is what the Hindus call atman and the Buddhists, nirvana, and Teilhard de Chardin speaks of the omega point. There is an immanent telos in evolutionary and involutionary processes in all manifestations of being, God in the shape of an "all-embracing chaotic attractor."[41]

According to Vedanta and Wilber's holon concept, one could deliberately interpret Still's "matter, motion, mind"[42] (which was definitely not intended) as follows (Table 1.10): as the dynamics of evolution are linked to increasing complexity and differentiation, something can go wrong at each individual evolutionary step, and new pathological patterns may develop. For example, emotional or mental pathological patterns may affect lower levels by displacing or suppressing biological factors. Differentiation may well overshoot its target and end up in dissociation instead of integration.

Adequate integral treatment must be able to classify pathological patterns and emerging dysfunctions and attribute them to the relevant evolutionary step. At a physical level, the disruptions are different from those at a biological or mental level. Consequential disruptions at the lower levels may annihilate all treatment options at higher levels, whereas the destruction of higher levels affects lower levels far less.

Atoms	Take in
Cells	Response to stimuli
Metabolic organisms (e.g., plants)	Rudimentary sensation
Protoneuronal organisms (e.g., Coelenterata)	Sensation
Neuronal organisms (e.g., annelids)	Awareness
Spinal canal (fish, amphibians)	Awareness/impulse
Brain stem (reptiles)	Impulse/emotion
Limbic system (lower mammals)	Emotion/pictures
Neocortex (primates)	Symbols
Complex neocortex (humans)	Notions (abstraction)

TABLE 1.11: Relationship between the outer objective (UR quadrant) and the inner subjective (UL quadrant) according to Wilber[43]

Model of all quadrants, levels, lines, states, and types (AQAL) according to Wilber

The holon concept is only one part of reality. It represents, as it were, the objective part of the holon. Its ideas are so universally valid (the smallest common denominator) that they apply equally to physical, biological, spiritual, or causal phenomena. However, this makes them inadequate as a model to accommodate the idiosyncrasies and properties of higher developmental stages, such as the spiritual level.

The holon concept is, as it were, an outside view of reality. The inner view is subjective and an inter-subjective experience. What is needed is an integral view that combines both perspectives. The brain is something external and objective, whereas the mind is something internal and subjective. The external can be described, but the internal can only be accessed by interaction and dialogue.

All stages we have gone through in evolution are still an active part of us, and yet they have become part of something bigger. Thus, single cells exist in us, forming tissue, etc. Due to integration, in a way, the inner views of cells, tissues, etc. are an integral part of us. Similarly, reptile instincts or sensations controlled by the limbic system (sexuality, fear, aggression, and hunger) are alive in us, as they are in lower mammals. They are part of us, but have been transformed and integrated into higher levels, thus making their power less absolute (Table 1.11).

According to Wilber, at least five areas of human experience must be considered for the understanding of the Cosmos (as well as for the understanding of disease, health, and treatment). They are quadrants, levels, lines, states, and types (AQAL – all quadrants, all levels). All experience can thus be described and classified as AQAL moments.

The four-quadrant model describes four inseparable dimensions or perspectives of "being in the world" for individuals. According to Wilber, the development of humans as well as the development of the world occurs simultaneously in all four quadrants (Figure.1.2): [44]

- Subjective efforts, experience, and awareness of the individual, summed up in the personal pronoun "I," upper left quadrant.

	Inside/outside within the quadrants	Routes of realization
Approach of the first person to the reality of the first person	UL, inside LL, inside	Phenomenology, introspection, meditation
Approach of the third person to the reality of the first person	UL, outside LL, outside	Developmental structuralism
Approach of the first person to the reality of the third person	UR, inside LR, inside	Biological phenomenology, autopoiesis, cognitive sciences Social autopoiesis
Approach of the third person to the realities of the third person	UR, outside LR, outside	Behaviorism, positivism, empiricism System theory, chaos and complexity theory

TABLE 1.12: Routes of realization with regard to the inside/outside concept of Wilber's quadrant model

- Objective structural, functional, or material/energetic equivalents, e.g., behavior, tissue structure, blood composition, physiology, individual gestures, subtle energies, etc., summed up in the pronoun "it," upper right (UR) quadrant.

- Inter-subjective action in a community of humans of equal depth, summed up in the pronoun "we," lower left (LL) quadrant.

- Corresponding inter-subjective external social structures, summed up in the pronoun "its," thought as a plural from, lower right (LR) quadrant.

In other words, all holons express themselves simultaneously in at least four aspects or quadrants. All quadrants must be taken into account in holistic therapy.[46]

Any disease or somatic dysfunction affects not only other holons in ascending and descending causal chains, but will express itself in all four quadrants. This means it has: (i) exterior-individual and objective "physiological and structural" representations; (ii) interior-individual, "emotional, mental, and spiritual," representations in experience and consciousness; (iii) interior-collective (cultural); and (iv) exterior-collective (social) representations. Any emotional disorder (upper left quadrant) will have an immediate effect on the neurochemical dimension (upper right quadrant). Treating

solely the dimension of the upper right quadrant would not take into account essential inner aspects (beliefs, emotions, and thoughts).

In traditional medicine, the treatment of individuals who are unwell is often reduced to chemical dynamics, whereas in current osteopathy, the perspective has often been narrowed to tissue dynamics. Although these perspectives are not necessarily wrong, they are incomplete. According to the AQAL model, there is no ontogenetic separation of psychological, structural–physiological, social, and cultural aspects in the osteopathic (somatic) dysfunctions and diseases. They form a complex, integrating all these perspectives. For example, a patient with a dysfunction of the quadratus lumborum and in the region of the cecum and certain unhealthy eating habits may suffer from emotional tension (for which the individual may compensate by eating unhealthily). The situation may be compounded by family problems, the loss of a job, and a general dismal social situation. Sorting out the mesentery and/or the quadratus lumborum may not be the wrong thing to do, but as single treatment, it would be inadequate because it is incomplete.

The inside/outside perspective of the quadrants

Furthermore, in his quadrant model, Wilber distinguishes eight main perspectives, thus dividing each

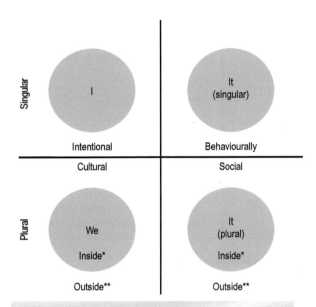

Singular

| Intentional | Behaviourally |

I

It
(singular)

Plural

We

It
(plural)

Inside*

Inside*

Outside**

Outside**

Cultural   Social

Figure 1.3
Four zones according to Wilber.[47]

quadrant into an inner and outer perspective. This differentiation may open up further research potential for osteopathy (Table 1.12 and Figure.1.3).

States are, according to Wilber, states of consciousness. Such states include ordinary states such as wakefulness, dreaming, and dreamless sleep, while more extraordinary states comprise meditative and drug-induced states of consciousness. The states are defined by the relevant levels (and the factors in all four quadrants) that an individual has reached in his/her development. The three stages are always present and accessible even to a toddler, whereas the (morphogenetic) potentials of the higher levels have not yet been realized. The achievements at each level will unfold through development only and turn into lasting qualities. States can only become lasting qualities if they run through several stages or levels.

Types are various forms of existence that allow you to exist and act at different levels of consciousness (e.g., as man or woman).

Explanation referring to a standard therapy situation

- UL (upper left) inside includes what happens phenomenologically between practitioner and client: thoughts, mental, and physical sensations.

- LL inside is the (inner) agreement between client and practitioner, their common "we."

- UL outside covers structures of consciousness and thus interpretation patterns used by the client to describe experiences during a session – of which the client is not necessarily aware, e.g., a guilt pattern along the lines "I have got this pain because I thought/did something bad."

- LL outside includes systemic/inter-subjective relation structures that formed between practitioner and client over one or several treatment sessions (again possibly without the parties being aware of them) that shape the content and sequence of treatment sessions, as may be demonstrated in a systemic list.

- UR inside looks at the manifestations of our perceptions, e.g., cognitive sciences, regarding subjective perceptions. Within the treatment scenario, this may apply to neurological complaints that affect perception.

- LR inside looks at the manifestation of what "holds together" a culture, such as the economy, religion, science, politics, etc., as described by the sociologist Niklas Luhmann.

- UR outside covers physiology as well as behavioral sciences and observations, such as the observation of client behavior.

- LR outside covers system theory, such as the (objectively observable) practitioner–patient treatment system and the effects changes in health legislation may have on it.

An osteopath who is aware of these perspectives when treating a patient will be able to see his/her action as part of a larger picture and evaluate their potential or limitations. The significance of so far neglected aspects will become evident, and treatment can be adapted accordingly.

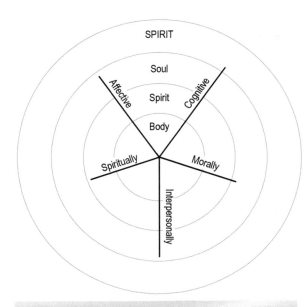

Figure 1.4
Lines of development according to Wilber.[48]

Lines or streams (Figure. 1.4) are the different dimensions or abilities of the self on its developmental path through the interior levels of growth or being. Over 24 such lines have currently been detected. They can develop in relative independence from each other. Thus, one developmental line may be highly developed, whereas another one is hardly detectable.

Two general categories of lines can be distinguished:

- Those related to the self, which are closely connected to the individual's identity, such as the sense of self (who am I?), moral (how do I relate to others?), and needs (what do I need?)

- Lines that represent talents and abilities, such as artistic abilities and kinesthetics.

Levels/steps or waves refer to ascending competence and complexity along the lines or streams, such as the cognitive ability to create images, symbols, concepts, and rules. The line of development in the individual will always follow this sequence of levels (pictures first, then symbols, followed by concepts, and then rules).

Initially, levels arise as evolutionary coincidences or creative, nondetermined novelties. Once they have emerged, they become cosmic habits through increasing repetition and are spread by morphic resonance and formative causation (passed on through own past, familial, subcultural, cultural, and supercultural patterns.) The shape and content of those steps is formed by the AQAL space. While the Vedanta philosophy distinguishes no more than 5 levels (Chapter 25), at least 12 levels (Chapter 18) of consciousness have been identified (in the spiral dynamics system), through which run 24 relatively independent lines of development.

Summary

Phenomenology in particular highlights a crucial aspect, namely that we can be conscious of ourselves through inner experience only. It also emphasizes that body and soul can become one where life is simultaneously experienced by body and soul in all its domains – in contrast to Descartes' separation of body and soul.[49] Once a disruption occurs in one of the essential domains of existence, it will disrupt the cohesion of all others. However, being holons, we are not only entities but also parts in a holonic hierarchy. Holarchic organization and its effects on human evolution have not been fully appreciated by phenomenology. This failure to acknowledge developmental dynamic aspects in human holons does not make this approach any more comprehensive or holistic.

The biomechanical approach regarding the unity of bodily functions, is a key concept developed by A.T. Still.[50] The procedures of osteopathy were founded on, and developed on, the basis of the structural/functional interactions taking place in the patient. This is where its therapeutic strength lies. The notion "functional" includes the objective physiological parameters of the upper right quadrant as well as consciousness aspects of the upper left quadrant. Thus, internal spiritual aspects interact with external tissues (form) or the inner spiritual world appertains to the external tissue complexity. Conversely, the external tissue dynamics are the outside of the internal spiritual, making the mind, to a certain extent, treatable by palpating the relevant tissue. However, the palpatory approach must be backed up by integrating the levels of self-experience in the patient, e.g., in a dialogue about the patient's experience, in the palpation process.

If approaches targeting the physical and biological aspects are uncritically applied to the direct treatment of internal, subjective levels, this will result in incoherence. Wanting to treat internal, subjective (consciousness-related) processes by manipulating brain or body tissue is like trying to alter a film script just by replacing paper, exchanging ink cartridges, and repairing the computer. It is certainly possible to establish contact with any tissue in the body and promote further integrative processes. However, do not expect too much of such an approach. If osteopathic treatment is to be effective at the level of consciousness, the laws of consciousness must be applied to osteopathic treatment. Where emotional levels are targeted, the laws of the emotional levels must be taken into account. A finely tuned range of methods is called for.

The existence of autopoiesis and interactive self-healing mechanisms, which have been partially backed up and interpreted by phenomenology, have been postulated. However, one often encounters reductionist interpretations and applications at the level of functional/structural interaction that do not take sufficiently into account the patient's subjective experience, or consciously include the subjective and inter-subjective world of the practitioner. The internal, subjective levels of a patient's experience are thus being reduced to their material tissue or energy aspects, such as somatic dysfunction, neurotransmitters, etc.

In addition, there is a tendency in modern osteopathy to reduce higher holons, such as humans, to their individual components (subholons). Instead of looking at human individuals from a perspective such as Wilber's AQAL model and treating them accordingly, practitioners see their patients as particularly complex machines with structural/energetic imbalances that need to be manipulated. This is not a wrong, but an incomplete, perspective, leading to inadequate treatment with reduced healing potential. Wilber's AQAL model resolves the artificial and arbitrary division into psychological, somatic, cultural, and social aspects or dysfunctions.

In osteopathy, the self-regulation of an organism is mainly interpreted at a biological level. In order to do justice to a patient's emotional, mental, and spiritual levels, this must be complemented by including the aspects of self-preservation, self-adaptation, self-immanence, and self-transcendence; therefore, increasing autonomy, differentiation, and increasing complexity (see above).

Another distortion may arise from transferring (mental/spiritual) realms of experience to lower (e.g., biological) realms of experience. Whether Still himself is guilty of such transfers from mental/spiritual levels to biological or physical levels (somatization, biologization, or physicalization) in his writings, can only be decided by taking account of his entire work. Quoting Still out of context may encourage such conclusions and may risk distorting his perspective, e.g., "The soul of man with all the streams of pure living water seems to dwell in the fascia of his body."[51]

Personally, I am convinced that Still included the spiritual level in his concept of interaction between form and function, although not in the highly differentiated form as is done today, e.g., mutual impact of psyche and soma. From a methodological point of view, whether he was of the opinion that the objective organization of matter represented the external, as opposed to internal/subjective consciousness, I cannot say. Neither could I come to a conclusion from his writings.

It seems to make sense to review osteopathic views and methods without prejudice and look at how holistic and integrated their approach is. It is not enough to postulate the unity of body, mind, and soul. Only a wider understanding of the socio-cultural environment in which osteopathy developed, as well as its philosophy, arts, and sciences, provides a basis from which osteopathy can tap into current trends in philosophy, medicine, and other sciences. This will help to develop the potential of Still's vision and refine, advance and enhance it.

Inadequate, un-reflected so-called renewals, or new inventions, in osteopathy without enough understanding of the roots of osteopathy on the one hand, as well as rigid, conservative dogmatism on the other hand, may be inadequate in the era of rationalism, as well from a post-rationalistic point of view, and inadequate for the development of a vibrant, integral osteopathy. The future of osteopathy will depend on its ability to leave dogmatism behind, put traditional views in perspective and integrate more comprehensive concepts.

In my view, the differentiated adaptation of the right and left quadrants in diagnostics and treatment seems to hold enormous potential. It would also mean a relaxation of the rigid practitioner–patient duality in terms of a subject–object relationship, something that has already been happening in osteopathic practice. Patients are no longer considered to be passive objects, but active agents in the therapeutic process. The shared experience of being (practitioner and patient in the therapeutic process) is already an integral part of functional osteopathy and is utterly desirable.

The removal of physical/mechanical blockages can be all the more profound and comprehensive, the more emotional, mental, and spiritual levels are part of the process. It is true that as an effect of the interaction between form and function, any change in form/matter is likely to have an effect on function as well as consciousness (which is part of functionality). However, whether the desired support for "the whole person" is likely to achieve its full potential depends on the integral understanding of a human being in all its dimensions, on which therapeutic interaction is based (e.g., on Wilber's AQAL model). Contact by palpation would then be able to elicit resonance at all levels involved. Otherwise, palpation would at best be translatory cosmetics and at worst invasive traumatology with therapeutically induced dissociation.

It is important to realize, in this context, that Still's metaphor of a "human machine" and the osteopath being a "mechanic" must be seen from the perspective of his time. Still was - like most Americans of the late 19th century - fascinated by technology. In his publications Still used metaphors that show a correlation to the industrial revolution.

"The one should be treated to take up more of the substances, and the other should be treated in such a manner as to cause him to burn up in the furnace of life all fuel sent there by Nature to keep it hot and in motion".

And: "Let us say that each person is a well organized city and reason by comparison that the city makes all the workshops necessary to produce such machinery as is required for the health and comfort of its inhabitants".

These metaphors indicate how Still converted his knowledge of machines to the human body.

"As Osteopathy is a science built upon the principle that man is a machine". [61,62,63]

The life machine was driven by some invisible vital force:[52] a concept deeply rooted in vitalism, as his chapter on biogens shows.[53] The osteopath as a mechanic acts on behalf of that vital force, to remove obstructions to the normal flow. He also postulated a dual entity of life and matter and a trinity of material body, spiritual being, and being of mind (see above).[54]

References

[1]Tagore, R., Sadhana – the Realization of Life, Macmillan, New York, 1916, p. 27

[2]Kuhn T., The Structure of Scientific Revolutions, University of Chicago Press, 1962

[3]Karger-Decker B., Die Geschichte der Medizin, Albatros, Düsseldorf, 2001 (available in German only)

[4]Bacon F., The Advancement of Learning, JM Dent & Sons, London, 1973

[5]McGovern J., McGovern R., Your Healer Within, Fenestra Books, Tucson, Arizona, 2003

[6]Levin D.M, Solomon G.F., The discursive formation of the body in the history of medicine, J Med Philos 10/1990;15(5); 515–537

[7]Personal communication by Kratky

[8]Stacher A., Warum fehlt der Dialog zwischen Schulmedizin und Komplementärmedizin. GAMED, 4/1996;8–12

[8a]Smuts J.C., Holism and Evolution. Macmillan, London, 1927

[9]IFAEMM - Reduktionistische und holistische Konzepte. http://www.ifaemm.de/B4_redho.htm

[10]Kratky, K.W., Complementary Medicine Systems: Comparison and Integration. In: Health and Human Development. Nova Science Publishers, 1 July 2008

[10a]Pischinger A., Das System der Grundregulation. 8. Aufl., Haug, Heidelberg, 1990

[10b]Heine H., Lehrbuch der biologischen Medizin: Grundregulation und Extrazelluläre Matrix, Hippokrates, Stuttgart, 2007

[11] Fischer L., Neuraltherapie nach Huneke. Hippokrates, Stuttgart 2001;49 (available only in German)

[12] Engel G.I., The need for a new medical model: a challenge for biomedicine. Science 1977;196;129–135

[13] McLaren N., A critical review of the biopsychosocial model, Austral New Zealand J Psychiatry 1998;31:86–92

[14] Boss M., Existential Foundations of Medicine and Psychology. Tr. S. Conway and A. Cleaves, Jason Aronson, Northvale, 1979

[15] Paulat U., Medard Boss und die Daseinsanalyse – ein Dialog zwischen Medizin und Philosophie im 20. Jahrhundert; Teetum, 2001

[16] Hannah T., What is somatics? Somatics 1986;5(4):4–8

[17] Husserl E., Cartesian Meditations, transl. b. Dorion Cairns, Springer, New York, 7th edition, 1988

[18] Boss M., Existential Foundations of Medicine and Psychology, Tr. S. Conway and A. Cleaves. Jason Aronson, Northvale, 1979

[19] www.isseem.org

[20] Bischof M., Energiemedizin – Heilkunst der Zukunft. Esotera 9/2000:20–25

[21] Kratky K.W., Complementary Medicine Systems: Comparison and Integration. In: Health and Human Development, Nova Science Publishers, 1 July 2008

[22] Wilber K., Sex, Ecology, Spirituality, Shambala Publications, Boston, Mass., 1995, 2000

[23] Wilber K., A Theory of Everything, Shambala Publications, Boston, Mass., 2001

[24] Wilber K., A Theory of Everything, Shambala Publications Boston, Mass., 2001

[25] Dippon M., Das holistische Menschenbild von A.T. Still: Man is a Triune. Eine Untersuchung des Ursprungs von man is a triune. Esslingen, SKOM, 2005

[26] Stark J., Still's Fascia. A qualitative investigation to enrich the meaning behind Andrew Taylor Still's concepts of fascia. Toronto. Thesis. Canadian College of Osteopathy, 2003

[27] Townbridge C., Andrew Taylor Still: 1828–1917. Thomas Jefferson UP, Kirksville, 1991;161

[28] Würhl P., Zur Übersetzung Grundlegender Konzepte von A. T. Still: Man is a Triune. DO-Deutsche Zeitschrift für Osteopathie 2005;2;31–33

[29] Pöttner, personal communication with Liem, 2005

[30] Stark J., Still's Fascia. A qualitative investigation to enrich the meaning behind Andrew Taylor Still's concepts of fascia. Toronto. Thesis. Canadian College of Osteopathy, 2003

[31] Seffinger M.A., Korr I.M., Osteopathic Philosophy. In: Ward R.C., Foundations for Osteopathic Medicine. Williams and Wilkins, Baltimore, 1997;5

[32] Wilber K., Sex, Ecology, Spirituality, Shambala Publications, Boston, Mass. 1995, 2000

[33] Varela F., (ed.) Sleeping, Dreaming and Dying. Wisdom Book, Boston, 1997

[34] Stark J., Personal communication, 3/2005

[35] Hulett G.D., Address to graduating class June 1903. J Osteop August 1903;241–246

[36] Schnucker R.V., Early Osteopathy in the Words of A.T. Still, Thomas Jefferson University Press, Kirksville, 1991;79

[37] Wilber K., Sex, Ecology, Spirituality, Shambala Publications, Boston, Mass., 1995, 2000

[38] Damasio A.R., The Feeling of What Happens, Harcourt Brace, 1999

[39] Porges S.W., The polyvagal theory; phylogenetic substrates of a social nervous system. J Psychophysiol 42(2)

[39a] Franz E.A., Gillett G., John Hughlings Jackson's evolutionary neurology: a unifying framework for cognitive neuroscience. Brain 2011;134(10);3114–3120

[39b] Jantsch, E., Die Selbstorganisation des Universums: Vom Urknall zum menschlichen Geist. DTV, München, 1982

[39c] Pischinger, A., Das System der Grundregulation. 8. Aufl., Haug, Heidelberg, 1990

[40] Teilhard de Chardin P., The Heart of the Matter, Harvest/HBJ, 2002

[41] Wilber K., Sex, Ecology, Spirituality, Shambala Publications, Boston, Mass., 1995, 2000

[42] Still A.T., J Osteop III(3):9;1896/Still A.T., J Osteop I(10):1; 1985

[43] Wilber K., Sex, Ecology, Spirituality, Shambala Publications, Boston, Mass., 1995, 2000

[44] Wilber K., Sex, Ecology, Spirituality, Shambala Publications, Boston, Mass., 1995, 2000

[45] Wilber, K., A Theory of Everything, Shambala Publications Boston, Mass., 2001

[46]Wilber, K., A Theory of Everything, Shambala Publications Boston, Mass., 2001

[47]Wilber, K., Integral Spirituality: A Startling New Role for Religion in the Modern and Postmodern World, Shambala Publications Boston, Mass., 2007

[48]Wilber, K., A Theory of Everything, Shambala Publications Boston, Mass., 2001

[49]Paulat U., Medard Boss und die Daseinsanalyse – ein Dialog Zwischen Medizin und Philosophie im 20. Jahrhundert; Teetum, 2001

[50]Comeaux Z., Somatic Dysfunction – a reflection on the scope of osteopathic practice. Manuscript for publication in Osteopathische Medizin, 2005:2

[51]Still A.T., Philosophy of Osteopathy, 1899, p. 165

[52]Still A.T., Philosophy and Mechanical Principles of Osteopathy. Hudson Kimberly Kansas, 1902, reprint by Osteopathic Enterprise, Kirksville, 1986, p. 184

[53]Still A.T., Philosophy and Mechanical Principles of Osteopathy. Hudson Kimberly, Kansas,1902, reprint by Osteopathic Enterprise, Kirksville, 1986, p. 251

[54]Still A.T., Philosophy and Mechanical Principles of Osteopathy. Hudson Kimberly Kansas 1902, reprint by Osteopathic Enterprise, Kirksville, 1986, pp. 16–17

[55]Ackerknecht, E. H., Therapeutics from the Primitives to the 20th Century. Hafner Press, New York, 1973.

[56]Gevitz, N., The Dos: Osteopathic Medicine in America. 2nd edition. Johns Hopkins University Press, Baltimore, 2004.

[57]Trowbridge, C., Andrew Taylor Still 1828-1917. 4th revised edition. Jolandos, Pähl, Germany, 2006.

[58]Still, A. T., Autobiography of A. T. Still. Revised edition. Published by the author, Kirksville, 1908.

[59]Sheldrake, R., Seven Experiments that could change the World. Inner Traditions, Rochester, Vermont, 2002

[60]Kaznacheyev, V.P., Michailowa, L.P., Ultraschwache Strahlung als interzelluläre Wechselwirkung (Russian), Nauka, Novosibirsk, 1981

[61]Still, A.T., The Philosophy and Mechanical Principles of Osteopathy. Kirksville, 1902, p. 292

[62]Still, A.T., Osteopathy Research and Practice. The Journal Printing Company, Kirksville, 1910, p. 14

[63]Still, A. T., Autobiography of A. T. Still. Revised edition. Published by the author, Kirksville, 1908, p. 90

The osteopathic object – reloaded

Peter Sommerfeld

Case history

Quite a few years back, I went to a seminar in philosophy dedicated to a book by Friedrich Nietzsche where he talks about the death of God.*,[1] The seminar focused on Martin Heidegger's re-questioning of Nietzsche's programmatic nihilism.[2] While attending the seminar, an uncanny feeling crept up on me that the nihilism debate might affect me, too, in my professional environment and I began to put that haunting feeling into words. In the resulting text, I accused osteopathy teachers and practitioners of veering toward "incomplete nihilism," as defined by Nietzsche. I argued that osteopaths invented a world beyond the material world, a counter-world to what they saw as the materialism of conventional medicine. This counter-world, I claimed rather discourteously, was nothing but a variation on the materialist theme, in which humans were assigned the role of biological or even physiological machines.

To give readers some idea of what I mean, here are a few examples. Nicholas Handoll (pp. 209, 213, 218)[3] describes our existence as human beings as nothing but "*crystals in a saturated solution,*" "*electromagnetic waves of photons in our body*" or even "*energy patterns that are recognized by the therapist.*" Talking of "work on tissue" or divine elements ("*the highest known element*") that express themselves in cerebrospinal fluid** would also fall into this category. Such dinky gems of psycho-spiritual syncretism can be found in abundance in the writings of William Garner Sutherland (pp. 33, 34):[4]

The "juice," [sic.] that invisible potency, the battery of the human body.

…He wants us to see this "copper tube" and the wire within, the potential. The principle is used in the material cable that carries messages across the Atlantic Ocean.

One might argue that those are just metaphors. Metaphors for what, may I ask? Sometimes they seem to stand for a kind of osteopathic cosmology or even culminate in an osteopathic version of the Bible, in which stories are transposed into history:

We have historical record. The waters were divided when the earth appeared. From the earth Man was created. The waters were divided! The fascia! Even the fascia is water, even the bony tissue is liquid.†

It would be interesting to see what "historical evidence" Sutherland uses to back up his statements – probably the fact that fasciae consist of water and bones are liquid – which takes us nicely back into the world of physically describable objects.

For Nietzsche, incomplete nihilism reveals a certain reluctance to deal with the essence of nihilism – a reluctance that may cause individuals to resort to substitute religions or substitute values. The void left by nihilism must be filled. Heidegger writes (p. 9):[2]

The now-empty authoritative realm of the suprasensory and the ideal world can still be adhered to.

…What is more, the empty place demands to be occupied anew and to have the god now vanished from it replaced by something else. New ideals are set up. That happens, according to Nietzsche's conception (Will to Power, Aph. 1021, 1887), through doctrines regarding world happiness, through socialism, and equally through Wagnerian music…

---

*"*Few of Nietzsche's statements have become as popular as this one*" writes Daniel Havemann.[1] Sentence number 125 in Nietzsche's compendium *The Gay Science* under the title The Madman (*The Gay Science* (Philosophical Classics) by Friedrich Wilhelm Nietzsche and Thomas Common, 2009).

**Compare with Still[5] p. 44. This remark was not particularly emphasized by Still,[5] but became a starting point for Sutherland to explore various counter-worlds and worlds that cannot be seen (compare with Sutherland,[4] p. 32 and passim).

†Sutherland[6] (p. 290) the emphasis on "historical" by myself (Peter Sommerfeld) and the emphasis on "Man" is from the original.

The materialism of conventional medicine (humans are nothing but an agglomeration of cells, the sum of physiological processes describable in physical terms, etc.) produces a gaping void, which is filled by osteopathy's deification of this same materialism. The deification of anatomy is probably the most prevalent form among traditional authors. The most recent variant of sticking to the materialist approach is simply by believing that it will be overcome in the paradoxes of quantum mechanics. This is what – amongst others – Handoll is guilty of. [††]

This is roughly the gist of what I wrote about incomplete nihilism in osteopathy. In my naivety, I sent the draft to a European professional organization of osteopaths, suggesting that this was a topic to be debated in public at a conference. What I did not realize at the time was the fact that this professional organization has been equipped with a kind of "police department for cultural sciences" that seemed to watch over the purity of osteopathic doctrine, protecting it from any subversive contamination. My paper was passed on to this cultural watchdog. The reply came immediately, accusing the author of incompetence, as is common practice among cultural scientists. I was told that the existentialism–nihilism debate, taken up by Heidegger and incompetently instrumentalized by me, had long been settled. The subject–object problem, on which my arguments were partially based, was no longer relevant. All this was water under the bridge and the problems I described no longer existed in osteopathy. To prove that this was the case, I was directed to Nicholas Handoll's book *The Anatomy of Potency* and its epistemological premises based on new insights from quantum physics that applied to all humans and osteopaths in particular.

I realized that I had touched on a sore point because Handoll's book is an excellent example, as far as my claims are concerned. However, I was in no mind to start a feud with the cultural police of a European professional organization. I came to the conclusion that no matter how strongly I felt about these issues, they either did not matter to the osteopathic community or it shared these feelings but preferred not to deal with them. Being accused of incompetence – well, that has happened to people of far higher standing. I certainly had rattled their cage and their response showed that they took me seriously.

[††]I would like to mention that my argumentation has found a lot of excellent support since Wührl.[7]

From then on, I took great care to smuggle my subversive thoughts past the culture police and had two versions published – one in a specialist journal[8] and another one under the title Über den Gegenstand der Osteopathie (About What Osteopathy is About) in the German edition of this book.[9] However, the translator who was working on my contribution ran into difficulty and I was contacted. I must admit that it is almost impossible to translate the text, given the clarity of the English language and the pragmatism of the Anglo-American culture. Besides, I also felt the German version could do with a revamp: being too clumsy, redundant, and complicated. However, the "uncanny" feeling I described earlier on has not gone away and something needs to be done about it.

How to reload

In my view, the urgency of the problem has increased over the past years and I feel that the topic I am writing about does not just affect osteopaths. Does osteopathy really differ from other healing professions in that respect? What is so special about the problems osteopaths face? Admittedly, osteopathy is continuously re-inventing itself, as are many other professions. This seems to be a social phenomenon. It has become trendy to re-invent yourself all the time. However, does that affect the essential problems we face in our work as osteopaths? Does it affect the situation where a patient comes to see an expert who – for whatever reasons – calls himself or herself an osteopath? The answer is no.

The problems we face are those of medicine in general if we agree to define medicine not just as the work of a physician. It is irrelevant whether osteopaths see themselves as working for or against, alongside or outside conventional medicine. I would even claim that questions of professional identity could be counterproductive when trying to find out what it is that we encounter in our daily work. Questions about identity always require inclusion and exclusion zones to be defined and encourage a discourse permeated by doctrine and ideology. Foucault (p. 132)[10] accurately observes that when facing a patient *"the prolix discourses of systems must be interrupted"* and he quotes Corvisart:[11] *"All theory is always silent or vanishes at the patient's bedside."* It does not matter to the patient how I define myself as an osteopath, nor does it matter how osteopathy sets itself apart from other healing disciplines. What matters to patients is whether we can help them in a situation that could be broadly described as clinical. A clinical situation is the classical encounter of doctor/therapist and patient. This is the background against which the question of the "object of osteopathy" is raised.

The osteopathic object in crisis?

It has to be said that raising the question of the object, in the context of our profession, is nothing short of a provocation. After all, in spite of all the craftsmanship-related analogies our founding father used, we are neither carpenters nor plumbers or engineers. We do not handle wood, metal, stone, or other matter. Which kind of "matter" matters in our case? The tissue? Do we indeed treat mere tissues, crystalline solutions, tides, potencies, or midlines? Isn't this the same as treating a broken leg or an infection? I would even go as far as saying that the metaphoric language used in osteopathy is a sham. It is trying to conceal the reality that osteopaths encountering patients is no different from the kind of reality reflected in ward-speak such as "Please could you attend to the 'liver' in ward 20." They might say instead "I have entered into a dialogue with the 'tissue' and, by being still, I managed to restore the unity of the potentials on ward 20."

I would go still further and claim that in some ways, conventional medicine is more honest than its complementary counterpart, as practiced by many osteopaths. When dealing with a representative of conventional medicine (assuming they exist and have not just been invented for argument's sake), at least patients know where they stand. Osteopaths, on the other hand, make patients believe they are safe in the paradise of a "humane healing method." Little do they know that even in osteopathy, they are usually assessed with the help of naïve materialist concepts and turned into manageable osteopathic objects. This is also true for concepts that do not meet all criteria of physicalism. In other words, even if I am convinced that my intention, imagination, and therapeutic flights of fancy or even my mere existence and patience have an effect on the patient – which sets its face against physicalism – it all comes down to physiology or physics, including quantum physics, on which osteopaths base their models. Osteopaths see themselves as the opposite of the narrow, reduced world of materialism and as part of a better, more humane, more truthful and, above all, more complete world. However, when we look more closely, we realize that osteopaths regard patients as physical objects, just as the imagined counterpart, the conventional physician, would. The conventional physician is being accused of materialism, while osteopaths use different ideas to replicate the very attitude they were trying to distance themselves from.

This becomes apparent especially in those osteopathic concepts that are deemed to be a long way away from the materialistic world view. Thus, cerebrospinal fluid is perceived as the *highest known element*, or 'liquid light' that may be sent into a patient's bones. The use of metaphors in sequence cannot divert from the underlying materialism, but leads back to it in the form of "element," "cerebrospinal fluid," "light," "liquid," etc. What makes this matter so contentious is that osteopathic practitioners seem to believe that they can manipulate physical objects with some paraphysical tricks (*potency, tide, breath of life*, etc.). The impression is given that osteopaths deal with a very special object when they talk about "energies," "fields," "rhythms," "waves," and "tides". The use of all those New Age tags cannot divert from the fact that the osteopathic object is talked about in a perverted form of physicalism. I am still waiting for an answer to my urgent questions: What do I treat? What is it that is affected by my action? What is standing, sitting, or lying opposite me in the treatment room? What do I deal with? What will I have to deal with?

The object – a never-ending challenge

All these questions are put to the test when facing a patient in a clinical situation. The ominous notions of energies, breaths, potencies, and tides are applied to what is in front of us and raise questions on the nature of being – those questions referred to in philosophy as ontology. The clinical situation brings us face to face with the nature of being – the abyss of ontology. Questions about physiology, psychology, or legislation are only secondary, and none of them can bridge the ontological abyss – whether the physiology of tissue, the activity of mirror neurons, or even an informed consent document to keep the evil spirits of jurisdiction at bay. They all go nowhere as long as we have not answered the question about what it is we are facing (a multicellular something with emotions perhaps) – a question asked from a more or less involved observer's perspective. The observer lets the object slide through his or her fingers, draws conclusions from findings, and finally begins treatment, working on tissue, for instance. The biddable object lets it happen. This is the pathos part in the word osteopathy – the object lets it happen.

We have now reached the point where we can safely replace the word "object" by "patient." According to Emmanuel Lévinas's ethical concept, the investigative observer is in the position of an individual who, out of metaphysical desire, forces the Other to become part of the individual's own world order, thus depriving the Other of primary alterity.

…sovereign reason knows only itself, that nothing other limits it. The neutralization of the Other who becomes a theme or an object – appearing, that is, taking its place in the light – is precisely his reduction to the same. (p. 43)[12]

Is that all we can do? In fact, we should ask: can we restrict ourselves to such limited action in a clinical situation? Should not our interest and commitment go beyond investigating an object for dysfunction, potencies, midlines, etc. that need to be dealt with?

Or, to put the question more urgently: does the Other not require us to do more? Traditional ontology, which looks at the essence of an object, is not much help here. The ontology we need cannot assign us the role of a neutral bystander. Its role is to wake us up, send a shiver down our spine and make us aware of the ethical precariousness of our situation as therapists.

I know some will argue that we need to keep a professional distance. Without professional distance, therapy could easily turn into manipulation. Agreed, but I would argue that keeping too much distance can lead to a cold, sober attitude that might fit the job description of a torturer as well as a medical professional. I know I am being a bit drastic here – please forgive me! Precisely because closeness and distance have such a pivotal role in osteopathic intervention, we must be alert to our object in a clinical situation and realize that our role is not just that of competent experts (that should be taken for granted), but comes with moral obligations. In other words, our usual explanations and arguments and the resulting action must stand up to scrutiny. This is what Lévinas calls ethics: *"We name this calling into question of my spontaneity by the presence of the Other ethics."*[12]

Furthermore, as individuals who must act within moral responsibilities, we are like acrobats without a net. Nobody can tell us with absolute certainty if we have done the right thing or not. If anybody could, this would be paramount to ethics on prescription, with our responsibilities following some kind of moral template. There is no way around the ultimate responsibility we have to accept. We must accept that we can never do enough by the standards of the Other. We can never be allowed to rest on our laurels. It is never enough, and our work is a continuous challenge. I am coming back to Lévinas, whose thoughts are homing in on this salient point:

Someone who expresses himself in his nudity – the face – is one to the point of appealing to me, of placing himself under my responsibility; henceforth, I have to respond for him. All the gestures of the other were signs addressed to me… The other who expresses himself is entrusted to me (and there is no debt in regard to the other, for what is due is unpayable: one is never free of it).[13]

Dawn of (the) bodies

I have been calling for an ontology that emphasizes the ethical precariousness of our situation. As far as the challenge represented by the Other is concerned (in our case the challenge resulting from the clinical situation), there seems to be no way around the works of Lévinas. He developed his concept of "alterity," which consistently focuses on the obsession with identification in Western philosophy.

There is, however, one topic which has become increasingly important to the cultural sciences over the last decade – it's the body. Luc Nancy's book *Corpus* has a key role in this discourse.[14] Nancy's approach is all the more interesting to us because he does not refute materialism (the body described by Nancy is a body of flesh and blood, a vulnerable body), while simultaneously focusing on the range of extraordinary ambivalences a body represents, and on the masses of bodies that make up our world. Nancy's notion of a body is not predefined, but sums up a whole world of confusion and unanswered questions. The question of what actually defines matter takes center-stage. It is no good to beat about the bush any longer – here is what it boils down to: how are we going to deal with those bodies? Nancy's book opens with the almost manic intensity of the well-known formula, repeated over and over in our history, to describe the ultimate sacrifice: *Hoc est enim corpus meum.* On reading, it conjures up an archaic scene, repeating itself again and again – the Greek hero Achilles circling around the walls of Troy, dragging Hector's corpse through the dust. What is it he is dragging through the dust behind his chariot?

This brings me back to my earlier questions as to where our continuous new challenges come from. Lévinas gives us the location or rather the non-location from where those challenges reach us – "the Other." Nancy[14] has the answer:

What is the space opened between eight billion bodies, and, within each one, between phallus and cephale, among the thousand folds, postures, falls, leaps and bounds of each? In what space do they touch each other and stray from each other, with none of them, or their totality, being absorbed into a pure empty sign of the self, into a body-of-sense? (p. 83)

This open space sends out a cry – the cry of bodies that open up and tear the space, turning it into a wide open space. Nancy[14] talks of the body's "areality," "*signifying the nature or specificity of an aire ('area')." "By chance,"* Nancy continues, *"this word also serves to suggest a lack of reality, or rather a slight, faint, suspended reality."* (p. 43)

In amongst the multitude of bodies, there is always one body that matters to us once we sit down in our treatment rooms. Many bodies cannot be described by the general term "body." What matters is always the one body, "This Very Body." This Very Body comprises the infinite uniqueness and uncanny singleness of our being. To quote Nancy:[14] "*The exceptionality of a body is common as such: substitutable for every other as unsubstitutable.*" (p. 93)

When we look at the individual body, refusing to ignore the infinite number of individual differences, we are stunned by the uniqueness and singleness of This Very Body, and that is exactly what we encounter as the object/subject in a clinical situation – regardless of how successfully it undergoes physically describable interaction or is kept at a distance by "professional attitude." Once we have been touched by This Very Body, it does not let go, it pursues us and keeps providing new challenges. You cannot carry it home in an anatomy or physiology book, clinical manual, or psychological compendium. "*Body is certitude shattered and blown to bits*" (p. 5) says Nancy[14] and again: "*There is nothing to decipher in a body – except for the fact that the body's cipher is the body itself …*" (p. 47)

This Very Body and the clinical situation

There is no easy way around it. This Very Body here and now rebels and has its demands. It demands that I give my utmost and I know that I will only be able to do it justice in a very limited way. This is my duty toward This Very Body, including my awareness that it will never be enough, I will never know enough, and I can never do enough.

This Very Body here and now is a pledge and command not to sit back and do nothing. It is the be-all and end-all of my actions in general and in particular in a clinical situation. What makes a clinical situation so special? This Very Body reveals itself in its frailty and refuses to be dealt with as a physical object that is at our disposition. This quality of not being at our disposition – that is what This Very Body is about. It is the core challenge we face in a clinical situation.

How do we respond to this challenge? What does This Very Body with its plea not to sit back want us to do?

Well, knowledge is a prerequisite – physics, biology, physiology, and anatomy, basic research and applied research may be relevant to This Very Body and must be at hand, but it is not the first priority. If knowledge were the first priority, This Very Body would be degraded to an exchangeable object, a piece of meat waiting in the slaughterhouse to be taken away. It would be turned into some general exchangeable body that could be addressed in a systematic way. In other words – knowledge, the epistemological domain, must be aware of its limitations when confronted with This Very Body in a clinical situation. If the knowledgeable person fails to accept this then they will take a position of power and dominate the clinical situation. The body will be turned into a meaningless object. A clinical situation, by contrast, requires something going beyond mere knowledge.

What I need to do as a therapist is to take seriously the appeal emanating from This Very Body – the appeal for utmost respect. This is precisely why I need to understand that all the fields of knowledge at my disposal can only help to shed light on certain aspects of This Very Body. This may be useful sometimes, but is by no means sufficient.

Our training and continuous professional development does not sufficiently take these requirements into account. For a professional group that claims to be osteopaths, it would perhaps be a good idea to spare a thought for this. One thing is certain. If we are to include the requirements of This Very Body in our professional training, it will be an arduous journey, but a worthwhile journey.

References

[1]Havemann D. 2009. "Gott ist tot". In: Ch Niemeyer (Hg.). Nietzsche Lexikon. Wissenschaftliche Buchgesellschaft, Darmstadt, S 133–134.

[2]Heidegger M. 2003. Nietzsche's Word "God is dead". Open source version.

[3]Handoll N. 2001. Anatomy of Potency. Executive Physical Therapy.

[4]Sutherland WG. 1990. Teachings in the science of Osteopathy, Rudra Press, Portland, Oregon.

[5]Still AT. 1986. (Reprint of 1902 edition). The philosophy and mechanical principles of osteopathy, Osteopathic Enterprise, Kirksville, Missouri.

[6]Sutherland WG. 1998. Contributions of thought: The collected writings of William Garner Sutherland, D.O., 2nd edition, Rudra Press, Portland, Oregon.

[7]Wührl P. 2006. Osteopathie, Quantenphysik, Offenbarung, Teil 1. Deutsche Zeitschrift für Osteopathie. 4:32–35.

[8]Sommerfeld P. 2005a. Osteopathie. Eine quasi-medizinische Spielart des unvollständigen Nihilismus? Versuch einer ontologischen Standortbestimmung. Osteopath Med. 6(4):17–21.

[9]Sommerfeld P. 2005b. Über den Gegenstand der Osteopathie. In: T. Liem (Ed.). Morphodynamik in der Osteopathie. Hippokrates. Stuttgart.

[10]Foucault M. 2010 (Reprint). The Birth of the Clinic. An archaeology of medical perception. Transl.: AM Sheridan, Routledge, London, NY.

[11]Corvisart J. 1808. Preface to the French translation of Auenbrugger: Nouvelle méthode pour reconnaîre les maladies internes de la poitrine, Paris.

[12]Lévinas L. 1991. Totality and Infinity: An Essay on Exteriority. Tansl.: A. Lingis, J. Wild, Kluwer Academic Publishers.

[13]Lévinas E. 2000. God, Death, and Time. Transl.: B. Bergo, Stanford University Press, Stanford, California.

[14]Nancy J-L. 2008. Corpus. Transl.: RA Rand, Fordham University Press, NY.

Biological rhythms and their significance in osteopathy

Maximilian Moser and Torsten Liem

Nature is not served by rigid laws, but by rhythmical, reciprocal processes.

V. Schauberger[1]

I think it would be difficult or even impossible to find a normal life process that is not subject to rhythmical fluctuations.

A. Bier (1933) quoted from W. Menzel[2]

Introduction

Our entire life is shaped by biological rhythms, as the human organism is subject not only to spatial, but also time structure. New research demonstrates how very important biological rhythms are for our wellbeing. These can provide many starting points in osteopathic treatment and go beyond the traditional form of manual synchronization with the body's rhythms (sometimes based on speculation), as the notion of the wholeness of the human body within a human time frame and interaction between them deepens.

It can in any case be assumed that a number of biological rhythms are characterized by feedback and self-regulation. It is possible that the components of the spectral element of chronomes (temporal wave patterns variable in the biosphere as well as in the physical environment) are subject to multiple intermodulations.[3] Particular biological rhythms, such as the circadian rhythm, should not be looked at in isolation, and disconnected from other phenomena of rhythm.

Rhythm is a universal organizational principle in nature. However, a central timing mechanism has so far not been discovered, although central oscillators seem to play a coordinating role. This is why the search for a central timer is no longer the focus of research, but rather questions of dynamic coordination between environmental and integrative rhythms.

The rigid model of the relationship between form and function has been complemented by a dialectic concept of the form–function relationship, in which multiple interdependent oscillatory processes are synchronized. One example is the intercellular oscillation process described by Jaeger and Goodwin, thought to be regulated by autonomous and non-autonomous processes within the cell and which has the ability to reproduce periodic gene property patterns during embryogenesis.[4]

Exploring and understanding the dynamic, synergic, and rhythmic processes that regulate equilibrium in humans can enhance the diagnostic and therapeutic potential of osteopathy. In the following, an overview will be given of rhythmic processes and their regulatory organization. This should provide a better insight into the organic order in humans.

The history of chronobiology – the science of biological rhythm

Practitioners of Chinese medicine were very aware that the different times of days had different qualities – assigning two hours in the day to each of the body's meridians.[5] The maximum time of a meridian corresponded to the minimum time of its complementary meridian. Recent research has confirmed that heart attacks, for example, occur most frequently around the maximum time of the heart meridian in Chinese medicine (between 11.00 a.m. and 1.00 p.m.), whereas the most frequent time for asthma attacks is the maximum time of the lung meridian (between 3.00 a.m. and 5:00 a.m.). This suggests that according to the Chinese organ clock, the maximum time for an organ coincides with the time of its greatest vulnerability.

As we know today, hormone levels vary throughout the day, controlling the circadian function of organs. The word circadian is derived from Latin circa (i.e., around) and dies (i.e., day) and was coined in the 1950s when it was discovered that the human body follows a cycle that is slightly longer than a 24-hour day. This was discovered when subjects were cut off from external timers such as daylight, e.g., in a bunker.[6] Incidentally, the middle of the 20th century was also the time when modern medicine became aware of rhythmicity in the human body. This rhythmicity was discovered while scientists were researching sleep, the patterns of which are only a partial aspect of the circadian rhythm. However, this has not been realized as yet by all medical sleep researchers.

Research carried out by Aschoff[7] in Andechs near Munich, Hildebrandt in Marburg[8] and Halberg in Minnesota[9] have made a significant contribution in shedding light on biological rhythms within the organism. Jürgen Aschoff identified chronobiological impulses such as light, the uptake of food, and the social environment, all of which help to integrate a person's daily routine into their environment.[10] He named them zeitgebers, a term that is now internationally used. Hildebrandt was one of the first to look at biological rhythms in a systemic context and to demonstrate that the various rhythms do not simply co-exist by coincidence, but are part of a larger temporal system with hierarchical as well as "democratic" structures. The resulting synergies resemble those observed between agonist and antagonist muscles and tendons. Hildebrandt has also the honor of discovering the significant effect of rhythms on human health.[11,12] His research as ergonomic physiologist and rehabilitation expert showed that the effectiveness of rehabilitation measures largely depends on restoring natural rhythms. Finally, Franz Halberg must be credited for demonstrating that the way rhythms develop through the day is a diagnostic and prognostic indicator of the severity and development of diseases. Thus, in hypertension, patients whose blood pressure decreases overnight (dippers) have a far better prognosis than those that show no such decrease (non-dippers) and whose circadian rhythm is weak or non-existent.[13]

Our description below will emphasize a systemic-context approach, as proposed by Gunther Hildebrandt, as this is of particular interest and value for the practitioner – especially the naturopathy and preventative medicine aspects.[14] Recent research also clearly confirms Hildebrandt's idea of the importance of rhythm for human health.

Rhythm as a basic constituent of life

Rhythm, regulation, and spatial-temporal coordination are fundamental constituents that generate order in life and aim to prevent the waste of energy. The rhythmical organization principle is universal in genotypic as well as phenotypic expression and metabolic regulation. It encompasses all life processes from fertilization, growth, homeostasis, and adaptive function to death.

Rhythm, form, and function

The phylogenetic as well as the ontogenetic development of form and function can be regarded as a continuous process of mutual interaction. Rhythm establishes order. Any further development of spatial order coincides with a higher degree of functional order. This is true at a molecular, cellular, macro-organism, or population level. Thus, cognitive organization is tied to oscillation dynamics, coordination, and self-adaptation of brain tissue.

The system of biological rhythms

Like any kind of oscillation, biological rhythms rely on polarity, i.e., there must be poles within the organism between which oscillation can take place. Such basic polarity is found, for example, in the autonomic nervous system between the sympathetic (S) and parasympathetic (P) branches. These control our ability to perform and to recover – daytime being largely controlled by the S and night-time by the P nervous system. The circadian rhythm was mentioned in 1799 by Hufeland[15] as a fundamental unit in biological time. This oscillation affects virtually all physiological and even some of the anatomical parameters of varying amplitude, such as heart rate, body temperature, hormone levels, immune system, and digestion parameters. Anatomic changes include body size and joint circumference. We are tallest in the morning roundabout 6.00 a.m. – which is also when our joints are most likely to be swollen – reducing mobility and adding to aches and pains. At about 8.00 p.m., we shrink to our smallest size. Counter-intuitively, this change in size is not – or not only – associated with the weight our skeleton must carry during the day. It has also been observed in test persons

Long-Wave Rhythms	Medium-Wave Rhythms	Short-Wave Rhythms
days to years	minutes to hours	milliseconds to seconds
affect the entire body	affect entire organs	affect cells and tissue
metabolism (e.g. wake/sleep rhythm)	rhythmical transport and distribution (respiration, circulation)	information system (nervous system)
Pendulum		vibration impulses (e.g. sawtooth waves)
under stress, frequency remains constant, amplitude varies	under stress, both frequency and amplitude vary*	under stress, frequency varies, amplitude remains constant
high-molecular weight proteins		ions (Na+, K+, Cl-)

*the higher the frequencies in the ultradian (several-hour) range, the more adaptable the rhythm

TABLE 3.1: Characteristics of Biological Rhythms

who followed a 2-hour rhythm of standing for 60 minutes and lying down for 60 minutes and were measured over 24 hours.

Good and healthy coordination of organ systems is characterized by good synchronization with exogenous timers/environmental factors for long-wave processes and good frequency and phase coordination of medium and short-wave endogenous rhythms. Disrupted synchronization may well be a symptom of disease. By the same token, lifestyles that disregard the natural order of endogenous rhythms and their external timers may create a predisposition for disease, whereas a lifestyle that conforms to the natural rhythm may be the foundation of good health.

The rhythmic functions of ultradian medium and long-wave processes are subject to synchronizing influences, which tend to keep them constant, in contrast to short-wave processes. Long-wave rhythms observed in the metabolism resemble the swing of a pendulum, incorporating complex processes and individual functions that are all coordinated, whereas short-wave rhythms in the nervous system are more sudden and tend to have an impulse wave pattern (Table 3.1).

Zeitgebers

Zeitgebers are physical or social cues that enable the human organism to adapt to external rhythms. Aschoff realized that light, and daylight in particular, is the most important.[16] Every morning at about 4.00 a.m., the human organism prepares for the new day and sunrise. The break of dawn triggers a whole cascade of physiological changes. It was long thought that the cue was passed on to the rest of the organism through the photoreceptors of the eye – cones and rods – that relay this cue. It became quite a sensation when a new type of photoreceptor cell in the inner retina was discovered in the 1990s. These photoreceptor cells are called intrinsically photosensitive retinal ganglion cells and contain a new type of photopigment: melanopsin. The photosensitive pigment had been previously identified in other animals and has a longer evolutionary history than the rhodopsin found in cones and rods. These photosensitive cells, which are related to ganglion cells with no specific visual function, complement the familiar photoreceptor cells. Unlike rods and cones, their efferent axons do not lead to the visual cortex in the occipital lobe, but straight to the suprachiasmatic nucleus and from there to the pineal gland. Even before their function was discovered it was known that the destruction of the suprachiasmatic nucleus, e.g., through cancer, resulted in severe disruption of the circadian and sleep rhythms. It is, therefore, not unreasonable to conclude that the suprachiasmatic nucleus coordinates the circadian rhythm. In addition, each body cell has its own circadian rhythm that is genetically controlled. Recent molecular research suggests that there is virtually no gene that is not subject to some circadian rhythm. There is oscillation throughout our body, coordinated by zeitgebers, the suprachiasmatic nucleus and interaction between the inner organs.

Health effects of rhythm disruptions

The discovery of circadian photosensitive cells was underpinned by other medical research that demonstrated that explicitly circadian-associated genes, such as PER2 and PER3 or CLOCK play an important part in retaining youthfulness and cancer protection. Epidemiological studies showed that breast cancer rates of female night and shift workers increased up to 70%,[17] while their male counterparts had prostate cancer rates increased between 40%[18] and 300%.[19] Animal tests showed that the deletion of just one of the known eight circadian coordination genes (PER2) resulted in the affected animals aging and dying much faster than the control group of genetically identical rats with all circadian control genes intact.[20,21] The rats still alive at the end of the trial all had cancer, in contrast to the genetically intact animals.

The new results on the youth-preserving and anti-cancer effects of intact circadian rhythms were published in a special edition of the renowned journal Cancer Causes Control,[22] prompting a statement from WHO (International Agency for Research on Cancer (IARC)), characterizing night and shift work "that involves circadian disruption [as] probably carcinogenic to humans."

The interplay of endogenous and exogenous rhythms

It was believed for a long time that the timer for CNS structures and neurohormonal cycles was located in the pineal body or in the hypothalamus. However, such a timer does not seem to exist. What has been found instead is a predominance of central oscillators. These have the ability to adapt the organism to environmental rhythms through synchronization.

For example, a modification of light and darkness periods causes distinct oscillations in the pineal body function. A few days after the modification of the light–dark rhythm, autonomous oscillations of many functions as well as unchanged adaptability of rhythms have been observed. Sinz comes to the conclusion that there must be a dynamic organization of functions, which is mediated by mechanisms of non-linear coordination.[23]

This raises the question as to whether there is dynamic coordination between environment-driven and integrating rhythms. This is not a relationship between an active and a passive element, but the coordination of self-excited cellular rhythms (synchronized throughout the tissue, organ, or organ system).

Although the rhythms vary in their significance, depending on magnitude of frequency, conclusions can be drawn from interaction patterns between the rhythms of organisms and the environment.[24]

Geophysical, ecological, and social environmental periodicities synchronize biological rhythms of cellular origin. However, there is also endogenous synchronization and coordination of multiple cellular, tissue, organ, organismic, or interorganismic oscillators and their frequencies (Figures 3.1 and 3.2).

External synchronization in the region of 10 Hz has often been observed. This is the range at which many biological oscillations occur (microvibrations, EEG alpha waves, hippus of the pupil, ciliary movements, nystagmus, or action potentials), which are synchronized with geophysical periodicities (seismic activity, variation in the magnetic field of the Earth – known as Schumann Resonance, infra-long waves). There are salient analogies between the temporal and amplitudinal behavior of minute-long pulsations in the magnetic field of the Earth and circaminute rhythms of organisms. However, no causal link has yet been established.

There are several sensory pathways that are supposed to sense temporal fluctuation immediately. Anochin presumes that when life develops, temporary sequences in the outer world, macrotime, is reflected as microtime in chemical processes and the structures and the organization of organisms.[25] These inner temporal structure patterns enable the organism to make probability forecasts about the outer world and to develop target-driven behavior.

In humans, the psyche seems to be able to make probability forecasts using biotic clocks and oscillatory

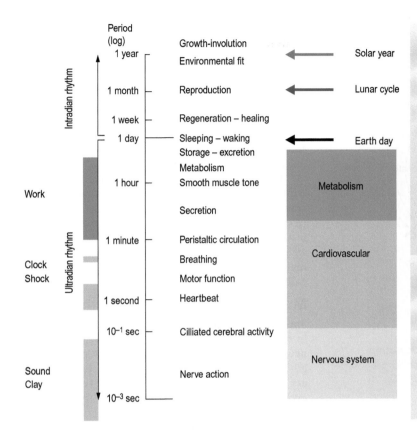

Figure 3.1

System of human core biological rhythms. The illustration shows the wide scope of biological rhythms, ranging from a thousandth of a second (bottom) to years (top). Virtually all physiological parameters in our organism oscillate in a daily or circadian rhythm (center). Above the circadian rhythm are the infradian rhythms, such as Earth day, solar year, or lunar cycle. These slower rhythms link us to the cosmic rhythms of the solar system, while below the circadian rhythm, the endogenic oscillations of ultradian rhythms are shown. These faster rhythms reflect the rhythmicity of the nervous (bottom), cardiovascular (center), and metabolic systems. The cardiovascular system connects the nervous system and the metabolic system and is also anatomically and chronobiologically placed between them. After Hildebrandt et al. 1998, Moser et al, 2006. ©HRI, 2014.

processes to reconcile the needs of the inner world with the outer world conditions, thus achieving satisfying regulation of the energy needs of the organism.[26] Humans could thus be enabled to develop hypotheses of the world based on "pre-emptive reflection," which would help control behavior.[27]

1 **Exorhythm:** this is a rhythmical oscillation of biological functions, controlled by exogenous factors, such as lighting conditions. Complete dependence on exogenous timers is only found at lower evolutionary stages.

2 **Exo–endo rhythms (circarhythms):** these are rhythmic processes generated by the organisms themselves, which are synchronized and regulated by periodically intervening environmental factors or incentives

(environmental timers). Such rhythmic processes continue to exist in an attenuated form once the exogenous timer has been eliminated: day and night, the circadian rhythms with their light-driven and social timers (affecting hormones, temperature regulation, metabolism, circulation, and respiration), the change of the seasons, annual rhythms (affecting the hormone metabolism, temperature regulation, metabolism, circulation, autonomic reactions, and hematopoiesis).

3 **Endorhythms:** an autonomous physiological rhythm, completely independent of exogenous timers. Such spontaneous rhythms, however, are coordinated with other spontaneous rhythms and organized in harmonic whole-number frequency and phase relations. Coordination occurs through

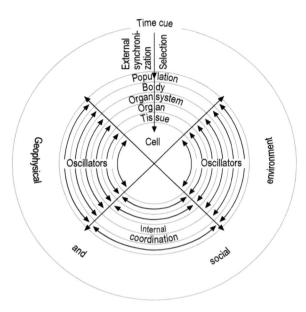

Figure 3.2
Secondary oscillators at different integration levels, excited by cellular primary oscillators.

reflexive interaction or magnetic effects between rhythmogenic centers within the central nervous system. When resting, coordination of rhythms and phase coordination of medium to short wave processes is more pronounced, whereas when active, rhythms may undergo frequency modulations. There are economic reasons for this. Coordination is particularly important in serially functioning systems, such as respiration and circulation. There is also coordination between autonomic and motor processes (e.g., gait and respiratory frequency).

Infradian rhythms

Figure 3.3 gives an overview of the entire system of biological rhythms – the upper part shows the three slower rhythms that place the human organism in its cosmic context, so to speak.

Infra-annual rhythm

Rhythmic population cycles in plants, animals, and humans are related to the exorhythms of sunspot activity with a mean length of 11.1 years.

Circannual rhythms

In temperate latitudes, we know seasons to be the result of the annual orbit of the Earth around the sun. The human organism undergoes a corresponding annual cycle, such as body weight. The "winter fat" we store in the autumn will reduce heat loss in winter. It would, therefore, be difficult and indeed counter-productive to start losing weight in autumn. In spring, however, many cultures observe a period of fasting, which helps to detoxify the body and reduce weight. Observing the circannual body rhythms can make weight watching easier and more physiologically compatible.

Menstrual rhythm/lunar rhythm

The orbit of the moon around the Earth and its position in relation to the sun produces the lunar phases, e.g., new moon, waxing crescent, full moon, and waning gibbous. The lunar rhythm has its place in evolutionary history and still has an effect on the reproduction cycles of virtually all marine life forms. Although in humans, the duration of the menstrual cycle suggests a link to the lunar cycle – around 28 days – there is little modern statistical evidence for this today. Many functional processes are synchronized via the date of menstruation, such as basal temperature, pulse frequency, subjective sensations, body weight, systolic blood pressure and blood pressure amplitude, instant and maximum force. In humans, menstrual rhythms are largely detached from the lunar rhythm, probably due to artificial lighting, which minimizes the awareness for lunar cycles. In men, periodic changes in the light sensitivity of the eye have been shown to coincide with lunar rhythms.

Weekly (circaseptan) rhythms

In humans, some functions showed a circaseptan rhythm that slightly deviates from the 7-day week. It is not usually regarded as a spontaneous rhythm, but a reactive periodicity (see below). Such rhythms usually stand in a harmonious whole-number ratio to spontaneous rhythms. The circaseptan rhythm has its evolutionary origins in a very old rhythmical order. Exogenous

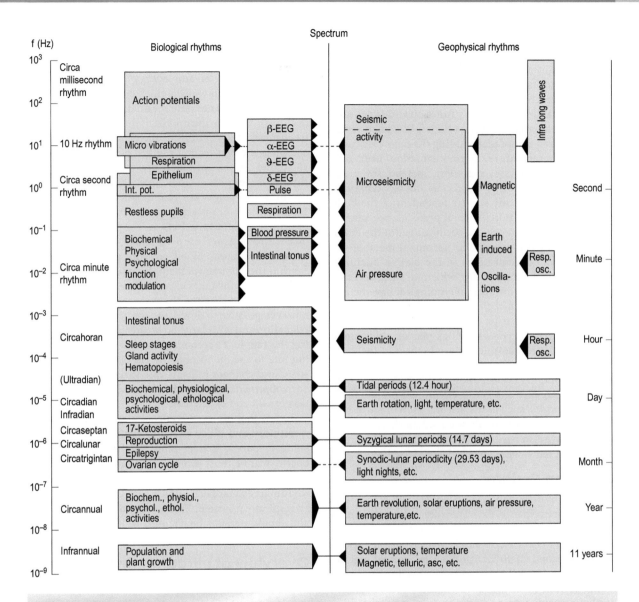

Figure 3.3
Corresponding preferred frequencies of biological and geophysical, lunar, or solar oscillations. They represent an evolutionary adaptation of structures within organisms to environmental periodicity.[28]

day rhythm cues (e.g., jetlag and certain lifestyles) have a clear impact on this rhythm, and it is thought that the circaseptan may be synchronized by exogenous (social) factors. In newborns, the predominance of a circasep- tan rhythm is gradually replaced by a synchronized day rhythm with larger amplitude, as the senses develop. The only circadian periodicity found in newborns was in the electric resistance of the skin.[29]

Day (circadian rhythms)

Day and night are determined by the rotation of the Earth around its axis. The circadian or day rhythm is the best-researched cycle in chronobiology.

There is practically no bodily function that is not subject to some fluctuation over 24 hours. Circadian variations have been recorded, including the following functions: body temperature, thermoregulation, heart and circulation, respiration, digestion, metabolism, renal function, composition of blood cells and blood plasma, physical strength, body size (independent of the body position), tissue turgidity, mental performance, performance of the sensory organs, performance of the brain, sensitivity to pain, mood, and hormonal metabolism. Thus, cortisol concentrations in the plasma fluctuate, depending on the time of day, which, in turn, acts as a main synchronizer for other physiological parameters, such as heart frequency, the strength of grip, rectal temperature, or the excretion of minerals.[30]

Plasma cortisol levels as well as plasma aldosterone levels and plasma renin levels are highest in the early morning (around 8.00 a.m.) and lowest at the beginning of the rest period (around midnight).[31–34] However, cortisol levels are also subject to circannual periodicity.[35] Other hormones, such as insulin and growth hormones have also been shown to follow circadian rhythms. Day rhythms have also been found in the heart frequency of mother and fetus, with a phase delay of one hour.[36]

Ultradian rhythms

Ultradian rhythms have a short wavelength and a periodicity shorter than a day. They are an expression of the body's own rhythm, with the fastest oscillations in the nervous system where single neurons fire at a speed of 1 millisecond (1000 Hz), and larger cerebral regions oscillating at 100 milliseconds (alpha rhythm) and over longer periods (delta and theta rhythm). As the fastest-oscillating part of our body, the nervous system also has the highest demand for energy. Energy is something the nervous system cannot generate by itself: it must have access to an external supply. In terms of energy consumption and metabolic activity per cubic centimeter, the nervous system is the most demanding in our body.

Where does the energy supply for the nervous system come from? It turns out that the metabolic system with the slowest oscillation provides energy for all other organ systems. Liver enzyme profiles reveal periodic changes over several hours, similar to the long-wave peristaltic movements of the intestine.

Energy generation and energy consumption mark two poles, between which a third system acts as mediator. This system is not only the anatomic middle, but its rhythms are also in the middle of the range of endogenic frequencies. The rhythms of the cardiovascular system comprise the one-second rhythm of the heartbeat, the 10-second rhythm of blood pressure, and the minute rhythm of peripheral blood flow. These cardiovascular rhythms also play a key role in osteopathy, where the 10-second rhythm is known as cranio-rhythmic input or primary respiratory rhythm. The periodicity is identical with blood pressure oscillations. Continuous measurement of systolic blood pressure yields a 10-second rhythm that modulates the pulse peaks. In respiration, a breath normally takes between 4 and 5 seconds, so the breath to blood pressure rhythm ratio is about 2:1. It is, however, possible to slow down the breathing rhythm in relaxation and with targeted breathing exercises, reducing the rate to 10 seconds. The slowing of the breathing rate to the blood pressure rhythm elicits dramatic structural changes in heart rate variability. These have been observed during meditation and during the recitation of OM and of hexameters.

Studies looking at the effects of osteopathy on the respiratory and blood pressure rhythms are currently being prepared. It is possible that the effect of osteopathy will be most profound if respiratory and blood pressure rhythms can be synchronized. The 10-second rhythm has so far been known as rhythm of the primary respiratory system. This name could be misleading and should perhaps be changed in light of the aspects mentioned above.

Overview of ultradian rhythms

- The Basic Rest-Activity Cycle (BRAC) is part of the body's metabolic cycles. Every 90 minutes on average, the rhythm, particularly in deep sleep, has been found to change. This pattern seems to persist in waking periods. Correlations in frequency between slower rhythms lasting several hours and day rhythms could be shown. The BRAC control center is located around the *Pons* and *Medulla oblongata*.

- Basic 1-minute rhythm of the smooth muscles. This is the predominant rhythm of smooth muscles, controlling the blood supply of skin, mucosa, and muscles as well as the basic rhythms of the hollow organs (e.g., the gastrointestinal tract). The basic 1-minute rhythm seems to involve the central nervous system as well as autonomous vasomotor rhythms.

- Third order waves. Naumenko and Moskalenko discovered oscillations of 1 per minute in the pressure of cerebrospinal fluid in the subarachnoid space.[37]

- Blood pressure rhythm. Variations in blood pressure were first discovered by Ludwig in 1847.[38] In 1865, Traube described a fluctuation of pulse pressure with a frequency similar to the respiration rhythm, which continued even when individuals held their breath. This was confirmed by Hering in 1869.[39,40]

The 10-second rhythm in blood pressure variation has a fluctuation range of 5–10 cycles per minute. The blood supply to the muscles is subject to fluctuations of 5–6 cycles per minute, which continue during muscle contraction.[47] These 10 second blood pressure fluctuations are regulated via muscle sympathetic nerve activity (MSNA) exercising a constrictive effect on the smooth muscles of the vascular walls of arterioles.[48] MSNA offsets the effect of local vasodilators during muscle contraction, presumably in order to maintain blood pressure within the muscle when blood supply may be temporarily diminished. MSNA is influenced by physical exercise, variation in cardiac rhythm and blood pressure as well as vestibular otolith stimulation, and its amplitude is reduced by estrogens.

The blood pressure rhythm may be phase-locked to the spontaneous respiratory rhythm.[49,50] Independent of the Traube/Hering investigations, Mayer observed similar oscillations at slower rates (0.6–5.4 cycles/minute) also called THM waves.[51] According to Schmidt (1996),[52] Mayer oscillations do not occur under normal conditions, but mainly in pathological physiological conditions, but this was not confirmed by Glonek.[53] THM oscillations are also being discussed as possible synonymous phenomena to the PRM rhythm. Thus, when investigating the PRM rhythm, phase-locking to respiration was observed.[54] Phase-locking in THM is also subject to variations over the day. Sinz distinguishes blood pressure fluc-

Fluctuations in Blood Pressure
1st Order synchronous with breathing
2nd Order Blood pressure rises with some delay after inhalation and falls after exhalation
3rd Order Traube-Hering Oscillations with a frequency of 10s. These include several respiration cycles
4th Order Variation in blood pressure within minutes. Circadian modulation with a drop in pressure at 3 o'clock in the morning

TABLE 3.2: Fluctuations in Blood Pressure

tuations of the first, second, third, and fourth order (Table 3.2).

It is assumed that rhythmic variations in blood pressure are caused by a range of factors.[55]

The vasomotor rhythm of vessels in the skin is also directly correlated to the blood pressure rhythm. The vasomotor rhythm frequency depends on body temperature. Within a temperature range of 28-30°C, the average period length is 7.5 seconds. An affinity to the breathing rhythm has been observed.

Rhythm in lymphatic vessels, as contractions of the thoracic duct, at a rate of 4–6 cycles per minute have been observed in humans. Cycles of 8–10 per minute in the lymphatic vessels of pigs and of male study participants standing motionless, while non-anesthetized sheep showed a rate of 1–30 cycles per minute.

- Cerebral pulsation (related to blood pressure and smooth muscle rhythms). During ultrasound examinations, centripetal pulsation rhythms were observed in the brain at a rate of 2–9 per minute,[56] and seem to be associated with the release phenomenon. Slower waves vary between 5 and 33 minutes. These are known as vascular energized waves (VEWs) and arise in closed and resonant systems of modeled cardiac and respiratory rhythms. Rhythmical changes in brain density and the shape of ventricles, following periodical movement patterns (VEWs), have been recorded in fast serial CT scans.

A slowly rolling wave moves through the cerebral parenchyma and pushes the CSF axially through the ventricles. This movement is interrupted when the breath is held. The wave sweeps through the body in regular intervals.[57]

The pulsating VEW movements seem to follow the 2–9 cycles per minute pattern encountered before, with periodicities of 56, 86, 150, and 224 seconds. This would also include 25–26 second rhythm waves, the above-mentioned "3rd wave." It is assumed that the underlying universal pulsation rhythm represents a base wave on which the 2–9 times per minute wave has been superimposed. The latter pulsation occurs in longer Respiratory rhythm. At rest, the spontaneous breathing rhythm has an average rate of 18 cycles per minute. It is significantly modified by extrinsic and intrinsic impulses, as well as long-wave day rhythms. It is part of a frequency pattern of ultradian rhythms. In humans, the relation between heartbeat and breathing is defined by the pulse–respiration ratio of 4:1, which can be observed during resting and deep sleep.

- Rhythmic modulation of the heart rate. Longer wave rhythms in particular have a frequency-modulating effect. This is reflected in the variability of heartbeat intervals. Many extrinsic and intrinsic factors elicit reactive frequency fluctuations that have repercussions on the frequency and phase coordination of other rhythms. Frequencies are also affected by the autonomic tonus (autonomic system).[58] Heartbeat frequency is modulated by the respiratory rhythm (respiratory arrhythmia). The frequency and phase coordination of the cardiac and respiratory rhythms becomes more pronounced in vagotonia and in resting positions.[59] Multiple modulations of circaminute rhythms have also been described.

- Arterial basic oscillation. In healthy individuals, the ratio of heart periodic duration and arterial basic oscillation duration is 2:1. This represents a response of the arterial system to the heartbeat.

- Microvibration (10–12 Hz in adults). Warm-blooded animals have not only various minute rhythms, but also a rhythmical microvibration with a frequency of 4–12 per second. The microvibrations seem to be,

at least to some extent, a neuromuscular response to the heartbeat – every single heart beat is echoed by a muted 10 Hz after- oscillation – apparently triggered by gamma motoneurons.[60]

Microvibrations are a persistent presence during sleeping and waking, only fading out several hours after death.[61] The amplitude, however, varies significantly, depending, for example, on the position of the individual. In space where supportive muscle tension is lower, active after-oscillations are significantly weaker.[62]

With increasing muscle tension, microvibrations increase and eventually turn into tremors. Recordings of microvibrations in the same individual at the same recording point show that the wave shape remains relatively constant. While resting, the frequency is predominantly in the alpha range (8–13 Hz) and under mental stress (during mental activity) in the beta range (13–20 Hz). The frequency also increases during fever. In epileptics and individuals in a state of anxiety, depression, or irritation, frequencies in the theta range (4–8 Hz) often occur. Microvibration is clearly affected by the autonomic system.[63] It is assumed that microvibration is responsible for maintaining body temperature, a sense of position in a resting body, and the continuous stimulation of the reticular formation in the muscles.[64]

- 40 Hz (gamma range) oscillations of the nervous system. There is a hypothesis about the coordination of various coded stimuli in the brain leading to an integral representation of objects. It is thought that this coordination process is brought about by 40 Hz gamma band oscillations generated in localized neural circuits, which set in at 8 months of age.[65]

- Rhythms known as primary respiratory rhythms. These rhythms are discussed here because of their role in osteopathic treatment. Various descriptions have been given of the primary respiratory and craniosacral rhythms, but their ontogenesis remains the subject of speculation. It remains to be seen whether the primary respiratory rhythm is an artifact, a rhythm in its own right, or has some correlation to other rhythms. It may be that it derives from respiratory, blood pressure, or metabolic cycles.
  - 10–14 cycles per minute: 4–6 second cycle (Magoun, oscillation)[66–72]

- 6–12 cycles per minute: 5–10 second cycle (Upledger)[73]
- 8–12 cycles per minute: 5–7.5 second cycle (Becker, Upledger)[74,75]
- 2.5 cycles per minute: 25 second cycle (Jealous)[76]
- 6–10 cycles in 10 minutes: 60–100 second cycle (Becker's "slow tide")[77,78]
- 1 cycle per 5 minutes: 300 second cycle (Liem, Lewer-Allen and Bunt et al.)[79,80]

In addition, Lewer-Allen, Bunt et al. observed during CT scans that there were periodical movement patterns affecting brain density and ventricles, i.e., cycles of 33 minutes (2000 second cycle).[81] No recorded palpations of the latter rhythm exist.

These and other rhythm descriptions are based on the palpatory experience of individual osteopaths, for example the 2.5 cycles per minute rhythm; on average values from palpation studies on the skull (10–14 cycles per minute); on average palpation results from intra-tester and inter-tester reliability studies; on studies of rhythmical motion in cerebro-cranial structures measured by various devices (sonography, CT, MRI); or on electromechanical measurements with simultaneous palpation (e.g., the 6–12 cycles per minute rhythm).

Measuring biological rhythms

Let us now look at the physiology of those oscillations in the human organism that probably form an important basis of our health. We are currently witnessing a fascinating paradigm change in biology and medicine: the concept of homeostasis, a tendency of the body to keep its parameters constant is being questioned, due to recent research results. It is now being replaced by the concept of homeodynamics, i.e.,[81a–g] panta rhei which means everything flows and oscillates in the body. The idea of oscillating life is much more easily reconciled with osteopathic approaches than the old homeostasis concept. The early Romantic poet Novalis wrote: "Any disease (is) a musical problem – its solution a musical solution" and "Musical relationships seem to be the most fundamental relationships in nature."[82] The musical oscillations of life are not just a metaphor, but can now be revealed by chronobiology. There is hardly any physiological parameter that is not subject to a day–night rhythm and is not integrated into the chronobiological system of periods and frequencies.[83-86] What

is particularly intriguing is the correlation that clearly exists between frequencies, time measures, and periods in music and ultradian rhythms observed in the human body.[87]

For a long time, such oscillations in the body were not easy to measure – which is probably one of the reasons why the phenomenon of biological oscillations was only discovered a few decades ago. Research into them was not considered to be serious science and only towards the end of the 20th century was their significance recognized. Many researchers still find it difficult to form a bigger picture out of the plethora of individual research results: the bigger picture of an organism structured and organized by time. However, it emerges that rhythms coordinate physiology and the many parts of the body can interact in ways so complex that we are only beginning to scratch the surface.[88,89] Time structures could be compared to an orchestra where agonist and antagonist rhythms cooperate and interact like the muscles and tendons in Vesalius's anatomy, organizing the course of life (Figure 3.4). While scientists are in the process of developing an anatomy of time, the first clues of histology of time seem to appear.[90,91] Microrhythms work in coordination with macrorhythms and there is clear evidence that the time structure of our organism is as complex as its spatial structure.

Our sense of vision makes us aware of space, but less so of time. We are only aware of time where time becomes space, as Richard Wagner says in his opera Parzifal. This happens, for example, in the annual rings of trees, but also in human kidney stones where layers reflect the circadian rhythms of uric acid concentration (Figure 3.5), and in the growth lines of tooth enamel (Figure 3.6).

The original significance and perhaps even the origins of music can still be observed in some traditional and Aboriginal cultures, Music made hard physical work easier, helped them to get into the swing of things and enjoy themselves.[96] Music accompanied all celebrations and sent children to sleep with lullabies. Physiological rhythms were expressed and enhanced by music. Life was music and African people from traditional societies cannot see the point of sitting for two hours in an opera house or a concert hall and listening to a performance with no interaction with the musicians. In their culture, a whole village becomes involved in dancing and making music.

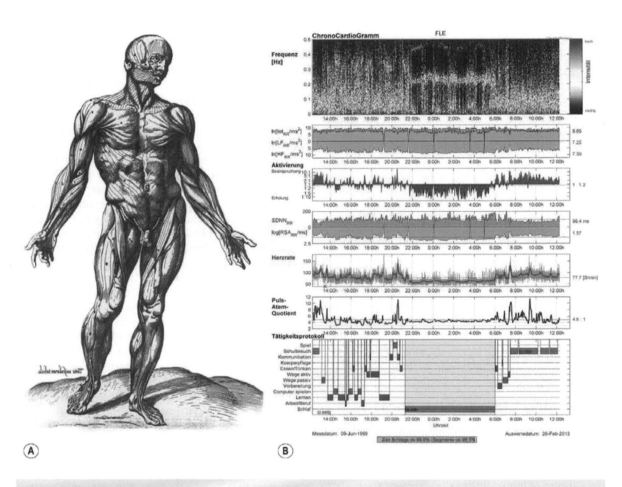

Figure 3.4
The human organism in space and time. While its spatial structure became a subject of research during the renaissance period (Andrea Vesalius), its time structure is still today a new and fascinating world.

Being excluded would be a punishment, as Bernd Bechtloff, percussionist in Hubert von Goisern's band, reported after touring Africa.

The link between music and human work used to be so strong that many traditional tools make perfect musical instruments, their size and weight helping to synchronize movement, heartbeat, and respiration. The rhythm of work itself generates rhythmical music at a human pace. In contrast to the rigid rhythm of machines that dominated the workplace later, those rhythms were flexible and had a swing to them.

The dance of the heart

The rhythm of the heart reflects the rhythms of many organs. Measuring heart rate variability (or better, 'heart rhythm flexibility') has therefore been a useful tool in establishing and analyzing body rhythms. Heart rhythm flexibility arises by interaction of the two polar

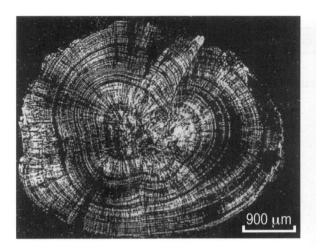

Figure 3.5
Life can leave spatial tracks of events modulated by time, such as tree growth. In kidney stones, increased nocturnal urea concentrations lead to rhythmic precipitations that can be seen as layers in the concrement. From Hildebrandt et al., 1998.[92]

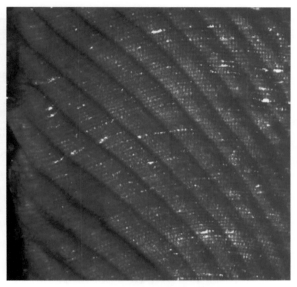

Figure 3.6
Retzius lines in human tooth enamel. They show how the tooth enamel built up not only over the day, but over a 7-day period. This is a fact that has been known for a long time,[93] but has only been further investigated by chronobiologists in recent years.[94] These lines or striae form during a modulated circaseptan growth period of cells before the teeth broke through. The circaseptan period is not a socially modulated week, but an endogenous rhythm over approximately 7 days. Similar cycles in the human organism have been observed in many healing processes. From Dean et al., 2001.[95]

controlling systems of the heartbeat – the sympathetic (S) and parasympathetic (P) nervous systems – and the sinus node, the local pacemaker. While the sympathetic system enables action and acceleration, flight and fight, the parasympathetic system has a slowing and cooling effect on the heart. It decelerates, enables recovery and protects from coronary heart disease and heart attack.[97]

A healthy heartbeat is slightly irregular: it does not march at a steady pace like a soldier, but oscillates around a mean rhythm, performing a dance. This phenomenon is described as heart rhythm flexibility, characteristic for periods of relaxation, recovery, and sleep. The need for recovery is a basic principle that distinguishes living organisms from machines. During periods of recovery, the organism renews itself, heals micro-lacerations, and rids itself of chemical metabolites. Recovery,[98] self-healing, and self-organization[99] are synonyms at different time scales. Recovery periods are characterized by intense rhythmicity and coordination. In a well-coordinated organism, physiological rhythms interact in harmony, resulting in short but thorough recovery periods. Rhythm saves energy and helps recovery.

During recovery phases, the organism is subject to particularly strong oscillations and the heartbeat is modulated by the P-mediated respiratory rhythm. The heart leans on the breath, so to speak, whereas under moderate strain, the heartbeat is ruled by a different rhythm, the S-mediated blood pressure. The heart is the hub of the organism, perfused by hormones circulating in the bloodstream, regulated by the sympathetic and parasympathetic nervous systems. This makes it the ideal organ for the visualization of homeodynamic oscillation processes in the body. ECG measurements

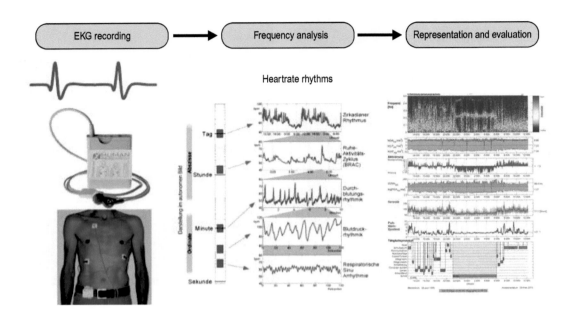

Figure 3.7
Measuring heart rhythm flexibility, frequency analysis and visualization in a Chronocardiogram. ©HRI, 2014.

can be taken continuously and non-invasively from the skin surface with no disruption to the body's physiology (Figure 3.7).

As briefly mentioned before, the visualization of the results of heart rhythm variability measurements is called a Chronocardiogram (from the Greek chronos which means "time" and graphein which means "to write").[100–102] In this view, the various rhythms appear as colorful timelines against a monochrome (blue) background. Rhythms that modulate the heartbeat, such as respiration, are shown as light lines or surfaces against the blue background.

If the heartbeat were absolutely regular, the surface in this Chronocardiogram would be monochrome blue. As soon as the heartbeat is modulated by other rhythms, such as respiration, blood pressure, or peripheral circulation, the surface of the Chronocardiogram shows crinkles at the location of the oscillations and becomes white (medium intensity), yellow, or even red (moderate to high intensity).

The method can be used as an easy system to produce a chronobiological profile of a night's sleep or, as sleep researchers would say, "the architecture of sleep" as an indicator of sleep quality.

Sleep architecture manifests itself in the Chronocardiogram in the way time is structured, i.e., quiet, restful periods rhythmically alternate with phases of chaotic autonomic activity (Figure 3.8). The latter seem to be dream periods, where the dreams wreak havoc on the autonomic rhythms.

Both elements – recovery and chemical renewal as well as processing and storing the day's events – show in the Chronocardiogram as the alternation between order in peaceful sleep and the chaos of REM (rapid eye movement) sleep stages. In a disrupted sleep pattern, the two stages alternate without any rhyme or reason and the cyclical sleep architecture of 90 minute long-wave periods fails to develop. Instead, there is an increase in irregular patterns with increased sympathetic activity. Good, undisturbed sleep, by contrast,

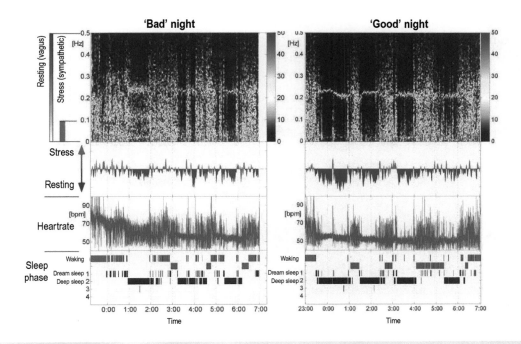

Figure 3.8

Chronocardiograms of a healthy subject during the first (left) and second (night) at a sleeping lab. The diagrams show – from top to bottom – Chronocardiograms, the balance of periods of tension and recovery, the heart rate and sleep stages, as derived from ECG monitoring.[102a] The differences in sleep quality and the more or less harmonious progression of the night are reflected in the differences in sleep architecture quality shown in the Chronocardiogram (based on data from the Universitätsklinik für Psychiatrie, Freiburg, Professor D. Riemann). © HRI, 2013.

produces a beautiful sleep architecture, reproducing what psychologists identified as the BRAC cycle.

Alternation between chaos and order is a major shaping force in life as well as art. Chaos leaves scope for freedom, unleashing creative qualities that would have no place in perfect order. However, permanent chaos would be exhausting and must be counterbalanced by order. Order provides security and stability, and built-in redundancy makes it more comprehensible and accessible. From that perspective, good sleep might be considered as the perfect work of art, bringing together chaos and order.[104,105] Chronocardiograms enable us to visualize and measure the quality of sleep, and the phases when the CSF canals are open (Figure 3.9). This autonomic sleep quality may even be more indicative of the recovery that takes place during sleep than the EEG

(cerebral activity) measurements traditionally used in sleep laboratories. While the latter only measures activity in the top three millimeters of the cortex, a Chronocardiogram also monitors activity in deeper brain stem areas and its effect on the heart.

Interaction of body rhythms

Biological rhythms are characterized by their systemic interaction and coordination, which can be observed during rest stages in particular. It has been observed in a group of subjects that over 24 hours their pulse–respiration ratio could vary between 2:1 and 7:1.

The diagram shows the trial participants in groups according to their pulse–respiration ratio, over a timeline of 24 hours. Individuals with a high pulse–respiration ratio decrease their ratio during sleep, whereas

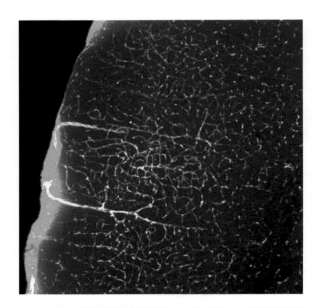

Figure 3.9
CSF canals opening up during the chemical deep-cleaning stages of deep sleep. These canals were first visualized and their function described in 2013.[103]

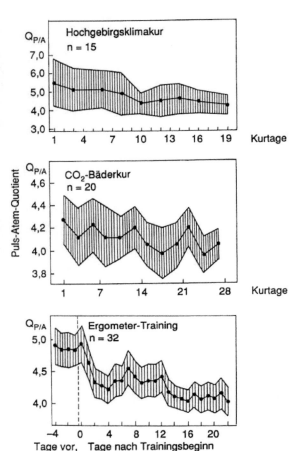

Figure 3.10
Pulse–respiration ratio in 89 subjects over a 24-hour day. Averages were taken of groups of individuals with a similar ratio. During the day, individual ratios ranged from 2:1 to 7:1, whereas at nighttime, all groups veered towards a universal 4:1 ratio (four heartbeats per breath). This is known as normalization effect, resulting in a very economical use of the body's resources. After Hildebrandt et al., 1998, 2013.[106]

those with a low ratio increase it. Thus, sleep has a remarkable normalizing effect, leveling out the pulse–respiration ratio at about 4:1. In the morning, the groups separate again and each individual goes back to the ratio of the previous day. In other words, the day/night pendulum swings between an individual and a universal pulse–respiration ratio. Further research showed that healing and recovery processes in health spa treatment or recuperation centers boost normalization, thus ensuring that the body works at its most economical. Such effects are likely to occur in osteopathic treatment as well and monitoring could be used to document success.

We know from research by Hildebrandt and colleagues that deep sleep stages not only enhance heartbeat–respiration correlations, but extend coordination to other rhythms. Blood pressure and peripheral blood flow rhythms also synchronize – veering toward a 4:1 ratio, which is a double octave in musical terms – for rhythms that follow one another.[107] While during the day, our organs follow their own individual music, they sing from the same hymn sheet at night. It is this consonance that has – in all likelihood – a significant

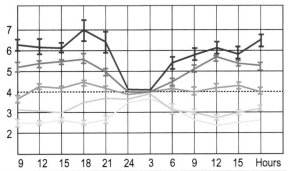

Pulse to breathing ratio

Figure 3.11
Changes of the pulse-respiration rate in a group of patients during various treatments. Regardless of what treatment was used, a universal trend toward a 4:1 pulse–respiration ratio can be observed. After Hildebrandt et al., 1998.

impact on our wellbeing and our health. Disruptions such as night and shift work result in serious health problems, including metabolic disorders,[108] heart disease,[109,110] and a substantially increased cancer rate.[111] Any holistic treatment should therefore aim at restoring rhythm and coordination. This can be measured and documented with state-of-the-art methods such as the Chronocardiogram.

Reactive periods

So far, we have been describing spontaneous rhythms the body generates to orchestrate our organ functions. There are, however, further oscillations that seem to develop particularly as a response to medium to severe stimuli and stress situations. Hildebrandt dubbed those "reactive periods" to distinguish them from spontaneous rhythms. Their frequency ranges lie between those of spontaneous rhythms – usually with a multiple integral ratio, i.e., 2:1, 3:1, 4:1, etc. with regard to the spontaneous rhythms.

Reactive periods can also be seen as a multiplication of existing spontaneous rhythms, providing additional rest and accelerating recovery. A practical example will illustrate this: our normal circadian rhythm encompasses 24 hours. In a relaxed organism, the body

temperature oscillates in a sinus wave between the sympathetic (higher daytime temperature) and parasympathetic-dominated (lower nighttime temperature) periods. If we are more tired than usual – perhaps due to lack of sleep during the previous night – we may experience an additional midday low. Our body temperature decreases and at two o'clock in the afternoon, we may want to take an afternoon nap. This has traditionally been interpreted as a postprandial slump: in other words, a consequence of a preceding meal. However, chronobiological rhythm research tells us that it is an underlying chronobiological phenomenon. Approaching the other pole of the circadian cycle (opposite the lowest body temperature at two o'clock in the morning), the organism inserts a resting point for recovery at two o'clock in the afternoon. Tiredness at that time of day is therefore not as much associated with a meal, as it represents a relay point that turns a 24-hour cycle into a 12-hour cycle to make up for the previous night's missing recovery time. The ratio between reactive periodicity (12 hours) and the basic rhythm (24 hours) is 2:1. Similar to a flute, where overblowing (blowing strongly) will produce an overtone at twice the basic frequency, the stressed organism will respond by frequency multiplication, in this case doubling the frequency. With further increase of stress, e.g., through shorter sleep periods, another multiplication may occur, resulting in three 8-hour periods or even four 6-hour periods, etc. In other words, tiredness and dips in performance will occur every 8, 6, etc. hours. Such changes in the "time organism" can therefore be chronobiological indicators of the level of stress an individual is exposed to.

Sports medical research has established that recovery progresses exponentially, i.e., recovery is greatest in the first minutes after exercising. This knowledge is harnessed in interval training, where exercise is broken up into short periods in order to achieve results much more quickly than with conventional continuous exercise. Our body has known it for ages.

Fast reactive periodicity (frequency multiplication) leads to a higher number of recovery phases, whereas slow reactive periodicity (period multiplication) prolongs recovery periods.

Within a reactive cycle, a wide range of multiple periods and submultiples may subdivide the predominant period. Periods may differ from one functional system to the other. The amplitudes of reactive periods are initially higher than those of spontaneous rhythms of a similar

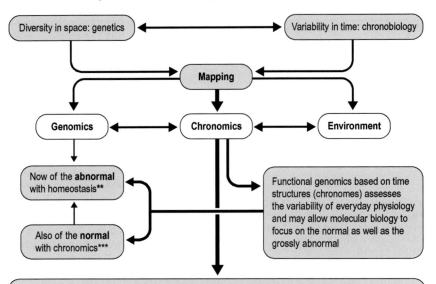

Figure 3.12
Diagram of the diversity in biological structure – diversity in space and time – the latter with complementary environment-time structures.[118]

range. Over time, however, amplitudes decrease, due to ongoing adaptation and compensation processes.

Phase shifts in reactive periods depend on key stimuli. Reactive periods occur within an organizational time framework (emergency schedule). Reactive periods with frequencies stretching over several hours (ultradian) reach their maximum amplitudes during the morning to decrease later in the day. Reactive periods usually follow a 12-, 8-, 6- or 4-hour pattern. These include 4-hour sleeping periods distributed over 24 hours to make up for lost sleep and the feeding rhythm of newborns fed on demand, where the need for food is the stimulus.

Similarly, A, B and C waves according to Lundberg[113] comprise the already described spontaneous rhythms as well as reactive periods, depending on their period length. When measuring ventricular CSF pressure, Lundberg observed three types of waves, which he named A, B and C waves. The A wave is a sustained increase of ventricular CSF pressure that occurs during pathological changes of the breathing pattern and is associated with a poor prognosis. The B wave is characterized by a change in ventricular CSF pressure occurring 0.5 to 2 times per minute during deep sleep or Cheyne–Stokes respiration. The peaks of the sinus curve coincide with hyperpnea and the troughs with apnea during Cheyne–Stokes respiration. C-waves coincide with Traube–Hering waves and have a frequency of approximately 6–7 per minute. They occur when ventricular CSF pressure is extremely high and are thus indicators of high intracranial pressure. According to Lundberg, C waves are physiological and a normal occurrence, but are barely measurable. They become only detectable when CSF pressure increases and with it the amplitude of the waves.

Studies of Cheyne–Stokes respiration showed that during hyperpnea, ventricular CSF pressure increases significantly and decreases during apnea.[114] These fluctuations occurred at a rate of once per minute, reflecting Lundberg's B wave. Very rarely could a C wave be found, with a frequency of 4–8 cycles per minute.

The finding that all functional systems within an organism react to systemic types of stress with a circaseptan (7-day) periodical response has practical implications. Such changes are orchestrated by the autonomic nervous system. Circaseptan reactive periods are initiated by a key stimulus. Their amplitudes usually decrease during the adaptive process. Thus, the crisis of the third day (i.e., approximately half of a seven day period) – a well-known phenomenon in health resort treatment – is a kind of oversteer.

Changes in the autonomic system are also mirrored in immunological processes. It has been known for a long time that the progression of disease often follows a pattern where critical events accumulate on the 7th, 14th, and 21st day. Various infectious diseases have a circaseptan development pattern. Hildebrandt observed a 7-day periodicity of fever peaks in children with scarlet fever: 7, 14, and 21 days after the first peak a new and hopefully much lower peak appears. This 7-day cycle seems to be common in many healing processes that have been researched. If, however, antibiotics are administered, the temperature decreases more rapidly and the 7-day cycle no longer exists. The question remains whether, in terms of future resilience of the entire organism, this is a good thing or not.

It seems plausible that the 7-day reactive periodicity of healing processes is derived from the 28-day lunar cycle – an evolutionary link to the days when our forebears were marine creatures. As mentioned earlier, many marine organisms follow a distinct lunar cycle pattern, which is reflected in lines in the chambers of nautilus shells and in shells of bivalves. Buildup and recovery are related processes and it comes as no surprise that the renewal rate of kidney cells after transplants is subject to reactive 7-day cycles. The same applies to young blood cells known as reticulocytes after induced oxygen starvation.

As practitioners, we may benefit from arranging weekly appointments with our patients, as this would allow us to take something like a stroboscopic view of the disease, at the same point in the 7-day disease cycle. Seeing patients after 7 days makes sense, not least because of the resonance effect that will be achieved, and activating the patient's self-healing forces in a 7-day rhythm.

Another reactive periodicity over 10 days has been observed, e.g., during recovery at a health resort. In contrast to the decreasing circaseptan rhythms, this "circadecan" effect increases until reaching the point of oversteer, usually on day 20. A circadecan response could be an indication to terminate the resort treatment.

Treatment through rhythm

Numerous studies have shown that adhering to a day rhythm by structuring the day, regular mealtimes and sleep patterns enhances health and quality of life even in individuals with pre-existing severe medical conditions.[115–117]

Although up to now we have only discussed the significance of a daily rhythm, we can already see that circadian research results can be applied in many ways to osteopathic medicine. It can be assumed that biological rhythms work like an orchestral score in the organism, coordinating the organs and their interaction so that they produce, process, or secrete the right chemicals at the right time. As long as the score is not flawed, the entire organism should function in a dynamic equilibrium – this is what we experience as health. If the score is flawed, the wrong chemicals will be produced at the wrong time and upset the organism. From an osteopath's view, this could be the herald of later disease. In fact, the onset or precursor state of many severe conditions is characterized by weakened or disrupted biological rhythms, such as the circadian rhythm. Weakened rhythms have been found in patients with depression, cancer patients, and individuals with burnout syndrome. This suggests that manual osteopathic treatment should be complemented with looking at the biological rhythms, e.g. by using Chronocardiograms.

Practical significance of rhythms in osteopathy

We can conclude that the world of biological rhythms permits new insights into the role of time in the human organism and can contribute to establishing a diagnosis, prognosis, and treatment of disease in humans. The harmonious interplay within the symphonic orchestra of our organs ensures health, wellbeing, and resilience, whereas disruptions can be early indicators or concomitant symptoms of disease. This opens up a new dimension – the dimension of time within the human body, and the heart with its beat variability is key to it – a part of reality hidden before our eyes for so long.[91]

Rhythmicity is a universal organizational principle throughout the organism

The human time organism not only establishes a schedule for organ functions, but also contributes to the efficient use of energy in the body. Virtually all of our sensory receptors work in phases, i.e., they only respond to change, whereas stimuli that remain the same lead to adaptation. Thus, change of rhythm has a major effect on proprioception in our body. Organ functions are stabilized and individual organs become aware of one another. This may also explain why the heart does not work as a continuous pump, but sends out blood in pulses. Chinese pulse diagnosis, and probably the heart too, can thus gather information about the function of our organs.

Including rhythm as the fourth dimension of our patients' body structure in our diagnostic considerations allows us to comprehend the wider context and patterns of phenomena and symptoms. The understanding of the wider context may reveal a deeper meaning of the phenomena. Thus, acute symptoms may be a resurfacing of suppressed processes, or they may be a stage on the way from chronic illness to healing. Looking at humans as dissipative, self-organizing systems that gravitate towards order and stability, alternating with phases of disorder (including certain disease symptoms) may deepen our insight (Fig. 3.3). The dialectic relationship between function and the oscillation dynamics of structures has already been explained.

There are many aspects of chronobiology relevant to osteopathy, some of which have not yet been sufficiently researched. They include:

1 The optimal time for treatment. The assumption is that during the first half of the day, the response to sympathicotonic stimuli will be far stronger than in the second half. Depending on the condition of the patient, the morning may be the time either to reinforce sympathicotonic stimuli or to induce a calm, vagally mediated response.

2 Harnessing endogenous rhythmic patterns to establish duration and structure of treatment. When treating acute conditions requiring several osteopathic treatment sessions throughout the day, the Basal Rest and Activity Cycle (BRAC) can provide guidance. This cycle was discovered by psychologists as oscillating in periods of 1.5–2 hours between vagally mediated deep sleep and sympathicotonic REM sleep. It extends into the day, where it can be observed as an attention span rhythm of 1.5–2 hours. Rehabilitation schedules should therefore be structured to follow this 1.5–2 hour pattern (or 45 minutes twice) of exercise, followed by approximately 30 minutes recovery time. This would exploit the BRAC resonance effects.

3 In general, physical activity plummets overnight and, depending on the patient's status, possibly again at around 2.00 p.m. The first of these sleep phases, in particular, is associated with a high point in immune

resistance, while the cardiovascular, digestive, and metabolic systems work at reduced capacity, yielding capacity to the immune system.

4 It is hard to find a body function that is not subject to rhythmical fluctuation in the course of a day. Under pathological conditions, these fluctuations often go beyond the normal range. Being familiar with the oscillating activity cycles of cells, tissues, organs, organ systems, and the entire organism is crucial for diagnosis and treatment, e.g., in menstruation-dependent headaches or rhythmical fluctuations of wellbeing, e.g., dependent on activity cycles, cortisol levels, etc.

5 Similarly, knowledge of periodical movement in the stomach and the small intestine, periodical movement of brain tissue, or of blood pressure fluctuation could be significant in palpatory diagnosis.

6 Rhythms, vibrations and oscillations in the tissues of an organism interact to create resonances amongst each other. Such processes transmit information and allow fine-tuning between organ systems. Ideally, body rhythms could express themselves quite freely, harmoniously, and symmetrically, depending on their place and type of origin. However, from birth, the body is exposed to multiple exogenous and endogenous influences that elicit numerous homeostatic and compensatory responses. If the body cannot balance out such influences, it adapts as best it can in a variety of ways. Such adaptive processes are supported by the homeostatic regulation of the various body rhythms. The specific patterns of rhythmic adaptation manifest themselves in the tissue structure, thus reflecting the changes in the body. Where, for example, continuous rhythmical expansion and contraction of tissue adapts to transitory acute stress or chronic tension patterns, corresponding asymmetries can be observed that reflect individual adaptation dynamics. Subtle variations in the quality and symmetry of rhythmical effects have diagnostic significance for the osteopath. Interaction between body rhythms can be assessed as well. Understanding palpable manifestations of rhythmical changes not only helps to locate a dysfunction but also enables us, with increasing experience, to distinguish between primary and secondary effects on the organism, acute and chronic problems and their emotional component, and to assess interaction between dysfunctions. Being able to diagnose interaction between structures and to put them in the context of the whole body and person, i.e., patterns of emotions, faith, and the cultural and sociobiological environment is a fundamental characteristic of osteopathic treatment. Osteopathic treatment focuses not on a single phenomenon, but on patterns emerging from the way it relates to other structures and energies, including self-awareness and the subjective experience of patients as well as their cultural, biological, and social environment and other relationship patterns.

7 Synchronization. The practitioner synchronizes with the patient's rhythms of respiration, language, gestures, and underlying tonus and (via palpation) with the rhythm of the tissues. This enables the therapist to share the patient's direct experience – a process that develops automatically once an empathetic relationship has been established between two humans. Conversely, the synchronization of a body's rhythm through general and specific techniques (e.g., in order to enhance the passing on of information in connective tissue) will result in more intense resonance. Thus, osteopathic treatment can support reorganization or integration into a higher order within the body.

8 Coherence. Phase similarities in various rhythms. Thus, in parasympathetic excitation, a coherence of medium wave rhythms was observed, e.g., respiration, heart frequency, and blood pressure. Osteopathic treatment that supports the release of fixed patterns in tissue, sensation, and belief conditioning as well as deeper relaxation and the establishment of higher order integration in the body probably encourages the development of coherence. This would be a topic worth investigating.

9 Chronodiagnostics. Our times are characterized by ubiquitous disruptions to biological rhythms, such as night and shift work, jet lag, artificial light facilitating nocturnal activity, thrillers on TV before bedtime, continuous time pressure, which all interfere with

and destroy our biological time organism. People usually are not aware that these are rhythm robbers. When advising patients on lifestyle, it is therefore important to identify rhythm robbers, based on measured parameters, so that the day schedule can be modified accordingly. This is where chronodiagnostics comes in. A Chronocardiogram will visualize disruptions to the time organism for the patient and help to select optimal treatment times. By the same token, a Chronocardiogram will visualize positive changes in the time organism, thus documenting the success of treatment, patient, and therapist.

10 Aging and biological rhythms. Biological rhythms are signs of vitality and, as such, will decrease in amplitude with aging. Studies of centenarians reveal that nearly all of them have a very regular lifestyle supporting their endogenous rhythms. Maintaining rhythm is a key element in anti-aging and the build-up of resilience and can be recommended to all patients. Disrupted sleep is generally a good indicator of disruption of overall rhythm and, in a healthy organism, disrupted sleep patterns will disappear with the re-establishment of a healthy day rhythm.

11 Future studies of response periods and integration time following osteopathic treatment will probably yield relevant results as to the optimal period between two treatment sessions. It seems that a period of rest should follow osteopathic treatment, during which enhanced frequency and phase coordination can take place. In German, this period of rest is known as "Lohnende Pause (rewarding break)," as it stabilizes the effects of the treatment.

12 Studies into possible correlations between the manifestation of disruptions/symptoms and rhythmical processes could provide further insights into patients' organizational patterns.[119]

13 Crisera's hypothesis[120] see also pp 60–233.

To ensure the coherent response of a body to various stimuli, there must be continuity at the levels of cells, tissue, and organs. Crisera surmises that a central rhythm is resonated by cells. This is what he describes as primary respiration (PR). This rhythm is thought to have the ability of synchronizing and combining varying numbers of physiological processes as functional units. Crisera also assumes that primary respiration originates in certain cell organelles: "In all probability, PR emerges within the crucial organelles, with special emphasis on the DNA, and propagated and transduced within the infrastructure of the cytoskeleton as wave harmonics."[121,122]

In the vertebrate subphylum, a corresponding vibration exists that depends on the development of the CNS and is generated by concentrically localized neurons that possess auto-oscillatory properties assembled into a vital network. The neurons are found in the reticular formation of the pons and the medulla. The vibration occurs as endogenous central pattern generators (CPGs) and has been described by Crisera as "craniosacral respiration."

It could be that this primary respiration/craniosacral respiration may be associated with the Basic Rest–Activity Cycle (BRAC).[123] This cycle has periods of 90–120 minutes (shorter in children) and its frequency is a multiple of the 24-hour day.

The quality of the central rhythm depends on the "long-range vibration" of the DNA.[124] The cytoskeleton acts as mediator of the vibration, eliciting physiological reactions within the cell. Whether these extremely fast vibrations can be picked up by palpation, however, is another question.

The considerations that follow may be fruitful for osteopathic work. There is, however, no hard evidence and we enter the realm of speculation.

Those cells expressing the largest proportion of their genome would have vibrations closest to the DNA vibration. Such processes seem to occur in neurons, which have self-oscillating properties – in particular in those that set the CPGs. Thus, respiratory neurons responsible for diaphragmatic breathing are described as primary because they create an endogenous rhythm independent from outside stimuli.[125] These CPGs are located in the pons and in the medulla where the BRAC is generated. They converge with CPGs such as those for the muscle tone or heart rhythm, which enables them to respond simultaneously to certain needs and extrinsic or intrinsic situations.

In phylogenetic terms, many biological rhythms seem to originate in protochordates, and then develop through the neuromeres of the rhombencephalon in vertebrates. There have been speculations whether pattern-generating cycles of recent developments such as voice, extensor muscle tonus, etc. could originate from the same hox gene that encodes the development of the rhombencephalon, which, in turn, generates the rhythm for cardiovascular circulation and thoracic respiration.[126] It could, therefore, well be that primary respiration was the first biological rhythm to develop in the early stages of life and that this later underwent changes during phylogenetic development so that integrated multi-rhythmic organisms emerged.

Living cells have three specific characteristics:

- A highly developed structural and temporal organization and coordination.

- The ability to extract and transform various forms of energy through metabolic processes in order to ensure growth, reproduction, the maintenance of structural integrity and mobility.

- Archetypes are stored in the DNA that manifest as instincts (that are genotype related) and as psychobiological engrams (instinctive behavior that may be modified by learning processes).

According to Crisera, the energetic system, also known as bioenergetic dynamics, which is tantamount to the inherent nature of life, can be divided into three components – structure, metabolism, and psyche. At its rudimentary level, this energy manifests itself as a bipolar force, an essential biological rhythm of expansion and contraction. Crisera describes the expansion–contraction ratio as the primary respiration quotient (PRQ). All psychological and physiological dynamics can be traced back to the PRQ. The PRQ generates a multiple of substates that code for specific psychophysiological conditions.

The tensegrity structures enable the exchange of energy vibrations within the cells via the cytoskeleton and are passed on through the extracellular matrix (via integrins) and the plasma lamellae of neighboring cells (via cadherins, selectins, and other cell adhesion molecules (CAMs)). It is thus possible to coordinate various physiological processes to enable the body to respond in unison to internal or external needs.

DNA in particular has low-frequency oscillations known as "breathing." Those long-ranged vibrations resonate at a particular frequency that stimulates specific genes that produce certain proteins.[127] According to Crisera, DNA breathing is the same as primary respiration.

A tensegrity intelligence system (TIS) is a resonating chain of intracellular elements coupled to the cytoskeleton that processes and transmits cytological information as mechano-electro-chemical transduction. Hence, the cytological architecture is "…an inert supportive framework" that converts "mechanical energy … into electrochemical responses." "Wave harmonics" has become an information system that affects DNA breathing, enzyme kinetics, mitochondrial activity, and the electrochemical properties of cell membranes.[128–131]

References

[1] Schauberger V: Nature as Teacher, Eco-Technology Vol. 2. Quotation also found on http://energy21.freeservers.com/schauberger.htm.

[2] Menzel W: Menschliche Tag-Nacht-Rhythmik und Schichtarbeit: Schwabe; 1962.

[3] Halberg F, Wang Z, Schwartzkopff O, Cornelissen G: Chronomik für die große Öffentlichkeit. Neuroendocrinology Letters Suppl 2003;1(24):74–83.

[4] Jaeger J, Goodwin BC: Cellular oscillators in animal segmentation. Silico Biol 2002;2(2):111–123.

[5] Stiefvater EW: Die Organuhr: Organmaximalzeiten der Akupunktur und 24-Stunden-Periodik. Heidelberg: Haug; 2006.

[6] Aschoff J, Fatranska M, Giedke H, Doerr P, Stamm D, Wisser H: Human circadian rhythms in continuous darkness: entrainment by social cues. Science 1971, 171(3967):213–215.

[7] Aschoff J: Circadian rhythms in man. Science 1965, 148(3676):1427–1432.

[8] Hildebrandt G, Moser M, Lehofer M: Chronobiology and Chronomedicine (in German). Weiz: gesundheitsleitsystem; 1998, 2013.

[9] Halberg F: Biological rhythms. Adv Exp Med Biol 1975, 54:1–41.

[10] Aschoff J, Poppel E, Wever R: Circadian rhythms in men under the influence of light–dark cycles of various periods. Pflugers Arch 1969, 306(1):58–70.

[11] Hildebrandt G: Outline of chronohygiene. Chronobiologia 1976, 3(2):113–127.

[12] Hildebrandt G, Moser M, Lehofer M: Chronobiology and Chronomedicine (in German). Weiz: gesundheitsleitsystem; 1998, 2013.

[13]Halberg F, Cornelissen G: Rhythms and blood pressure. Ann Ist Super Sanita 1993, 29(4):647–665.

[14]Hildebrandt G, Moser M, Lehofer M: Chronobiology and Chronomedicine (in German). Weiz: gesundheitsleitsystem; 1998, 2013.

[15]Hufeland CW: Macrobiotics or the art of extending human life (in German). Stuttgart: A.F. Macklot.

[16]Aschoff J: Circadian rhythms in man. Science 1965, 148(3676):1427–1432.

[17]Moser M, Schaumberger K, Schernhammer E, Stevens RG: Cancer and rhythm. Cancer Causes Control 2006, 17(4):483-487.

[18]Erren TC, Pape HG, Reiter RJ, Piekarski C: Chrono-disruption and cancer. Naturwissenschaften 2008, 95(5):367–382.

[19]Kubo T, Ozasa K, Mikami K, Wakai K, Fujino Y, Watanabe Y, Miki T, Nakao M, Hayashi K, Suzuki K, et al: Prospective cohort study of the risk of prostate cancer among rotating-shift workers: findings from the Japan collaborative cohort study. Am J Epidemiol 2006, 164(6):549–555.

[20]Fu L, Lee CC: The circadian clock: pacemaker and tumour suppressor. Nat Rev Cancer 2003, 3(5):350–361.

[21]Lee CC: Tumor suppression by the mammalian Period genes. Cancer Causes Control 2006, 17(4):525–530.

[22]Moser M and Stevens R: Special section on Cancer and Rhythm, in: Cancer Causes and Control 2006, 17 (4), pp. 483-621.

[23]Sinz R: Zeitstrukturen und organismische Regulation. Berlin: Akademie Verlag; 1978:75 (in German only).

[24]Sinz R: Zeitstrukturen und organismische Regulation. Berlin: Akademie Verlag; 1978:114.

[25]Anochin PK: Beiträge zur allgemeinen Theorie des funktionellen Systems. Jena: Fischer; 1978 (in German only).

[26]Jantzen W: Transempirische Raume-Sinn und Bedeutung in Lebenszusammenhängen. http://members.aol.comfbasaglialmuhlh97.html.

[27]Hildebrandt G, Moser M, Lehofer M: Chronobiologie und Chronomedizin. Stuttgart: Hippokrates; 1998, 2013 (in German only, but it may be worth looking at http://pulse.embs.org/Past_Issues/2008January/Moser.pdf).

[28]Sinz R: Zeitstrukturen und Organismische Regulation. Berlin: Akademie Verlag; 1978:114.

[29]Hellbrügge T, Ehregut-Lange J, Rutenfranz J, Stehr K: Circadian periodicity of physiological functions in different stages of infancy and childhood. Annals of the New York Academy of Sciences 1964; 117(1):361–373.

[30]Lemmer B: Chronopharmakologie. Stuttgart: Wissenschaftliche Verlagsgesellschaft; 1984:27.

[31]Williams GH, Cain JP, Dluhy RG, Underwood RH: Studies of the control of plasma aldosterone concentration in normal man. I. Response to posture, acute and chronic volume depletion, and sodium loading. J Clin Invest 1972;51(7): 1731–1742.

[32]Michelakis AM, Horton R: The relationship between plasma renin and aldosterone in normal man. Circ Res 1970; 27:185–194.

[33]Kaulhausen H, Muhlbauer W, Benker W, Breuer H, Vetter H: Circadian rhythm of the renin-angiotensin-aldosterone system. Z. Klein. Chem. Klein. Biochem. 1974;12(5):268-269

[34]Pongratz G, Zietz B, Gluck T, Scholmerich J, Straub RH: Corticotropin-releasing factor modulates cardiovascular and pupillary autonomic reflexes in man: is there a link to inflammation-induced autonomic nervous hyperreflexia? Ann NY Acad Sci 2002;966:373–383.

[35]Haus E, Halberg F: Circaannual rhythm in level and timing of serum corticosterone in standardized inbred mature C-mouse. Environment Res 1970; 3:81–106.

[36]Halberg F, Wang Z, Schwartzkopff O, Cornelissen G: Chronomik für die große Öffentlichkeit. Neuroendocrinology Letters Suppl 2003;1(24):74–83.

[37]Moskalenko YE: Cerebral pulsation in the closed cranial cavity. Izv Akad Nauk SSSR 1964;4: 620–629.

[38]Ludwig C: Beiträge zur Kenntnis des Einflusses der Respirationsbewegungen auf den Blutumlauf im Aortensystem. Arch Anat Physiol 1847:242.

[39]Traube L: Uber periodische Tatigkeitsanderungen des Vasomotorischen und Hemrnungs-Nervenzentrums. Cbl Med Wiss 1865; 56:881–885.

[40]Hering E: Über Atembewegungen des Gefäßsystems. Sitzung b. d. k. Akad DW math. Naturw. 1869;60: 829–856, Table III.

[41]Kitney RI: An analysis of the nonlinear behavior of the human thermal vasomotor control system. J Theor Biol 1975;52:231—248.

[42]Burch GE, Cohn AE, Neumann C: A study by quantitative methods of the spontaneous variations in volume of the finger tip, toe tip, and posterior—superior portion of the pinna of resting normal white adults. Am J Physiol 1942;136433—447.

[43]Chess GF, Tam RMK, Calaresu FR: Influence of cardiac neural inputs on rhythmic variations of heart period in the cat. Am J Physiol 1975;228:775—780.

[44]Hyndman BW: The role of rhythms in homeostasis. Kybernetik 1974;15:227—236.

[45]Akselrod S, Gordon D, Ubel FA, et al.: Power spectral analysis of heart rate fluctuation: A quantitative probe of beatto-beat cardiovascular control. Science 1981;213:220—221.

[46]Akselrod S, Gordon D, Madwed JB, et al.: Hemodynamic regulation: Investigation by spectral analysis. Am J Physiol 1985;249:867—H875.

[47]Larsson SE, Cai H, Oberg PA: Percutaneous measurement by laser-Doppler flowmetry of skeletal muscle microcirculation at varying levels of contraction force determined electromyographically. Eur J Appl Physiol Occup 1993;66(6):477—482.

[48]Nakata A, Takata S, Yuasa T, et al.: Analysis of heart arterial pressure, and muscle sympathetic nerve activity in normal humans. Am J Physiol 1998;274:1211—1217.

[49]Portaluppi F, Smolenslcy MH (ed.): Time-DepentE7 Structure and Control of Arterial Blood Pressure. Proceedings of a conference. Ferrara, Italy, September, 10—12. 1995. Ann NY Acad Sci 1996;783:1—342.

[50]Sinz R: Zeitstrukturen und organismische Regulation. 7: Berlin: Akademie Verlag; 1978: 328.

[51]Mayer S: Über spontane Blutdruckschwankungen. Sitzung b. d. k. Akad. D. W. math. Naturw. 1869;67:281—305.

[52]Schmidt JA: Periodic hemodynamics in health and disease. Heidelberg: Springer; 1996.

[53]Glonek T: personal correspondence: 27.12.2004.

[54]Magoun HI: Osteopathy in the Cranial Field. 3rd ed. Kirksville: Journal Printing Company; 1976:40.

[55]Sinz R: Zeitstrukturen und Organismische Regulation. Berlin: Akademie Verlag; 1978:366.

[56]Allen K, Lewer, Goldman H: Phasic pressure characteristics of the cerebrospinal system. South African J Surgery 1967.

[57]Lewer-Allen K, Bunt EA, Lewer-Allen CM, Sorek S: dynamic studies of the human craniospinal system -7H9 don: Janus Publishing Company; 2000:5.

[58]Moser M, Lehofer M, Sedminek A, Lux M, Zapotoczky HG, Kenner T, Noordergraaf, A: Heart rate variability as a prognostic tool in cardiology. Circulation. 1994;90:1078—1082.

[59]Sinz R: Zeitstrukturen und Organismische Regulation. 7: Berlin: Akademie Verlag; 1978: 328.

[60]Gallasch E, Rafolt D, Moser M, Hindinger J, Eder H, Wiesspeiner G, Kenner T: Instrumentation for assessment of tremor, skin vibrations, and cardiovascular variables in MIR space missions. IEEE Trans Biomed Eng 1996, 43(3):328–333.

[61]Rohracher H, Inanaga K: Die Mikrovibration, Bern: Hans Huber; 1969, 91—94, 100.

[62]Gallasch E, Moser M, Kozlovskaya IB, Kenner T, Noordergraaf A: Effects of an eight-day space flight on microvibration and physiological tremor. Am J Physiol 1997, 273(1 Pt 2):R86—92.

[63]Rohracher H, Inanaga K: Die Mikrovibration, Bern: Hans Huber, 131, 132.

[64]Rohracher H, Inanaga K: Die Mikrovibration, Bern: Hans Huber, 43-61, 72ff.

[65]Csibra G, Davis G, Spratling MW, Johnson MH: Gamma oscillations and object processing in the infant brain. Science 2000;290:1582—1585.

[66]Woods JM, Woods RH: A Physical Finding Related to Psychiatric Disorders 1961;60: 988—993.

[67]Magoun HI: Osteopathy in the Cranial Field. 3rd ed. Kirksville Journal Printing Company; 1976:25.

[68]Becker RE; Craniosacral trauma in the adult. Osteopathic Ann 1976;4(8):43—59.

[69]Lay E: Cranial field. In Ward RC. (ed.): Foundations f: - Osteopathic Medicine. Baltimore: Williams and 1997:901—913.

[70]Lay EM, Cicorda RA, Tettambel M: Recording of the cranial rhythmic impulse. JAOA. 1978;78(10):149.

[71]Wirth-Patullo V, Hayes KW: Interrater reliability of craniosacral rate measurements and their relationship with subjects and examiners heart and respiratory rate measurements. Phys Ther 1994; 67(10):1526—1532.

[72]Nelson KE, Sergueef N, Lipinski CM, et al.: Cranial rhythmic impulse related to the Traube-Hering-Mayer comparing laser Doppler flowmetry and palpation. J A Osteopath Assoc 2001;101(3):163–173.

[73]Upledger JE, Vredevoogd JD: Craniosacral Therapy, Eastland Press 1983.

[74]Becker RE: In: Brooks RE (ed.). Life in motion: The osteopathic vision of Rollin E. Becker. Portland: Stillness Press;1997:120.

[75]Upledger JE, Vredevoogd JD: Craniosacral Therapy, Eastland Press 1983, p.205.

[76]Jealous J: Emergence of originality – A biodynamic view of osteopathy in the cranial field. 1997;12:35 (lecture script).

[77]Becker RE. In: Brooks RE (ed.). Life in motion: The osteopathic vision of Rollin E. Becker. Portland: Stillness Press;1997:122.

[78]Nelson KE, Sergueef N, Lipinski CM, et al.: Cranial rhythmic impulse related to the Traube-Hering-Mayer comparing laser Doppler flowmetry and palpation. J A Osteopath Assoc 2001;101(3):163–173.

[79]Liem T: Lecture OFM Munich 1998.

[80]Lewer-Allen K, Bunt EA, Lewer-Allen CM, Sorel S: Hydr:- dynamic studies of the human craniospinal system. Lc 7 don: Janus Publishing Company; 2000:5.

[81]Lewer-Allen K, Bunt EA, Lewer-Allen CM, Sorel S: Hydr:- dynamic studies of the human craniospinal system. Lc 7 don: Janus Publishing Company; 2000:5.

[81a]Bertalanffy Lv, Beier W, Laue R: Biophysik des Fliessgleichgewichts Braunschweig: Vieweg, 1977.

[81b]Maturana HR, Varela FJ: Autopoiesis and Cognition: The Realization of the Living. Boston Studies in the Philosophy of Science 1980; 42.

[81c]Moser M: Between Chaos and Order – Considerations on the Emergence of Shape and Form. In: Karl Toifl (Ed.): Chaos Theory and Medicine: Self Organisation in the Complex System „Man" (In German), 1999.

[81d]Moser M, Frühwirth M, Bonin D von, Cysarz D, Penter R, Heckmann C, Hildebrandt G: The Autonomic Picture (ChronoCardiogramm) as a Method to Portray the Rhythms of the Human Heartbeat (in German). In: Peter Heusser, Hrsg. Hygiogenesis, Peter Lang, Bern, 1999, 207–223.

[81e]Prigogine I, Nicolis G, Babloyantz A: Nonequilibrium problems in biological phenomena. Ann NY Acad Sci 1974; 231(1):99–105.

[81f]Moser M, Fruhwirth M, Kenner T: The symphony of life. Importance,interaction, and visualization of biological rhythms. IEEE Eng Med Biol Mag 2008; 27(1):29–37.

[81g]Moser M, Kripke DF: Insomnia: More trials needed to assess sleeping pills. Nature 2013; 493(7432):305–305.

[82]Novalis H, Friedrich von: Die Enzyklopädie – Die Philosophischen Wissenschaften. 1798/1799.

[83]Aschoff J: Circadian rhythms in man. Science 1965, 148(3676):1427–1432.

[84]Hildebrandt G, Moser M, Lehofer M: Chronobiology and Chronomedicine (in German). Weiz: Gesundheitsleitsystem; 1998, 2013.

[85]Moser M, Penter R, Fruehwirth M, Kenner T: Why life oscillates – biological rhythms and health. Conf Proc IEEE Eng Med Biol Soc 2006, 1:424–428.

[86]Proceedings of the Why Life Oscillates—biological rhythms and health: 2006.

[87]Moser M, Fruhwirth M, Kenner T: The symphony of life. Importance, interaction, and visualization of biological rhythms. IEEE Eng Med Biol Mag 2008, 27(1):29–37.

[88]Hildebrandt G, Moser M, Lehofer M: Chronobiology and Chronomedicine (in German). Weiz: Gesundheitsleitsystem; 1998, 2013.

[89]Strogatz S: Synchron – Vom Rätselhaften Rhythmus der Natur: Berlin Verlag; 2004.

[90]Moser M, Fruehwirth M, Penter R, Winker R: Why life oscillates – from a topographical towards a functional chronobiology. Cancer Causes Control 2006, 17(4):591–599.

[91]Moser M, Fruehwirth M, Kenner T: The symphony of life - Importance, interaction and visualization of biological rhythms. IEEE Eng Med Biol Mag 2008, 27(Jan–Feb):29–37.

[92]Hildebrandt G, Moser M, Lehofer M: Chronobiology and Chronomedicine (in German). Weiz: Gesundheitsleitsystem; 1998, 2013.

[93]von Asper H: Über die braune retziusche parallelstreifung im schmelz der menschlichen zähne. Schweiz Vjschr Zahnheilkunde 1916, 26; 275–314.

[94]Dean C, Leakey MG, Reid D, Schrenk F, Schwartz GT, Stringer C, Walker A: Growth processes in teeth distinguish modern humans from homo erectus and earlier hominins. Nature 2001, 414(6864):628–631.

[95]Dean C, Leakey MG, Reid D, Schrenk F, Schwartz GT, Stringer C, Walker A: Growth processes in teeth distinguish modern humans from homo erectus and earlier hominins. Nature 2001, 414(6864):628–631.

[96]Bücher K: Arbeit und Rhythmus. Leipzig: Hirzel; 1899.

[97]Moser M, Lehofer M, Sedminek A, Lux M, Zapotoczky HG, Kenner T, Noordergraaf A: Heart rate variability as a prognostic tool in cardiology. Circulation 1994, 90(2):1078–1082.

[98]Hildebrandt G, Moser M, Lehofer M: Chronobiology and Chronomedicine (in German). Weiz: Gesundheitsleitsystem; 1998, 2013.

[99]Maturana HR, Varela FJ: Autopoiesis and Cognition: The Realization of the Living Boston; 1980.

[100]Moser M, Frühwirth M, Semler I, Lehofer M: Heart rate variability in sleep medicine – the autonomic picture of the heart (in German). Wiener Klinische Wochenschrift 2000, 112(5):18–19.

[101]Proceedings of the Why Life Oscillates – biological rhythms and health: 2006.

[102]Moser M, Fruehwirth M, Kenner T: The symphony of life – Importance, interaction and visualization of biological rhythms. IEEE Eng Med Biol Mag 2008, 27(Jan–Feb):29–37.

[102a]Rechtschaffen A, Kales A: A manual of standardized terminology, techniques and scoring system for sleep stages of human subjects. Nr. 204, US Dept. of Health, Education, and Welfare, Public Health Services-National Institutes of Health, National Institute of Neurological Diseases and Blindness, Neurological Information Network, 1968.

[103]Xie L, Kang H, Xu Q, Chen MJ, Liao Y, Thiyagarajan M, O'Donnell J, Christensen DJ, Nicholson C, Iliff JJ, et al.: Sleep drives metabolite clearance from the adult brain. Science 2013, 342(6156):373–377.

[104]Moser M, Fruhwirth M, Kenner T: The symphony of life. Importance, interaction, and visualization of biological rhythms. IEEE Eng Med Biol Mag 2008, 27(1):29–37.

[105]Moser M, Fruehwirth M, Penter R, Winker R: Why life oscillates – from a topographical towards a functional chronobiology. Cancer Causes Control 2006, 17(4):591–599.

[106]Hildebrandt G, Moser M, Lehofer M: Chronobiology and Chronomedicine (in German). Weiz: Gesundheitsleitsystem; 1998, 2013.

[107]Raschke F: Chronobiological viewpoints of respiratory regulation. Wien Med Wochenschr 1995, 145(17–18):435–439.

[108]Holmback U, Forslund A, Lowden A, Forslund J, Akerstedt T, Lennernas M, Hambraeus L, Stridsberg M: Endocrine responses to nocturnal eating – possible implications for night work. Eur J Nutr 2003, 42(2):75–83.

[109]Karlsson BH, Knutsson AK, Lindahl BO, Alfredsson LS: Metabolic disturbances in male workers with rotating three-shift work. Results of the WOLF study. Int Arch Occup Environ Health 2003, 76(6):424–430.

[110]Knutsson A: Health disorders of shift workers. Occup Med (Lond) 2003, 53(2):103–108.

[111]Moser M, Schaumberger K, Schernhammer E, Stevens RG: Cancer and rhythm. Cancer Causes Control 2006, 17(4):483–487.

[112]Hildebrandt G, Moser M, Lehofer M: Chronobiology and Chronomedicine (in German). Weiz: Gesundheitsleitsystem; 1998, 2013.

[113]Lundberg S: Continuous recording and control of ventricular fluid pressure in neurosurgical practice. Acta Psych et Neurol Scand 1960;149;36, 81–193.

[114]Miller JD: Intracranial pressure monitoring. Arch Neurol 1985;42:1191–1193.

[115]Mormont MC, Levi F: Cancer chronotherapy: principles, applications, and perspectives. Cancer 2003, 97(1):155–169.

[116]Innominato PF, Levi FA, Bjarnason GA: Chronotherapy and the molecular clock: Clinical implications in oncology. Adv Drug Deliv Rev 2010, 62(9–10):979–1001.

[117]Moser M, Penter R, Fruehwirth M, Kenner T: Why life oscillates – biological rhythms and health. Conf Proc IEEE Eng Med Biol Soc 2006, 1:424–428.

[118]Halberg F, Wang Z, Schwartzkopff O, Cornelissen G: Chronomik für die große Öffentlichkeit. Neuroendocrinology Letters Supplem 2003.

[119]Szmelskyi AO: A retrospective survey of the predictive value of biorhythm theory in acute patients

presenting in osteopathic practice. Comp Med Res 1990; 4(2):35–38.

[120]Crisera PN: The cytological implications of primary respiration. Medical Hypothesis 2001;55(1):40–51.

[121]Chou KC: Low frequency vibrations of DANN molecules. Biochem J 1984;221:27–31.

[122]Pienta KJ, Coffrey DS: Cellular harmonic information transfer through a tissue tensegrity-matrix system. Med Hypothesis 1991: 34:85–88.

[123]Llinas RR: The intrinsic electrophysiological properties of mammalian neurons: Insights into central nervous system function. Science 1988; 242:1654–1664.

[124]Fröhlich H: The Genetic Code as Language. In: Fröhlich H (ed): Biological Coherence and Response to External Stimuli. Berlin: Springer, 1988.

[125]Arshavsky YI, Deliagina TG, Orlovsky GN: Pattern Generation. Curr Opin Neurobiol 1997;7:781–789.

[126]Bass AH, Baker R: Phenotypic specification of hindbrain rhombomeres and the origins of rhythmic circuits in vertebrates. Brain Behav Evol 1997; 50:3–16.

[127]Fröhlich H: The Genetic Code as Language. In: Fröhlich H (ed): Biological Coherence and Response to External Stimuli. Berlin: Springer,1988.

[128]Dayhoof J, Hameroff SR, Lahoz-Beltra R, Swenberg CE: Cytoskeletal involvement in neuronal learning: a review. Eur Biophys J 1994; 23:79–93.

[129]De Loof A: The electrical dimension of cells: The cell as a miniature electrophoresis chamber. Int Rev Cytol 1986;104:251–351.

[130]Hameroff SR, Watt RW: Information processing in microtubules. J Struct Biol 1997;118:94–106.

[131]Tuszynski JA, Trpisová B, Sept D, Brown JA: Selected physical issues in the structure and function of microtubules. J Struct Biol 1997;118: 94–106.

Physical principles

Lorenz Fischer

Modified from Part I, Propädeutik, in: Fischer L: Neuraltherapie nach Huneke, 2nd edn. Stuttgart: Hippokrates; 2001.
We are simultaneously a part and the whole, observer and observed in a single united whole.

J.C. Payan (Personal communication)

Modern physics and biology

Introduction

The philosophical paradigm which, following Descartes, views body and soul as separate, and classical physics with its Newtonian laws, have long tended to create in scientists the assumption that every process in the inhabited and uninhabited world could be analyzed into individual mathematical and mechanical concepts (reductionism). This approach excludes everything that does not directly have to do with the question at issue. When dealing with complex problems, a series of partial solutions is assembled, using linear equations. Linear equations permit transfer to other systems; generalizations and predictions can be made (determinism). Anything that is unique or individual is inaccessible to classical science. This type of science is nonetheless necessary in many fields (technology, acute medicine) in order to achieve progress of a targeted, specific kind (and major successes have been achieved). This does not mean that the approach should be seen as right in principle in all fields (e.g., chronic disease, complex natural phenomena).

It is an illusion, therefore, to believe that the way to arrive at understanding and predictability in respect of everything in nature is simply to isolate and investigate the minutest components and subsystems, and reassemble the results in the manner of a mosaic. Ultra-small components (subatomic particles) and their simple properties and interactions are inadequate to explain complex natural phenomena; it constantly becomes necessary to postulate further particles with increasingly complicated properties to complete the picture. Here, classical science with its focus on the particular comes up against its boundaries; the more comprehensive the explanatory capacity of the model tries to be, the more complex the model becomes, and the more the model itself requires explanation.[1] The arrival of quantum theory and mathematical chaos theory made clear that reductionism cannot achieve its goal without error and that predictability is impossible in nature. Non-linearity, positive feedback and indeterminism hold sway in complex natural phenomena and in living organisms (though linearity and negative feedback do determine matters in certain "islands of order"). Everything hangs together and the "whole is more than the sum of its parts." By the late 19th century, Newton's laws were already beginning to be shaken; for an idealized system consisting of just two bodies (e.g., earth and moon), Newton's equations yield precise solutions, but if a third body is added, then astonishingly the only way to deal with the situation is by using the mathematical method of gradual approximation. This is accurate enough to be applied in practical technology, but Henri Poincaré recognized that the problem of multiple bodies is not linear, and saw the possibility that, as a result of positive feedback, the tiniest gravitational effect from a third body (an asteroid, for example) could under certain circumstances throw a planet completely out of its usual orbit. Unfortunately, inadequate attention was initially paid to this discovery. A few years later, however, the Newtonian laws were shaken once again, by quantum physics (Max Planck), and by Einstein's early work on the theory of relativity.

Quantum theory teaches that an objective description of nature is impossible; the observer is always involved in the experiment (see section on Quantum physics).

Matter in the usual sense no longer exists; particles are now simply positions with a large field of force.

Einstein's theory of special relativity produces a completely new concept of space and time. One of its conclusions is the principle of mass–energy equivalence: matter is a form of energy:

$E = mc^2$ (energy (E) equals mass (m) multiplied by the square of the speed of light).

Einstein's theory of general relativity, a new theory of gravity, began in 1915 to supplant Newton's law of gravity, which was not universally valid. According to Einstein, gravity is the consequence of the bending of space-time. Significant discoveries by other researchers were also made, and in the course of time it became possible to describe natural processes in terms of the following four elementary forces:

1 The strong nuclear force

2 The weak interaction (spontaneous radioactive decay and neutron decay)

3 The electromagnetic interaction

4 Gravitation.

It remains the dream of physicists to unite all four elementary forces in a single theory. The difficulty lies in the fact that it has not so far been possible to establish a link between quantum mechanics and general relativity. Dirac (1928) and later Feynman (Nobel Prize 1965) did however succeed in uniting special relativity and quantum mechanics. This successful theory was given the name "quantum electrodynamics" (QED). It uses the interaction of electrons with light (photons) to describe all natural processes except gravitation and radioactivity. The whole of chemistry can also be described by this means.[2]

Feynman always took pleasure in questioning established laws of logic and mathematics. His quantum theory is beyond any "common sense" understanding – even for Feynman himself – but it functions excellently, and with a degree of precision hardly equaled by anything before it.

In the 1970s, Georgi succeeded in bringing together all the elementary forces except gravitation and reduce them to a common denominator.

Theories to unite all four elementary forces contained up to 26 dimensions, but had still not achieved the breakthrough. Recently, however, "superstring" theory has given rise to fresh hope: space-time is a network of ribbon-like strings, whose lowest oscillatory state is the basis of all elementary particles.[3] In other words: the many different particles in nature, and also the four elementary forces, are simply different resonance vibrations (energetic states) of the strings.

The modern physical theories of such as David Bohm, Burkhard Heim, and Rupert Sheldrake represent a further type of unified theory;[4–6] they postulate fundamental levels (dimensions) "behind" those of matter and energy. These dimensions cannot be measured by any of the scientific methods available to date, although they can to some extent be calculated by means of mathematical models.

In general, in the dimension of matter and energy ("normal" space-time) the speed of light (photons) is held to be the most rapid means for the transport of information. Now, however, these additional levels ("dimensions") are potential patterns of structure and information for normal space-time; they link it "network" fashion into a whole. In this way, every point in the system is informed about the whole, without any time delay (so in this case faster than the speed of light). The names of these coordinating, "directing" levels outside normal space-time differ from one author to another: "structure and information pattern," "quantum field," and "morphogenetic fields." Alain Aspect has given a practical demonstration of the existence of such fields or patterns by means of an inspired experiment (described in the section on Quantum theory). This new direction in physics and science confirms the correctness of the holistic view of regulation medicine, a category that includes osteopathic medicine.

Summary

Classical, reductionist, and deterministic science (especially Newtonian physics) cannot adequately describe natural processes. To do this requires the additional statements of modern physics. These lead to a holistic – we might say, more appropriate – way of looking at nature, which also corresponds to regulation medicine. However, this by no means implies that modern physics is able to describe all phenomena of nature.

Quantum physics

In 1900, Max Planck discovered that absorption of light does not happen evenly, but rather in portions (particles, or quanta).[7] Building on this, one of the most successful theories of the last hundred years was developed: quantum theory, concerned with the motions and energies of atomic and subatomic particles. In essence it deals with the interaction of light (synonyms: electromagnetic waves/radiation, photons) with matter. It is able to explain all the subsidiary fields of physics – except gravitation – and the whole of chemistry.[8]

To express this another way: with the exception of the mysterious force of gravitation, the whole physical and "chemical" world can be described in terms of interaction between photons and electrons. This very broad applicability and precision of quantum physics hides the fact that it cannot be understood using hitherto known concepts of logic. There are often several paradoxical, even mutually contradictory solutions to the equations, and the decision comes only with the act of observation. This fact is underlined by statements from quantum physicist and Nobel Prizewinner Niels Bohr ("Anyone who is not shocked by quantum theory has not understood it") and Richard Feynman ("You don't understand quantum theory; you only get used to it").

Classical physics (and biology) had made constant progress by applying reductionism (see previous section) and determinism (predictability) and separation of the subjective and objective. Quantum physics then remorselessly revealed the fact that nature cannot adequately be described in this way; there had to be a revolution, a complete rethink. Most of those who use quantum physics, however, do not seem to know all that this highly exact scientific theory in fact involves:

The observer effect

In quantum physics, the subject/object distinction is no longer possible; we cannot separate observer and observed. Depending on the design of the experiment, light can be represented either as a wave or as a particle. Niels Bohr recognized early on that subatomic "particles" do not adopt their clearly defined properties until someone observes them. The act of observation also influences the result, changing the position and speed of a "particle."[9]

More than one hundred years ago, Michelson and Morley demonstrated by experimental measurement that, contrary to common sense expectation, the speed of light does not depend on whether one is moving with or against the beam of light. Einstein tested and confirmed the fact that the speed of light is indeed constant and the same for all observers. The "price" he had to pay for this was to abandon absolute standards in the measurement of length and time: a moving clock runs faster; measuring rods in motion shrink. Adopting this enables the theory to be maintained and everything to be precisely measured in technology. It is exciting, however, to reexamine such apparently clear facts; Meyl, for example, suggests the following: he allows time to remain constant and postulates the field dependence of light.[10] Now, if the constant nature of the speed of light postulated by Einstein does not exist, we would not be able to observe or measure this.[11] If a light source moves toward or away from a detector, the speeds will be added or subtracted.[12] However, in the beam of light the fields that influence the speed of the light, the detector, and the measurement technician are superimposed.[13,14] Therefore the technician will always observe and measure identical speeds of light, and falsely demonstrate a constant speed of light.[15]

Everyday experience often shows how objectivity can be called into question. Here is a simple experiment: We have learned that a particular electromagnetic spectrum produces a particular color. This spectrum is captured by the retina, transmitted to a specific area of the brain, and we perceive a color: red, or blue, and so on. If I wear a red pullover in an office with strip lighting (short wave electromagnetic spectrum), then go into the dark corridor where there is little light, and then outside into the open where there is a setting sun, (longer wave electromagnetic spectrum), each time the total light spectrum (mix of frequencies) experienced by my retina on looking at my pullover is different, yet I see the same red of the pullover in all three places. Therefore, it is not only the light spectrum emanating from a particular color that determines the color we recognize; it is at least equally due to experience and the structure of our nervous system. Maturana[16] says in this connection that it is possible to establish a correspondence between the naming of colors and states of neuronal activity, but not to establish one with wavelengths. It is only the individual structure of the person that determines what pattern of neuronal activity is produced by what stimuli.[17] The problems encountered in experimental particle physics (which include the structure of the particle detector) are similar (as mentioned above). Therefore, there is no "world out there" with us as objective observers. We are integrally part of this world and are ourselves bound up with what we are measuring. Another analogy might be the unity of patient and practitioner in osteopathy. In addition, we can recognize that "our world" is a whole, and that we can never separate out one element of that whole and perform experiments on it without error.

One of the conclusions to be drawn from this is that the holistic and individual view of regulation medicine has a modern scientific context.

Rethinking the concept of matter

Matter, as we would normally understand it, no longer has any place in quantum theory, as was already the case in Einstein's theory of relativity. Subatomic "particles" are not little spheres that can be isolated, but a complicated network of interrelated energy in which everything is connected and interwoven with everything else.

Researchers worldwide constantly seek the smallest components, ever smaller subatomic particles, which could in the reductionist view be reassembled to recreate the whole. However, in experimental particle physics, observation, measurement, and theory are more strongly interwoven than people might think.[18,19] This forces a reassessment of what is meant by "matter." Subatomic particles are not "substance" or actual entities in themselves. They cannot be captured independently of their interaction with the measuring apparatus; in other words, they do not exist independently of the measuring apparatus.[20] What this means is that the assumed subatomic particles only come into existence as a consequence of the properties of the particle detector, after the waves that belong to a total quantum system have "collapsed."[21] In the "quantum world" it is not possible to isolate particles from the complex interrelated whole without error.

Indeterminism

It will help to begin with an explanation of determinism: in Newtonian physics, with mechanical time, limitless space, and dead, inert matter, determinism (predictability, the capacity to be determined) applies. In other words, there is a linear relationship between cause and effect. This is transferable to other (non-living) systems and reproducible.

Quantum physics reveals that this relationship of cause and effect no longer applies at the atomic and subatomic level (indeterminism).

This was demonstrated by Heisenberg's uncertainty relation: it is never possible to measure the position and speed of a subatomic particle simultaneously. The experimenter must therefore decide which to measure: position or speed. When we have defined the position, we can no longer say anything about the future path of the particle (and vice versa). The predictability of classical physics can no longer be assumed. Many scientists see this uncertainty in a negative light, but in essence it is an expression of an infinitely close connection between present and future, in which, in a dynamic process of interactions, every point in a system is always informed about the whole (holographic view).

Niels Bohr adopts a similar view: precisely because the unobserved particles exhibit uncertainty, they can never be conceived as discrete entities that can be isolated, but only as parts of a large, holistic system. David Peat,[22,23] Fred Alan Wolf [24] and Rupert Sheldrake[25] had the revolutionary idea that it was this indeterminism at the quantum level that provided the basis for the influence of spirit on matter. Improbable as it may seem, in the case of "unobserved" subatomic particles, no "decision" has yet been made.

Non-locality

Here too it will help to begin by clarifying locality in classical Newtonian physics: two masses influence each other only when they are in "local" relationship to each other. This interaction happens by way of fields: gravitational field, electromagnetic field, and the fields of the strong and weak interactions in the subatomic sphere. The forces diminish with increasing distance and the speed of transmission is limited to the speed of light.

As against this, "non-locality" states that there exist correlations between particles that do not decrease with increasing distance, and are not bound to fields.[26] Alain Aspect demonstrated experimentally in 1981[27] that photons communicate without any time delay, i.e., more quickly than the speed of light. This observation supports the theory of the British physicist David Bohm[28] that there is a "quantum potential" outside the dimensions of space and time measurable by physics. The quantum potential determines the position and speed of the elementary particles and links them in a network. In this way, every particle is informed about the others without any time delay (faster than at the speed of light). Since the mathematics of "normal" quantum physics is linear so that each of the equations produces several paradoxical solutions, Bohm was trying to restore order by introducing the mathematically non-linear, "chaotic" quantum potential. (Here we see another example of the paradox of "order through chaos"). By doing so he showed that everything is connected with everything else, with endless feedback, and that there is no room left for chance.[29-31] Bohm thus managed to complete quantum physics, which even Einstein saw as incomplete, and lent support to the holographic principle (every part possesses the entirety of the information; every part knows – irrespective of distance – what any other part is "doing"). This is the end of the exclusive validity of the reductionism of the classical sciences – in quantum systems things cannot be separated: there are no isolated systems.

Seen in this way, somatotopies ("pictures" of the entire body on the ear, the sole of the foot, or the mucosa of the mouth, etc.) no longer seem so strange to us. Further insights are provided by "fractal geometry" (see section on Chaos theory).

Quantum physics and biology (examples)

According to Popp,[32] there is a field of electromagnetic waves (biophotons) in the interior of the cell. This is coherent (wave trains are coherent when there is a phase relationship between them, unchangeable in time, at any and every point in space, after the principle of laser light which is capable of carrying information). The fields of all individual cells are linked with each other; in association with the field of the ground system this produces a common biophoton field that permeates the entire organism and, in cooperation with material structures, coordinates a great variety of different processes.[33,34] In this way information can reach every part of the body at the speed of light. Even the smallest, targeted changes in the biophoton field, such as those produced by osteopathic manipulation or a neural therapy injection at the right place, can have a great effect on biochemical processes, blood flow, muscle tone, etc.[35,36] Exogenous electromagnetic influences (e.g., living near a radio transmitter) can also affect our biophoton field. Here the determining factor appears to be not necessarily the quantity but the frequency pattern, which encounters a different biophoton field in every individual and so causes different disturbances.

The experiment carried out by Kasnacheyev and Michailova[37] provides an example of a disorder of the "quantum physics" kind: two closed glass flasks contain the same cell cultures. The bases of the flasks are in contact with each other. The cell culture in one flask is infected with a virus. If the base of the flask consists of normal glass (impermeable to UV radiation), the cell culture in the second flask does not sicken. However, if quartz glass is used (which is permeable to UV radiation), the other cell culture does sicken, even though not a single virus particle can pass from one (sealed, enclosed) flask to the other. The explanation: disease signals in the UV range (electromagnetic impulses, biophotons) penetrate the quartz glass and "infect" the healthy cell culture. This example indicates that even in the case of infection it is not the matter of the microorganism that determines the disease, but its quantum physical information.

Experiments performed by Cyril W. Smith and Jean Monro[38,39] demonstrate that particular electromagnetic oscillations can produce the same allergic reaction as contact with allergens.

Living organisms, therefore, are influenced on a fundamental level by electromagnetic interactions (quantum physical processes). Molecular processes are among the events directed in this way.[40,41] Since modern quantum physics knows only linking of the holistic kind, it is an important basis on the most fundamental level in self-organizing processes in the body, as will be seen later in dissipative structures.

Summary

Quantum physics in its most complete and precise form knows only wholeness and not "subsystems" capable of being isolated and assembled. In this, it stands in contrast to classical physics (reductionism, determinism). It is taken into consideration in holistic regulation medicine.

Chaos theory

This will be better understood if we begin with an explanation of linearity and non-linearity. In linear equations – one of the most essential principles of classical Newtonian physics – a particular cause produces a particular effect. The result is reproducible and transferable to other systems; generalization is possible. All this is no longer given in non-linear systems. Feedback is an essential feature of non-linear equations: in mathematical terms, positive feedback (or "iteration") means that parts of the equation are repeatedly multiplied by themselves. The result will depend strongly on the starting conditions (individuality!). In a non-linear equation, the slightest change in one variable can drive the system in a completely new, unexpected direction. Reproducibility and unambiguous, linear predictability (determinism) are no longer given in chaos theory, whose essential characteristics are non-linearity and feedback. This is consistent with the fundamental statements of quantum physics.

Chaos theory is a new area of research in mathematics and physics. Chaos research is involving an interdisciplinary association of various disciplines such as physics, geometry/mathematics, biology, economics, meteorology, etc. It is a theory of complex, non-linear systems, able to provide a more realistic description of natural processes than can be achieved by classical, linear, idealized physics which is really only applicable to islands of order in the midst of non-linear, "chaotic," complex systems. In contrast to classical physics and linear mathematics, chaos theory is able to describe such things as the (unique) shape of a tree, the fall of a leaf, or the complexity of a cloud. This is because non-linear phenomena predominate in nature.[42–45]

In 1960, the meteorologist Edward Lorenz solved changes in the earth's atmosphere by using non-linear equations. In order to test this for the purposes of weather forecasting, he reentered the same data for temperature, wind direction, etc. into the computer, and to save time entered the figures to only three decimal places instead of the more precise six places he had previously. Despite this minute change the result was an entirely new weather system. The "blame" for this lies with positive feedback and non-linearity, which are significant features of dynamic systems in nature. Positive feedback massively strengthens the minutest change. This gave rise to the saying that the flap of a butterfly's wings can influence the overall weather situation, in ways that are dependent on the starting conditions.

Unambiguous predictions are no longer possible, however, by this means, faithful as it is to nature and reality. One associated reason is the fact that open, interlinked systems react extremely sensitively to the most minor stimuli at particular points of divergence (bifurcations) as a result of internal feedback. At these bifurcation points, phase transitions or transitions to other "attractors" occur. Here, the system has the possibility of choice for new states of order. The minutest external stimuli, such as an osteopathic manipulation applied in the right place, can drive the system into a different bifurcation branch. The starting conditions are always taken into account. If the stimulus is too strong it destroys the dynamic "structure." This new perspective in mathematics and physics opens up the possibility of bringing "old" principles of regulation medicine (the principle of the smallest appropriate "quantities," the Arndt–Schultz Law, Ricker's pathology of related structures, etc.) up to date. Prigogine also uses this kind of mathematics to explain his "dissipative structures".

Fractals

From the end of the 1960s onward, the mathematician Benoit Mandelbrot published studies on a new way of looking at forms in nature.[46,47] Classical geometry is simply unable to describe such things as clouds, leaves, the branches of the bronchial tree, the circulatory system of the blood, coastlines, etc.

Taking as an example the length of the coast of Britain, Mandelbrot showed that the length varies according to the distance from which it is observed.[48] If we measure it from an aircraft at a great height, all we need to do is to add up simple lines. If we sail around the coast in a boat, taking into account all the tiny bays and bays within bays, the length of the coastline gradually increases. As we look at it in ever finer detail, we find that the same shapes recur over and over at ever smaller scale, and that this seems to continue infinitely, down through small projections of the cliffs to the atomic and subatomic level of the coastline. In other words, it is simply impossible to produce a quantitative measurement of the coastline: it is infinite! It is only possible to give a qualitative description of its shape. This picture of what is in principle the same form down to the smallest details can be described by non-linear mathematics with feedback. Nature knows not only lines and levels (two-dimensions), etc. but also broken dimensions not represented by whole numbers (fractals). In doing so, Mandelbrot brought quantitative measurement into question and demands a qualitative description by means of the fractal dimension. For the British coastline, this is 1.26.

The "living world" is also full of fractals. West and Goldberger calculated that the structure of our lungs corresponds to the laws of fractal geometry.[49] In nature no two fractals are the same (clouds, trees, ferns, cauliflower, etc.). So it appears that the individual complex systems in nature contain the form of their appearance in detail down to ever smaller scales.[50,51] These statements by a new branch of science must have consequences for biological systems. From this perspective the idea of "pictures" of the entire human body on the ear or sole of the foot, etc. (somatotopies) need no longer seem illogical. The importance of the starting conditions in chaos theory and the fact that no two fractals are quite the same are also consistent with the statements made by regulation medicine ("no two patients are the same").

The message of fractal geometry that everything contains "all in all" lends support to holographic views such as those of the physicist David Bohm (see previous section), Burkhard Heim[52] and Rupert Sheldrake.[53]

Solitons

Waves whose stability is determined by non-linear interactions are called solitons. This single statement demonstrates how inseparably order and chaos (non-linearity, feedback, and stability) are interwoven in nature.

Normal waves (e.g., linear radio waves) are for the most part reflected at boundary layers. Solitons, however, can "tunnel" through boundary layers and arrive on the other side without loss, thanks to non-linear effects. They are neither true light nor a mere matter of excited atoms, but a non-linear combination of both.[55]

Examples

Although soliton oscillations should be seen as the model, some interesting aspects arise: soliton oscillations may have far-reaching importance in biological systems as information transmitters. Nerve impulses, for example, may consist of soliton oscillations. The nerve concerned needs to possess a kind of "memory" for the interactive propagation of neural solitons:[56] the neuron appears to store impulse frequencies ("information") that it has previously carried, in a holographic fashion. Back in 1924, Ricker predicted on the basis of experiment that the peripheral autonomic nervous system would also be found to have a kind of memory. In other words, the soliton theory may be a modern scientific explanation for the results obtained by Ricker. The neural soliton theory also offers interesting insights that may help explain the "field of disturbance"

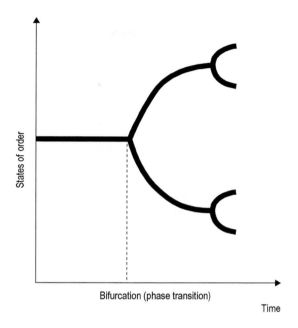

States of order / Bifurcation (phase transition) / Time

Figure 4.1
Dynamic systems with positive feedback are extremely sensitive to phase transitions. The minutest stimuli of the appropriate kind produce new states of order that cannot be precisely predicted. From Fischer, 2001.[54]

phenomenon (first strike, second strike). (See later in this chapter.)

The soliton theory may also be an aspect to consider with regard to information transfer in the acupuncture meridians. Here, old information would always be included as a result of the required positive feedback. Such considerations render earlier theories of an "ancient layer," proposed by Scheidt, as relevant once more.

Summary

The interpretation offered by chaos theory and fractal geometry in biological systems confirms many of the holistic and individual approaches in regulation medicine. Further, non-linear chaos theory shows that appropriate tiny quantities of energy can have enormous effects. These insights, applied professionally in various holistically oriented therapies, can be integrated into practice when treating the non-linear human body and person.

Thermodynamics

Thermodynamics of closed systems

In this context the input of energy (e.g., gas in a closed vessel) means an increase in entropy (i.e., disorder). Following every change in energy input, over time, a thermodynamic equilibrium is established. The processes are reversible (reproducible). Thus energy input in a closed, classical thermodynamic system means destruction of structure. There is no room here for the emergence of new states of order by the input of energy. Too much consideration is, unfortunately, still paid to this type of thermodynamics in biological systems. Strictly speaking, the classical laws of equilibrium thermodynamics apply only to non-living systems. Life, the living structure of order, is only possible at far remove from thermodynamic equilibrium (see the following text).

Thermodynamics of energetically open systems (non-equilibrium states)

In open systems (e.g., in living organisms that exchange energy and matter with the environment) the situation looks completely different: the situation here is far from thermodynamic equilibrium. The processes are irreversible. In accordance with the laws of chaos theory, which is of course non-linear, a "decision" has been made at every bifurcation point in favor of one or other of the possible directions (states of order). This decision can be influenced, perhaps, by osteopathic manipulation, for example, or another appropriate form of information and energy. The sensitivity to the minutest disturbances (appropriate energy input) and instability of the states of a system at the bifurcation points is the prerequisite for the emergence of new structures.[57]

Thus appropriate energy input favors the emergence of dynamic structures (new states of order). In 1979 the Nobel prizewinner Ilya Prigogine[58] devised the concept "dissipative structures" (from the Latin "dissipare" which means to "distribute"): the energy that effects the transformation into a certain state of order is well-nigh instantaneously distributed as information over the entire system and links all the parts into a whole.

The studies on dissipative structures showed that they involved a kind of self-organization of chemical reactions. We might see this as an experimental demonstration of the non-linear thermodynamics of energetically open systems. The most important conclusion from this is that such a system must be able to operate as a whole, and Prigogine states that every molecule must be informed about the state of the whole. This calls to mind the holistic field concept from the section on quantum physics, and brings us back to the holographic view. Once we are aware of such connections we can no longer dismiss as "unscientific" such phenomena as Huneke's frequently observed "flash phenomenon" (Sekundenphänomen) or those encountered in osteopathy. Many rhythmic physiological processes in the body are "dissipative structures" and as such capable of explanation in terms of mathematical chaos theory. One example of an oscillatory system in this sense is glycolysis. Our ground substance can also be seen as a dissipative system. The systems are coupled to each other.

Summary

Thermodynamics of closed systems (non-living systems):

- Linear mathematics

- Input of energy means increase of entropy

- Establishment of equilibrium

- Reversible.

Thermodynamics of energetically open systems (living organisms/biosphere):

- Non-linear mathematics (feedback, chaos theory)

- Input of energy means new structures (dissipative structures)

- Far-from-equilibrium states

- Irreversible.

The ground substance of our bodies can be regarded as a dissipative system. The energy that brings about the transformation into a particular state of order is instantaneously distributed as information over the entire system and links all the parts into a whole. It seems entirely practicable that such processes might play a role in osteopathic medicine.

Non-linear, irreversible thermodynamics with dissipative structures that react in a holistic manner further demonstrates that the only way to regard living beings is in holistic terms.

References

[1]Kiene H: Komplementärmedizin – Schulmedizin. Stuttgart: Schattauer; 1994.

[2]Feynman RP: QED: The strange theory of light and matter. Princeton University Press; 1985.

[3]Kaku M, Trainer J: Beyond Einstein, Oxford: OUP; 1997.

[4]Bohm D: Wholeness and the implicate order. London: Routledge and Kegan Paul; 1980.

[5]Heim B: Elementarstrukturen der Materie. Einheitliche strukturelle Quantenfeldtheorie der Materie und Gravitation, vols. 1 and 2, Innsbruck: Resch; 1984.

[6]Sheldrake R: Seven experiments that could change the world. New York: Riverhead Books; 1995.

[7]Schubert M, Weber G: Quantentheorie, Grundlagen und Anwendungen. Heidelberg: Spektrum; 1993.

[8]Feynman RP: QED: The strange theory of light and matter. Princeton University Press; 1985.

[9]Kaku M, Trainer J: Beyond Einstein. Oxford: OUP; 1997.

[10]Meyl K: Elektromagnetische Umweltverträglichkeit, Part 1. Villingen-Schwenningen: Indel; 1996.

[11]Meyl K: Elektromagnetische Umweltverträglichkeit, Part 1. Villingen-Schwenningen: Indel; 1996.

[12]Meyl K: Elektromagnetische Umweltverträglichkeit, Part 1. Villingen-Schwenningen: Indel; 1996.

[13]Falkenburg B: Teilchenmetaphysik, 2nd edn. Berlin: Spektrum Akad. Verlag; 1995.

[14]Meyl K: Elektromagnetische Umweltverträglichkeit, Part 1. Villingen-Schwenningen: Indel; 1996.

[15]Meyl K: Elektromagnetische Umweltverträglichkeit, Part 1. Villingen-Schwenningen: Indel; 1996.

[16]Maturana R, Varela FJ: The tree of knowledge: The biological roots of human understanding. Boston: Shambhala Publications; 1987.

[17]Maturana R, Varela FJ: The tree of knowledge: The biological roots of human understanding. Boston: Shambhala Publications; 1987.

[18]Falkenburg B: Teilchenmetaphysik. 2nd edn. Berlin: Spektrum Akad. Verlag; 1995.

[19]Van Fraassen BC: The semantic approach to scientific theories. In: Nersession. 1987:105.

[20]Falkenburg B: Teilchenmetaphysik. 2nd edn. Berlin: Spektrum Akad. Verlag; 1995.

[21]Falkenburg B: Teilchenmetaphysik, 2nd edn. Berlin: Spektrum Akad. Verlag; 1995.

[22]Briggs J, Peat DF: The turbulent mirror. New York: Harper & Row; 1989.

[23]Peat DF: Synchronicity: The bridge between matter and mind. New York: Bantam; 1987.

[24]Wolf FA: The new physics of body, mind and health. New York: Macmillan; 1986.

[25]Sheldrake R: Seven experiments that could change the world. New York: Riverhead Books; 1995.

[26]Kratky KW, Wallner F: Grundprinzipien der Selbstorganisation. Darmstadt: Wissenschaftliche Buchgesellschaft; 1990.

[27]Aspect A: Expériences basées sur les inégalitées de Bell. J. Physique. 1981;42:63–80.

[28]Bohm D: Wholeness and the implicate order. London: Routledge and Kegan Paul; 1980.

[29]Bohm D: Wholeness and the implicate order. London: Routledge and Kegan Paul; 1980

[30]Briggs J, Peat DF: The turbulent mirror. New York: Harper & Row; 1989.

[31]Mainzer K: Symmetrien der Natur. De Gruyter, Berlin; 1988.

[32]Popp FA: Neue Horizonte in der Medizin, 2nd edn. Heidelberg: Haug; 1987.

[33]Bischof M: Biophotonen. Frankfurt: Zweitausendeins; 1995.

[34]Popp FA: Neue Horizonte in der Medizin, 2nd edn. Heidelberg: Haug; 1987.

[35]Klima H: Der Organismus als offenes Netzsystem. In: Stacher, A, Bergsmann, O. Grundlagen für eine integrative Ganzheitsmedizin. Vienna: Facultas; 1993.

[36]Popp FA: Neue Horizonte in der Medizin, 2nd edn. Heidelberg: Haug; 1987.

[37]Popp FA: Neue Horizonte in der Medizin. 2nd edn. Heidelberg: Haug; 1987.

[38]Bischof M: Biophotonen. Frankfurt: Zweitausendeins; 1995.

[39]Smith CW et al.: The emission of low intensity electromagnetic radiation from multiple allergy patients and other biological systems. In: Jezowska et al. (ed.): Photon emission from biological systems. Singapore: World Scientific; 1987.

[40]Feynman RP: QED: The strange theory of light and matter. Princeton University Press; 1985.

[41]Popp FA: Neue Horizonte in der Medizin, 2nd edn. Heidelberg: Haug; 1987.

[42]Briggs J, Peat DF: The turbulent mirror. New York: Harper & Row; 1989.

[43]Klima H: Der Organismus als offenes Netzsystem. In: Stacher A, Bergsmann O. Grundlagen für eine integrative Ganzheitsmedizin. Vienna: Facultas; 1993.

[44]Kratky KW, Wallner F: Grundprinzipien der Selbstorganisation. Darmstadt: Wissenschaftliche Buchgesellschaft; 1990.

[45]Mainzer K: Symmetrien der Natur. De Gruyter, Berlin; 1988.

[46]Briggs J, Peat DF: The turbulent mirror. New York: Harper & Row; 1989.

[47]Mandelbrot B: How long is the coast of Britain? Science. 1967;156:636.

[48]Mandelbrot B: How long is the coast of Britain? Science. 1967;156:636.

[49]West BJ, Goldberger AL: Physiology in fractal dimensions. American Scientist. 1987:7–8.

[50]Briggs J, Peat DF: The turbulent mirror. New York: Harper & Row; 198.

[51]Mainzer K: Symmetrien der Natur. De Gruyter, Berlin; 1988.

[52]Heim B: Elementarstrukturen der Materie. Einheitliche strukturelle Quantenfeldtheorie der Materie und Gravitation, vols. 1 and 2, Innsbruck: Resch; 1984.

[53]Sheldrake R: Seven experiments that could change the world. New York: Riverhead Books; 1995.

[54]Fischer L: Neuraltherapie nach Huneke. 2nd edn. Stuttgart: Hippokrates; 2001.

[55]Briggs J, Peat DF: The turbulent mirror. New York: Harper & Row; 1989.

[56]Briggs J, Peat DF: The turbulent mirror. New York: Harper & Row; 1989.

[57]Kluge G, Neugebauer G: Grundlagen der Thermodynamik. Heidelberg: Spektrum; 1994.

[58]Prigogine I, Stengers I: Dialog mit der Natur – neue Wege wissenschaftlichen Denkens. Munich: Piper; 1981.

5

Neurobiological principles

Lorenz Fischer

Modified from Part I, Propädeutik, in: Fischer L: Neuraltherapie nach Huneke, 2nd edn. Stuttgart: Hippokrates; 2001.

Cybernetics

The basic principles of cybernetics can be traced back to the works of Norbert Wiener from 1948 onward.[1] Living organisms are open systems, which exchange energy and matter with the environment.[2] The maintenance of flow equilibrium and dynamic states of order far from thermodynamic equilibrium requires innumerable interlinked regulatory loops.

Definition

Cybernetics is the science of control and information. Its basic principles are homeostasis and economy. Its smallest unit is the regulatory loop. When there is any change or disturbance of the controlled variable, the regulator is "informed" by a sensor (actual value). It then compares the actual value with the desired value (set point) and causes the necessary correction to be made. The set point does not have to be constant, and can be identical with the controlled value of another regulatory loop.

Formulated in mathematical terms, the regulator can operate proportionally, but is also capable of differentiation and integration. A mixing principle is usually applied, e.g., if a muscle makes known its location at that moment to the central nervous system, it simultaneously informs it of its speed of motion (the time differential quotient).

There are regulators with negative feedback (e.g., simple hormonal thyroid regulation). This serves to stabilize a particular state of order. The advantage is that of stability; the disadvantage that it is not very adaptable, and remains inflexibly in a particular state with a constant set point.

Alongside these there are also regulators with positive feedback (as encountered for example in the non-linearity of dissipative systems). This serves to destabilize an old state of order and develop new dynamic states of order. The advantage here is the great adaptability and the disadvantage the instability. It even provides a way of integrating mathematical chaos theory (non-linearity, positive feedback) into cybernetics.

The regulatory loop systems can oscillate. The switching of a system from one functional state to another is the transient response. The quality of control is a function of transient behavior:[3–5]

Normal:

- Muted transient behavior

- → Short time, slight energy loss: principle of economy.

Pathological:

- Periodically distorted, labile transient behavior (excessive, with subsequent fluctuations)

- A periodically distorted, sluggish transient behavior (delay or failure to achieve regulatory goal)

- → Loss of time and energy; no economy principle.

Distortion may be brought about, for example, by stress to the ground system caused by heavy metals, field of disturbance, or segmental stresses, among other influences. Over time the distorted regulatory loop systems become exhausted in an equivalent way to the adaptation syndrome described by Selye, producing regulatory disturbance or blockade. This can result in disease. This kind of problem can be treated causally or, in the ideal situation, prevented, by osteopathic treatment.

One point that became clear when discussing the quantum level is the impossibility of separating subject (observer) and object. Likewise, that separation is absent on the biological level. Matter and consciousness, body and spirit, soma and psyche (the "observer effect") cannot be separated one from the other; instead they correlate with one another throughout the entire world of phenomena.

Summary

Cybernetics is the science of control and information. Its basic principles are homeostasis and economy. The smallest unit is the regulatory loop.

Pischinger and Heine's "ground system"

Introduction

Definitions (according to Heine):

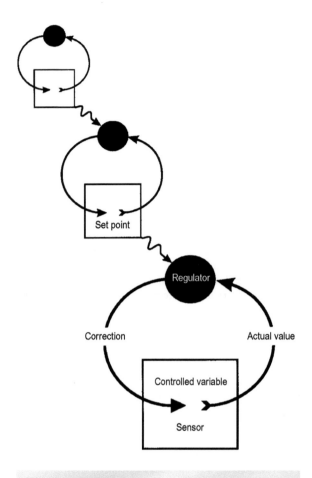

Figure 5.1
Interlinked, mutually dependent regulatory loops. From Fischer, 2001.[54]

- Ground substance (i.e., matrix): a mesh of high polymer sugar protein complexes containing proteoglycans, glycosaminoglycans (most importantly hyaluronic acid), structural coproteins (collagen, elastin), and meshwork proteins (fibronectin, laminin). Also contained within this is also water, some of which is ordered in a particular spatial arrangement, ions, etc.

- Ground system: the ground substance plus cellular, humoral, and neural components.

- Ground regulation: local regulatory capacities of the ground system plus the superior level neural, hormonal, and humoral regulatory systems.[6]

The system of ground regulation permeates the entire extracellular space. It is a functional unit ("ubiquitous synapse"). Every point in the organism is linked with every other via the ground system, which has priority over all organ parenchymal cells. It is responsible for nutrition, defense, and information. The meaning of "information" is more than just the transfer of messages by means of nerves and hormones; the ground substance has the capacity in its own right to channel and store information. This is extremely important especially in chronic disease: the organs' parenchymal cells only operate properly when the ground system is morphologically and functionally intact. As a result, chronic diseases of

With regard to regulatory loops of the primarily neural (also humoral) kind we should not forget that in both the transfer of information and energy, as implied by quantum physics, is still present. This means that there is an additional "independent" quantum physical information network in the ground system (photon/electron interactions). This can operate considerably more rapidly than anything achieved at the speed of nerve conduction or enzymatic processes.

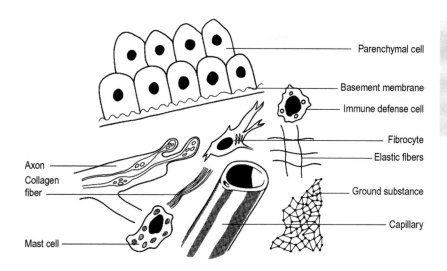

Parenchymal cell

Basement membrane

Immune defense cell

Fibrocyte

Elastic fibers

Axon

Collagen
fiber

Ground substance

Capillary

Mast cell

Figure 5.2

The ground system according to Pischinger and Heine (schematic representation). From Fischer, 2001.[54]

organs and systems often develop – if not genetically determined – as a consequence of a dysfunction of the ground system. A dysfunction can arise as a consequence of a great variety of problems affecting the ground system – usually indeed several.

This view is in opposition to Virchow's cellular pathology, which looks to classical Newtonian physics. Here the search is mainly for unicausal, linear relationships of cause and effect, thus a direct pathological effect – and also healing effect – on the (parenchymal) cell itself. In acute diseases, this is entirely appropriate and successful. In chronic diseases, whose origins are usually multicausal, this principle fails. The only way to understand the informative processes in the ground system is by drawing on modern physics and cybernetics.

These two viewpoints (the complex, multicausal, non-linear influences affecting the ground system versus the unicausal, linear view involving Virchow's cellular pathology and molecular biology) should not be seen as mutually exclusive. When we take too one-sided a view, this can tend to hinder real progress.

Energetic aspects

The sugar–protein complexes of the ground substance are under tension because of their negative charge, as the charges repel each other. This provides a "scaffold" and enables some of the water to be bound, ordered in a fluid crystal manner. Certain ions and metabolites have the effect of creating structure; others the effect of breaking

structure down.[7,8] At body temperature, around 60% of the water is present in fluid crystal form.[9] The structure of this water appears to some extent to obey the laws of fractal geometry.[10] Physiological and also pathological information can be transmitted and stored in the fluid crystals. At higher body temperatures, there is some dissolution of fluid crystals, and in this way pathological information (as in the case of virus infections) can be re-extinguished. Using medication to bring down fever may not therefore be helpful in every case.

The protein–sugar complexes of the ground substance form a "molecular sieve."[11] This sieve has a certain mechanical and electrical pore size, depending on the ultrastructural and energetic state of the ground substance.[12] Pore size is determined by such factors as the size and concentration of the proteoglycans, pH value, electrolyte concentration, etc. This provides a means of governing which substances are able to pass from the capillaries into the parenchymal cells of the organs: the "transit stretch."[13]

The ground substance has a base electrostatic tonus.[14] Any change in the ground substance results in changes in the potential. This brings about a change in the pattern of electromagnetic oscillation, an effect of which is that it is transmitted to the glycocalyx (the sugar film on the surface of the cells) as information (e.g., via membrane "second messengers" such as cAMP). This stimulates intracellular responses resulting in protein synthesis by DNA/RNA.

Changes in the potential differences can also produce other effects: the variations can cause oscillation of structures within the ground substance and dipole elements of the cell membrane.[15] The result of this, according to Fröhlich, is certain electromagnetic resonance frequencies.[16,17] These exhibit a high degree of coherence (see section: Modern physics and biology). There is therefore extremely rapid, wide-ranging, independent information available in the ground system, which is also independent of neural or hormonal signals. Such transmission of information can even be seen as a line of supraconduction into the fluid crystals of the ground substance. The amount of energy required would, for reasons of quantum physics, be minute.

In response to the appropriate energy (corresponding electromagnetic frequency pattern) the ground system can react holistically within fractions of a second (as a dissipative system).

From the point of view of thermodynamics, the ground substance is an energetically open system. The structures therefore oscillate far from equilibrium. The fact that it is a dissipative structure (see section: Modern physics and biology) means that an appropriate input of energy (information) can be distributed practically instantaneously across the entire system, bringing about a change in structure (e.g., in the ordered state of the water). Here too, in accordance with the laws of chaos theory, the sensitivity to tiny appropriate amounts of energy is extremely high, particularly at phase transition points (bifurcation points).

According to Bergsmann,[18] impulses of short duration cause partial depolarization of the proteoglycans. This is resolved immediately in healthy systems by restoration of the charge. Appropriate impulse stimuli can produce an autocatalytic chain reaction of partial depolarizations. The resulting electromagnetic oscillations can exhibit a far-reaching effect in the ground system.

The fasciae, which are so important in osteopathy, can be seen as a highly specialized form of the ground system (this is particularly the case with collagen). Collagen fibers can be regarded as electrical dipoles. A change in pressure (osteopathy!) of the collagen produces electrical signals.[19] These can replicate like an avalanche in the ground system.

If there is a field of disturbance, we are dealing with impulses of the minutest duration which can over long periods of time result in lability of the cybernetic

regulatory loops and even alter the ultrastructure of the ground system.[20]

This capacity of the ground system to oscillate and this electrolability also offer an explanation for the feeling of being "under the weather" and the effect of "electrosmog."[21] These effects become all the more clear when we realize that the ground system surrounds the nerve bundles of the vessels in cylinder-like form ("Heine cylinders"); in this way they reach the surface of the body and are able to act as "receivers" (the "Heine cylinders" pierce the fasciae).

The ground substance therefore has an independent capacity to transmit and store information – one to which too little consideration has so far been paid in conventional, allopathic medicine. Humoral and neural regulatory loops must also of course be included, and there is therefore also a connection to the brainstem via capillaries and the network of autonomic nerves.

The complex, cybernetic interpenetration of all regulatory systems serves to maintain structure and homeostasis. These complex dynamics have the advantage of great adaptability. The initial effect of pathogenic information (e.g., brought about by a field of disturbance) is simply lability of the cybernetic regulatory loops (disturbance of regulation). It is only after a longer time interval that functional disturbance occurs, potentially with structural disturbance of parenchymal organs "downstream."

Leukocytolysis

The physiological degradation of leukocytes is important if the regulatory function of the ground system is to operate efficiently.[22] Degradation substances include lymphokines, cytokines, prostaglandins, hormones, and neuropeptides. This broad spectrum of degradation substances ensures that a wide range of different kinds of regulation will be affected.

One of the "points of entry" addressed by regulation therapies is stimulation of physiological leukocytolysis. In the case of "regulatory blockade" (see below), such stimulation is no longer possible.

Stress of the fibroblast–macrophage system/ground system

The protein–sugar complexes making up the ground substance are synthesized by fibroblasts. Their breakdown is the work of macrophages. Normally, synthesis and breakdown are in equilibrium. In certain

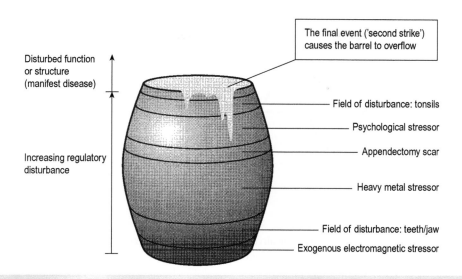

Disturbed function
or structure
(manifest disease)

Increasing regulatory
disturbance

The final event ('second strike')
causes the barrel to overflow

Field of disturbance: tonsils

Psychological stressor

Appendectomy scar

Heavy metal stressor

Field of disturbance: teeth/jaw

Exogenous electromagnetic stressor

Figure 5.3

Stress (examples) and decompensation of the ground system (represented symbolically as a barrel). From Fischer, 2001.[54]

situations (e.g., stress, field of disturbance, heavy metals), fibroblasts produce an "excess" of protein–sugar complexes.[23] The unphysiologically structured ground substance that results has a smaller pore size,[24] which hinders the free flow of information. There is at the same time a change in the base electrostatic tonus, which in turn produces a different "resonance base" for incoming electromagnetic signals. This alters both the cybernetic incoming oscillatory behavior and the processing of information.

The ground system has the autonomous ability to compensate a certain amount of stress. However, if further stress is added to this "previously impaired" terrain, the ground system can decompensate (the "barrel overflows"). This means that, in certain circumstances, a quite minor additional event such as a viral infection, scar, etc. may trigger chronic disease. This process is the "second strike" described by Speransky.[25]

Regulatory blockade

Excessive stress on the ground system (e.g., by fields of disturbance or heavy metals) blocks the autonomous

regulatory processes (see previous section). The system is then no longer capable of regulation to combat external pathological stressors (e.g., susceptibility to infection). Further, a ground system that is changed in this way ("regulatory blockade") is also unable to respond to various healing stimuli.

Regulatory blockades can also be triggered by medication: high-dose administration of corticosteroids, repeated antibiotic therapy, psychopharmaceuticals, cytostatic drugs, etc.

Nonspecific reactions in the ground system

A normally functioning ground system reacts holistically and nonspecifically to a whole range of different stress factors, initially with the "alarm reaction" described by Selye. This is stimulated irrespective of the type of stressor involved: physical, biochemical, infectious, or psychological. The reaction consists of three stages: shock, countershock, and recovery. In the analysis made by Hoff,[26] the shock stage corresponds to sympatheticotonus, and the countershock stage

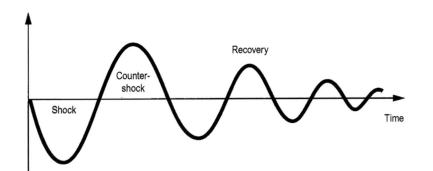

Figure 5.4
Selye's "alarm reaction": nonspecific reaction in the ground system to qualitatively very varied stressors. From Fischer, 2001.[54]

to parasympatheticotonus. Rhythmic biophysical, humoral,[27] and cellular changes occur[28] as this sequence of stages progresses. The purpose served by this rhythmicity is that of a nonspecific defense mechanism. The alarm reaction cannot be stimulated in regulatory blockades. Another possible situation is that the alarm reaction can "remain stuck" in the shock or countershock stage, depending on previous or additional stressors, forcing the body into constant compensation work. If the noxious stressor (e.g., infection) persists, then, according to Selye, following a period of resistance, a stage of resistance is followed by one of adaptation or exhaustion.

The ground system reacts holistically in the way described, but the reaction is not necessarily a unified one. The reason for this may, for example, be that the initial energetic state is different in one stressed region (segment) as compared with others; stress of the ground system is in the first instance most intense locally/segmentally ("first strike"). Stressors may be myogeloses, restricted joints, infections, etc. If additional stressors impact elsewhere in the body ("second strike"), the previously stressed segment experiences most additional stress from the renewed nonspecific, holistic ground system reaction. What may now be seen to happen here is disease affecting "downstream" organs; it is at this stage, then, that nonspecific reactions in the ground system have led to "specific" pathology of an organ.

Summary

The ground substance (matrix) contains (among other components) high polymer sugar–protein complexes. Contained in this is water, some of which is ordered in fluid crystal arrangement. This provides a morphological and energetic basis for it to have its own transmission and storage of information. The ground system consists of the ground substance plus cellular, humoral, and neural components.

The ground system has the following tasks: support, nutrition, nonspecific defense, adaptation to changed conditions, information storage and transmission, etc. It is a functional unit and present throughout the whole body (even in organ clefts) ("ubiquitous synapse"). Osteopathic dysfunctions and also impulses delivered in osteopathic treatment can reach every part of the body via the ground system (and sympathetic nervous system).

Ricker's pathology of related structures

Virchow's cellular pathology, which in terms of the etiology of diseases and disorders involves a static, reductionist view based on findings at the level of the cell and organ, remains to this day the basis for scientific medicine. It has enabled great successes to be achieved in acute medicine and, for example, certain infectious diseases. However, this approach falls down when dealing with most chronic conditions.

In contrast to Virchow's cellular pathology, Ricker's pathology of related structures represents a dynamic approach. It sees the etiology and pathogenesis of a very varied range of diseases as lying in a pathological stimulation of the perivasal sympathetic nervous system. The ground substance is altered as a result of circulatory disturbances, and it is this that then brings about the cellular pathological effects in the "downstream" parenchymatous organs. In other words, in Ricker the cell comes at the end, not the beginning, of the pathological events.[29–31] Pischinger and collaborators later confirmed this theory, which states in principle that no organ cell can develop "acquired" disease without dysfunction of the "upstream" ground system (which includes the capillaries and end structures of the autonomic nervous system).

Ricker demonstrated experimentally that the pathological stimulus needed for cellular pathology to develop does not, in the primary instance, take hold at the cell itself but rather the sympathetic nervous system.[32,33] Astonishingly, it is immaterial whether this stimulus is physical, chemical, or microbial in nature. The response evoked from the perivasal sympathetic nervous system is not qualitative but quantitative (the impulse frequency is different). This stimulus response is produced according to Ricker's law of levels:[34,35] weak stimuli lead to vasodilation and acceleration of the circulation, medium stimuli to ischemia and strong stimuli to stasis and exit of leukocytes, erythrocytes, etc. The results are changes in the ground system and finally also in the parenchymal organ cells.

If the irritation of the perivasal sympathetic system was layered and of long duration, Ricker found in addition results such as hyperplasia or necrosis of parenchymatous tissue.

Even if the irritation of the sympathetic system happened way back in the past, it seems that this can in some unexplained way be stored, and a renewed stimulus can cause an exaggerated response.[36,37] This is reminiscent of the "second strike" described by Speransky, the older layer described by Scheidt, and even chaos theory in dissipative systems. It can even be helpful to look to this aspect as a theoretical basis for what happens in relation to fields of disturbance. The same intensity of stimulus can produce a response that varies according to the individual.

The sympathetic nervous system therefore seems to have a kind of "memory" for pathological stimuli. According to this, a stimulus that causes inflammation, which may be of many different kinds, begins in the primary instance by affecting the sympathetic nervous system, which transmits the irritation. It follows that when treating pain and inflammation in acute pancreatitis, for example, the logical therapy is regulation of the sympathetic system (by local anesthetic at the celiac ganglion).

There is probably no pathophysiological process that does not involve the autonomic nervous system, in particular the sympathetic system, as the transmitter of the irritation.[38] Seen in this experimentally proven light,[39] it is logical to begin treatment by way of regulation of the sympathetic nervous system. Holistic methods such as osteopathy "automatically" involve the autonomic nervous system in therapy.

Summary

Ricker demonstrated experimentally that there is a relationship between acquired cellular pathologic changes and the perivasal sympathetic nervous system (and thus also the ground system). Treatment methods that are holistic in orientation can produce a change in the individual irritability of the sympathetic system, which is present everywhere. This influences the "downstream" systems of the ground substance and parenchymatous organs and also muscle tonus.

Speransky's neuropathology

The Nobel prizewinner Pavlov (1904) realized that the nervous system governs and directs all physiological processes. He proved that it is the nervous system alone, in its supraordinate position, that co-ordinates all organ functions, taking into account also the environmental conditions. All biological processes can be altered from the starting point of the nervous system.[40] The conclusions resulting from Speransky's inspired experiments[41] are listed briefly below. They correspond remarkably with the basic tenets of modern physics.

- The nervous system is supraordinate and controls humoral and biochemical regulatory loops and cellular reactions.

- The primary point at which all stimuli impact is the nervous system, even when the secondary effect is to stimulate humoral, cellular, or biochemical processes.

- No isolated, self-contained processes occur in the nervous system (taken to include the ground system as a "ubiquitous synapse"). (This corresponds with the pronouncements of quantum physics and the assumptions of non-linear, feedback, dissipative systems).

- The nervous system tends to react as a whole entity. Changes remain stored for an extraordinarily long

RICKER
(Perivascular
sympathetic
nervous system)

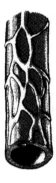

PISCHINGER
(Ground system)

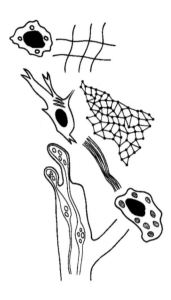

VIRCHOW
(Cellular
pathology)

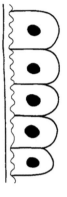

Figure 5.5

Different views of the routes leading to disease and healing:

Ricker – primarily via perivascular sympathetic nervous system;* Pischinger – primarily via the ground system;* Virchow – primarily by noxious agents or healing molecules affecting the parenchymal cells. *The parenchymal cells are only secondarily affected. From Fischer, 2001.[54]

time as information. New information is implanted onto this, triggering reactions that are dependent on the stored "older" information; this evokes parallels with Scheidt and with Ricker's pathology of related structures (see earlier in this chapter). This in turn is reminiscent of the positive feedback of modern mathematical chaos theory, which is particularly appropriate in describing biological systems.

- The quantity of the stimulus is more important than its quality in the holistic reaction of the nervous system described here (bearing in mind, however, the individual nature of the reaction in different patients). In principle, therefore, it becomes almost irrelevant for the course of the reaction whether the stimulus is physical, chemical, or infectious in nature. At first glance this seems astonishing. Nevertheless it corresponds to the course of events in the perivascular sympathetic nervous system described by Ricker, and those in the ground system that were later described by Selye and Pischinger.

- Speransky demonstrated experimentally in animals that irritation of *any* part of the peripheral or central nervous system can be the point of origin both for pathogenic and for healing mechanisms.

- "Disease is the body's response to stimulus under the directing influence of the nervous system" (Speransky).

- The pathogenic stimulus can emanate from any point in the nervous system. There, it can become a "focus" (field of disturbance), from which the emission of minute pathological impulses occurs. This leads to a changed state of tonus of the entire autonomic nervous system. Over time, a great range of different diseases and disorders can develop as a result, depending on individual predisposition ("weak spot").

- The "remote" disease can usually be healed by eliminating the stimulus (the focus) at its point of origin.[42,43] However, it may happen that the disease takes on an autonomous course of its own, depending on the individual stimulus threshold and the duration of the stimulus, so in effect becoming "decoupled" from the field of disturbance.

- Every body appears to have the capacity to cope with a number of stressors (including fields of disturbance) by regulatory means. However, if an additional stress occurs at the point when "the barrel is almost full" (even if the stimulus in question is tiny), the barrel will overflow and disease symptoms will appear. This final stimulus that causes decompensation by the autonomic nervous system is referred to as the "second strike" in terms of Speransky's pathology. Since this second strike arrives on top of different previous stressors in different bodies, the same stimulus can produce different diseases affecting the particular "weak spot" of the individual, and these of course differ from one individual to another. That weak spot may be a segmental reflex complex that has been made labile by a pre-existing field of disturbance ("first strike").

- Speransky's experiments imply that the (autonomic) nervous system is supraordinate to the humoral system. This means, for example, that toxic substances only exert a pathological effect when they trigger information in the nervous system.

- Some examples from Speransky's experiment that illustrate this point are: tetanus toxin exerts the most marked toxic effect when injected at a site that has the most nerve endings. Alternatively: no tetanus disease is generated if the toxin is injected together with procaine. Neural inhibition of the Sanarelli–Shwartzman phenomenon may also be mentioned in this connection.

Summary

The nervous system is a supraordinate one that "oversees" and controls all processes.

The theory of the "second strike" states that prestressed systems can decompensate in response to a repeat of stress (i.e., develop into manifest disease).

The autonomic nervous system

General

The autonomic nervous system is a functional unity. It is seen as falling into two divisions, the sympathetic and parasympathetic branches, whose afferent and efferent signals regulate the function of all organs. Sympathetic tonus is raised in stress or major physical exertion (acceleration of heart rate and respiratory frequency, increased sweat production, lessening of intestinal motility, increased level of alertness, etc.). Raised parasympathetic tonus has the opposite effects and serves above all to produce general regeneration.[44-46]

With its network of ultrafine fibers, the autonomic nervous system permeates the ground substance. (The sympathetic system permeates the whole of the body, while the parasympathetic system is absent in the limbs and abdominal wall). Its main task lies in the maintenance of a constant internal environment and co-ordination of organ functions, apparently by means of the cybernetic principles of homeostasis and economy. This requires the constant input and processing of information. The hormonal system is also involved in this, both peripherally (the ground system) and centrally (the hypothalamus). The autonomic nervous system has several levels of integration, linked with each other in vertically ordered feedback loops:

1 The autonomic periphery (ground system)

2 The peripheral-spinal level ("segmental reflex complex")

3 The rhombo-mesencephalic level (medulla oblongata, pons, reticular formation, tectum of the midbrain, etc.): cardiovascular functions, vigilance, rhythmicity, activity of gamma motor system, etc.

4 The diencephalic level (thalamus, hypothalamus)

5 The cortical level (limbic system, psychological phenomena in somatic diseases, etc.).

On the occurrence of a peripheral stimulus, it is initially the lowest integration level, the ground system, that tries to deal with it by regulating it. If the stimulus continues or increases in intensity, the next integration level up becomes involved. This separation into different integration levels is made in order to clarify what is happening. In actual practice every component system is probably informed about the entirety (holographic view).

The central autonomic system

The central ganglia of the sympathetic and parasympathetic nervous systems are located in different sections, thoracolumbar in the case of the sympathetic nuclei, and cranio-sacral in that of the parasympathetic nuclei. The thoracolumbar sympathetic and sacral parasympathetic nuclei lie in the lateral horn of the spinal cord. The parasympathetic nuclei in the brain stem include the Edinger–Westphal nucleus (visceral nucleus), the salivatory nuclei, and the dorsal vagal nucleus.

The peripheral autonomic system

Sympathetic nervous system: myelinated (white) preganglionic fibers run from the lateral horn along the ventral root to the sympathetic trunk, via the white ramus communicans. The fibers mostly make synapses in these ganglia (paravertebral ganglia), after which the fibers are unmyelinated. All the nerve fibers returning via the gray ramus communicans to the spinal nerve are also unmyelinated (gray). In the thoracic section, the paravertebral ganglia of the sympathetic trunk are regularly organized.[47] The thoracic region contains 10–11 ganglia, and the lumbar and sacral region each about 4 ganglia. Distally the "end of the line" is the ganglion impar, which lies medially, ventrally to the coccyx. In the cervical region there are three paravertebral ganglia: the superior cervical ganglion, the middle (variable), and the inferior cervical ganglion; the inferiormost cervical ganglion usually merging with the superiormost thoracic ganglion to form the cervicothoracic (stellate) ganglion. Fibers run through the ganglia of the sympathetic trunk (paravertebral ganglia) to the prevertebral ganglia, as they are called, the most important of which lie ventral to the vertebral column and ventral and lateral to the abdominal aorta (e.g., the celiac ganglion). These prevertebral ganglia lie within large nervous plexuses that also contain parasympathetic fibers. They synapse here and then branch out (according to the principle of divergence) to the organs. This arrangement makes it easier to provide osteopathic regulation of the internal organs by applying treatment at ganglia.

The sympathetic nervous plexuses continue cranial to the superior cervical ganglion, on into the head region, and for the most part along the arteries. There is no development of a white ramus communicans in the cervical sympathetic nervous system. Instead, in the neck region there is a gray ramus communicans with connections to the spinal branches of the cervical spinal cord and to several cranial nerves: the hypoglossal nerve, glossopharyngeal nerve, vagus nerve, and the superior and inferior laryngeal nerves.[48]

Parasympathetic nervous system: in contrast to the sympathetic nervous system, the ganglia of the parasympathetic branch are usually situated close to their target organs or even inside them (intramurally). The fibers of the cranial parasympathetic nervous system run, in various cranial nerves, to the ganglia in the head region (the ciliary, pterygopalatine, otic, and submandibular ganglia). At the synapses in these ganglia there is a transition to the cranial parasympathetic fibers. Sympathetic and autonomic sensory afferent and proprioceptive fibers also pass through these ganglia, but without synapse. The sacral parasympathetic nervous system also sends its axons along the ventral roots; they leave the relevant sacral foramina with the cauda equina and run to the pudendal nerve. From here, as pelvic splanchnic nerves, they enter the prevertebral plexus (the superior and inferior hypogastric plexuses and vesicoprostatic or uterovaginal plexus). These plexuses also contain sympathetic fibers.

The terminal branching of the autonomic nervous system

The nerve fibers do not terminate directly at the parenchymal cells of the organ, but in the ground system. There are no precisely defined autonomic nerve endings in the periphery, but rather, according to Stöhr, Reiser, and van der Zypen[49] a terminal reticulum: a fine neurofibrillary mesh without endings. This appears to be integrated into the ground system with almost no evident transition. According to van der Zypen[50] the transmission of a stimulus can occur at lightning speed at any point in the autonomic mesh. Also, since the ground system and sympathetic nervous system are everywhere present, this stimulus can also reach anywhere, even beyond any segmental order.

Summary

The autonomic nervous system is a functional unity. It co-ordinates all organ systems according to the internal and external conditions present at that moment.

The terminal branching of the autonomic nervous system to create a terminal reticulum produces a "seamless" transition into the ground system. This provides further scientific substantiation for holistic information therapies.

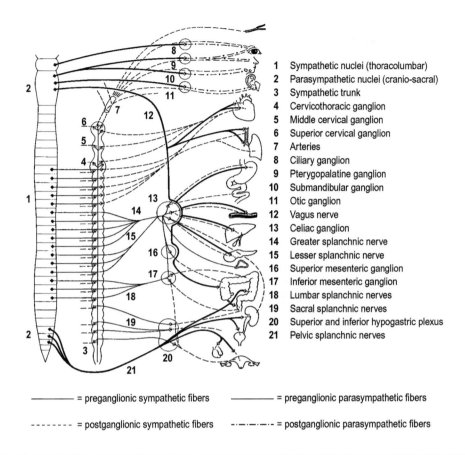

1 Sympathetic nuclei (thoracolumbar)
2 Parasympathetic nuclei (cranio-sacral)
3 Sympathetic trunk
4 Cervicothoracic ganglion
5 Middle cervical ganglion
6 Superior cervical ganglion
7 Arteries
8 Ciliary ganglion
9 Pterygopalatine ganglion
10 Submandibular ganglion
11 Otic ganglion
12 Vagus nerve
13 Celiac ganglion
14 Greater splanchnic nerve
15 Lesser splanchnic nerve
16 Superior mesenteric ganglion
17 Inferior mesenteric ganglion
18 Lumbar splanchnic nerves
19 Sacral splanchnic nerves
20 Superior and inferior hypogastric plexus
21 Pelvic splanchnic nerves

———— = preganglionic sympathetic fibers   ———— = preganglionic parasympathetic fibers

- - - - - = postganglionic sympathetic fibers   -·—·—·- = postganglionic parasympathetic fibers

Figure 5.6
Topography of the autonomic nervous system (simplified, schematic representation). From Fischer, 2001.[54]

The extended segment concept

It is primarily – though not only – the autonomic nervous system that is responsible for "breaking out of" the segmental order that usually applies. An understanding of the connections listed below helps to explain reflex phenomena that have so far defied explanation. A "segment" of the spinal cord is generally understood to refer to one vertebral "slice" of the cord together with the gray matter and roots belonging to it that together make up a spinal nerve pair. The spinal nerves (with their various qualities of fiber) supply a particular region of the body, the peripheral segment, so that the peripheral segment is a projection of a spinal cord segment in a particular body region. This is composed of:

1 The segmental (radicular) innervation of the skin (dermatome)

2 The segmental (radicular) innervation of the muscles (myotome)

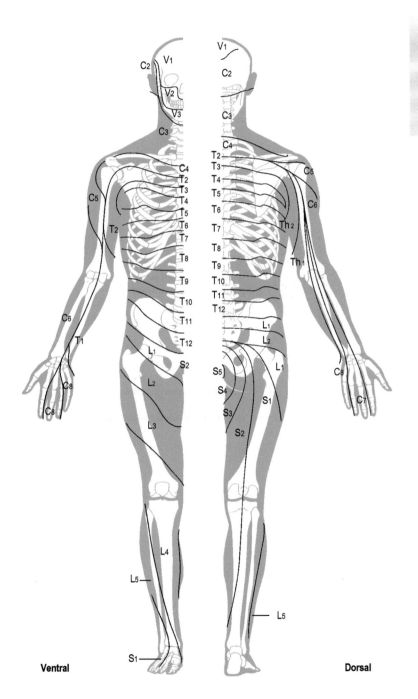

Ventral

Dorsal

Figure 5.7

Usual segmental order: sensory and radicular innervation of the skin (dermatomes). From Fischer, 2001.[54]

3 The segmental (radicular) innervation of the periosteum/bones (sclerotome)

4 The segmental (radicular) innervation of the viscera (viscerotome).

A spinal cord segment such as this creates a reflex inter-switching between the skin, muscles, bones, and internal organ in all directions. The sympathetic nervous system and sympathetic trunk play a major role in this, as regards both the afferent and the efferent pathways. Connections exist in all directions: a viscerocutaneous reflex path (head zones), a cutivisceral reflex path, a viscero–somato-motor one, and so on. Bergsmann and Eder described this interconnection (which is also influenced by descending pathways from the brain) as a segmental regulatory or "segmental reflex complex."[51,52]

Pain and the sympathetic nervous system

It is particularly in relation to pain that we see how the sympathetic nervous system extends the boundaries of the segment. An illustration of the kind of vicious circle that builds up in the "segmental reflex complex" can be given using the example of nociceptors: nociceptors are thin, plexiform terminal branches of sensory nerves, unmyelinated or with little myelin. They report tissue damage and pain (nociceptive = sensitive to damaging tissue change). Nociceptors are distributed throughout the body, and are even present in internal organs. Irritation of nociceptors is not necessarily reported as pain (if below the threshold). Nociceptive processes are only expressed as pain when the consciousness is "in the loop."[53,54] A reflex response is almost always triggered, however. This is expressed in the form of symptoms such as changes in blood flow, increased skin turgor, and hyperalgesia of particular skin areas, disturbed regulation of the internal organs relating to the metamer or segment and muscle hardness (which may be associated with trigger points).

This "package response" to incoming signals of any structure belonging to that segment can be explained as follows: afferent (especially nociceptive) signals from the skin, the muscles, and the internal organ converge at the same cell of the dorsal horn.[55-60] The skin zones, for example, related to the organ as a result of this convergence of afferent signals may be referred to as "head zones" of the particular organ.[61] Once the dorsal horn

cell has received impulses from one or more structures, onward transmission is divergent, toward the skin, muscles, and internal organ (and also to the brain). In this way sympathetic and motor neurons may for example be excited simultaneously. The vicious circle is still further intensified, given the inevitable assumption that sympathetic efferent signals in the periphery increase nociceptor activity: under pathophysiological conditions, "sympathetic-afferent coupling" can occur, in which sympathetic fibers in the periphery couple with afferent neurons. Sympathetic nervous system blockade causes this kind of pain to disappear (author's own experience and Baron, 1998[62]). The sympathetic nervous system can also exert a causal effect not only in inflammation-related pain but also in the development of the inflammation. This was demonstrated by Spiess[63] as long ago as 1906. Results from clinical practice confirm this understanding, as do those of recent research.[64,65]

From this alone, various logical points of approach on the part of reflex therapies can be derived. The segment concept needs to be extended yet further in addition to the segmental reflex described above (unfortunately still far too little regard is paid to this in diagnosis and therapy):

- Dermatome, myotome, and sclerotome do not correspond exactly.

- There are overlaps in neural supply.

- A single muscle and internal organ are supplied by more than one segment.

- The sympathetic nervous system is divided up in a remarkable way: the nuclei of the sympathetic system are not distributed along the entire spinal cord,[66] but only its central section (C8 to L3), and the sympathetic supply to the entire body comes from here. There are therefore very great differences between the segmental allocation of somatic and sympathetic innervation, especially in the head limb regions.[67,68]

- The element of the sympathetic system that runs to the periphery along with vessels and peripheral nerves additionally disrupts the usual segmental divisions.

- Irritation of the ganglia demonstrates the extraordinarily wide area supplied, with the appearance of a

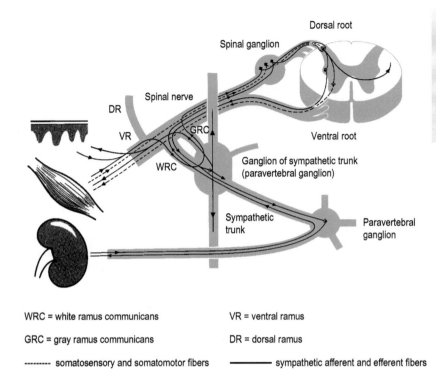

Dorsal root

Spinal ganglion

Spinal nerve

DR

VR

GRC

WRC

Ventral root

Ganglion of sympathetic trunk
(paravertebral ganglion)

Sympathetic
trunk

Paravertebral
ganglion

Figure 5.8
Reflex transmission from
skin, muscles, and internal
organs. Schematic,
simplified diagram. From
Fischer, 2001[54].

WRC = white ramus communicans   VR = ventral ramus

GRC = gray ramus communicans   DR = dorsal ramus

-------- somatosensory and somatomotor fibers   ———— sympathetic afferent and efferent fibers

great range of symptoms: in the case of the stellate ganglion, it covers the upper quarter of the body, and in the case of the celiac ganglion, a large proportion of the abdominal organs.

- The spine is often involved in the development of the syndrome even when the primary disturbance is "peripheral" (peripheral locomotor apparatus, internal organ): at first through restriction of a motion segment, and later through the appearance of degenerative changes. As a result, over time there can even be a change of side. The Flechsig ground bundles (fasciculi proprii) of the spinal cord and connections of the sympathetic nervous system (interganglionic ramus communicans) that cross between sides may possibly also play a part in this. In this way, if symptoms persist for a long time the contralateral side can be affected involving a segmental reflex complex. (Perhaps, when further neurophysiological insights are available, such considerations may be able to

contribute to some extent to explaining what is happening in the field of disturbance).

- The reaction of the musculature to nociceptive irritation coming from the skin, internal organ or locomotor apparatus is not an "individual muscle" reponse, of muscle hardness and weakness, but always that of an entire kinetic muscle chain (extending over several segments) whose function is to produce a complex movement programmed in the reticular formation (gamma motor system) and learned in childhood. Neural transmission here is suprasegmental (via interneurons, etc.). Along the length of these kinetic muscle chains, pseudoradicular symptoms and trigger points are found:
  - Pseudoradicular syndrome as described by Brügger:[69,70] pain, weakness, hypertonus, shortening, and autonomic symptoms (vasomotricity, hyperhidrosis, dysesthesias) of that kinetic muscle chain.[71-74] If this emanates from the spinal column,

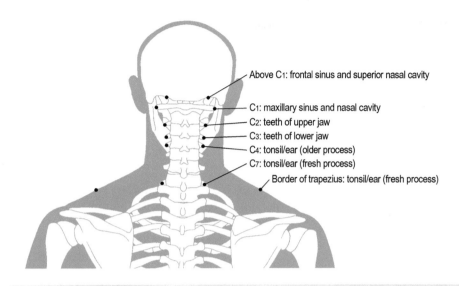

Above C1: frontal sinus and superior nasal cavity
C1: maxillary sinus and nasal cavity
C2: teeth of upper jaw
C3: teeth of lower jaw
C4: tonsil/ear (older process)
C7: tonsil/ear (fresh process)
Border of trapezius: tonsil/ear (fresh process)

Figure 5.9
The Adler–Lange pressure points. From Fischer, 2001.[54]

it is additionally designated "spondylogenic." In this case too, the main responsibility for the symptoms appears to lie with the sympathetic nervous system.

- Myofascial trigger points are also situated in this functional unit of the kinetic muscle chain. There are painful sites in the muscles either at rest or on movement, or only in response to pressure. The referred pain projected and communicated from the trigger point corresponds to the pseudoradicular symptoms and is also located within this kinetic muscle chain.

- There is an interesting connection with acupuncture that deserves to be mentioned here; the musculotendinous meridians of acupuncture also follow the kinetic chains.[75,76] Also, according to Melzack, the trigger points correspond to acupuncture points to the extent of 71%.[77]

- The Adler–Langer pressure points also deserve mention under the heading of the extended segment concept. Ernesto Adler[78] repeatedly found points in the nape of the neck that were tender to pressure, and related as follows (and as confirmed many times in clinical practice): nasal sinuses – inferior border of the occiput and C1; maxilla and dental region – transverse process C2; mandible and dental region – transverse process C3; tonsils – in the region of the superior/anterior border of the trapezius (Fig. 5.9). Painful areas are also found here when there is disease of the internal organs, with the signals being transmitted via the phrenic nerve. Langer expanded the list of these points and differentiated them further:[79] In particular the transverse process of C4 is tender to pressure in the case of old processes affecting the ears and tonsils, and the transverse process of C7 in that of fresh processes affecting these.

We can attempt to explain these connections, which were found empirically, as follows: sympathetic afferent fibers are also present everywhere in the head region. In the neck region, although there is no white ramus communicans developed, there is a gray ramus communicans that leads to cervical spinal nerves, and in this way local increase in tonus of the neck muscles can occur. Other possible explanations are: the afferents via the trigeminal nerve – from, for example, the nasal sinuses and the teeth – terminate in the region of the trigeminal nucleus; this region extends into the cervical spinal cord to the level of C2/C3 (nuclei tractus spinalis) and itself has connections to the anterior horn cells of the cervical spinal cord. Consequently, in disorders of the teeth and nasal sinuses there will often be irritation of various kinds (restrictions, tenderness to pressure, etc.) in segments C1 to C3. Over time, more distally located segments can also be affected, because, as pointed out by Lewit,[80] one of the most frequent reasons for restriction of a vertebral segment is restriction in another segment.

Afferent fibers from cranial nerve XI (the glossopharyngeal nerve, including the tonsillar branches!) and from cranial nerve X (vagus, including afferents from the pharyngeal plexus!) terminate at the dorsal nucleus of the vagus nerve and nucleus of the solitary tract. The region of the nuclei of the solitary tract extends into the cervical spinal cord, and there are also connections with the spinal nucleus of the trigeminal nerve. This offers an explanation for irritation in the cervical spine region in tonsillitis and pharyngitis.

Motor root cells of the glossopharyngeal nerve are also situated together with those of the vagus and accessory nerves in the nucleus ambiguus, whose spinal process extends far into the cervical spinal cord. It is only logical for there to be common efferent signals and their existence could cast further light on what happens in connection with a field of disturbance. In addition there are connections from the accessory nerve to spinal nerves of the cervical spinal cord.

Overstrain of the eyes often produces irritation, especially suboccipitally as far as C3. A frequent finding in this case is transverse processes that are tender to pressure. One explanation for this phenomenon could be the function of the medial longitudinal fasciculus, which (among other things) links nuclei of the muscles of the eye with motor nuclei in the upper cervical spinal cord (to C3).

The same symptoms are often found in painful diseases of the eye. The linking structure in this case could be the trigeminal nerve with its spinal nucleus, which extends down as far as C2/C3. Sympathetic afferents must also be involved.

- In diseases of the upper abdomen and chest, autonomic afferents via the phrenic and vagus nerves additionally extend the segment concept.

Summary

- The skin, locomotor apparatus, and the related internal organ are linked as one unit in terms of nerve impulse transmission ("segmental reflex complex"). The main agent of this is the autonomic nervous system.

- The muscles react, not as a single muscle with muscle hardness and weakness, but as a kinetic functional chain. Pseudoradicular symptoms and trigger points with referred pain are also found along this chain.

- The spine is also involved in the segmental reflex.

- The territory supplied by the ganglia, and by the perivasal sympathetic nervous system, further extend the segment concept.

- Neuroanatomical transmission mechanisms offer an explanation for the fact that disturbances of the nasal sinuses, teeth, tonsils, oropharynx, and eyes cause irritation in the cervical spine region.

The gate control theory of Melzack and Wall

Targeted injections of local anesthetics have longlasting effects on pain and functional disturbances, as is evidenced in practice. The pharmacological effect does not provide the explanation. One of the links in the chain of explanatory models is the gate control of Melzack and Wall.[81] This theory relates to the "entry control" of afferents before they synapse with the transmission cells in the dorsal horn. The afferents consist of somatic (thick) and autonomic (thin) nerve fibers. Both types give off collaterals to cells in the gelatinous substance, which lies on the dorsal horn like a cap and is responsible for

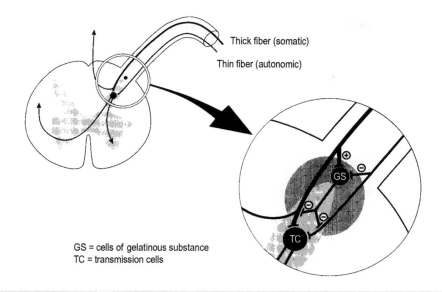

Thick fiber (somatic)

Thin fiber (autonomic)

GS = cells of gelatinous substance
TC = transmission cells

Figure 5.10
The gate control theory of Melzack and Wall. From Fischer, 2001.[54]

intensifying the incoming pain signals ("gate open") or diminishing them ("gate closed"). Melzack and Wall postulate the following course of transmission (Fig. 5.10): if the cells of the gelatinous substance are activated, they inhibit both fiber types by a feedback process. If thick fibers are stimulated, then, via collaterals, they activate the cells of the gelatinous substance. This brings about presynaptic inhibition, and the gate closes. The process is different if thin fibers are stimulated: their collaterals inactivate the cells of the gelatinous substance, and it is then no longer able to produce presynaptic inhibition. The gate is therefore open, and pain impulses can pass unhindered. This occurs on the one hand via central positive feedback, and on the other by directly feeding into the "segmental reflex complex" to produce a vicious circle: pain – muscle tension – ischemia – increased pain.

The aim of therapy must therefore be to close the gate. Given the course of transmission this can happen in either of two ways: activation of the thick fibers, or inhibition of the thin fibers.

Many other inhibitory processes besides the presynaptic inhibition postulated by Melzack and Wall occur at the secondary neurons; they are therefore postsynaptic. Such models supplement but do not contradict the gate control theory.

Summary

Methods such as osteopathy have a beneficial effect on the dorsal horn gate control ("gate closed"). This consequently hinders pathological processing of pain, both in the central nervous system and in the segmental reflex complex.

References

[1]Wiener N: Kybernetik oder Regelung und Nachrichtenübertragung in Lebewesen und in der Maschine. Düsseldorf: Econ; 1963.

[2]Lullies H, Trincker D: Taschenbuch der Physiologie, vol. 1. Stuttgart: Fischer; 1974.

[3]Bergsmann O, Bergsmann R: Projektionssymptome, 2nd edn. Vienna: Facultas; 1992.

[4]Dosch P: Lehrbuch der Neuraltherapie nach Hunecke, 14th edn. Heidelberg: Haug; 1995.

[5]Stacher A, Bergsmann O: Grundlagen für eine integrative Ganzheitsmedizin. Vienna: Facultas; 1993.

[6]Heine H: Lehrbuch der biologischen Medizin. Stuttgart: Hippokrates; 1991.

[7]Buddecke E: Grundriss der Biochemie. Berlin: De Gruyter; 1974.

[8]Pischinger A: Das System der Grundregulation, 8th edn. Heidelberg: Haug; 1990.

[9]Buddecke E: Grundriss der Biochemie. Berlin: De Gruyter; 1974.

[10]Eisenberg W, Remer U, Trimper S, et al.: Synergie, Syntropie, nicht lineare Systeme. Book 1 Dynamik und Synergetik. Leipzig: Verlag im Wissenschaftszentrum; 1995.

[11]Heine H: Lehrbuch der biologischen Medizin. Stuttgart: Hippokrates; 1991.

[12]Heine H: Lehrbuch der biologischen Medizin. Stuttgart: Hippokrates; 1991.

[13]Heine H: Lehrbuch der biologischen Medizin. Stuttgart: Hippokrates; 1991.

[14]Pischinger A: Das System der Grundregulation, 8th edn. Heidelberg: Haug; 1990.

[15]Bergsmann O, Bergsmann R: Projektionssymptome, 2nd edn. Vienna: Facultas; 1992.

[16]Bischof M: Biophotonen. Frankfurt: Zweitausendeins; 1995.

[17]Popp FA: Neue Horizonte in der Medizin, 2nd edn. Heidelberg: Haug; 1987.

[18]Bergsmann O, Bergsmann R: Projektionssymptome, 2nd edn. Vienna: Facultas; 1992.

[19]Athenstaedt H: Pyroelectric and piezoelectric property of vertebrates. Ann. New York Acad. Sc. 1974;238:68–110.

[20]Pischinger A: Das System der Grundregulation, 8th edn. Heidelberg: Haug; 1990.

[21]Bergsmann O: Grundsystem, Regulation und Regulationsstörung in der Praxis der Rehabilitation. In: Pischinger A: Das System der Grundregulation, 8th edn. Heidelberg: Haug; 1990.

[22]Pischinger A: Das System der Grundregulation, 8th edn. Heidelberg: Haug; 1990.

[23]Heine H: Lehrbuch der biologischen Medizin. Stuttgart: Hippokrates; 1991.

[24]Heine H: Lehrbuch der biologischen Medizin. Stuttgart: Hippokrates; 1991.

[25]Speransky AD. A Basis for the Theory of Medicine. New York: International Publishers; 1943.

[26]Dosch P: Lehrbuch der Neuraltherapie nach Huneke, 14th edn. Heidelberg: Haug; 1995.

[27]Imoberdorf R et al: Die Akutphasereaktion. In: Therapiewoche Schweiz. 1995;11:34–38.

[28]Heine H: Lehrbuch der biologischen Medizin. Stuttgart: Hippokrates; 1991.

[29]Barop H: Lehrbuch und Atlas der Neuraltherapie nach Huneke. Stuttgart: Hippokrates; 1996.

[30]Barop H: Neuraltherapie nach Huneke aus der Sicht der Relationspathologie Rickers. In: Aktuelle Beiträge zur Neuraltherapie nach Huneke, vol. 15. Heidelberg: Haug; 1994.

[31]Ricker G: Pathologie als Naturwissenschaft – Relationspathologie. Berlin: Springer; 1924.

[32]Barop H: Neuraltherapie nach Huneke aus der Sicht der Relationspathologie Rickers. In: Aktuelle Beiträge zur Neuraltherapie nach Huneke, vol. 15. Heidelberg: Haug; 1994.

[33]Ricker G: Pathologie als Naturwissenschaft – Relationspathologie. Berlin: Springer; 1924.

[34]Barop H: Neuraltherapie nach Huneke aus der Sicht der Relationspathologie Rickers. In: Aktuelle Beiträge zur Neuraltherapie nach Huneke, vol. 15. Heidelberg: Haug; 1994.

[35]Ricker G: Pathologie als Naturwissenschaft – Relationspathologie. Berlin: Springer; 1924.

[36]Barop H: Lehrbuch und Atlas der Neuraltherapie nach Huneke. Stuttgart: Hippokrates; 1996.

[37]Ricker G: Pathologie als Naturwissenschaft – Relationspathologie. Berlin: Springer; 1924.

[38]Barop H: Lehrbuch und Atlas der Neuraltherapie nach Huneke. Stuttgart: Hippokrates; 1996.

[39]Ricker G: Pathologie als Naturwissenschaft – Relationspathologie. Berlin: Springer; 1924.

[40]Speransky AD. A Basis for the Theory of Medicine. New York: International Publishers; 1943.

[41]Speransky AD. A Basis for the Theory of Medicine. New York: International Publishers; 1943.

[42]Dosch P: Lehrbuch der Neuraltherapie nach Huneke, 14th edn. Heidelberg: Haug; 1995.

[43]Speransky AD. A Basis for the Theory of Medicine. New York: International Publishers; 1943.

[44]Clara M: Das Nervensystem des Menschen. Leipzig; Barth; 1942.

[45]Monnier N: Physiologie und Pathophysiologie des vegetativen Nervensystems, vols 1 and 2. Stuttgart: Hippokrates; 1963.

[46]Wilson-Pauwels L, Stewart PA, Akesson EJ: Autonomic nerves. Basic science, clinical aspects, case studies. London: B. C. Decker Inc, Hamilton; 1997.

[47]Kahle W: Nervensystem und Sinnesorgane. Stuttgart: Thieme; 1976

[48]Van der Zypen E: Anatomie des sympathischen nervensystems, VASA, vol. 6. 1977; 2:115–123.

[49]Van der Zypen E: Elektronenmikroskopische befunde an der endausbreitung des vegetativen nervensystems und ihre deutung. Acta. Anatom. 1967;67:431–515.

[50]Van der Zypen E: Elektronenmikroskopische befunde an der endausbreitung des vegetativen nervensystems und ihre deutung. Acta. Anatom. 1967;67:431–515.

[51]Bergsmann O, Bergsmann R: Projektionssymptome. 2nd edn. Vienna: Facultas; 1992.

[52]Tilscher H, Eder M: Reflextherapie. 2nd edn. Stuttgart: Hippokrates; 1989.

[53]Handwerker HO: Einführung in die Pathophysiologie des Schmerzes. Berlin: Springer; 1999.

[54]Zieglgänsberger W: Central control of nociception. In: Mountcastle VB, Bloom FE, Geiger SR (ed.): Handbook of Physiology – the Nervous System: Baltimore: Williams & Wilkins; 1986.

[55]Haschke W: Grundzüge der Neurophysiologie unter dem Aspekt der integrativen Tätigkeit des ZNS. Jena: Gustav Fischer; 1986.

[56]Pothmann R: TENS-Transkutane Elektrische Nervenstimulation in der Schmerztherapie. 2nd edn. Stuttgart: Hippokrates; 1996.

[57]Schäfer M: Physiologie und Pathophysiologie des Schmerzes. Therapeut. Umschau. 1999; 56:426–430.

[58]Travell JG, Simons DG: Myofascial Pain and Dysfunction, vols I+II. Baltimore: Williams & Wilkins; 1982.

[59]Wolff HD: Neurophysiologische Aspekte des Bewegungssystems. 3rd edn. Berlin: Springer; 1996.

[60]Zimmermann M: Die Neuraltherapie im Licht Neuerer Erkenntnisse der Neurobiologischen Forschung. In: Neuraltherapie, vol. 2, Stuttgart: Hippokrates; 1984.

[61]Zimmermann M: Die Neuraltherapie im Licht Neuerer Erkenntnisse der Neurobiologischen Forschung. In: Neuraltherapie, vol 2, Stuttgart: Hippokrates; 1984.

[62]Baron R, Jänig W: Schmerzsyndrome mit Kausaler Beteiligung des Sympathikus. Springer: Anästhesist; 1998;47:4–23.

[63]Spiess G: Die Bedeutung der Anästhesie in der Entzündungstherapie. München: Med. Wschr. 1906;8:345–351.

[64]Baron R, Jänig W: Schmerzsyndrome mit Kausaler Beteiligung des Sympathikus. Springer: Anästhesist; 1998;47:4–23.

[65]Raja SN, Meyer RA, Ringkamp M, Campbell JN: Peripheral Neural Mechanisms of Nociception. In: Wall PD, Melzack R (ed.). Textbook of Pain. 4th edn. Edinburgh: Churchill Livingstone; 1999.

[66]Van der Zypen E: Anatomie des sympathischen nervensystems, VASA, vol. 6. 1977;2:115–123.

[67]Fischer L: Myofasciale Trigger-Punkte und Neuraltherapie nach Huneke. Erfahrungsheilkunde. 1998;3:117–126.

[68]Zimmermann M: Die Neuraltherapie im Licht Neuerer Erkenntnisse der Neurobiologischen Forschung. In: Neuraltherapie, vol. 2, Stuttgart: Hippokrates; 1984.

[69]Brügger A: Die Erkrankungen des Bewegungsapparates und Seines Nervensystems. Stuttgart: Fischer; 1980.

[70]Brügger A: Lehrbuch der Funktionellen Störungen des Bewegungssystems. Brügger, Zollikon und Benglen; 2000.

[71]Bergsmann O, Bergsmann R: Projektionssymptome. 2nd edn. Vienna: Facultas; 1992.

[72]Brügger A: Die Erkrankungen des Bewegungsapparates und Seines Nervensystems. Stuttgart: Fischer; 1980.

[73]Thurneysen A: Liegen die Meridiane in den Muskeln? Akup. Theor. u. Prax. 1982;10:217–220.

[73]Travell JG, Simons DG: Myofascial Pain and Dysfunction. Band I+II. Baltimore: Williams & Wilkins; 1982.

[75]Bergsmann O, Bergsmann R: Projektionssymptome. 2nd edn. Vienna: Facultas; 1992

[76]Thurneysen A: Liegen die Meridiane in den Muskeln? Akup. Theor. u. Prax. 1982;10:217–220.

[77]Melzack R et al.: Trigger point and acupuncture points for pain. Pain. 1977; 3:3–23.

[78]Adler E: Störfeld und Herd im Trigeminusbereich, 4th edn. Heidelberg: E. Fischer; 1990.

[79]Langer H: Die Adler-Langer'schen Druckpunkte als Mittel zur Störfeldsuche. In: Dosch P (ed.). Aktuelle Beiträge zur Neuraltherapie nach Huneke, vol. 15, Heidelberg: Haug; 1994.

[80]Lewit K: Manipulative Therapy: Musculoskeletal Medicine. Edinburgh: Elsevier; 2010; 20.

[81]Melzack R, Wall PD: Pain mechanism. A new theory. Science 1965;150:971.

6

The effect of formative and regulatory forces on living organisms

Torsten Liem

Nature makes use of the biodynamic form of movement, which is the biological prerequisite for life coming into being.

V. Schauenberger[1]

Introduction

Morphology is the study of the shape and structure (configuration or (inner) construction of an object or system) of organisms; it deals with the observation and description of organisms and their classification, in terms of their shape and also with the developmental dynamic changes. Their phenotypic expression is determined by environmental influences as well as by genotype; this is so both for ontogenetic and phylogenetic dynamics. The process by which shape emerges (morphogenesis) is still not fully understood, so that many aspects remain hypothetical.

The organism – an autopoietic entity

According to the modern systems theory approach in biology, the existence of life brings about a break in symmetry through the appearance of autopoiesis. The autopoietic entity – a self-renewing system – is distinguished by a certain autonomy over its environment, and to a great extent acquires its size and shape independently of the environment that sustains it.

Life itself and the human body in particular behave as an open system, which organizes itself as a system and operates far from thermodynamic equilibrium. This requires energy transfer to be assured within the system and also needs to take account of information as a central parameter.

The creation of borders enables living systems to maintain their inner order by separating themselves off from the entropy of the environment. It is via this border that sensory and motor communication between the inner world of the organism and the external world takes place, and it is here that the exchange of matter,

energy, and information (i.e., the distinguishing characteristic of an open system) occurs.[2]

One of the most fundamental laws of self-organization (where "organization" is defined as the relations between the component parts of a system) is the mutual correspondence of structure and function; this is also one of the main principles of osteopathic treatment. (Structure, according to Jantsch, refers not only to spatial arrangement but to the ordering of processes in spatial and temporal terms. Maturana defines it as consisting of the components and relations that make up a united entity, and by which its organization is generated.) This correspondence, being fairly freely flexible, offers grounds for the possibility of achieving a genuine balance of the autopoietic entity; alternatively, that a system might evolve in conjunction with its environment.[3]

Living systems as self-reproducing (autocatalytic) entities are cyclically organized, i.e., in a closed circle (hypercycle model). In this closed circle of transformation or of catalytic processes, the structure is renewed by exchanging parts of the system while maintaining the organization of the whole.[4]

The development, motion, and meaning of shape: the field of activity for osteopathy

The question of osteopathic treatment and the practice of touch receives new impetus as we consider the issues of shape, energy, and information. What it is that determines the specifics of shape and structure, and the field in which osteopathy operates? How are energy (in both the vitalist and the scientific sense) and information stored in living tissues and organisms and how are they transmitted between them? What mechanisms maintain the integrity of the body as a whole, and what physiological or pathophysiological processes are triggered within it by external stimuli? Because it is a dissipative system (see pp. 74, 77, 80, 238, 321.), information can be transmitted within it so as to reach all parts of it in an extremely short time. It is usually not so much a case of the amount of energy as the organization of that energy. A decisive question in treatment is how to assist the reorganization of the energy and information in the body as a whole.

Field properties appear to have a regulatory and controlling function from reproduction, growth, and regeneration through to death and to ensure maintenance of the organic whole.

Speaking of these fields, Burr says:

This starts with the simplest living forms, runs upwards through all life to the most complex form we know – man – and then extends outwards into space... It must also extend from the heart of the smallest atom to those gigantic forces which keep the planets in their orbits, which govern the stars in their courses and which regulate the feverish race of the most distant galaxies towards the outer reaches of space. Burr, 1991[5]

The body constantly experiences its own existence and that of the external world. These two worlds exist simultaneously, both independent and in interaction with each other, interwoven by way of rhythmic processes of exchange and integration, forming a dynamic continuity of reality in the body as a whole.

Since Einstein, the strict distinction of matter and energy can no longer be held to be valid, and we might instead see matter as condensed energy. The characteristics of matter in general and body tissue in particular are determined by the way in which energy is distributed, and by the organizational pattern of the energy. The way in which the energy is organized or disorganized, and the way in which the information or misinformation is transmitted in the energy continuum, determines who and what we are and our perception of ourselves and the world.[6]

The underlying assumption would need to be the existence of a dynamic interrelationship and a physical and energetic continuity between the practitioner's hand and the surface layer of the skin, through the whole body down to the nucleus of every cell. The effect here is not only that of the hand contact itself as a catalyst for spontaneous reactions of healing and harmonization, but also the synchronous presence in the same space, or spatial nearness, of practitioner and patient, the interpersonal interrelationship between them and the intention of the practitioner.

It will become clear from the following sections that the prime aim in osteopathy should not simply be the manipulation of a particular bone, organ, or other tissue alone, but also the harmonization of the fields in which the bone or organ and person, who is more than the sum of component parts, are organized and develop.

Morphogenetic fields

The existence of a morphogenetic field was first proposed by Hans Driesch in 1892 after he observed that, if the first division of fertilized sea urchin eggs was disturbed, both daughter cells developed normally and independently. According to his vitalist approach there is an inherent vital force in every organism that determines its shape. This approach is based on Aristotle's concept of entelechy: the concept of the goal achieved by the activity itself.

In 1910, Boveri also developed a concept of the morphogenetic field, and in the early 1920s three biologists elaborated models that attributed the development of tissue to certain "fields": Alexander Gurwitsch,[7–9] Hans Spemann,[10] and Paul Weiss.[11] Gurwitsch initially described these fields as 'Kraftfelder' and 'Geschehnisfelder', fields of force in which events occur in a coordinated manner, and made reference to the embryonic development of tissues and to the functions of regulation and regeneration in this very early period of development.

Structuralist approaches in embryology were formulated by authors such as Waddington, D'Arcy Thompson,[12] René Thom,[13] and Brian Goodwin. These authors characterized a field as a spatial order of specific relationships, in which the state adopted by each and every part is jointly regulated by the state of neighboring parts. Waddington[14] postulated that morphogenetic fields operate by means of physical and chemical forces.

Whilst Waddington's and Thom's contributions lie mainly in the description of morphogenetic dynamics (Waddington's catastrophe theory and Thom's mathematical topography), Goodwin seeks possible explanations for the meaning and purpose of these fields, and sees in them archetypical and timeless forms (corresponding to the ideas of Plato) that are true for all time and are then become manifest in the course of the ontogenetic and phylogenetic development.[15]

Morphogenetic fields, according to Goodwin, are above all chemical–mechanical–genetic fields.[16] The viscoelastic properties of gels provide another explanatory model. These fields operate as forces that, on the basis of their own organization in space and time, direct shape and organization in the development of cells, microorganisms, plants, and animals. Biosystems also appear to possess a fundamental quality of coherence, which enables them to regulate metabolism. The coherence of quantum emission thus directs all processes in the protoplasm.

The interaction of mechanical and electrical influences produces mechanical intracellular pulsations in the macromolecules, the nucleic acids, and the cell membranes and leads to coherence. This is based on the transport of stored energy. If stress factors have lowered the state of order in the biosystem, it tries to regain its highest state of coherence.

Morphogenetic fields exert an effect in the nanometer range. Molecules and supramolecular structures are mechanically deformed by morphogenetic fields; leading to a change in chemical potentials and electrical, electromagnetic fields. These altered fields in turn influence molecular reactions. The oscillation frequency of these structures in the non-equilibrium range is very large, e.g., in the range of several minutes. The oscillation of individual cell components has a much higher frequency.

Electrical, magnetic, and electrodynamic fields

According to Becker[17] – whose work has significantly influenced the field of energy medicine – at the deepest level in all living organisms, electrical and magnetic forces direct processes of growth and healing in those organisms. Intercellular communication takes place by means of low frequency oscillations.[18]

Electrical fields can be subdivided into electrostatic, electrodynamic, and electromagnetic fields. Alternating electromagnetic fields are used for diagnosis by electroencephalogram (EEG) or electrocardiogram (ECG). The propagation of low frequency membrane potential oscillations in extracellular spaces appears to be partly responsible for the production of the EEG. It is not only the components of atoms that are held together by electromagnetic fields, but also molecules, cells, organs, and actual organisms.

To give examples, electrical fields are generated by the transmission of nerve impulses or produced in other membrane systems by different electrolyte potentials either side of the membrane. Constant electrical fields have been measured in humans, with four groups being identified: those with an electrical field of 2, 2–4, 5–6, and 10 mV. In women of childbearing age this potential changes every month for 24 hours, according to Burr,[19] increasing at the time of ovulation; in men it remains constant.

The electromagnetic field of the heart remains detectable a few meters from the body, although the significance of this is still unknown.[20] The heart's changes are therefore shared with the whole body. Oschman[21] demonstrated that each organ has its own biomagnetic field and that these fields are interrelated, creating multilayered resonances and an exchange of information.

Burr[22] also established that "electrodynamic fields" play an important role in the organization of body structures, in the control of growth, and the morphogenesis of living creatures.

For him, the field is the most important matrix for the development of shape in living entities, with fields providing direction for the flow of energy in the organism, creating patterns of organization. The electrodynamic field involved is to a degree determined by its atomic, physical, and chemical components, and the field then to a degree controls the organization and orientation of these components.

Experiments have even found the incorporation of the specific individual fields into larger ones and the influence of external forces on these fields; one example is the influence of sunspots on the electrodynamic fields of trees. It also proved possible to produce distinct, reproducible changes in these fields by means of feelings induced by hypnosis.

Neurons grown on culture medium react to the tiniest electrical fields.

In a field strength of only 0.1 and 1 V/mm, osteoclasts migrate to the positive electrode and osteoblasts to the negative electrode. Different cells from the same tissue can therefore react differently to the same electrical signal.[23] At the same time their longitudinal axis aligns itself at right angles to this field; this is accompanied by cytoskeletal shape changes.

Electrical fields produce a marked change in the polymerization of proteins, e.g., in the formation of spindle fibers.[24] The transcription of genes in salivary cells of the fruit fly is stimulated after a 15–45 minute exposure to weak, pulsing electromagnetic fields.[25]

Static and oscillating magnetic fields influence cell growth and various other cell functions, such as changes in the outflow of calcium (Ca^{2+}) ions in cells and tissue.[26]

The perineural system, older in evolutionary terms, has a low voltage current that controls repair processes in the body. This system reacts to magnetic fields. During injury, a positive injury potential develops in the form of an electrical direct current; damaged body tissue is therefore positively charged against the rest of the body. This declines again after two days, after the separated nerve endings have reconnected with the skin cells (neuroepidermal junction), and is replaced with a negative charge. During the growth of the blastema, the potential at the injury site becomes highly negative, eventually returning to its potential before the injury.[27] The low-voltage current of perineural structures regulates the development and the growth of embryonic and adult tissue, tissue repair, and many other processes.[28]

According to Barr, melanin causes a change in acoustic and electrical energy fields. Melanin is acting as an amorphous semiconductor in physiological regions of neuronal electrical potentials. Barr postulates that the direct current of the peripheral glial system is controlled by neural crest melanin and that the direct current of the central nervous glial system is controlled by the melanin system of the brain stem.

The ground substance also exhibits a basic electrostatic tone and appears to have a central role in the transmission of electromagnetic effects in the body.[29] If changes occur in the ground substance, this causes variations in potential, resulting in a changed pattern of electromagnetic oscillation. This can be passed into the cell by the cell membrane as biochemical information. It is also possible for variations in potential to cause oscillation of structures in the ground substance and the cell membrane. Electromagnetic resonance frequencies[30] with a high degree of coherence could function as an information system in the ground system. According to Bischof (1995),[31] all the water of the body could be understood in its entirety, together with the proteoglycans of the ground substance, as a giant fluid crystalline molecule. Seen from this perspective, the classical anatomical structures appear as something abstract, while living tissue stands out for its constant interaction and dynamic behavior. In the ground substance (operating as a dissipative structure), even the most minor influences are instantly transmitted to the whole of the ground substance, and can lead to a change in structure (Bergsmann in Bischof, 1995).[32]

In this way, both somatic dysfunctions and osteopathic treatment could take effect throughout the body via the characteristics of the ground substance described.

The bodies of organisms generally respond more to weak magnetic fields than to weak electrical ones. Fluctuating magnetic fields trigger electrical currents in the body. Static fields affect them by causing magnetically sensitive molecules, such as those in membranes, to align themselves according to the field and because these reflect endogenous electrical currents. Membrane lipids therefore belong to the class of fluid crystals that are particularly prone to align themselves in electrical or magnetic fields.

Oscillating magnetic fields can accelerate chemical reactions that are taking place. Endogenous electrical currents align themselves at right angles to the direction of a static magnetic field. There are clear indications that certain electromagnetic oscillations produce similar or even identical effects as exposure to an allergen (Smith et al. 1987 in Bischof 1995).[33]

Smith[34] demonstrated that the activity of trypsin changes when it is placed between the poles of a strong magnetic field or between the palms of a "healer's" hands. The effect caused by the hands was comparable to the strength of a magnetic field of 10^{-4} Gauss.

Zimmermann,[35] investigating therapeutic touch by trained practitioners in a state of relaxation, recorded electromagnetic waves with a frequency of 0.3–30 Hz and a maximum of 7–8 Hz. This could not be detected for test subjects who were not practitioners of a healing profession.

Seto et al.[36] were also able to measure these electromagnetic fields in the case of trained practitioners. They recorded field strength of 10^{-3} Gauss with a mean frequency of 8–10 Hz. In comparison to this the heart, the strongest producer of electromagnetic fields in humans, produces a field of only 10^{-6} Gauss.

It was also found that practitioners of Qigong can emit infrared radiation from their hands that brings about stimulation of cell metabolism.[37] Similar results are also quite likely to be found especially in the functional and morphodynamic categories of osteopathic approaches.

Effects were also achieved, not only by means of the hands, but by pure visualization when plant growth was influenced over a distance of 900 km, and an effect was also obtained on cloud formation in a cloud chamber.[38] There are even some records stating that A.T. Still, founder of osteopathy, was able to detect over distances of many kilometers whether a patient's condition had improved.[39]

Biophoton fields

The concept of biophotons was introduced by Popp in 1976.[40]

He quotes an example of light emission by biological systems described by Popp and Ruth, which:

- is constantly emitted by all living organisms;

- exhibits an intensity of the order of a few photons to some hundred photons per second and per square centimeter;

- appears continuously in the part of the spectrum upward of 260–800 nm;

- occupies all phase space cells almost equally, far from thermodynamic equilibrium, the statistics conforming to Poisson distribution;

- proceeds from coherent quantum states; and

- can be understood as the outcome of the hyperbolic decay function of delayed luminescence.[41]

Faulty functional organic, cellular, and molecular regulation of tissues leads to a "squeezing" of the tissue radiation of microwaves and infrared radiation, into the visible range of the spectrum.[42]

Alexander Gurwitsch[43] first conducted investigations into biophoton emission; Popp and coworkers[44] produced the first scientific demonstration that ultraweak photon emission does occur in animal and plant cells.

In studies of mammalian cells from rats, cats, cows, dogs, humans, etc. light-induced photon emission (IPE) was recorded. This varied from 4–100 photons per 10^4 cells, depending on cell type. The highest IPE values were obtained from cells of fibroblastic origin.[45]

The beginning of the death of organisms is accompanied by a steep increase in light emission. Intracellular microtubules also have a capacity to conduct biophotons. These are assumed to have directional functions in the cell.[46]

Studies of *Daphnia* (a genus of water flea) demonstrated that there are long-range interactions between organisms. The photon emission varies periodically with cell number and indicates a relationship to the average separation distances between individual organisms.[47]

The effects of various growth factors on the proliferation of skin fibroblasts also correlate with ultraweak photon emissions.[48] DNA has also been identified as a source of biophoton emission. DNA is viewed as an exciplex laser system that is able to achieve a stable state, far from thermodynamic equilibrium.[49]

It was demonstrated experimentally that all external perturbations such as changes in temperature or exposure to light operating on the exciplex model can be seen as a shifting of the working parts of the system, which leads to a diversity of nonlinear responses in biophoton emission.[50]

Biophoton emission therefore correlates with the functional states of cells and organisms and changes in response to external stimuli.

Previous studies have shown that these emissions have a high degree of coherence, on the grounds of photocount, spectral distribution, decay behavior following light stimulation and their capacity to penetrate optically dense materials. There is simultaneous coherence in a broad band of frequencies.[51] These effects are characteristic of the intrinsic coherence within living systems.

According to Popp's biophoton model, all the light of all the cells of a multicellular organism forms one light field that permeates and surrounds the organism. The maintenance of this light field occurs away from thermodynamic equilibrium. Because of its coherence, the photon field possesses a high degree of order and thus the property of structured matter, storing and transmitting information.[52] The fact that the biophoton emission of each organism reacts specifically to light stimulation is therefore unsurprising.[53]

Since the coherent biophoton field lies at the borderline with laser light, it is able to switch to and from either side of this distinction. It can alternate back and forth between a chaotic state and an ordered/coherent one. Bischof distinguishes two kinds of coherence: one is the opposite of chaos and the other a higher state of coherence that comprehends both these opposites (the chaotic and the ordered/coherent state) and regulates the switching between them.[54]

Popp demonstrated how the biophoton field is responsible for intercellular communication and also communication between organs and organ systems. He even believes that the exchange of information between animals, plants, and humans by means of the biophoton field may be possible. Biophoton fields thus have an organizing, regulatory and pattern-forming effect on organisms. From this could be concluded that atoms as well as cells and complex organisms are the result of coherent interactions of sunlight on the earth.[55]

Morphogenetic fields according to Sheldrake

In contrast to Goodwin's deterministic explanatory model, which sees shape as "given" for all time, Sheldrake sees a possibility of development in morphogenetic fields, which he conceives as having physical reality. However, he extends previous explanatory models in that he assumes these fields to be determined, not by mathematical or Platonic arguments, but by the actual shape of similar organisms of the past. This means that a shape that has come into being exerts a causal effect on all subsequent similar shapes (i.e., shape-giving causation, similar to Aristotelian formal causation).

What is shape? The material shape of a human individual develops, matures, renews, and maintains itself and is then destroyed again by death. The total amount of energy and matter in the world is not thereby changed; what might be said to have changed is the way in which this energy and matter in the world is organized.

"Shape" is material in the sense that the bone of a forearm, a fascia, or a muscle, for example, is material; however, shape in itself is not material. According to Rupert Sheldrake[56] the matter and energy of which things consist can be present in many different shape. Consequently it is not possible to explain shape simply in terms of material or energetic constituents. Shape, then, according to Sheldrake, exists on the one hand over and above the material components that give it its appearance, and on the other hand only finds expression as the organization of matter and energy. Sheldrake draws the conclusion that, for modern physics, matter consists of rhythmic processes, of bound and structured energy within fields.

In his hypothesis as to the causes responsible for the creation of shape, he takes the view that there is such a thing as "morphic resonance," based on similarities; that is, on the idea that the greater the similarity of an organism to previous organisms, the stronger the morphic resonance. Further, the more there were of such similar organisms in the past, the greater their cumulative influence. He stresses that this resonance does not depend on an energy transfer in the physical sense, but represents a non-energetic transfer of information. Morphic resonance is thus seen as operating quite independently of energy. The feature that it has in common with existing physical hypotheses is that both are based on rhythmic patterns. On every level of living organisms, we encounter rhythmic oscillations and cyclic and periodic motions.

Morphic resonance comes about when the patterns of rhythmic activity of structures resemble each other. This can influence subsequent structures and ensure that the future development of organisms occurs in continuity with the shape such organisms have already acquired. According to Sheldrake, this influence is not limited by place or diluted by distance in space or time. Sheldrake quotes experiments that support this assumption; for example, if rats anywhere in the world find their way out of a particular maze, other rats at any other place in the world find their way out of the same maze more quickly. Morphogenetic fields are therefore "probability structures, in which the influence of the most common past types combines to increase the probability that such types will occur again."[57] Nature therefore re-employs effective patterns and strategies (basic holons), once found, as building blocks in further stages of development – using them, however, in larger and more comprehensive contexts, so transcending the bounds of separateness. He sees these probability structures as being evidenced both in phylogenesis and ontogenesis.

Sheldrake's hypothesis does however give rise to certain objections:

1 It is questionable whether a cause that gives rise to the creation of shape and is claimed to influence energy and matter can in fact operate without any kind of energetic causation. This would at the very least contradict the laws hitherto known and accepted which govern the way in which shape and energy are linked.

2 Sheldrake denies that any archetypal potential given, or timeless and unchanging categories might be causatory factors in the creation of shape; instead he

expresses the view that all creation of shape can be traced to previous development and creative emergence. Wilber, however, points out that Sheldrake's model does contain certain archetypal *a priori* categories: energy is causally influenced by energy, and shape is causally influenced by shape; this is the essential meaning of development and creativity. He suggests that some unchanging deep structures do appear to exist archetypally, as it were, for this Cosmos. In contrast, specific surface structures are everywhere, distinctive, and developed.[58]

3 There needs at least to be some qualification of Sheldrake's concept of a cause for the creation of shape that is entirely independent of place, in that the majority of known examples of transmission of information occur in a manner that is bound to time and place.[59] The further investigation into this phenomenon suggested by Sheldrake could cast additional light.

4 Further discussion is needed as to whether morphic resonance as proposed by Sheldrake might not result in increased uniformity, in contrast to the greater variety encountered in nature.

5 Another point of criticism according to Cramer is that Sheldrake quotes no concrete conditions for the phenomenon he describes, and that his choice of an imposing name for his observed phenomenon might indeed impress the lay person, but does not actually explain anything.[60]

Finally, it should be noted that Sheldrake himself speaks of this hypothesis of the formgiving cause as not yet fully developed. At the same time he does try to encourage further, experimentally repeatable studies.[61]

The emergence of shape through vortex patterns according to Edwards[62]

The contemporary mathematician L. Edwards studied the development of shape mainly in association with vortex* patterns, extending his investigations into the development of embryological shape.[63] He sees the emergence of embryological shape as the perfect creation of a spiritual universe, which assumes shape according to the laws of mathematics.

He addressed among other issues the question as to what form the geometrical calculations might produce if the axis of the airy vortex lay asymmetrically in relation to the axis of the bud transformation of a plant bud. For this calculation he selected six airy vortices from a common field. Their common axis was placed parallel to the axis of the bud transformation, but shifted to one side. Taking the graphic representation of these calculations, and evaluating various cross-sections, produced a clear resemblance to the invagination process that takes place during the development of the mesoderm in the third week of gestation. Even when the parameters were varied, for example by moving the vortex or the orientation of the axes to each other, the result still resembled an embryonic form. These forms, viewed in sequence, are reminiscent of various stages of embryonic development.

By using a simple movement of a vortex, transformed by "egg transformation" (a certain set of mathematical calculations), it became possible, for example, to describe the general shape of a developing embryo. A certain positioning of the vortex (and of the resulting transformations) produced a remarkable similarity to the general form of a developing embryo. If these calculation models are applied to the uterus – which, like the egg and the flower bud, exhibits a good path curve form in the first weeks of pregnancy – a clear relationship or similarity is found between the biological reality (the shape of the actual stage of development of the embryo) and the geometric cross-sections obtained from certain calculation processes (Fig. 6.1).

Edwards postulates that the development of seeds and avian embryos can be traced to the shape of the bud and the egg (in the sense of an operative, active shaping force). Shape could then be demonstrated as an active force for (initial or subsequent) development by the general sequence of formative gestures in embryonic development, by means of these geometric transformation processes. In line with this thinking, Edwards tries to represent neural tube formation in geometric terms. A constant increase in the width of the vortex, as in graphic representations of neural tube formation, produces growth of the two sides toward each other until eventually they meet and fuse (Fig. 6.2).

---

*"Vortex" refers to a flowing eddy that draws in energy as an effect of the vacuum generated at its center.

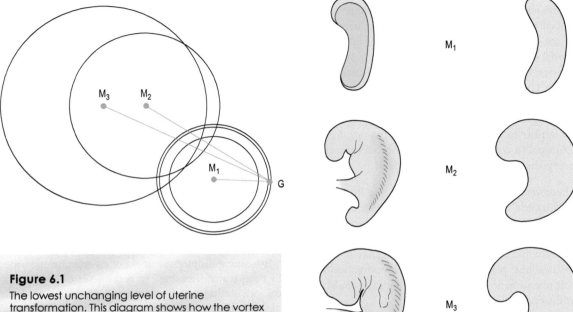

Figure 6.1

The lowest unchanging level of uterine transformation. This diagram shows how the vortex must intersect to produce the main formative gesture of the developing embryo. The double circle shows the widest part of the uterus, the typical point of implantation for the ovum (point G in the wall of the uterus). The vortex striking upwards from below with its axis turning like a simple cone centered on point G.

The rest of this diagram shows the horizontal plane through the pointed end of the uterus. Successive points at which the vortex axis will cut this bottom invariant plane of the uterus transformation are represented by M1, M2, and M3. The first position of the vortex (M1) (form of the very early embryo) will have its axis very close to the pointed end of the uterus itself.[63]

Figure 6.2

(A) Embryonic development. (B) Cross-sections produced from the tendencies of the vortex, as presented in Figure 6.1. M1 on the left: very early embryo with amniotic sac. M2 on the left: 24-somite embryo (28 days). M3 on the left: 37-day embryo.[63]

The widest vortex produces a shape that achieves the closing of the tube. All that is needed to produce this remarkable transformation geometrically is to have an airy vortex (transformed by uterus transformation, i.e., the increased curvature of the uterus at the beginning of pregnancy) increase its radius.

Another possible way of achieving this result (with minor deviations) would be to retain the same radius and move the vortex, from above to below, from below to above, or inward from both sides.

In order to convert the process of neural tube closure (beginning at the middle and proceeding cranially and caudally) into geometric terms, we need to think of two vortices approaching each other from opposite directions: from above to below and from below to above, or inward from right and left. The process of neural tube closure according to Edwards could be interpreted metaphorically as follows: the first vortex from the past, the second from the future; or, the first vortex communicating the unconscious element of our being and the second, the conscious.

The golden section

The golden section, golden mean, or golden ratio is a principle of dynamic of spatial arrangement describing

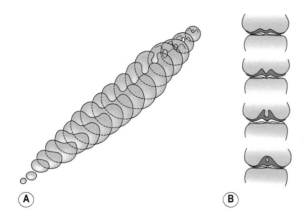

Figure 6.3

(A) Cross-section of particular vortices, arranged one behind the other. (B) Diagram of neural tube formation.

a constant principle of division or ratio of the whole and the part. György Doczi defines it as the proportion whereby the smaller part stands in the same ratio to the larger part as the larger part does to the whole; this is expressed by the formula A:B = B:(A+B)[64]

The principle that becomes evident here is the one that determines the Fibonacci numbers: 1, 2, 3, 5, 8, 13, 21, 34, 55, etc. The quotient of adjacent elements is close to 1.618... (the golden ratio or golden section).[65]

This ratio is the most irrational of all irrational numbers, which can be described only by approximation as an infinite number. It is a unique ratio, since there is only one point on any line that divides it into the two unequal parts, which stand in that unique ratio to each other.[66]

This division proportion ensures that the whole always continues to resonate in the part, so that it remains present and effective. "The force of the golden section to create harmony stems from its unique capacity to combine different parts into a whole in such a way that every part maintains its identity and is at the same time subsumed without remainder into a greater whole."[67] As an example of this, in the variety of the human anatomy there is an astonishing correspondence in the size ratios of various bones in males and females.[68]

These harmonious ratios exist in the measurements of the human body and are repeated in those of individual limbs. Thus the hand is a kind of microcosm that reflects the macrocosm of the body.[69] Even in the gravitational resonance of the planets in our solar system, we see the golden ratio.[70]

For Cramer, the golden ratio is a kind of harmony at the border between order and chaos, the expression of which could correspond to the subjective perception of beauty: beauty, typified by that fine line between order and chaos, or in that border region where "a dynamic system is just able to avoid chaos."[71] This comes into being as it were in dynamics hovering in that transitional region between the dissolution of all order into chaos and solidification into symmetry and order.[72]

Cramer further says that structures built according to the golden ratio have the best chance of survival if they are disrupted. They can resist the incursions of chaos for longest.[73] They are located at the ideal fulcrum between rigidity and openness, between the individual and the infinite, between unity and multiplicity, and between dissolution and solidification.

Is it not the goal of all osteopathic treatment to bring the body as a whole into contact with this fulcrum by whatever means?

Summary

The properties of morphogenetic fields, electrodynamic, biophoton, and other such fields, offer some possible explanations for the effects and origins of somatic dysfunctions as well as the way in which osteopathic treatments work on the body as a whole. Whether and in what way these aspects are consciously incorporated into osteopathic treatment remains a highly individual matter; to date they feature only here and there in the normal teaching curriculum. Some osteopaths claim to be able to perceive some aspects of these field phenomena. At present it is only individual experiences that are taught.[74-76] Systematic investigations and studies of these phenomena in association with osteopathic treatment methods are needed.

Closing remarks

The form of the Cosmos is that of a process, whose time modus varies continuously. The world in which we live is one of continuing creation, in which structures are constantly coming into being and passing away. Structure-forming, cyclic passages of time, rhythms, oscillations, and reversible processes act to maintain the system. Cramer nevertheless remarks that all this is in reality simply biding time, each system circulating for just so long as it is current, until it reaches the point of chaos.[77] This must happen, because although these cyclic passages of time can remain stable for a long time, sooner or later perturbations and their own inner incongruities make them unstable. Symmetry is broken, and all cyclic motion, wave motion, or oscillation enters a state of spatial and temporal discontinuity; something new emerges, only to a limited extent predictable. This course is neither reversible nor repeatable, and expresses the uniqueness of every living being.

Matter, including macroscopic matter, is always made up of frequency, rhythmicity, and waves. According to Cramer, depending on the way in which we approach it, we encounter matter either by striking against it (as a corpuscle) or by oscillating along with it (as a wave). Matter in that latter sense is therefore capable of resonance and can interact with other matter by resonance of waves.[78] According to Cramer, then, even non-biological matter is in some degree living.

The ability of osteopathy as a resonance therapy to work in a regulatory manner upon homeostasis in the body as a whole is surely not a privilege reserved to it alone, since resonance is in a sense the form of interaction as such by which all space–time structures are able to make a connection with each other.[79] Over the years that it has been in existence, osteopathy has however developed a great variety of different manual treatment methods that take account of both the corpuscle and the wave character present in tissue. These methods are able to exert a regulatory effect on order. Their holistic character emerges from a deep understanding of the dialectic interaction and functional relationship between order and chaos, health and the symptoms of disease. Seen in this light, the patient's symptoms and somatic dysfunction can be viewed as a chaotic situation; a phase of instability, which can potentially stabilize into new, higher patterns of order or alternatively lead to regression and a tendency to dissolution (in which the higher is subsumed into the lower) in the patient. The boundaries of osteopathic action apply in cases where regulatory methods are no longer able to turn around a tendency to dissolution (regression); that is, when this cannot be achieved without massive invasive medical intervention.

The world of phenomena that surrounds us, which of course includes the body tissues that we touch in our work as osteopaths, are not rigid and "set" but rather temporary phenomena, the expression of circumstances and forces interacting one with another. Everything depends on an endless multiplicity of dependencies and other factors.

It could be helpful for the further development and extension of experience-oriented diagnostic and therapeutic processes in osteopathy to draw on methods that seek to understand these determining factors; this would include both systematic, rational methods and also mystic methods of perception and comprehension. We should bear in mind that the field properties discussed in this chapter are only the external, objectifiable dimension of individuals' existence in the world, and are inseparably linked with inner, subjective, and intersubjective dimensions as well as external, collective (i.e., social) ones.

Technical skill is important. Nevertheless, we should avoid limiting healing potential by excessive focus on technical performance.

Healing is not simply a one-way process directed from the practitioner to the patient. The conscious participation of all concerned in the healing process also seems to be extremely important, as is an empathetic insight into the way that symptoms are related and into the interlinked mutual relationship and evolutionary dynamics of all life forms.

References

[1]Schauenberger V: Nature as teacher. Bath: Gateway Books; 1998:9.

[2]Maturana HR, Varela FJ: Der Baum der Erkenntnis. Die biologischen Wurzeln menschlichen Erkennens. Bern: Goldmann/Scherzverlag; 1987:53.

[3]Jantsch E: Die Selbstorganisation des Universums. Munich: Hanser; 1992:75.

[4]Jantsch E: Die Selbstorganisation des Universums. Munich: Hanser; 1992:64.

[5]Burr HS: Blueprint of Immortality. 5th edn. Essex: Saffron Walden; 1991:114.

[6]Davis W: Energetics and Therapeutic Touch. In: Heller M (ed.): The flesh of the soul: the body we work with: Selected papers of the 7th Congress of the European

Association of Body Psychotherapy, 2–6 September 2001, 59.

[7]Gurwitsch A: Die Vererbung als Verwirklichungsvorgang. Biol. Centralblatt. 1912;32:458–486.

[8]Gurwitsch A: Über den Begriff des embryonalen Feldes. Arch. Entwicklungsmech. Org. 1922;51:383–415.

[9]Gurwitsch A: Über Determination, Normierung und Zufall in der Ontogenese. Arch. Entwicklungsmech. Org. 1910;30:133–193.

[10]Spemann H: Die Erzeugung tierischer Chimären durch heteroplastische embryonale Transplantation zwischen Triton cristatus u. taeniatus. Arch. Entwicklungsmech. Org. 1921;48:533–570.

[11]Weiss P: Principles of development. New York; Holt; 1939.

[12]Thompson D'Arcy W: On Growth and Form. London: Cambridge University Press; 1961.

[13]Thom R: Structural stability and morphogenesis. Massachusetts: W.A. Benjamin; 1975.

[14]Waddington CH: Fields and gradients. In: Locke M: Major problems in developmental biology. New York: Academic Press; 1966:105–124.

[15]Wilber, K. Sheldrake's theory of morphogenesis. *Journal of Humanistic Psychology*, 1984 24 (2)1

[16]Goodwin BC: What are the causes of morphogenesis? Bioessays. 1985;3(1):32–36.

[17]Becker RO. Cross Currents. The Promise of Electromedicine, the Perils of Electropollution. Torcher, Los Angeles 1990.

[18]Adey W, Lawrence A: Nonlinear Electrodynamics in biological systems. New York: Plenum Press; 1984.

[19]Burr HS: Blueprint of Immortality. 5th edn. Essex: Saffron Walden; 1991:49.

[20]Stroink G: Principles of cardiomagnetism, Advances in Biomagnetism (ed. Williamson, et al.) New York: Plenum Press;1989:47–57.

[21]Oschman J: Readings on the scientific basis of bodywork energetic and movement therapies. Dover; 1997.

[22]Burr HS: Blueprint of Immortality. 5th edn. Essex: Saffron Walden; 1991:33.

[23]Ferrier J, Ross SM, Kanehisa J, Aubin JE: Osteoclasts and osteoblasts migrate in opposite directions in response to a constant electrical field. J. Cell Physiol. 1986; 129(3):283–288.

[24]Meggs WJ: Enhanced polymerization of polar macromolecules by an applied electric field with application to mitosis. J. Theor. Biol. 1990;145(2):245–255.

[25]Goodman R, Bassett CA, Henderson AC: Pulsing electromagnetic fields induce cellular transcription. Science. 1983;220:1283–1285.

[26]Mohamed-Ali H, Scheller M, Hetscher J, et al.: Action of a high frequency magnetic field on the cartilage matrix in vitro. Bioelectrochemistry and Bioenerget. 1995;37:25–29.

[27]Becker RO: Cross currents, the perils of electropollution, the promise of electromedicine. New York: Jeremy P. Tarcher/Putnam; 1990.

[28]Barr F: Melanin – The organizing molecule. Medical hypotheses. 1983;11:111–140.

[29] Bischof M: Biophotonen. Das Licht in unseren Zellen. Frankfurt: Zweitausendeins; 1995.

[30]Popp FA: Neue Horizonte in der Medizin. Heidelberg: Haug; 1987.

[31]Bischof M: Biophotonen. Das Licht in unseren Zellen. Frankfurt: Zweitausendeins; 1995.

[32]Bischof M: Biophotonen. Das Licht in unseren Zellen. Frankfurt: Zweitausendeins; 1995.

[33]Bischof M: Biophotonen. Das Licht in unseren Zellen. Frankfurt: Zweitausendeins; 1995.

[34]Smith J: The influence of Enzyme growth by the "laying-on-of hands". Academy of Parapsychology and Medicine, Dimensions of Healing Symoposium proceedings, Los Altos, California; 1972.

[35]Zimmermann J: Laying-on-of-hands healing and therapeutic touch: A testable theory. BEMI currents. J. Bio-Electro-Magnetics Institute. 1990;2:9–17.

[36]Seto A, Kusaka C, Nakasato S, et al: Detection of extraordinarily large bio-magnetic field strength from human hand. Acupuncture and Electro-Therapeutics Research International Journal. 1992;17:75–94.

[37]Muesham D, Markov M, Muesham P, et al.: Effects of QiGong on cell free myosin phosphorylation: preliminary experiments. Subtle Energies. 1994;5:93–108.

[38]Miller RN, Reinhart PB, Kern A: In: Kinnear W (ed.): Thought as energy. Los Angeles, California: Science of Mind Publications; 1972.

[39]Pickler EC: Early impressions of Dr. Still. JAOA. 1921;5:244.

[40]Popp FA: Biophotonen. Heidelberg: Verlag für Medizin. Dr. Ewald Fischer; 1976.

[41]Beschreibung des Internationalen Instituts für Biophysik, Neuss, 2002.

[42]Popp FA: Biologie des Lichts. Grundlagen der ultraschwachen Zellstrahlung. Berlin: Parey; 1984. Popp FA: Biophotonen. Ein neuer Weg zur Lösung des Krebsgeschehens. Schriftenreihe Krebsgeschehen, vol. 6, 2nd edn. Fischer, Heidelberg 1984.

[43]Gurwitsch AG: The mitogenic rays. Bot. Gaz. 1925; 80:224–226.

[44]Popp FA, Ruth B, Bahr W, et al.: Emission of visible and ultraviolet radiation by active biological systems. Collective Phenomena. 1981;3:187–214.

[45]Van Wijk R, van Aken H, Mei W, et al.: Light-induced photon emission by mammalian cells. J. Photochem. Photobiol. 1993b;18(1):75–79.

[46]Hameroff SR, Smith SA, Watt RC: Nonlinear electrodynamics in cytoskeletal protein lattices. In: Adey WR, Lawrence AF (ed.): Nonlinear electrodynamics in biological systems; 1984.

[47]Galle M, Neurohr R, Altmann G, et al.: Biophoton emission from Daphnia magna: a possible factor in the self-regulation of swarming. Experimentia. 1991;47:457–460.

[48]Niggli HJ, Scaletta C, Yu Y, et al.: Ultraweak photon emission in assessing bone growth factor efficiency using fibroblastic differentiation. J. Photochem. Photobiol. 2001;64(1):62–68.

[49]Popp FA, Nagl W, Li KH, et al.: Biophoton emission. New evidence for coherence and DNA as source. Cell. Biophys. 1984;6(1):33–52.

[50]Gu Q, Popp FA: Nonlinear response of biophoton emission to external perturbations. Experientia 1. 1992;48:1069–1082.

[51]Popp FA, Nagl W, Li KH, et al.: Biophoton emission. New evidence for coherence and DNA as source. Cell. Biophys. 1984;6(1):33–52.

[52]Bischof M: Somatische Intelligenz. Homo Integralis-Zeitschrift für Integrales Bewusstsein und die Zukunft des Menschen. 1999;3:27–38.

[53]Musumeci F, Scordino A, Triglia A: Delayed luminescence from simple biological systems. Rivista di Biologia. 1997;90:95–110.

[54]Bischof M: Somatische Intelligenz. Homo Integralis-Zeitschrift für Integrales Bewusstsein und die Zukunft des Menschen. 1999;3:27–38.

[55]Bischof M: Biophotonen. Das Licht in Unseren Zellen. Frankfurt: Zweitausendeins; 1995.

[56]Sheldrake R: Morphic resonance and the habits of nature. London: Collins; 1988.

[57]Sheldrake R: Morphic resonance and the habits of nature. London: Collins; 1988:109.

[58]Wilber, K. Sheldrake's theory of morphogenesis. Journal of Humanistic Psychology, 1984 24 (2)1

[59]Wilber, K. Sheldrake's theory of morphogenesis. Journal of Humanistic Psychology, 1984 24 (2)1

[60]Cramer F: Symphonie des Lebendigen. Frankfurt am Main: Insel; 1996:14,19,30,205.

[61]Zänker KS: Zellkommunikation und die Theorie morphischer Felder. In: Dürr HP, Gottwald FT: Rupert Sheldrake in der Diskussion. Bern: Scherz; 1997:65.

[62]Edwards L: Vortex of life. Edinburgh: Floris books; 1993:168–202.

[63]Edwards L: Vortex of life. Edinburgh: Floris books; 1993:168–202.

[64]Doczi G: Die Kraft der Grenzen. 6th edn. Stuttgart: Engel & Co; 2005:14,27,119.

[65]Cramer F: Chaos und Ordnung – Die komplexe Struktur des Lebendigen. Frankfurt am Main: Insel; 1993:201,205f.

[66]Doczi G: Die Kraft der Grenzen. 6th edn. Stuttgart: Engel & Co; 2005:14,27,119.

[67]Doczi G: Die Kraft der Grenzen. 6th edn. Stuttgart: Engel & Co; 2005:27.

[68]Doczi G: Die Kraft der Grenzen. 6th edn. Stuttgart: Engel & Co; 2005:27.

[69]Doczi G: Die Kraft der Grenzen. 6th edn. Stuttgart: Engel & Co; 2005:14,27,119.

[70]Cramer F: Symphonie des Lebendigen. Frankfurt am Main: Insel; 1996:14,19,30,205.

[71]Cramer F: Chaos und Ordnung – Die komplexe Struktur des Lebendigen. Frankfurt am Main: Insel; 1993:202.

[72]Cramer F: Symphonie des Lebendigen. Frankfurt am Main: Insel; 1996:14,19,30,205.

[73]Cramer F: Symphonie des Lebendigen. Frankfurt am Main: Insel; 1996:14,19,30,205.

[74]Fulford R: Liem's course notes; 1994.

[75]Jealous J, Jealous J: Liem's course notes 1996 to 2001; 2004.

[76]Liem T: Kraniosakrale Osteopathie. 3rd edn. Stuttgart: Hippokrates; 1998.

[77]Cramer F: Symphonie des Lebendigen. Frankfurt am Main: Insel; 1996:14,19,30,205.

[78]Cramer F: Symphonie des Lebendigen. Frankfurt am Main: Insel; 1996:32.

[79]Cramer F: Symphonie des Lebendigen. Frankfurt am Main: Insel; 1996:14,19,30,205.

7

Regulative forces in embryology

Torsten Liem

…differentiation is an undivided biodynamic process that occurs during development…

E. Blechschmidt[1]

…According to its own rhythm (sequence of processes) and its own type (juxtaposition of parts) the organic life-process builds for itself the body from substances that it absorbs from the world outside.

K.E. von Baer, 1864

Introduction

In phylogenetic and ontogenetic terms the system or the organism is characterized by a particular type of organization. This determines a particular type of exchange, of uptake and breakdown of information, energy, and matter with the outside world. The phylogenetic organizational patterns form preferences for specific patterns of change in the periphery (see pp. 9f., 97) or in the environment surrounding the organism at specific time points in ontogenesis.

Ontogenetically, in line with the surrounding environment, particular individual structural formations become possible. Bacteria, for example, invariably express certain receptors on their surrounding membrane, while other receptors are present only when the environment around them possesses specific qualities.[2] Developmental steps within ontogenesis are dependent upon previous organizational stages in the framework of ontogenesis. Thus, each previous developmental step also has a structure-determining effect for the subsequent developmental stage. Each subsequent developmental construct evolves from the previous one. In this sense, life unfolds by interacting and coming to terms with the surrounding environment. Genetic organization and information can be understood only as part of these dynamics and cannot be considered in isolation from them.

Genomes are factors that – together with other nongenetic factors – determine which structures may develop, but not at what point in time or where. It is not merely the activation or inhibition of genes that is a decisive process for the development and function of a cell, but also the coupling of this process to morphogenetic fields. These morphogenetic fields appear to function as mediators between genotype and phenotype. Just as the cell (and not its genome) works as the unit of organic structure and function, so the morphogenetic field (and not the genes or the cells) is seen as a major unit of ontogeny whose changes bring about changes in evolution.[3]

To date, little is known concerning the interaction between genes and morphogenetic fields. Additional reference to scientific theories of complexity and nonlinear dynamics is essential to drive forward the exploration of constraints at the level of genetic networks and of morphogenesis.[4] The location as well as the timing of structure formation is dependent on these fields. There is feedback with the organism as a whole and with the developmental state of the organism.

Blastomeres of the zygote (1–8 cells) possess all the developmental potential of the organism as a whole and are therefore also referred to as omnipotent or totipotent cells. A whole embryo can still develop from them. Cells of the morula (8–32 cells) are termed pluripotent because they are still able to differentiate into different cell types. Differentiation into the trophoblast and the embryoblast takes place in the blastocyst (64–200 cells). The embryoblast cells are pluripotent. With the appearance of the primary germ layers the cells are then only multipotent. They can develop into cell types of the different tissues but no longer into cell types of other organ systems. Later some cells (for example, in the bone marrow, skin, olfactory and intestinal epithelium, and brain) retain these multipotent characteristics. These are termed somatic stem cells.

In the blastula stage and the earliest gastrula stage a tissue that has been transplanted from one region to another or even to another embryo will develop in line with its new surroundings. By contrast, transplantation at a later stage after embryonic determination results in the tissue developing in line with its origins, i.e., cells transplanted from an arm bud to the head will lead to the formation of an arm in the head region.[5]

While chemical morphogens have not been found, nonlinear vector fields are assumed to be the cause of these processes. The behavior of the tissues in this respect is consistent with that of liquid crystalline structures.[6]

Liquid crystalline properties of living organisms

Living systems not only *behave* like liquid crystals but may also be regarded as such. According to Ho,[7] the key to the long-term memory of living organization resides in the physicochemical properties of living matter, and these properties are formed, in particular, by the liquid crystalline structures of living matter. The liquid crystalline state is inherent in all the major constituents of living matter: lipids of cellular membranes, DNA, and all proteins, e.g., cytoskeletal proteins, muscle proteins, etc.

The liquid crystalline phase is a state of matter that is in between solid and liquid; hence, it is termed a mesophase. Unlike those in true liquids, the molecules in liquid crystals are aligned in a certain direction, and unlike true crystals, liquid crystals are flexible, malleable, and responsive. There are different kinds of liquid crystals: some are more like liquids while others more closely resemble solids. Unlike mineral crystals, however, the more solid liquid crystals are quite dynamic, and they depend on energy input.[8]

According to Ho, the liquid crystalline structure of living matter is responsible for axis formation during embryonic development. The major polarizing axis is the anterior–posterior axis. This is the main axis of molecular orientation for the entire organism.

Ho and co-workers have mapped the early embryonic organizational patterns of the fruit fly, and recorded the periodicities of these patterns. They found that the full body pattern becomes progressively determined over the course of two hours. It is suspected that electrodynamic forces are involved in the patterning of liquid crystalline structures.[9]

Influence of electromagnetic fields

Burr assigned to "electrodynamic fields" a key role in the organization of body structures, and in the control of the growth and morphogenesis of living creatures. Having identified the axis with the highest voltage gradient in a frog's egg and an unfertilized salamander egg, Burr was able to detect the future direction of growth of the nervous system.[10] However, the frog's egg should not be taken as a representative example for the development of symmetry in higher animals and humans.

Extremely weak pulsing electromagnetic fields are able to induce gene transcription.[11] Thus it has been demonstrated that electrical fields can reactivate old genome sections no longer utilized by evolution. A "primeval" form that had become extinct 100 years before was hatched from the eggs of farmed rainbow trout that had been exposed to a weak electrical field.[12] Exposure of early *Drosophila* embryos to weak, static magnetic fields during the period when cryptic pattern determination processes are taking place resulted in characteristic body pattern abnormalities in larvae hatching 24 hours later.[13] Profuse electrical signals have been recorded from fruit fly embryos during the earliest stages of development.

Influence of light

Certain frequencies of UV light that is emitted from dividing cells have a stimulatory effect on the division of other cells. Despite the many differences between morphogenesis and biophoton emission, these two groups of events share the properties of non-additivity, delocalization, self-focusing, and several others that are related to field phenomena. To a large extent, the field properties of the biological systems are associated with a set of oscillations of different time periods.[14]

Influence of tension fields

Blechschmidt had already postulated that positional development determines development of shape and this in turn determines structural development. In his view, the submicroscopic components of these processes are movements, known as metabolic movements, with chemical, physical, and morphological characteristics. Metabolic movements of particles that are ordered submicroscopically are contained in metabolic fields. The movements of particles in these fields always occur against resistance on the part of their surroundings and therefore, according to Blechschmidt, represent real work in a physical sense: a performance or an achievement specific to the individual.[15] He consequently regards cell aggregates and organs as locally modified force fields. The growth processes are based on precisely coordinated, inductive interactions of the tissues involved.

The formation of the gut, nervous system or sensory organs is associated with an ordered folding of epithelial tissue. Tension fields or mechanical tensions of the morphogenetically active epithelia are responsible for the fact that constant structures are sustained over lengthy embryological development periods. Experimental modification of these fields, e.g., a reduction in tension, results in chaotic morphogenesis. In contrast, a directed tension leads to correction.[16]

Beloussov has formulated a hypothesis in which he postulates self-regulation of the process of morphogenesis. Biomechanical feedback between patterns that actively generate mechanical stress and passive stress, such as stretching and/or compression, results in an initially exaggerated response by embryonic tissues.[17,18] He has hypothesized that the embryonic development periods represent a succession of mutually linked hyper-restoration responses. Embryonic tissue that has been taken out of its original state due to external mechanical force is thought to overreact initially as it attempts to return to its original state. When tissue is tensed, over-relaxation therefore takes place to begin with as the tissue overreacts to stretching initially in the form of compression.[19] Ventral ectodermal explants taken from *Xenopus laevis* embryos during early gastrulation were artificially stretched by Beloussov and co-workers, either using two opposite concentrated forces or using a distributed force that was applied to the inner layer of the explant. These modes of stretching reflect different mechanical situations that occur during normal development. Two main types of mechanical response to the applied tensions were recorded. Initially, after 15 minutes, a substantial proportion of the explant cells exhibited a concerted movement toward the closest point of the applied stretching force (i.e., tensotaxis). Later, in response to both concentrated and distributed stretching, there was a re-orientation of the trajectories of most cells perpendicular to the stretching force. The cells started to intercalate between each other, both horizontally and vertically. This was accompanied by extensive elongation of the outer ectodermal cells and by reconstruction of cell–cell contacts. The intercalation

movement led first to a considerable reduction in the stretch-induced tension and then to the formation of peculiar bipolar "embryoid" shapes. The type and intensity of the morphomechanical responses did not depend on the orientation of the stretching force in relation to the embryonic axis.[20] Using a polarizing microscope to study *Drosophila* embryos, Ho and co-workers were able to interpret their molecular structures and also to follow the dynamic processes within the living organism. They were even able to discern traces of the pre-patterning of the body plan.[20] The most dramatic changes were seen in the embryos shortly before they hatched (Box 7.1).

Blastula stage

The account that follows is based largely on Bischof's description of the formation of the embryo.[21] Research indicates that the crucial organizing principle in the early embryogenesis of *Drosophila* is based less on particular local interactions and more on global field

---

Box 7.1

Causes of growth movements[1]

- Electromagnetic fields (induction of gene transcription/effect on liquid crystals)

- UV light frequencies (stimulation of cell division)

- Contact guidance

- Contact inhibition

- Chemotactic mechanisms and recognition molecules

- Formation of glial or connective tissue guiding structures (nerves, myoblasts)

- Genetic information

- Sheldrake's theory of morphogenetic fields?

---

[1]According to Liebermann-Meffert, modified by Liem.

mechanisms.[22] Goodwin has further established that in the blastula stage development is characterized by a typical pattern that appears to follow mathematical laws and points to underlying harmonic laws. Bischof additionally concludes that the phenomena in question must be electromagnetic fields.

Cleavage of the ovum begins with indentation along specific lines. These lines may be understood as cell division lines of least resistance.

The cleavage planes are constant, independent of the size of the sphere. Thus, according to Bischof, the harmonic functions have holographic properties. A function of one part of the sphere can be restored by any other part of the sphere, in line with the property of an embryo in the blastula stage. All forms of a living organism have their cause in the field properties of living states. According to Bischof, Popp had already explained the mitotic spindle during cell division in terms of the structure of the field.

The further dynamics of the cleavage process in the blastula stage are, according to Goodwin, determined by the dialectic between surface fields and fields in the cell interior. As a result the cell organelles are brought into a specific arrangement during cell division. The fields in the cell interior activate the surface fields that in turn trigger cell division along certain nodal lines. The divided cells then call forth a new field in the cell interior, which produces a new surface field. This process essentially repeats itself as it unfolds in a systematically altered context. Bischof describes this process as non-linear.

Transition to the gastrula stage

Here we are dealing with the transition from a hollow cell ball to an initially bi-layered and then tri-layered structure (germ layers). This happens as a result of an inward folding of the cells. According to Goodwin, the replacement of the cleavage field by a new field in gastrulation happens due to the increasing destruction of order resulting from a frequency increase of the surface field and an increase in incoherence due to progressive cell division. The new field is associated with the formation of a polarizing anterior–posterior longitudinal axis.

Bischof describes the subsequent process as the formation of partial fields. This is also characterized by the increasing specialization of the cells, in the course of which they lose their omnipotence. The cells no longer merely submit to the differentiation tendency of their surroundings or to the field of the organism as a whole but they develop an active field of their own within them. However, because of bias in successive symmetry-breaking events, the dynamic coupling between the different mechanisms involved in development appears to restrict or reduce the choices available to the system.[23]

Jaeger and Goodwin[24,25] have described an oscillatory process within cells which functions as a developmental clock whose periods are tightly regulated by cell-autonomous and non-autonomous mechanisms. A spatial pattern is generated as a result of an initial temporal ordering of the cell oscillators freezing into spatial order as the clocks slow down and stop at different times or phases in their cycles.

When applied to vertebrate somitogenesis, this means that the cellular oscillator model is able to reproduce the dynamics of periodic gene expression patterns observed in the presomitic mesoderm. Different somite lengths can thus be generated by altering the period of the oscillation. There is evidence to suggest that the dynamic principles of sequential segmentation might be equivalent throughout the animal kingdom.

References

[1]Blechschmidt E, Gasser RF. Biokinetics and Biodynamics of Human Differentiation. Springfield, Illinois: Charles C. Thomas; 1978:xiii.

[2]Koshland DE Jnr. Bacterial chemotaxis in relation to neurobiology. Ann Rev Neurosci 1980;3:43–75.

[3]Gilbert SF, Opitz JM, Raff RA. Resynthesizing evolutionary and developmental biology. Dev Biol 1996;173:357–72.

[4]Goodwin BC. The life of form. Emergent patterns of morphological transformation. CR Acad Sci III 2000;323:15–21.

[5]Harrison RG. Experiments on the development of the fore limb of Amblystoma, a self-differentiating equipotent system. J Exp Zool 1918;25:413–461.

[6]Ho MW. The Rainbow and the Worm. 2nd edn. Singapore: World Scientific Publishing Co.; 1998.

[7]Ho MW. The Rainbow and the Worm. 2nd edn. Singapore: World Scientific Publishing Co.; 1998:170.

[8]Ho MW. The Rainbow and the Worm. 2nd edn. Singapore: World Scientific Publishing Co.; 1998:177.

[9]Ho MW. The Rainbow and the Worm. 2nd edn. Singapore: World Scientific Publishing Co.; 1998:181.

[10]Burr HS. Blueprint for Immortality. 5th edn. Saffron Walden: CW Daniel; 1991:61.

[11]Goodman R, Bassett CA, Henderson AS. Pulsing electromagnetic fields induce cellular transcription. Science 1983;220:1283–1285.

[12]Ciba-Geigy AG. Verbessertes Fischzuchtverhalten. Patent EP 0351.357;1989.

[13]Ho MW, Ross S, Bolton H, Popp FA, Li XX. Electrodynamic activities and their role in the organization of body pattern. Journal of Scientific Exploration 1992;6:59–77.

[14]Beloussov LV. Morphogenetic fields: outlining the alternatives and enlarging the context. Riv Biol 2001;94:219–35.

[15]Blechschmidt E. The Ontogenetic Basis of Human Anatomy. Berkeley, California: North Atlantic Books; 2004:62.

[16]Beloussov LV. The dynamic architecture of a developing organism. Dordrecht: Kluwer Academic Publishers; 1998.

[17]Beloussov LV, Kazakova NI, Luchinskaia NN, Novoselov VV. Studies in developmental cytomechanic. Int J Dev Biol 1997;41:793–799.

[18]Beloussov LV, Luchinskaia NN. Biomechanical feedback in morphogenesis, as exemplified by stretch responses of amphibian embryonic tissues. Biochem Cell Biol 1995;73:555–563.

[19]Beloussov LV, Luchinskaia NN, Stein AA. Tension-dependent collective cell movements in the early gastrula ectoderm of *Xenopus laevis* embryos. Dev Genes Evol 2000;210:92–104.

[20]Ho MW. The Rainbow and the Worm. 2nd edn. Singapore: World Scientific Publishing Co.; 1998:165.

[21]Bischof M. Biophotonen. Das Licht in unseren Zellen. Frankfurt: Zweitausendeins;1995:240 ff.

[22]Hunding A, Kauffman SA, Goodwin BC. *Drosophila* segmentation: supercomputer simulation of prepattern hierarchy. J Theor Biol 1990;145:369–384.

[23]Goodwin BC, Kauffman S, Murray JD. Is morphogenesis an intrinsically robust process? J Theor Biol 1993;163:135–144.

[24]Jaeger J, Goodwin BC. Cellular oscillators in animal segmentation. In Silico Biol 2002;2:111–123.

[25]Jaeger J, Goodwin BC. A cellular oscillator model for periodic pattern formation. J Theor Biol 2001;213:171–181.

8

Role of mechanical stresses in embryonic development

Lev V. Beloussov

Introduction

At any of its stages, embryonic development of all the animal organisms (and human beings) is associated with extensive and highly ordered movements of their constituent parts. These may be components of an egg cytoplasm (which start to change their positions immediately after fertilization), the individual cells of an early embryo (which can rotate and shift in respect to each other) or, at the more advanced stages, the entire embryonic layers consisting of no fewer than several hundred cells. In this review, we will deal mostly with this last category of morphogenetic movements. These may be roughly divided into two categories. The first category is a rearrangement of freely moving cells that can easily exchange their cell neighbors. This is exemplified by a cell intercalation, that is, the insertion of single cells and entire cell rows between each other.[1] One of the most important embryonic structures, the notochord, which creates the main body axis in all of the vertebrate animals, is built in this way. The second category corresponds to the changes in geometry of embryonic layers that consist of a large number of tightly connected cells. The layers can, in a highly precise way, change their curvatures by creating tubes, pockets, vesicles, and so on. Virtually all the organs of vertebrate animals and human beings (e.g., a gut with all of its derivatives, a central nervous system, sensory organs, etc.) are formed in this way.

While performing any of the above movements, embryonic cells overcome certain mechanical resistances and, therefore, produce mechanical work. In several cases it was possible to measure this, e.g., an amphibian embryo, during the formation of a neural tube (a rudiment of the central nervous system), wastes 8×10^{-3} erg of mechanical energy and overcomes a resisting force of about 4×10^{-7} N. At first glance, this force is very small. However, dividing it over the area onto which it is applied (which is also very small) we get values ranging between 10^2 and 10^4 N/m^2. For comparison, the pressure applied by a skier to snow is about 10^3 N/m^2 (see Beloussov[2] for more details).

The ratio of a force to the area to which it is applied is called the mechanical stress. In mechanics three main kinds of stresses are distinguished: tensile stresses (generated by stretching a body), pressure stresses (generated by its compression), and shear stresses (caused by the shift of the body parts in opposite directions). The bodies that maintain (do not relax) measurable stresses during short periods after force application are called elastic, while those immediately relaxing the stresses are qualified as plastic. Correspondingly, elastic bodies, contrary to the plastic ones, maintain what is called the residual stresses.

Shape-forming capacities of the elastic and plastic bodies are quite different. While plastic bodies (such as a piece of a plasticine) can take and maintain any shape imposed by external forces for an indefinite time period, elastic ones possess a much more restricted set of shapes which, to a great extent, depend upon the initial geometry of a body. As a rule, these shapes are quite regular and may be rather complicated, even if the acting force is homogeneously applied (Figure 8.1). Another property of elastic bodies is that while being stretched in one direction, they become compressed perpendicularly (so-called Poisson's deformation). In this way a single tension force produces an orthogonal deformation pattern. Also, elastic bodies, contrary to plastic ones, have a property that can be qualified as "holistic": a deformation of any part of such a body will be perceived, due to elastic stresses, by all the other parts. Thus, it would be strange, if a living body, during its evolution, did not select such simple and effective tools for making precise shapes.

However, until recently only a few authors (among them D'Arcy Thompson)[4] paid any serious interest to the mechanical properties of developing organisms. For

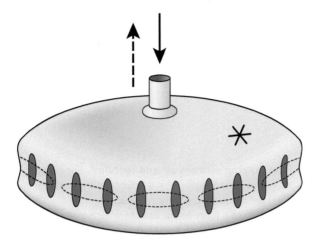

Figure 8.1

Inflation (solid arrow) of a flattened balloon generates on its surface a series of vertical folds, while its deflation (dotted arrow) produces a series of horizontal folds. In each case, the number of folds is quite precise and depends upon the balloon's geometry. This shows how a regular, complicated pattern can be created by applying no more than one force. From Martynov, 1982, with the author's permission.[3]

most biologists this approach seemed to be an oversimplification of a biological reality. In this context a prophetic statement, made more than a century ago by a German anatomist, is worth remembering: "To believe that a heredity governs the development of organisms without using mechanical tools is a kind of a non-scientific mysticism."[5] In the last few decades, however, the situation changed considerably and it became widely accepted that mechanical stresses are among the main regulators of many cellular and morphogenetic processes (reviews: Alt et al. eds,[6] Beloussov,[2] Gordon,[7] and Cowin[8]). A special branch of embryology, studying the generational and morphogenetic roles of mechanical stresses in developing embryos, has emerged and is often called embryo- or morphomechanics.

Morphomechanics deals with two main questions. First, what are the devices used by embryonic cells for producing mechanical stresses? And, second, what is their morphogenetic role?

Molecular machines for producing stresses

Over the last few decades a number of special molecular devices within cells have been discovered, called molecular or protein machines. These machines transform the chemical energy of ATP hydrolysis, firstly, in the intramolecular mechanical stresses and, secondly, by releasing these stresses into the movements of molecular parts, individual molecules, and entire supramolecular structures. We will not discuss here the intimate mechanisms of these events (see Alberts et al.).[9] Rather, we will focus on those mechanical stresses that affect the entire cell and the cell collectives. Here are the main ones:

1 Generation of osmotic turgor pressure in the cavities and vacuoles. A main factor in plant growth and morphogenesis, this also plays an important role in animal development. Lower marine invertebrate animals, such as sponges and coelenterates, grow by periodically pumping water in and out of the cell vacuoles and intercellular spaces.[10,11] For the development of higher animals and human beings it is crucially important to maintain proper turgor pressure within the primary body cavity,[12] the cavity of the neural system, the eye chamber,[13] and so on. If such a pressure is released, either experimentally or as a result of pathologies, the development of the corresponding rudiments becomes highly abnormal. Several refined mechanisms, some of which are located in cell membranes, regulate the osmotic pressure within cells and cavities.

2 Contractile forces cause myosin-mediated antiparallel sliding of actin microfilaments. This is the mechanism of muscle contraction. In all the cells, including embryonic ones, there are structures similar to miniature muscles. They are located usually just beneath cell membranes. Due to a cooperative contractile activity of many adjacent cells, these forces produce extensive deformations of cell layers. They are the main factors of animals' morphogenesis.

3 Directed pushing forces. Microfilaments are able not only to contract, but also to elongate actively,

producing pushing forces that extend cell protrusions. However, the main source of directed pushing force within cells are the so-called microtubules, tiny tubules of 24 nm in diameter and consisting of a glycoprotein, called tubulin. Similar to actin filaments, microtubules are actively elongated (due to the addition of new tubulin subunits) and overcome mechanical resistance. Mutually overlapping microtubule arrays, bound with a motor protein (the kinesin), push apart cell poles during mitotic divisions, thus providing the main force for proliferative growth (so-called proliferative pressure).

It should be emphasized, that the molecular machines which produce mechanical stresses are themselves mechanosensitive.[14–16] This is achieved in different ways. An important role is played, for example, by so-called mechanosensitive ionic channels in cell membranes that are activated by stretching and permit several kinds of ions to penetrate inside a cell or to leak outside. So-called focal junctions, supramolecular conglomerations linking extracellular matrix via the cell membrane to a cytoskeleton are probably the most important cell mechanosensors.[17,18] As a result, an entire cell together with its nucleus creates a mechanically integrated entity with all the other cells of an organism.[19,20] As we will see later, this is of primary importance for development of embryos and for the viability of their cells.

Patterns of mechanical stresses in developing embryos

As mentioned above, to properly understand morphogenetic mechanisms, it is very important to know what the mechanical properties of embryonic tissues are: if they are similar to plastic bodies, any shape is equally possible and embryos are mere "toys" in the hands of external deforming forces. Hence, in order to produce regular shapes these (shapes) should be set quite precisely. Correspondingly, such a mode of morphogenesis requires a lot of "information." On the other hand, if embryonic tissues possess elastic properties, the set of shapes is much more restricted and, hence, the direction of development is much more "canalized" or robust. Under these conditions even non-precisely settled forces produce quite definite shapes (Figure 8.1).

Over the past 70 years the presence of substantial residual stresses of tension and compression has been revealed in embryonic and adult tissues of practically all

animal species studied: Cnidaria (lower invertebrates),[21] *Drosophila*,[22] sea urchins,[23] fish,[24] amphibians,[25,26] and hens.[27,28] On a descriptive level (without experimental approval), the detailed patterns of mechanical stresses in human embryos were postulated by Blechschmidt and Gasser.[29] For the medically oriented, it is of interest to know that substantial residual stresses were detected in embryonic hearts[30,31] and adult arterial walls, even in the absence of blood pressure.[32] The main function of the connective tissue cells, the fibroblasts, is also to permanently maintain the collagen fibers in a stressed state.[33]

In most of the works cited above mechanical stresses were detected by precisely localized partial dissections of embryonic tissues and tracing immediate deformations of dissected parts. This permitted the registering of both tensile and pressure stresses. For example, if a certain tissue area has, beforehand, been under tension, it will contract after the dissection, while if it was under pressure, it will expand. If the stresses are different in the different layers of a tissue piece, the tissue will change its curvature after the dissection, and so on.

As a result, it appears that mechanical stresses in embryonic tissues are arranged according to quite definite patterns, which are mostly created by the "tension lines" (files of stretched cells) crossing embryonic tissues and by the tension nodules (meeting points of these lines). The patterns remain topologically constant during long time periods corresponding to those known in embryology as gastrulation, neurulation, and so on. This means that during these periods no new tension lines and/or nodules are formed (Figure 8.2).

Role of mechanical stresses in embryonic morphogenesis, cell viability, and gene expression

In different species the initiation of development is associated with setting up tensile stresses on the egg or embryo periphery. Such is the formation of a contractile cortical layer immediately after activation of egg development[34] and the re-tension of area opaca of a hen's embryo immediately after the start of incubation.[35]

Artificial relaxation of tensile stresses always leads to grave developmental abnormalities (even in spite of an irresistible tendency of a living tissue to restore the relaxed tensions). Release of hydrostatic pressure in the gastral cavity of a *Hydra* bud,[10] blastocoel of amphibian embryos,[36] or eye chamber of a hen

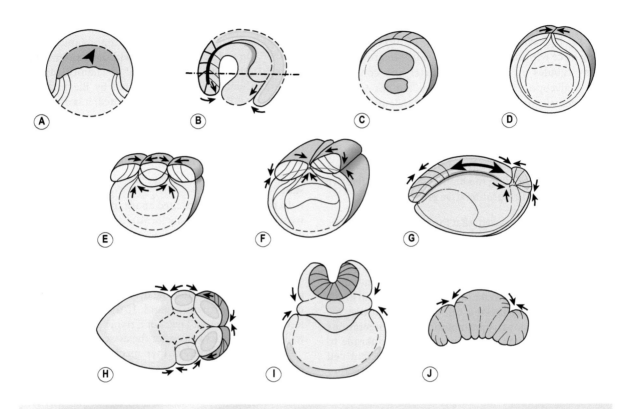

Figure 8.2

Maps of mechanical stresses for several successive periods of a frog's (*Rana temporaria*) development. A: late blastula; B, C: midgastrula; D–F: different cross-sections through early neurula stage embryos; G–I: late neurula/early tail-bud stage; J: a fragment of embryonic tissue 10–15 min after its extirpation from a neurula stage embryo. This time was enough for *de novo* formation of a tensile pattern relaxed during the dissection of the fragment. Heavy contours indicate the mostly pronounced tension lines, dotted contours indicate dispersed tensions, fine lines indicate poorly tensed surfaces. Dense double-headed arrow in "G" points to a longitudinal pressure stress that is taking place in the dorsal embryonic wall (notochord + neural plate). Filled arrowhead in "A" is the turgor pressure within the blastocoel. Small converging arrows point to the main stress nodules. Note the topological differences between the successive maps. From Beloussov et al., 1994.[38]

embryo[13] arrests further development of the corresponding rudiments. Relaxation of circumferential tensile stresses on the surface of amphibian embryos leads to several kinds of morphological malformations: formation of abnormal protrusions, disturbance of bilateral symmetry, partial fusion of the rudiments, and sometimes to a complete disorder in their arrangement.[37–39] There is a notable, extensive increase in morphological variability in embryos relaxed at certain crucial stages (especially at the beginning of gastrulation) (Figure 8.3). Most of these abnormalities can be avoided if restoring tensions in 1–2 h after relaxation. If the direction of the dominating tensions is changed, the axial organs become correspondingly

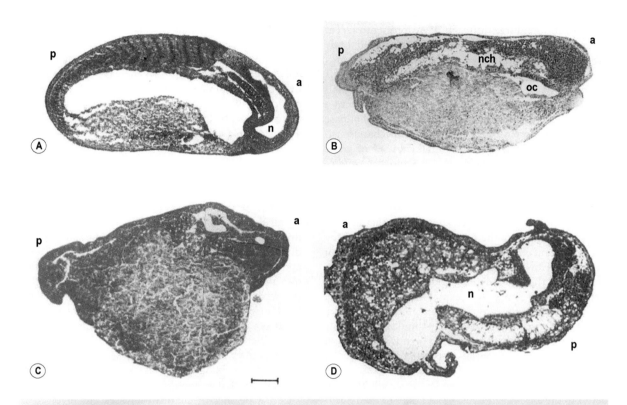

Figure 8.3

Abnormal amphibian (*Xenopus laevis*) embryos (B–D) obtained by relaxing circumferential tensions at the late blastula–early gastrula stages, as compared to a normal sample (A). Notice the variability of abnormal shapes. a, p: anteroposterior axis; n: neural tube; nch: notochord; oc: oral cavity. From Beloussov et al., 1990.[37]

reoriented.[40] The capacity for such reorientation is stage-specific and disappears in advanced embryos. Next, if artificially creating a gradient of tensions (that is, making them more concentrated at one pole of a sample in relation to the opposite) embryonic cells start to move in a concerted way upwards along the tension gradient.[41] Such an experiment reproduces a situation typical of normally developing embryos because most of the tensions in embryonic bodies are organized in a gradient-like fashion.

Several decades ago it was discovered that cell shape (always associated with tensile stresses) plays a direct role in synthetic cell activity, including DNA synthesis.[42] Recent investigations provide important contributions in the field of cytomechanics. By cultivating single cells on small "islands" of adhesive substrate it was discovered that to remain alive a cell should have a space in which to spread (self-tensed). Otherwise (when placed on too small an island) a cell switches on an apoptotic program and dies.[43] This indicates that mechanical stresses are among the necessary components of signaling pathways rescuing a cell from apoptosis and providing its normal functioning. Such a suggestion perfectly fits the modern views that claim "pathways that involve predominantly protein components may signal in a semi-solid fashion with minimal free diffusion."[44] According to recent views, even intracellular water possesses solid body properties due to its highly ordered structure.[45] Accordingly, a large list of so-called second messengers, that is enzymes involved in the transmission of various signals from the extracellular matrix and cell membrane to a cell nucleus, various tyrosine-kinases, phospholipase C, and RAS proteins were found to be mechanosensitive.[7] Along with that, a substantial number of genes were found to be mechanosensitive too.[46–48] Studies dealing with a developmentally important twist gene were carried out recently on *Drosophila* embryos.[49] This gene is involved in morphogenesis of an anterior part of embryonic gut – the so-called stomodeum that is compressed normally by the adjacent region of expanding gut. In mutant embryos, with no expansion, twist is not expressed. However, several minutes of artificial compression of the stomodeum region by a micro-needle were enough to renew twist expression. A direct target of a pressure force was found to be a protein, b-catenin, which is allowed, by mechanical stimulus, to migrate from the cell membrane towards the nucleus where it activates *twist*, and probably also other developmental genes required for invagination of a stomodeum.

Also worth mentioning is the fact that cells respond better to the changes in stress values than to their absolute magnitudes.[50] Sometimes very small but rapid force changes are enough to evoke a cell response. For example, under microgravity conditions Ca^{++} concentration within cells is changed in a few seconds under the actions of forces that do not exceed 10^{-7} N (and strains not exceeding 1 nm per cell).[51]

Mechanical stresses and developmental feedback

In the embryonic development of all organisms, why do we see arising a regular succession of morphological structures? Why does any given shape of an embryo transform at a definite moment in time into another one, no less regular and even more complicated? We still do not have a satisfactory answer to these fundamental questions, which are important not only for theoreticians, but also for those involved in bioengineering projects. Meanwhile, there is increased agreement about the broadest conceptual basis on which a future theory of embryonic development can be erected: this is a theory of a self-organization, an interdisciplinary branch of

science created in the last decades of the twentieth century. This theory (for its popular and biologically oriented review see Ball[52]) claims that complicated systems, far removed from thermodynamic equilibrium, may not only remain ordered but also increase their complexity if their dynamic components are interlinked by so-called non-linear feedback. Non-linearity means that the components' interactions are associated either with a considerable enhancement, or, on the contrary, with an inhibition. It is plausible to suggest that embryonic development belongs to a vast realm of self-organizing processes. What should then be its main feedback links? Modern developmental biology suggests two kinds of responses to this question. In the first viewpoint, which is called chemokinetical, the most important feedback links are established among the production, splitting, and diffusion of two kinds of chemical substances: activators and inhibitors.[53] It is assumed that the activators diffuse over much shorter distances than the inhibitors, and so the activating feedbacks are short range ones while the inhibitory feedbacks belong to long range interactions. There is a large family of models of this kind that reproduce different color patterns and other kinds of biological "tapestry." However, they meet serious difficulties if applied to morphogenetic processes with a pronounced and complicated geometry.

Can it be that mechanical stresses are involved in morphogenetic feedback links so that a self-organization includes an essential mechanical component? A first, clear demonstration of such a possibility was given by Harris et al.[54] They observed that if seeding the fibroblast cells onto elastic substrates, which the cells themselves are able to stretch, an initially homogeneous cell spreading is exchanged in quite a regular pattern, consisting of cell clusters connected by files of stretched cells (Figure 8.4). No such patterns were observed in the case of non-deformable substrates. Hence, what we have here is a mechanical-based self-organization of cell aggregates. The authors postulate[55] that this is due to the combination of short-range positive feedback (providing a further increase in cell–cell contact areas in already condensed cell groups) and long-range negative feedback (exemplified by a stretching of a substrate due to cell traction).

Somewhat later quite a similar model for a very ubiquitous morphogenetic process, namely the segregation of an initially homogeneous cell layer into the domains of columnar and stretched cells, has been suggested.[56]

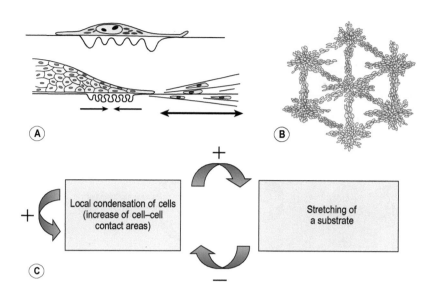

Figure 8.4
Experiment by Harris et al.[31] and its interpretation. (A) A schematic presentation of a single crawling fibroblast (above) and a multicellular fibroblast cluster (below) which shrink the underlying substrate (folds) and hence stretch the peripheral area (shown to the right). (B) The resultant patterns consisting of cell clusters and files of stretched cells. (C) A scheme of the involved feedback (see text for comments). From Harris et al. (1981),[31] with the author's permission.

In this model short-range positive feedback was provided by so-called contact cell polarization, that is a mutual support of columnarization in the domains of adjacent cells, while long-range negative feedback was similar to a previous model stretched by already columnarized cells (Figure 8.5). The model effectively reproduces a proportional segregation of an epithelial layer into different domains, even under different absolute dimensions, and not very precise initial conditions. Hence, it has the property of robustness, which is important for any morphogenetic model.

None of the above models is broad enough to describe the overwhelming diversity of morphogenetic processes, including those associated with substantial geometric changes. Through searching for such a model, Professor J. Mittenthal, from Illinois University, and I[2,38] suggested the hypothesis of hyper-restoration of mechanical stresses (HR hypothesis) that is formulated as follows: a cell or a tissue piece, after being shifted by an external force (either introduced artificially, or exerted by another part of the same normally developing embryo) from its initial stress value, develops an active mechanical response, which is directed towards restoring this stress value, but as a rule overshoots it in the opposite direction.

The main idea of the HR hypothesis is illustrated by Figure 8.6: if a sample is stretched by an external force, it tends to reduce the value of a stretching stress up to developing an active pressure stress (Fig. 8.6A). If, on the contrary, it is relaxed or further compressed by an external force, its response will be directed towards re-stretching itself, which can be achieved by a tangential contraction of some of its cells (Fig. 8.6B).

There are several sets of evidence, both on the single cell level and that of multicellular collectives, which are in favor of the HR hypothesis. At the single cells level, we will mention just two examples:

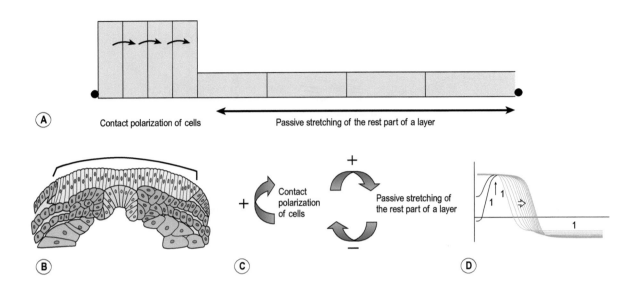

Figure 8.5
Model of the segregation of an initially homogeneous cell layer with fixed ends (black spots in A) to the domains of columnarized and flattened cells. (A) A dynamical scheme. (B) An example of a neural plate (with boundaries indicated by brackets) segregated from the surrounding ectoderm. (C) A scheme of the involved feedback. (D) A succession of modeled shapes. Horizontal axis: length of a layer; vertical axis: height of cells. Starting from a local polarizing perturbation (arrow, contour 1–1–1) and a zero cell height throughout the entire layer we come to a stable segregation of the domains of extensively columnarized and flattened cells.

1   The growing neurons transform tensile stresses to those of an internal pressure.[57,58]

2   If an intercellular tension is increased by disruption of microtubules then the increased stress value is rapidly diminished by a subsequent enlargement of cell–cell contact.[15]

The most obvious cases of the hyper-restoration (HR) response in multicellular embryonic tissues are as follows:

1   A usual response to a stretching is cell intercalation. This refers to producing an extensive internal pressure with the same direction as the previous stretching. In other words, a piece of embryonic tissue tends to transform its passive stretching to the active pressure-mediated elongation taking place just in the stretching direction.

This reaction is used in a stretch therapy for bone trauma and the orthopedic procedures for elongating abnormally short bones.[59] In these kinds of treatments a continuous stretch, even if painful, was reported to give much better clinical results than a direct surgical insert of a bone or artificial material without stretching. Correspondingly, the amount of post-stretching relaxation (which it is possible to measure by special devices) is a most suitable criterion of a successful cure. All of this perfectly fits the expectation of HR hypothesis.

2   A widespread reaction to the relaxation of tension is, as mentioned above, the columnarization of single cells and the entire domains of coherent cells. Another one is exemplified by cell migration inside a sheet. Through both of these mechanisms the relaxed tension is hyper-restored.

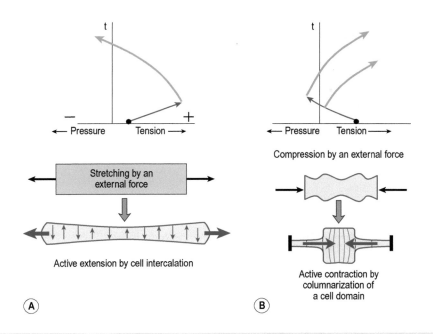

Figure 8.6

Stress hyper-restoration (HR) responses in the case of stretching (A) and relaxation/compression (B). Upper row: HR loops; horizontal axes: stress values; vertical axes: time; fine lines: external forces; solid curves: active responses. Lower row: examples of HR reactions in cell layers – cell intercalation in response to stretching and cell contraction in response to relaxation/compression.

It is morphogenetically important that both HR relations are linked with each other by positive feedback. For example, if part A of a cell layer is actively contracted, it will stretch an adjacent part B and trigger, according to HR hypothesis, cell intercalation in the latter. Now an actively expanded part B will relax or even compress part A, stimulating its further contraction, and so on. In such a way, a cell layer will become segregated into the domains of contracted and stretched cells.

Another property of HR relations is that they are very sensitive to the geometry of a cell layer. For example, a cell layer is slightly bent (curved) by an external force and, as a result, the concave part of the layer will be compressed (or at least relaxed), while the convex part is stretched (Figure 8.7A1). In which way will the HR tendencies now be expressed? If a layer cannot straighten back in a spring-like manner, the following

should be expected: the concave side with relaxed/compressed cells, in order to (hyper) restore the initial tension, will either contract tangentially their free surfaces, or/and migrate to the convex side (centrifugally). Correspondingly, the cells of the convex side should enlarge their outer surfaces, either by the insertion of new portions of plasma membrane, or by getting more cells from the opposite surface. In any case, both processes will enhance each other and be directed towards the active increase of the passively initiated curvature (Figure 8.7A2). This will automatically produce areas of an opposite curvature on the flanks of a given maximum curvature, which themselves should also pass from the passive to the active state, producing the next curvature maxima of the opposite sign on their periphery, and so on. In such a way, any mechanically active epithelial layer tends to be folded. The number, shape,

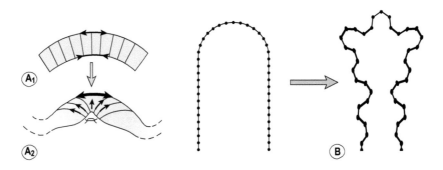

Figure 8.7

Active curvature increase and its morphogenetic consequences. (A) Transformation of a passive bending (A$_1$) to an active one (A$_2$) due to extension of a convex surface, contraction of a concave surface and a concave–convex cell migration (arrows). (B) A model transformation of a smooth surface to a regularly folded one (see Beloussov and Grabovsky[60] for a detailed explanation). Points represent kinematically independent units (and not necessarily single cells).

and location of the folds would depend upon the geometrical and mechanical properties of a layer (and, correspondingly, the epigenetic and genetic factors affecting these properties). By setting up the different parameter values, these processes can be modeled and the resultant shapes compared with the real ones (Fig. 8.7B; see Beloussov and Grabovsky[60] for more details).

In general, one may hope that knowledge of HR relations is not only of theoretical interest, but can be also used for bio-engineering. For example, if one needs to concentrate cells along a certain axis, it might be enough to stretch a sample along this axis. Similarly, if required to produce an amount of columnarized cells (which are, in many cases, biochemically much more active than the flattened ones) a tissue piece should be relaxed.

Further reading

Lev V. Beloussov (with a contribution by Andrei Lipchinsky) (2015). Morphomechanics of Development. Springer Cham, Heidelberg.

References

[1]Keller, R. (1987). Cell rearrangements in morphogenesis. Zool. Sci. 4: 763–779.

[2]Beloussov L.V. (1998). The Dynamic Architecture of a Developing Organism. Kluwer Academic Publishers, Dordrecht, Boston, London.

[3]Martynov, L.A. (1982). The role of macroscopic processes in morphogenesis. In: Mathematical Biology of Development (A.I., Zotin, E.V., Presnov, eds) Nauka, Moskva, pp. 135–154 (in Russian).

[4]Thompson, D'Arcy (2000). On Growth and Form. Cambridge Univ. Press, Cambridge.

[5]His, W. (1974). Unsere Korpersform und das physiologische Probleme ihrer Entstehung. Leipzig, F. Vogel.

[6]Alt, W., Deutsch, A., Dunn, G. (eds) Dynamics of Cell and Tissue Motion. Birkhauser, Basel, Boston, Berlin. 1997.

[7]Gordon, R. (1999). The Hierarchical Genome and Differentiation Waves: Novel Unification of Development, Genetics and Evolution, Singapore & London: World Scientific & Imperial College Press.

[8]Cowin, S.C. (2000). How is a tissue built? J. Biomech. Engineering 122: 553–569.

[9]Alberts, B., Bray, D., Lewis, J., Raff, M., Roberts, K., Watson, J.D. (2002). Molecular Biology of the Cell (4th edition). Garland Publishing, Inc., New York, London.

[10]Wanek, N., Marcum, B.A., Lee, H.T., Campbell, R.D. (1980). Effect of hydrostatic pressure on

morphogenesis in nerve-free hydra. J. Exp. Zool. 211: 275–280.

[11]Beloussov, L.V., Labas, J.A., Kazakova (1993). Growth pulsations in hydroid polyps: kinematics, biological role and cytophysiology. In: Oscillations and Morphogenesis (L. Rensing ed.). Marcel Dekker. N.Y., Basel, Hong Kong. pp. 183–193.

[12]Stern, C. (1984). A simple model for early morphogenesis. J. Theor. Biol. 107: 229–242.

[13]Coulombre A.J. (1956). The role of intraocular pressure in the development of the chick eye. J. Exp. Zool. 133: 211–226.

[14]Banes, A.J., Tsuzaki, M., Yamamoto, J., Fischer, T., Brigman, B., Brown, T, Miller, L. (1995). Mechanoreception at the cellular level: the detection, interpretation and diversity of responses to mechanical signals. Biochemistry and Cell Biology 73: 349–365.

[15]Pletjushkina, O.J, Belkin, A.M, Ivanova, O.J, Oliver, T., Vasiliev, J.M, Jacobson, K. (1998). Maturation of cell-substratum focal adhesions induced by depolymerization of microtubules is mediated by increased cortical tension. Cell Adhesion and Communication 5: 121–135.

[16]Kaverina, O., Krylyshkina, K., Beningo, K., Anderson, Wang, Yu-Li, Small, J.V. (2002). Tensile stress stimulates microtubule outgrowth in living cells. J. Cell Science 115: 2283–2291.

[17]Chrzanowska-Wodnicka M., Burridge K. (1996). Rho-stimulated contractility drives the formation of stress fibers and focal adhesions. J. Cell Biol. 133: 1403–1415.

[18]Riveline, D., Zamir, E., Balaban, N.Q., Schwarz, U.S., Ishizaki, T., Narumiya, S., Kam, Z., Geiger, B., Bershadsky, A. D. (2001). Focal Contacts as Mechanosensors: Externally Applied Local Mechanical Force Induces Growth of Focal Contacts by an mDia1-dependent and ROCK-independent Mechanism. J. Cell Biol. 153: 1175–1185.

[19]Ingber, D.E., Dike, L., Hansen, L., Karp, S., Liley, H., Maniotis, A., McNamee, H., Mooney, D., Plopper, G., Sims, J., Wang, N. (1994). Cellular tensegrity: exploring how mechanical changes in the cytoskeleton regulate cell growth, migration and tissue pattern during morphogenesis, Int. Rev. Cytol. 150: 173–224.

[20]Maniotis, A.J., Chen, C.S., Ingber, D.E. (1997). Demonstration of mechanical connections between integrins, cytoskeletal filaments, and nucleoplasm that stabilize nuclear structure. Proc. Natl. Acad. Sci. USA 94: 849–854.

[21]Krauss, Ju.A, Cherdantzev, V.G. (1995). A primary epithelization of cells in the early morphogenesis of a marine hydroid, Dynamena pumila L. Ontogenez (Russ. J. Devel. Biol.) 26: 223–230.

[22]Kiehart, D.P., Galbraith, C.G., Edwards, K.A., Rickoll, W.L., Montague, R.A. (2000). Multiple forces contribute to cell sheet morphogenesis for dorsal closure in Drosophila. J. Cell Biol. 149: 471–490.

[23]Beloussov L.V., Bogdanovsky S.B. (1980). Cell mechanisms of embryonic regulations in sea-urchin embryos. Ontogenez (Sov. J. Devel Biol) 11: 467–476.

[24]Cherdantzeva, E.V., Cherdantzev, V.G. (1985). Determination of a dorso-ventral polarity in the embryos of a fish, Brachydanio rerio (Teleostei). Sov. J. Devel. Biol. 16: 270–280.

[25]Beloussov, L.V., Dorfman, J.G., Cherdantzev V.G. (1975). Mechanical stresses and morphological patterns in amphibian embryos. J. Embryol. Exp. Morphol. 34: 559–574.

[26]Jacobson, A.G., Gordon, R. (1976). Changes in the shape of the developing vertebrate nervous system analyzed experimentally, mathematically and by computer simulation. J. Exp. Zool. 197: 191–246.

[27]Bellairs, R., Bromham, D.R., Wylie, C.C. (1967). The influence of the area opaca on the development of the young chick embryo. J. Embryol. Exp. Morphol. 17: 197–212.

[28]Beloussov, L.V., Naumidi, I.I. (1977). Contractility and epithelization in the axial mesoderm of chicken embryos. Ontogenez (Sov. J. Devel Biol) 8: 517–521.

[29]Blechschmidt, E., Gasser, R.F. (1978). Biokinetics and Biodynamics of Human Differentiation. Charles C. Thomas Publisher, Springfield, Illinois.

[30]Omens, J.H., Fung, Y.C. (1990). Residual strain in rat left ventricle. Circ. Res. 66: 37–45.

[31]Taber, L.A. (1995). Biomechanics of growth, remodeling and morphogenesis. Appl. Mech. Rev. 48: 487–545.

[32]Vaishnav, R.N., Vossoughi, J. (1987). Residual stress and strain in aortic segments. J. Biomechanics 20: 235–239.

[33]Harris, A.K., Stopak, D., Wild, P. (1981). Fibroblast traction as a mechanism for collagen morphogenesis. Nature 290: 249–251.

[34]Detlaff, T.A. (1977). Establishment of organization of a mature egg in amphibians and fishes. In: Modern Problems of Oogenesis (Editorial Board) Moskva, Nauka, pp. 99–144 (in Russian).

[35]Kucera, P., Monnet-Tschudi, F. (1987). Early functional differentiation in the chick embryonic disc:

interactions between mechanical activity and extra-cellular matrix. J. Cell Sci. Suppl 8: 415–432.

[36]Beloussov, L.V., Ermakov A.S. (2001). Artificially applied tensions normalize the development of the relaxed Xenopus laevis embryos. Ontogenez (Russ J. Devel Biol) 32: 288–294.

[37]Beloussov, L.V., Lakirev, A.V., Naumidi, I.I., Novoselov, V.V. (1990). Effects of relaxation of mechanical tensions upon the early morphogenesis of Xenopus laevis embryos. Int. J. Dev. Biol. 34: 409–419.

[38]Beloussov L.V, Saveliev S.V, Naumidi I.I, Novoselov V.V (1994). Mechanical stresses in embryonic tissues: patterns, morphogenetic role and involvement in regulatory feedback. Intern. Rev. Cytol. 150: 1–34.

[39]Ermakov A.S., Beloussov L.V. (1998). Morphogenetical and differentiation consequences of the relaxation of mechanical tensions in Xenopus laevis blastula. Ontogenez (Russ. J. Devel. Biol.) 29: 450–458.

[40]Beloussov, L.V., Lakirev, A.V., Naumidi, I.I. (1988). The role of external tensions in differentiation of Xenopus laevis embryonic tissues. Cell Diff. and Devel 25: 165–176.

[41]Beloussov, L.V., Louchinskaia, N.N., Stein, A.A. (2000). Tension-dependent collective cell movements in the early gastrula ectoderm of Xenopus laevis embryos. Dev. Genes Evolution. 210: 92–104.

[42]Brunette, D.M. (1984). Mechanical stretching increases the number of epithelial cells synthesizing DNA in culture. J. Cell Sci 69: 35–45.

[43]Huang S., Ingber D.E. (2000). Shape-Dependent Control of Cell Growth, Differentiation, and Apoptosis: Switching between Attractors in Cell Regulatory Networks. Experimental Cell Research 261(1): 91–103

[44]Hunter, T. (2000). Signalling – 2000 and beyond. Cell 100: 113–127.

[45]Watterson J.G. (2004). Enzyme function: random events or coherent action? http://www.1sbu.ac.uk/water/

[46]Iba, T., Sumpio, B.E. (1992). Tissue plasminogen activator expression in endothelial cells exposed to cyclic strain in vitro. Cell Transplant. 1: 43–50.

[47]Resnick, N., Collins, T., Atkinson, W., Bonthron, D.T., Dewey, C.F., Jr, Gimbrone, M.A., Jr (1993). Platelet-derived growth factor B chain promoter contains a cis-acting fluid shear-stress-responsive element. Proc. Natl. Acad. Sci. USA 90: 4591–4595.

[48]Chiquet, M. (1999). Regulation of extracellular matrix gene expression by mechanical stress. Matrix Biology 18: 417–426.

[49]Brouzes, E., Farge, E. (2004). Interplay of mechanical deformations and patterned gene expression in developing embryos. Curr. Op. Genetics & Devel 14: 367–374.

[50]Suter, M.D., Errante, L.D., Belotserkovsky, V., Forscher. P. (1998). The Ig superfamily cell adhesion molecule, apCAM, mediates growth cone steering by membrane-cytoskeletal coupling. J. Cell Biol. 141: 227–240.

[51]Jones, D., Leivseth, G., Tenbosch, J. (1995). Mechano-reception in osteoblast-like cells. Biochem and Cell Biol. 73: 525–534.

[52]Ball, P. (2001). The Self-Made Tapestry. Pattern Formation in Nature. Oxford University Press, Oxford.

[53]Meinhardt, H. (1982). Models of Biological Patterns Formation. Academic Press, N.Y.

[54]Harris, A.K., Stopak, D., Warner, P. (1984) Generation of spatially periodic patterns by a mechanical instability: a mechanical alternative to the Turing model. J. Embryol. Exp. Morphol. 80: 1–20.

[55]Oster, G.F., Murray, J.D., Harris, A.K. (1983). Mechanical aspects of mesenchymal morphogenesis. J. Embryol. Exp. Morphol. 78: 83–125.

[56]Belintzev, B.N., Beloussov, L.V., Zaraisky A.G. (1987). Model of pattern formation in epithelial morphogenesis. J. Theor. Biol. 129: 369–394.

[57]Dennerly, T.J., Lamoureux, P., Buxbaum, R.E., Heidemann, S.R. (1989). The cytomechanics of axonal elongation and retraction. J. Cell Biol. 109: 3073–3083.

[59]Buxbaum, R.E., Heidemann, S.R. (1992). An absolute rate theory model for tension control of axonal elongation. J. Theor. Biol. 155: 409–426.

[59]Ilizarov, G.A. (1984). Stretching stress as a factor exciting and supporting the regeneration and growth of the bone's and soft tissues. In: Structure and Biomechanics of the Skeletal-Muscular and Heart-Vessel Systems of Vertebrates. Kiev, Ukraine Rep. Conference, pp. 38–40 (in Russian).

[60]Beloussov, L.V., Grabovsky, V.I. (2003). A geometro-mechanical model for pulsatorial morphogenesis. Computer Methods in Biomech. and Biomed. Engineering 6: 53–63.

9

Developmental patterns and adaptive organization of body functioning: How tissue memorizes information

Patrick van den Heede and Anne Jäkel

Introduction

Is there, besides the classical cognitive aspect of memory, a reason to define other kinds of memory? What are the morphological domains that are responsible for tissue memorization? Are there histological, molecular, purely chemical or physical aspects that contribute to the definition of tissue memory? Of what use could this memory be to the diagnosing and treating osteopath?

The exact knowledge of embryonic stages and fetal development can be of great value for the understanding of the subtle relationships between tissue differentiation and organ development. These could, at least partly, explain the complex interferences between symptoms and causality that most therapists generally are looking for in a rather linear model of disease interpretation. The study of morphology seeks to clarify the relationships that exist between embryonic polarities and adult body organization and orientation. It also helps to understand the subtle relationships that are present between molecular, electrical and mechanical interferences during cell differentiation and its determinations. Furthermore, it makes use of the knowledge on tissue, structure, and organ development and its final determination and function in the adult body.

A couple of reservations apply here, in order to make the content of this chapter clearer. Some representations, such as cellular pathways involving growth factors and cytokines, have been simplified. Hence, certain complex interactions are not explained in full detail. Furthermore, some of the described research results are derived from non-human life forms such as newts, fish, and others; hence, the application of these findings onto human embryos should be done with caution. For instance, the comparison of the very homogenous human ovule with polar structured non-human egg

cells is only viable to a certain extent. The same applies to the process of gastrulation in the newt, being initiated by the cells of the dorsal lip of the blastopore, in contrast to the gastrulation of the human embryo.

Function and memory

Function is an adaptive and evolutionary memory. What do osteopaths treat when they touch a specific part of the body? They may claim that their intervention is meant to improve function. The problem remains that only the structure "knows" how to support the function that the osteopath aims to improve, and that is expressed by particular symptoms, such as a lack or decrease in function. Does the structure rely on an actual state of expression? Does it remember the cause of the dysfunction, and what are its tools to rebalance the disorder into a different kind of 'order'?

The easiest way to know how something 'functions' is to explore how it may have worked during other states of evolution. This could be investigated in relation to the time of evolution for the same and other parts of the body. It can also be explored in relation to the same and other species. The actual function not only holds the 'history' of its own evolution and maturation, but also the story of integrated information related to epigenetic, cognitive, emotional and traumatic inputs and conditioning.

The questions remain how far and in which way the brain, as the epicenter of consciousness, is dependent on its relationship with other body parts and how the 'periphery' of the whole body structure could participate in increasing or eliciting specific parts of memory and consciousness. Brain, consciousness, and memory have been and still are extensively studied. In contrast, the phenomenon of memory within the structural elements supporting our general physiology and the vitality of the brain remains rather unclear. This is largely due to the fact that until now rather little has been invested in research investigating tissue and cellular memory. Hence, in the world of morphogenesis and differentiation processes during early stages of life one has to presume how structure is established by using inductive and differentiating processes that support a genetic and epigenetic landscape.

When studying morphogenesis extensively and by following the final determinations of morphogenetic processes to organogenesis and even further during postnatal development, one could propose that every step in the differentiation of tissue and organ is related to, and supports a specific time/space pattern[1]. The related pattern can itself be considered a specific function. Each of these time related events serves as a stepping stone for further stages of development and establishment of definite function. This would imply that each of these milestones in pre- and postnatal differentiation and derivation of a specific structure can be considered a function itself. This is in line with the hypothesis of E. Blechschmidt[2] who postulated that each intermittent stage of embryological and fetal development should be considered as an adaptive function, supporting the needs of organ maturation and the developing fetus.

One can also ask whether in postnatal life a definite function really exists. The body, as an open biological system, is constantly exposed to changing information. It seems rather evident to consider the actual function as a summation of earlier integrated functions, such as those of tissue, morphogenesis, structure and form, which are stored in patterns and being combined with new adaptive patterns. Each of these functions is related to definite memorized stages and developmental differentiation during the embryonic and fetal maturation process on different levels of structure specification, which support increasingly complex functions during postnatal life. All these processes express specific histological, morphological and functional adaptive features that contribute to further refinement of a specific developing structure. In some way, there seems to be no definite function as long as the body is capable of exchange.

The function and the form seem to be related to certain structural laws. The outcome is a definite function that supports the physiology and homeostatic adaptation, and increases the possibility of interaction of the individual with the external environment. This can be called adaptive consciousness of the structure. Specific

emphasis is placed on the 'intermediate tissue', known in embryology as the mesenchyme. Here, many transformative and adaptive processes take place during morphogenesis and organogenesis. It forms the core tissue between most of the morphostatic and morphodynamic processes during embryogenesis, and it is also the organizing tissue for most of the space occupying processes during organogenesis (Figure 9.1).

The fibroblasts are at the core of the mesenchymal adaptive and transformative processes, and can act as constructive tools but can also render older embryological patterns of adaptation during periods of tissue and organ deterioration. They are like a working bench by which transformative inputs on a molecular and chemical level are interpreted and restored in the tissues by changes in the constellation of the extracellular matrix (ECM) (Figure 9.2).

At first, the 'unspecific mesenchyme reaction' is organised by storing primary information, which later on, in case of deteriorating processes (i.e. inflammation) can be recalled and re-installed during advanced stages of development and adult function. The myocardium, for instance, can rely on such a mechanism called 'hibernating myocardium'. The complex interference of the fibroblast with the ECM during normal and inflammatory processes is shown in Figure 9.3.

Fibroblasts can be considered inspectors and organizers of the specific and unspecific reactions of the mesenchyme by which it is turned on in an adaptive or in a regressive way. The mesenchyme is able to tune into a transformative state, but it can also regress into a more protective state of tissue and functional organization. In a certain way it displays *the real cellular balance* by which, at one and the same time, the molecular, chemical and mechanical properties of the tissue and its immediate environment can be altered. A.T. Still proposed that the fascia was the meeting place between the nerves, the arteries and the lymphatic vessels and that it covers the whole body[4]. By 'fascia' he not only meant the mechanical strands that linked organs and bones to each other, but that all mesenchyme and epithelium could be considered as belonging to the big family of the connective tissue.

The osteopath knows that the art of osteopathy is depending on the degree of cooperation that can be elicited within the tissues he is working with. It relies for a major part on the way it can cooperate with the principles and forces of the body. One of the big tools of

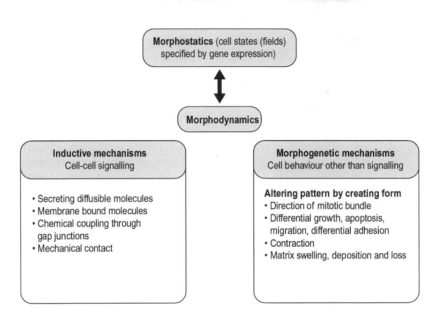

Figure 9.1

Morphodynamic and morphostatic properties of developing tissue (both processes are running simultaneously and are complementary), and specification of mechanisms that determine the morphodynamic interferences during patterning

the osteopath is the way by which he can offer a fulcrum to the body, hence being able to establish the right point of balance.

With regards to fibroblasts and their capability of organizing the vast area of mesenchymal tissue in the body, one should also consider their ability of establishing a deep cellular balance, organizing the reaction of the mesenchyme, either in a specific or nonspecific way. The fibroblast represents one of the first elements reminding us that the body possesses an efficient way for *memorizing* and *recalling (re-expressing)* the stages it went through during morphogenesis and organogenesis. It also relativises the 'pride' of the osteopath claiming that he did some good work on the body. What the osteopath can do is give 'the right fulcrum at the right time and the right place', or 'once the hands are on the body, the body is in command', as Anthony Chila has proclaimed in his numerous courses[5]. The balance that is installed depends mainly on the story that is memorized by the fibroblast and the initiation of a specific or unspecific mesenchymal reaction. A small part is contributed and experienced by the osteopath who serves as a witness of this intimate exchange.

The fulcrum seems to be the entry point into the tissue, and the story of the tissue is expressed and governed by all kinds of biological principles and reaction patterns of thermodynamic, chemical and biomechanical nature. Most of the time the osteopath interprets those events as a 'release' which is accompanied by deep breath, loosening of tight tissue and deepening of motion or increased range of motion.

R. Becker[6] proposed that only the tissue 'knows', and that the symptom ignores the cause. A lot of time and osteopathic practice is needed in order to understand these secrets. It is clear that an osteopath who has an excellent knowledge of the stages of different body structures during different morphogenetic and organogenetic episodes possesses a tool for transferring

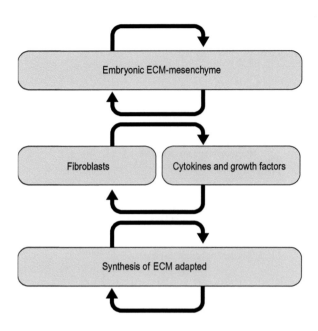

Figure 9.2

The importance of fibroblasts as organizers and modulators of the ECM and mesenchymal reaction modalities, and their influence on growth factors and cytokines

an alteration of a physiological state into a subsequently altered mesenchymal reaction. When the osteopath is finely tuned into the tissue he should also be capable of relating the symptom to preceding stages of body structuring during its earlier development. This could be considered as a kind of etiological study that reaches back into the embryological period and which reinforces the diagnostic intuition of the therapist. The art of palpating and interpreting the tactile findings is related to an extensive field of information that also implicates the memory of the tissue. In a certain way the osteopath is gathering information that spans the whole life of the individual and that even includes prenatal development. By further investigating what is meant by memory, one can presume that it can be part of different units of life-supporting and -expressing processes and forms. Memory should be interpreted as stored or patterned energy that can play an important role in

supporting different types of vital processes and that can be used in a repetitive way (Figure 9.4).

The support can be provided by basic material particles (chemical molecules and bonds), by molecular arrangements and exchanges as well as by frequencies and phases organized by electrical and electrochemical processes or fields. On the whole, a vast array of possibilities for evoking and integrating parts of memory is created. All of the constellating parts of a physiological unit can be seen as a source of memory. The biophysical, biochemical and physiological properties of the structure/function relationship all contain pieces of information that rely on the integrative and interfering patterns found in the most elemental units of matter that is supporting life. Memory belongs to matter but it can also be expressed as a frequency, a development of phases, or retained as an electromagnetic field potential.

The osteopath has to take into account all of these parameters when interpreting a certain structure he is synchronizing to. This can be compared with a 'zooming in' process by which the hand and the mind of the osteopath can be confronted with the gross unit of shape and matter, or with the infinitesimal particles that support only the energetic level (cells, molecules, and atoms). When the living matter of the body is handled, one can certainly distinguish different memories stored at different levels of density of the structure/function relationship expressed in different physiological subunits (Table1).

Construction of the basic body plan

Embryological concepts and laws

Introduction

The definition of the different stages of embryological development depends on the tools used for studying embryology. The historical development of embryology as a science offers a wide range of definitions of developmental principles and laws, which are important for understanding the basics of developmental biology. The first most influential observations with regard to embryological development were made in the second half of the 19th century. Embryology developed from a purely observational into a molecular and experimental science during the late 20th and early 21st century. It nowadays includes genetic manipulation and cloning.

The tools for observation gradually changed, from 'the naked eye observation' to using microscopes,

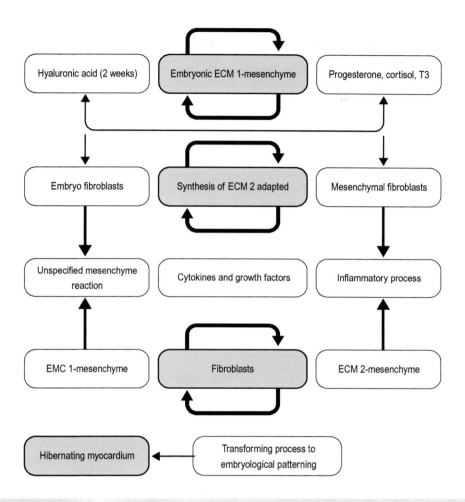

Figure 9.3

Complex interference of fibroblast activity during normal and inflammatory processes, using differentiation programs that were patterned during embryogenesis (adapted from Heine[3])

ECM1: primary mesenchyme dependent on epithelio/mesenchymal transition or from mesodermal layer; ECM2: differentiated mesenchyme that supports definitive function or that is ready to undergo mesenchymal/epithelial transition; T3: tri-iodiothyronine

electron microscopes and *in vivo* as well as *in vitro* observation and experimentation employing different types of imaging. Although these new technologies offer more advanced insights into evolutionary processes most of the laws and principles defined during the past two centuries are still valid. They not only combine the great laws of evolution and genetics, but they also describe the principles of the interrelation between structure, form and function. They help to understand the basics of tissue regeneration and deterioration.

Matter memory	Matter contains the crystallized form of rhythms and atomic/molecular constellations that are condensed in a particular way. Matter contains geometrical patterns, density and affinity.
Tissue memory	Tissue can be considered living matter (structure/function) that has the capability of expressing parts of the qualities of its constellating parameters in specific rhythms and phases of particular processes, governed by the laws of thermodynamics, biophysics and quantum dynamics.
Morphogenetic memory	Morphogenetic information belongs to the domain of phylogenetic and ontogenetic transmission of the laws of survival and adaptation governed by specific sets of genes and epigenetic factors.
Cognitive memory	Cognitive memory is the conscious/subconscious capability of the mind for memorizing, recalling and modifying units of experience stored and retained in a highly ordered brain function and aimed at recognizing identical processes or at organizing/re-organizing the environment.
Matrix memory	Matrix memory can be conceived as the most fundamental part of the integrative network to and from the brain. It constitutes a vast array of membrane proteins and lipids that offers an ultrasensitive landscape within the body by which information is transmitted to the brain in an ultra-rapid way, even faster than the fasted nerve pathway. At the same time, it displays a field of sophisticated interaction where all kinds of information can be combined, enhancing and supporting the vital states of the body (vegetative, autonomous, subconscious) and relieve the conscious activity of the brain of excessive survival strategy.

TABLE 9.1: Types of memory that can constellate the creation of a mental image for the osteopath

The secrets of structure-form-function interrelationship are stored in the subtle domains of tissue structure, organization, exchange and origin. Both observational and experimental embryology contribute to a constant renewal of the insights gained by genetics and *in vitro* and *in vivo* experiments during different embryological stages. For the osteopath, it is important to remember that the principles of osteopathy belong to the principles of life. The secret of life and body plan is already apparent and integrated into the successive stages of development of form and structure. In the adult, these different processes are partially repeated in anatomical, physiological, biochemical and biomechanical exchanges.

Within the 'historical' and experimental progression in the embryological studies, where the embryo is seen as developing from germ to a differentiated form (invertebrate, vertebrate, and mammal) in a linear fashion, there exists also the possibility for studying the embryo as a dynamic exchange between 'fields of evolution'. This would mean that one could study a particular tissue outside its linear evolution within the general body plan (stages of evolution), where the tissue becomes a biodynamic field of biomechanical exchange, organization and hierarchy.

Biodynamic principles integrate morphogenetic and epigenetic, chemical and mechanical exchange as the basis for the generation of an integrated body plan and function. The general body plan can be considered as a linear process of molecular morphogenetic events, but it can also be studied from the viewpoint of continuous dynamic exchange between different 'patterns' and organs modulated by constant interference between morphogenetic and epigenetic factors.

Within the biodynamic aspect of embryology, the body plan is considered a 3-dimensional event in which biomechanical elements participate as well as pure cell/tissue differentiation occurs, guided by biochemical factors. The developing body becomes an individualized organism that expresses an organization in time (4-dimensional). Events and stages such as induction, synchronicity and polarity cannot only be considered as

Memorizing life

Memory: a physical unit/holon
Memory: a frequency bit
Memory: a space/time unit
Memory: a physiological unit
Memory: an organ/tissue
Memory: a cognitive process
Memory: a retainment or a recall
Memory: an electrical field
Memory: a wave pattern
Memory: a work out of phases
Memory: an EMF (Electromagnetic field)

Figure 9.4
Complex interference of different types of memory will compose the definite reaction pattern of the individual at a particular moment during life

passages in evolution but also represent 'moments' with a persistent value that partially can be recapitulated in the adult during normal and pathological processes.

It is evident that the process of patterning is a time/space event of close interference between the genomic information that is quite definite, with epigenetic factors being concentrated and active in the extracellular matrix. Hence, quite a stable informative genomic pattern interferes within the extracellular matrix with epigenetic factors that constitute time/space-related information for the genetic pattern. The genomic information itself can only be adapted by some specific cells, which apparently are capable of changing their genetic information by means of a specific enzyme - the recombinase enzyme. Some neuroblasts and lymphoblasts display this capability during their lifetime.

The following flowchart displays the close relationship between the genetic core (the genetic program functioning as an original 'blueprint', representing the greatest probability for optimal morphogenesis and subsequent function), adaptive cells and the interference field, known as the ECM (Figure 9.5).

Principles and laws in 'historical' perspective

Historical research findings with regard to the embryological principles provide an insight into the processes that embryologists and other researchers went through for defining the 'laws of life energy'. S.F. Gilbert[7] synthesized the following framework during the stages of embryological research and development that can be used for the studies of morphology:

- Laws of origin
- Laws of causality
- Organization of axes in relation to the body plan
- Pre-patterning and patterns in the organization of the embryo
- Morphogenetic factors and molecules

The laws of origin

K. von Baer made the first important observation and definition of an embryological law in the first half of the 19th century[8]:

'During the development of animals and multicellular species the cells that originate from cell divisions of the ovum are organized in distinct layers:

- the ectodermal layer, offering the serosal substrate
- the endodermal layer, resulting in the construction of the mucosal substrate
- the mesodermal layer, providing the vascular substrate

Generally, particular organs or structures always develop from the same layers for every animal species observed:

- the ectoderm provides the anlage for the skin and the nervous system
- the endoderm constructs the internal covering of the digestive tract and its associated glandular organs
- the mesoderm contains the substrate for blood, blood vessels, muscles, connective tissue, kidney's, gonads .... and the skeleton'.

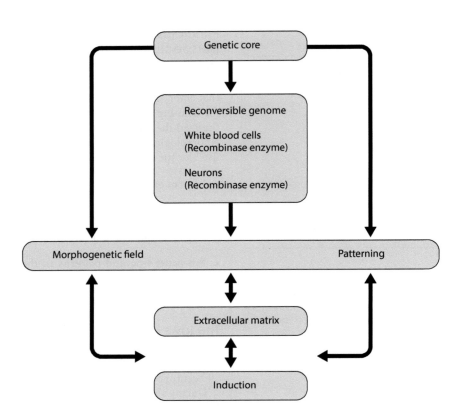

Figure 9.5
Patterning as a space/time molecular event

These findings could be defined as a multi-layered origin of form and function.

Another interesting observation was that all species, at a certain time point during their development, pass through developmental stages of lower ranked species.

Consecutive to these observations *'the laws of embryological resemblance'* were defined. The main conclusion from these observations was that each individual being recapitulates the phases of phylogenesis during its own ontogenesis, which was defined and described in different ways by subsequent authors:

• A parallelism between the stages of ontogenesis and phylogenesis was described (Law of Meckel-Serrèz).

• Darwin stated that it was not completely true that a developing being makes its ontogenetic evolution by passing through stages of lower ranked species (The origin of species 1855).

• Haeckel certainly influenced the embryological thoughts most profoundly and long lasting by stating that ontogeny is a recapitulation of phylogeny. He defined his observations as *the theory of recapitulation* (The biogenetic law).

Today we know that each embryological stage is not a recapitulation of an ancestral form. Biomolecular research findings underline the definition of ontogenesis as being a transition of subsequent developmental stages which resemble developmental characteristics of other phyla during their specific morphogenetic stages.

The laws of causality

In the late 19th/early 20th century scientists started more and more to be interested in the cause of form and structure building. The pure establishment of consecutive series of changing modalities in form and structure was not in the center of interest any more, as opposed to the mechanism by which changes were induced and developed.

Each structure in an organism undergoes a consecutive series of transformations, depending on:

- cell proliferation
- cell elimination
- cell transformation[9]

Two general concepts were defined:

- tissue structure displays *a gradient of development*
- *an organizer* is needed for coordinating cell proliferation, elimination and transformation

These two concepts can only come to life if a certain polarity is already found in the basic pattern of the cell. The axes of polarity for the future organism were thought to be already present in the ovum, long before differentiation of the embryo starts. The nucleus was found to be localized close to the superior pole of the cell in *the animal hemisphere*, together with the polar bodies. The vitellus was abundant in the lower hemisphere, which was called *the vegetal hemisphere*. This main organization is respected during future development of the fertilized ovocyte and guided by excretion of substances (later defined as morphogenes).

The principle of regulation was defined by S. Hörstradius during his research on the embryological development of the sea-hedgehog[10]. He remarked that at the vegetal pole there was a concentration of micromeres during the normal cell divisions. Hörstradius stated that:

- the quantity of these factors was of primal importance
- that a balance between the animalizing and vegetal tendencies was needed before a larva could develop in a normal way

Later, the 'micromeres' were defined as morphogenes.

The organization of axes in relation to the body plan

H. Spemann stated that the formation of the axial organs was the most important event during the early development of the vertebrate embryo[11]. He established that the cells at the dorsal lip of the blastopore constituted '*the organizing center*' for the individuality of the embryo. The blastopore appears as an invagination at the posterior part of the vegetal hemisphere during gastrulation and initiates the development of the ectodermal layer, after which neurulation starts. The anterior-posterior (a-p) axis of the future embryo was proposed to be already established in the female gamete during ovogenesis, which was supported by the asymmetry of the ovocyte.

The substances that play an important role in the construction of the future organism are produced by the genome of the gamete. These substances are concentrated in the cytoplasm in accordance with a well-defined order, which conditions the cephalad-caudal axis.

The point of entry of the spermatozoid determines the dorsal-ventral axis of bilateral symmetry. The generation of the dorsal-ventral coordinates is of major importance for conditioning the mesodermal germ layer and the nervous system.

Maternal proteins produced by the follicular cells and deposited in the vitelline envelope before ovogenesis determine the dorsal-ventral polarity. The dorsal versus ventral developmental factors interfere during the development of the neural tube as well as between the dorsal and ventral aspect of the blastula and gastrula. They also exert a reciprocal inhibitory pattern on the intrinsic facilitation of their opponent proteins.

The formation of the axial organs depends on substances localized in the dorsal region of the embryo. The main conclusion of Spemann's findings was that the a-p axis precedes the formation of the primitive streak, *confirming that geometry exists before form is laid down in structure.*

Spemann made a distinction between an autonomous and dependent differentiation. The dorsal lip of the blastopore seemed to be the center for differentiation of all axial organs. Later on Spemann stated that not only was it the center of differentiation but also 'the organizing center'. This center induces the neurulation phase after the formation of the three fundamental layers of the embryo. This phenomenon (neurulation) defines the start of the organization of the embryo and the development of the organs, which will materialize the a-p axis.

Other researchers, such as W. Vogt distinguished between primary and secondary induction[12]. Fertilization was considered primary induction. It elicits an ordered cascade of secondary induction responsible for form and structure. This secondary induction was called *morphogenesis*. Cells depending on the secondary induction react and organize themselves following a pre-existing plan. For the first time the term '*pre-pattern*' was mentioned.

The role of the organizer is restrained to the structure responsible for organizing the a-p axis. This axis is already determined in the ovocyte during ovogenesis. By means of the preliminary organization of the ovum (a-p axis) an inevitable cascade of secondary induction can occur that forms the embryo.

The dorsal lip of the blastopore contains the capability for organization and induction.

It remained to explore whether maternal or dynamic factors, i.e. chemical or physical influences, mediate the induction. If the determining factor was of a chemical nature, it should be found at the level of the organizer or the inductor. Spemann established that the induction of the new embryo was not dependent on one single substance, but two different types of factors. One factor is able to induce the neural structure. The other factor was thought to act on the mesodermal tissue[13]. Researchers such as Toivonen-Saxen published the hypothesis that during normal development these two factors are distributed in two different gradations[14]. One factor is distributed in an a-p direction (mesodermal component). The other factor is spread in a dorsal-ventral direction (neural component). The distribution of these two factors establishes a biochemical duality in the mechanisms responsible for the generation of the a-p and dorsal-ventral axis. The a-p axis develops with the aid of mesodermal components. The dorsal-ventral axis is generated by neural components.

It seems that 'neural induction' by 'the center of Spemann' is preceded by the induction of the mesodermal layer. The dorsal mesoderm has the function of the 'organizer' and 'inductor' of the nervous system, but a primary impulse is needed to start up this organogenesis. It was established that the mesoderm is activated by the dorsal endoderm. This center is situated higher up than the center of Spemann.

It was P. Nieuwkoop who discovered the role of the dorsal endoderm that influenced the organizing center of Spemann[15]. The new center was called 'the center of Nieuwkoop'. Mesodermal cells only seem to be produced when cells of the animal pole are associated with cells of the vegetal pole.

A new order was described:

- the dorsal blastomeres are capable of inducing the development of the axial organs (notochord and somites)

- the ventral and lateral blastomeres activate the generation of blood, associated vessels and the connective tissue

Based on these findings, a provisional conclusion was made:

- The mesoderm is formed by cells in the marginal zone, which is influenced by 'a mesoderm induction factor' dependent on the endoderm

- The endoderm itself displays two distinct impulses:
  - an impulse for a dorsal developmental pattern; i.e. the notochord
  - an impulse for a ventral developmental pattern: i.e. blood and blood vessels

- A third factor elicits the formation of the somites, the kidneys and the gonads. This chemical signal is related to the activation of the dorsal mesoderm (center of Spemann) and is distributed following a dorsal-ventral gradient, influencing the development of the striated muscle and of the kidney

Different factors of peptidergic nature have been discovered and described as activators of the mesoderm: PGF (Peptide growth factor), FGF (Fibroblast growth factor), TGF (Transforming growth factor) bèta, Activine A. They function as a 'passe partout' (a general accessory tool for activation or inhibition of a certain cellular program) and have varying effects dependent on the cell with which they interact.

Besides the fact, that the neurulation process needs an inductor of mesodermal origin (center of Spemann), another interesting fact has been established. When there is absence of a specific activator, the ectoderm is capable of an 'auto-neurulation'. This process most likely is activated by BMP4 (Bone morphogenetic protein). At the same time, the ventral developmental pattern continues to be activated, but seems to be dependent on a specific activator (analog to Activine A). In turn, this same activator is inhibited by two proteins of the notochord, noggin and chordin, which are associated with the center of Spemann.

Based on these findings, the following conclusions can be made:

- The organizer facilitates the dorsal developmental pattern

- The ventral structuring depends on the specific induction protein BMP4

- BMP4 is inhibited by two proteins issuing from the center of Spemann

It is important for the osteopath to understand the interdependence of the different induction phases as this could mean that perhaps also in the fully grown individual a 'hidden' hierarchy still exists, in function interdependence as well as in space/time organization. An example may clarify this statement: The autonomy of the enteric nervous system is nowadays established and accepted; it can be considered as a second brain. This 'brain' is not only able to function almost independently but also influences the autonomy of the central nervous system. The key can be found in the fact that before actual nerve activity was generated, the endoderm, as a germ layer, already was capable of determining induction, orientation and position of the neuroectoderm. Concerning space/time the body's structure and form is dependent on early patterns on which the definite functional forms and structures are built.

Pre-patterning and patterns in the organization of the embryo

It was W. Vogt who first mentioned the term 'pre-patterning' to summarize findings of migrating colored mitotic cells being capable of creating a mosaic structure of distinct regions in the developing embryo. Apparently, these cells corresponded to a pre-existing organization of cells. The induction of these cells seemed to respond to morphogenetic stimuli, which he considered responsible for what he called 'secondary induction'. The patterning of the embryo seems to be organized around a predetermined body axis. The major part of this axis is defined by maternal genes activated during ovogenesis. The development of the ovocyte starts in the anterior part of the female gamete called *the germarium*.[16]

This germarium contains germ cells, which undergo further divisions and in turn produce identical germ cells and cells destined to produce the ovocyte. Subsequent cell divisions occur in a longitudinal way and a concentration of germ cells lying ahead of the definitive ovocyte which is surrounded by follicle cells can be distinguished. One can make a distinction between a germinating cell lineage (germ cells and ovocyte) and a somatic or non-germinal lineage. The germ cells produce the major part of the cytoplasm and the mRNA, of which, after fertilization, proteins are generated in a specific sequence. The proteins as well as the mRNA are of ovocyte origin. They are stored in the cytoplasm.

These structures are determinative during the initial phases of the generation of the axes of polarity. About 50 maternal genes interfere with the establishment of the a-p and dorsal-ventral axes.

L. Wolpert studied the pre-patterning organization of the embryo.[17] Cells obtain an 'identity' in relation to their placement along a certain body axis and depending on their genetic information. They receive information about their position (positional value) and they are able to interpret this information, depending on their genetic determination. Consequently, a cell belonging to the endodermal, ectodermal or mesodermal cell layer will interpret an identical position differently. These cells react to the gradient of a substance capable of activating or inhibiting the activity of the genes contained by the cells.

The concentration of this substance varies along the co-ordinating axis of the embryo. A cell placed at a certain point of this axis will recognize its position in relation to the whole of the body organization. This substance acts as a morphogen in the establishment of the pattern. The frontier between different cell groups is probably delimited by the difference in the concentration of this particular morphogen.

The interpretation by a cell of its positional value is facilitated by concentration gradients, and its activation depends on the threshold, under or above which the answers of the mitotic cells will be different. By this means, well-demarcated zones of cell groups are created.

Morphogenetic factors and molecules

One of the major interests of embryology was to study the origin of polarity in the embryo and finding the different axes of the body that determine its definite development and internal references.

By studying the fruit fly, *Drosophila melanogaster*, three types of maternal genes have been identified which organize the a-p axis during gastrulation:

- Genes that organize the anterior region of the early larva

- Genes which are responsible for the posterior region

- Genes organizing the polarity of the anterior and posterior extremities

The 50 maternal genes that interfere with the establishment of the a-p and dorsal-ventral axes all possess their specific mRNA that produces specific proteins. For the a-p axis the proteins working on the anterior part are called *bicoid*. Those for the posterior part are called *nanos*. These proteins interfere along the a-p axis of the ovum in a decreasing gradient, with the concentration of bicoid being greater at the anterior part of the axis and almost not existent at the posterior part. For nanos the reverse can be stated. Interestingly, the extremities are also associated with a specific gene, which is called *torso*.

It activates the production of specific proteins, such as *acron* (anterior) and *nelson* (posterior). This gene is not transcribed by the cells of the ovum itself but by the follicle cells.

It is obvious to conclude that the extremities may develop in association with the activation of different types of genes compared to the central line. One has to remember that genes governing the a-p axis and their protein production belong to the germinal cell lineage, and that genes belonging to the follicle cell, i.e. the somatic cell lineage of the mother, govern the extremities.

The influence of the genetic program on the development of different body domains

It is evident that a great deal of embryonic development occurs under tight genetic control. Genetics have been well studied in invertebrates, such as the fruit fly *Drosophila melanogaster*, over many years. Starting in the early eighties, more and more molecular embryological studies have been conducted in the field of embryologic development and some evidence exists that similar molecular and developmental mechanisms are the basis for the fundamental aspects of early embryogenesis both in Drosophila and in humans.

In the earliest stages, the dorso-ventral and antero-posterior axes are established by actions of a series of maternal effect genes.

Once the oval-shaped embryo is developed, it undergoes a series of three sequential steps that result in the segmentation of the entire embryo along an antero-posterior axis.

Three different types of genes govern these three steps:

- *gap genes* which subdivide the embryo into broad regional domains

- *pair rule genes* which are involved in the formation of individual body segments

- *segment-polarity genes*, which work at the level of individual segments and are involved in their antero-posterior organization[18]

These three kinds of genes can be considered morphogenes because they prepare the organogenesis at an early stage: i.e. at the level of patterning and structuration.

A large family of homeotic genes, which facilitate the development of specific structures, governs the specific and regional characteristics of each segment. Recent molecular research has shown that the homeotic genes are arranged along the chromosome in a strict order and that this order corresponds to the topography of their expression in the body. Within the homeotic genes there is a highly conserved region called the homeobox. This homeobox produces a 61-amino acid homeo domain protein segment, which acts as a transcription factor.

Humans possess a large number of homeobox genes, which are found in four clusters on four different chromosomes. There exists a connection between certain agents affecting morphogenesis and the activation of homeobox genes. Retinoic acid, FGF and TGF-beta all activate different clusters of homeobox genes.

In general, one can presume that genes are implicated in three important evolutions during embryogenesis: patterning, histo-morphogenesis and cyto-differentiation. The patterning genes are morpho-genetic genes which determine spatial domains without anatomic specificity, they supply or determine the information about position. The genes of histo-mopho-genesis control the processes in space and time and the quality of cell metabolism.

The genes of cyto-differentiation induce multipotent cells into a specific cell lineage.

The homeotic genes seem to be the masterpiece of the general body organization and structuration. Their expression is regulated by the nucleic receptors of *retinoic acid*.

Retinoic acid intervenes not only in the workout of the general body axes but also contributes to organogenesis by organizing the patterning and the information of neural crest cells during their definitive determination and specification.

Other morphogenetic genes, such as that for the peptide *Sonic hedgehog (Shh)* also contribute to differentiation of general body axes. Shh determines the antero-posterior axis of the upper and lower extremities, the dorso-ventral axis of the neural tube and the right-left axis of the body. All cells derived from the same fertilized ovocyte are genetically identical, hence it is the work of the genes to select specific information in their genetic arsenal to establish region specific and segmental specific function. The homeobox genes (*Hox-genes* in humans) seem to play a capital role in these specifications.

Globally one can propose that retinoic acid plays a crucial role in the morphogenetic patterning during embryogenesis and organogenesis. By acting as a specific ligand, it activates nuclear receptors, such as RAR (retinoic acid receptor) and CRABP (cellular retinoic acid binding protein). Interestingly, the crucial role of retinol (a derivative of vitamin A) was observed in certain anomalies, such as fetal deficit of vitamin A. Anomalies of the eye, diaphragm, respiratory tract, and urogenital and myocardial deficiencies are sometimes combined, wholly or partially, in this syndrome.

Another interesting observation is that already in early embryogenesis Hensen's node functions as a source of retinoic acid production and secretion. Reti-

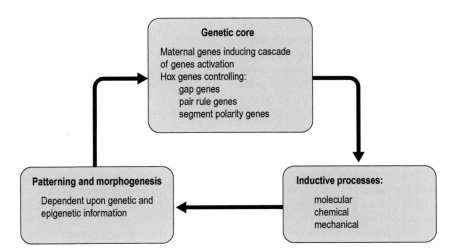

Figure 9.6

The genetic core is influenced by a successive battery of genes interfering with the triblastic organization of the future embryo, with patterning events that are synchronously occurring together with early inductive processes that happen at cellular level noic acid receptors seem to be indispensable for the ontogenesis of the mesectoderm. The mesectoderm is a sub-population of cells originating from the cephalic neural crest that generates mesenchymal cells, which help to construct an important part of the base of the heart, the chondroid and osteoblastic cells of the cranium and the face and the connective tissue of the thyroid, thymus and parathyroids. Arterial anomalies are usually accompanied by positional anomalies of these glands.

The following model can help to understand the different molecular events during embryogenesis and organogenesis that support the process of time and space related patterning (Figure 9.6).

Electrical and molecular factors in patterning and morphogenesis

Polarity as the first possible axis

The male genome seems to be more important for the development of the external layers of the embryo during the nidation phase, whereas the female genome determines the inner world of the fertilized ovum. This presents a qualitative distinction between the respective functions of the male and female information so far as the future embryo is concerned. Already before fertilization, a certain orientation of the primitive ovocyte seems to be apparent. During the first meiotic stage, a part of the material found in the nucleus of the cell is sequestered and eliminated towards the cell surface as the first polar body, which could possibly function as a first attracting pole to which the cell material is orientated.

A further polar body is secreted during the second meiotic division of the fertilized ovum. This polar body could be determining the orientation of the animal or vegetal pole of the blastocyste. Also, the sperm cell is able to segregate part of its cell content which could represent a third polar body. The place of entry of the spermion co-determines the embryonic/ab-embryonic axis (defined by the cell clusters which will form the later animal pole/vegetal pole) of the body. Apparently, an inherent polarity is already present during the meiotic and first mitotic phase of the ovum. It permits a certain organization of the cell around a central line for the development of nuclear divisions and cell multiplication. The initial polarization of the ovum seems to be dependent on the molecular concentration of metabolic compounds in the cell. They accentuate an eccentric position of the cell nucleus.

The intrinsic polarization and orientation is at the same time used as an orientation device for directing the zygote towards a metabolic pole outside the ovum, with the spermion helping to orientate the embryonic/ab-embryonic axis.

It is important for the osteopath to consider the non-differentiated or totipotential cell mass of the ovum and the zygote as a field of molecular and ionic compounds that interact by attractive poles. These attractive fields are governed by osmotic, ionic gradients that already organize micro-currents in the fluid and electrical environment of the first cells.

Polarity seems to be organized by an aggregation of cellular compounds that are able to modify the molecular and ionic concentration within the cell and its direct environment.

This could imply, that the first cell (the ovocyte) already 'knows' the intrinsic mechanism to polarize itself by segregation of the first polar body. It could also indicate that polarization is an indispensable event to provide structure to undifferentiated matter (molecular and ionic compounds).

This would mean that besides the structure-function relationship, also well known as one of the osteopathic principles, there exists an ultra-cellular world where electrical fields and currents determine the backbone for structure and shape. Consequently the osteopath should consider that disturbances in the electrical field of the body not only could be conceived as effects of traumatic, inflammatory or infectious episodes but that the electrical field in itself could be a disturbing factor for normal functioning or structuring processes.

In other words, the electrical field precedes the structuring process and guides its functioning. The following relationships should be considered in order to understand where the dysfunction in the body has started: undifferentiated matter – electrical field and currents – fluid currents – structuration – function – motion as an electrical and fluid outcome.

Two other consequences should be considered: Could it be that polarization organizes matter? Could it be that environmental fields orientate the intrinsic field of our body and that they are also capable of disturbing it? It seems clear that atmospheric changes or food imbalances profoundly interact with the normal polarization of cells. Should the metabolic process not be conceived as an electrical field? Do fluids and ionic exchange organize the chemical exchange in the gut not for a major part? Based on those assumptions, the osteopath perhaps may have to re-consider his therapeutic impact on the patient by seeing himself as a possible electrical field that more or less balances ionic and fluid gradients towards normality: *a balanced field of electrical exchange* where structure and function start optimizing their expression.

Genetic plan of embryogenesis

Genes are important for the generation of the fundamental body plan; they are involved in three important evolutions during embryogenesis:

- patterning

- histo-morphogenesis

- cyto-differentiation

All cells of the first mitotic phases are genetically identical and totipotential.

Homeotic genes determine the selection of appropriate cells and the program of their differentiation in the first instance. They act as selecting genes and are concentrated in specific domains of some chromosomes known as the homeodomain. One of the transcript substances used to inform the blastomeres is retinoic acid. Cells appear to have specific retinoic acid receptors (RAR), which are linked to a protein (RABP) that is capable of coupling the retinoic acid to receptor elements in the cell nucleus, which interact with cell division and DNA multiplication. Retinoic acid is also functioning as a 'fluidizer' in tissue reactions. One of the most explicit places where retinoic acid is secreted is at the Hensen's node. Here it organizes the major cell migrations towards the sites of intense morphogenesis. The linea primitiva and Hensen's node function as an important organizer for lateralization processes starting out from a formative midline. Each interference with tissue by manual or mechanical means could favor this primary process and give the body a subsequent impulse to reorganize the periphery in reference to the midline.

Body axis and lateralization

The linea primitiva represents the earliest manifestation of the generation of a basic body axis. It is evident that polarization processes of the zygote already precede this event.

The most remarkable feature is that at Hensen's node two morphologically different cell layers manifest, with epiblasts displaying a columnar population of cells and the hypoblasts showing a cuboid form. The cuboid cells of the hypoblast layer all possess cilia which introduce a leftward movement of the liquid in the vitelline vesicle. The structuring proteins generating this movement are dyneines and kinesines, which facilitate mobility of the cilia and the transport of organelles and protein complexes along the microtubules. They activate the rotation of the cilia that induces the displacement of the vitelline liquid.

A trophic factor is secreted into this cavity which is transported to the left part of the Hensen's node and which facilitates the activation of the morphogenetic genes by ligand/receptor interaction.

The cytokines of the TGF - beta family of growth factors, lefty 1 and lefty 2, as well as nodal cytokines are exclusively secreted by the cells of the left part of the embryo around the node. Lefty 2 and nodal cytokines are temporally inhibited because they tend to construct the right body plan. More caudally or parallel to the nodal flux, other signaling molecules are in use, such as Shh and retinoic acid (AR).

AR signaling seems to be implicated in a later stadium of migration of the neural crest cells or possibly during the post-migratory phase of the ontogenesis of the cardiac neural crest cells. It is at this time that the left/right axis of the body plan is constructed.

One can speculate that when the general left/right axis is not respected the visceral organization displays a tendency to a generalized isomerism, with the organs developing towards the midline of the body. Left and right isomerism are described, or a polysplenic or asplenic syndrome, respectively.

On a molecular and cellular level one can describe the lateralization process as being organized in three steps:

- Determination of the right-left body axis

- Asymmetric expression of signaling molecules

- Asymmetric morphogenesis

It is clear that beside the generation of a ventral/dorsal midline which creates a functional axis of the early body plan, there exists a general lateralizing tendency of organ positioning which is activated by structuring proteins and signaling molecules around or in the node and parallel to the primitive line. The tendency of a general isomerism, i.e. to develop towards a more or less complete symmetry, can be interpreted as an attempt to approaching the midline. This can be interpreted as an establishment of an equilibrium between laterality and the central axis, indicating a failure in molecular and protein signaling of the central line of the body. It seems evident that any disturbance in signaling, positioning or in the space/time process of the organogenesis will have its repercussion on adult body posture and functioning. In the osteopathic context, one could presume that "the twig" is already bent early during gastrulation.

The notochord and its influence on the neural tube

As long as the notochord, a rod-shaped cord of cells on the dorsal aspect of the embryo which defines the primitive axis of the body, stays in contact with the base of the neural groove and neural tube, it will exert a dorsalizing effect on the development of the peri-ependymal neurons. This indicates that it has a trophic and organizing influence on the final structure and shape of the neural tube.

In a later stage of development, the notochord loses its direct contact with the neural tube. The cells of the basal lamina of the neural tube continue to have a dorsalizing influence on neuron migration. The notochord in turn concentrates the chordal mesoderm around its axis and becomes an attracting pole for the lateralization and ventralization of the paravertebral and prevertebral ganglia. This attraction prepares the proximal part of the ventral pathway for migration and structuration of most of the peripheral motor- and sensorial neurons and of the vegetative nervous system.

The distal part is organized by visceral development and all structures converge towards the anterior part of various kinds of tissue of different origin. The different copulae and symphyses are the anatomical witnesses of this anterior, circumductive migration of the major vascular and nervous structures. Two major pathways influence the central dorsal signaling: towards the head or towards the periphery. The nervous and the vascular system both display a central ascending/descending and a peripheral posterior/anterior trajectory.

In conclusion, the interweaving of both functions creates a subtle and precise landscape for transmission of fluid and electrical information towards the periphery and the anterior part of the body, supposing that the electrical and vascular signaling informs other functions concentrated at the anterior part of the body. Major parts of the lymphatic and endocrine systems seem to be organized around a 'potential' anterior midline organization.

Memory in body functioning: osteopathic considerations

Structure and function are reciprocally interrelated

The interaction of function and structure in pre-natal patterning is one of the most important items studied in embryology. Until today, little has been published on transient functions of organ pre-forms and their relationship to definite function and position after birth. The structure/function relationship is one of the basic principles of osteopathy (i.e. the third principle as stated in 'The foundation for osteopathic medicine' of the AOA)[19].

It is commonly accepted that structure is needed in order to have function. This contradicts a statement by W.G. Sutherland who advocated that function exists before structure.

Equally, Blechschmidt[20] stated that each embryological structure is already a function.

The idea behind these two affirmations is that embryological development should be seen as a structuring by life, rather than creating life by structure.

Different authors have studied the principles of life from a molecular viewpoint[21] and taking account of physical forces, i.e. thermodynamics[22,23]. The assumption is that life needs the flow of energy for its structuring and patterning. The exchangeable energy creates the possibility of the shape, which sooner or later will integrate the original (originating) function that was 'dissipated' in form of free stereo-isomers of organic molecules, amino acids and minerals. Numerous biogenic compounds could be synthesized with nothing more than sparks of energy flow[24]. Prebiotic life seems to be organized as an ancestral 'metabolic complex' that created protocells and other forms[25].

The complexity of the inner organization, established by cell crowding, created the need for exchange mechanisms from the inner of the cell towards the outer layers and for immediate communication with the cell environment. These mechanisms were the precursors of transmembrane ion pumps and channels, themselves being precursors of more complex patterns of signaling, and they served as the neuro-endocrine signaling pathways of the systemically organized organism. The influence of the surrounding electrical fields on cell-behavior, form and polarity has been extensively studied in metazoans, ovocytes, blastocytes and gastrulating cells[26]. All seem to display the possibility of being influenced by minimally changing electrical fields, which are capable of altering polarity, and by electrophoresis of the cell membrane and the content of the cell.

If one wants to understand the claims made by W.G. Sutherland that function exists before structure then the physical laws of origin of life need to be taken into account. Embryology has always been studied from an 'anthropocentric' point of view, although man, as a living form, can only be considered being a part of life. Early embryologists went in search of the origin of men by studying the origin of species. They were not in search of the origin of function. Even nowadays, we are still influenced by 'the laws of embryological resemblance' (K. von Baer)[27] and the embryological recapitulation theory (C. Darwin and E. Haeckel)[28]. Studying molecular 'forms' still aims at understanding the function of structure but not life in function.

It could be proposed that embryological patterning not only serves to create and support adult forms of function but also continues to transform adapted patterns of function to more effective function as life continues. The mechanism of transformation of function is not solely dependent on a transformation of structure because learning processes for instance do not necessarily change the neurological substrate per se, rather than the patterning of the structure. Hence, function is not completely dependent on structure but on the quality, the kind of energy that is generated or released by the mechanism. One should consider the possibility that patterning is probably more a question of energy storage at different molecular levels (i.e. within proteins, amino acids, nucleic acids) than information purely bound to a certain anatomical form or physiologically supporting structure. Energy bound to macromolecules is stored in the form of vibration or electrical units, which create a space and time pattern that is applicable to specific transformations created by altering life circumstances or demands of survival.

Embryological processes seem to be more organized by genetic information, but on the other hand the amino acids that were generated via nucleic acids are in turn already space-time units organized by energy flow on the highest storage level (vibration and electrical energy). That is what Mae Ho means: 'Energy flow organizes the system and in its turn the system organizes the flow.'[23]

On a macroscopic anatomical level, one can observe the same laws of adaptation to the rules of life. Organs that change in position or shape do not necessarily indicate an involution of life, rather than a progression of life into another order of function.

As Hinrichsen proposed with regards to the heart: 'The heart is descending until senescence.'[29] Embryological patterning may not only serve as support for adult function but also continues its intrinsic transformational proceedings of patterns until death.

The patterning can be considered a silent exchange between function/structure until a novel function manifests itself. There is no definite structure in the body, even as there is no steady heart or brain function.

How could structure remain unchanged if functions are multivariable over the life span?

The answer may be that there exists a cycle between free circulation and dissipating energy that can modify the patterning that was laid down in the structure/function relationship.

This is essential to function, which not only displays a patterning dependent on structure but also constitutes an intrinsic space/time relationship. Speaking of prenatal patterning, one can remark that there are two stages to consider. The first stage would be tissue differentiation (i.e. gastrulation), elicited by the need of a specific exchange of ions and molecules (gas exchange, osmotic exchange) between different compartments, such as the amniotic cavity, coelom and vitelline vesicle. The second stage refers to tissue differentiation which structures a form of specific integrated function. The tissue that creates support and directs all kinds of exchanges is the mesenchyme, by means of epithelio-mesenchymal and ecto-mesenchymal exchanges.

The *prenatal period* can be seen as a stage of tissue information and organization, depending on genetic and epigenetic influences exempt from gravitational forces. The *postnatal period* is related to a time scale during which genetic influences decrease, and are replaced by epigenetic and gravitational factors. *Adult life* expresses a balanced interchange between function and structure, giving the opportunity for refinement or decline in function and subsequent alteration in structure.

When questioning the process of ageing one should also take into account the duality between structure and function: i.e. is it the deterioration of structure that impedes function, or is it the decline in function, which determines the deterioration of structure?

Senescence should be considered an altered state of function rather than a decline in function by loss of structure. Life can be regarded as a balance of function dependent on different types of environments that are composed of parts of our biological sphere (Figure 9.7).

Function is a continuous process of energy passing through matter, adapting to patterns of information more or less continuously in the conformation of the structure it composes.

As the twig is bent, so grows the tree

Minimal changes in function require structure to adapt; changes in structure impede the inserted function of the original patterning. This process can be perceived as an adaptation or a loss of original capacity to interfere with the inner or outer environment.

The conclusion would be that the structure presents a 'balancing role' between the function and the inserted pattern, therefore representing a tool used by function to achieve its aims.

Function is structured such that it permits itself to be expressed and re-expressed in a repetitive way. Part of the function seems to be 'memorized' in the di-electric bonds within the structure of proteins and collagen bonds. Structure is in fact a memorized geography of integrated function.

It seems evident that structure serves function in 'memorizing' its tools. Original structure, i.e. 'balanced' structure can support original patterning, such as original potency expresses itself by way of balanced momentum between function and structure. Probably the organism struggles for conservation of its original potency; for that reason it needs free tissue, free energy and a kind of determined chaos[30].

Thermodynamic, electrodynamic and electromechanical laws of energy conservation seem to play a

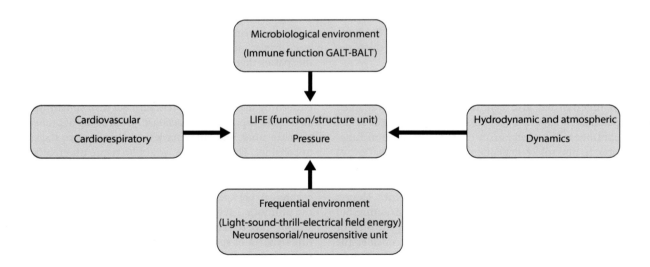

Figure 9.7
Life is organized and expressed by different biological and biophysical parameters.
GALT - Gut-Associated Lymphoid Tissue. BALT - Bronchus-Associated Lymphoid Tissue

crucial role between function and structure in a living organism[5]. It is noticeable that any structure that takes on or creates form is an 'imprinted' pattern of function. Conception is already a pattern; embryogenesis, organogenesis, birth, all of these episodes represent an increasing summation of inserted patterns. They are imprinted in decreasing or increasing order by means of genetic and epigenetic information.

Ultimately, form is shaped by its inherent function/structure relationship (i.e. biofeedback loops of segmentally organized biomechanical, visceral, and immune-endocrine patterns).

To find the patterns the osteopath should support the structure in its balanced tension to get in contact with the original function (i.e. energy transformation), inserted into a specific pattern that withholds a specific time/space unit. This procedure elicits non-segmental reactions based on free-energy exchange and on biodynamical principles. Here, the balanced state of a structure contains more basic information than the organized patterns, belonging to the segmented construction of body function.

The osteopath can communicate with the imprinted pattern by supporting it in its original confrontation with the laws of life. These laws are dependent on:

- *Genetic-epigenetic patterning and pre-patterning*
  Pre-patterning is dependent on the laws of polarity, laterality, molecular concentration gradients, and morphogenetic fields.

  Example: Intra-uterine environment: i.e. rhythmic information of the intra-uterine environment by vascular, hormonal, maternal-placental and placental-fetal exchange, maternal infections during pregnancy.

- *Perinatal circumstances*
  Descent of the baby and presentation of the head in the pelvic girdle of the mother, pattern of the birth process, postnatal care giving of the baby by the delivery team, including doctors and midwives – all these are important factors that determine later reaction patterns of the baby.

  Also gentle handling of the baby by the parents, for example by changing diapers, are important for determining the way in which the child will react to physical contact and social interference later on in life[31].

  Example: Cesarean section: By lack of compression during the passage through the birth canal, the decompression forces may be insufficient, not procuring enough volume or resiliency to some tissues or organs. Compression of the spleen seems necessary for freeing oxygen-rich blood that supports the re-organizing cardio-vascular circulation for a short time. Tissues such as the peritoneum or pleurae may remain in a more or less 'retracted' state instead of a dynamic resilient physiology of their collagen-elastin substrate. It seems evident that the osteopath should be able to recognize such compressed patterns and subsequently provide physiological compression, facilitating a more dynamic pattern of tissue response.

It should be noted that an 'imprinted' pattern is not necessarily a 'traumatized' pattern. In a traumatized pattern, the structure no longer serves the original imprinted function but rather expresses an impeded or deteriorated function. This changed pattern will predispose to dysfunction by altering the movement, motion or tension in the structure and by this means falsify the reflex patterns organized by the nervous and biomechanical units of the body.

A dysfunction of a structure does not need this hierarchical organization of the body autonomy to induce an accident-prone 'behavior' of the organism. The whole organism, i.e. body and body consciousness, is organized as a coherent field, implicating that a 'tissue dysfunction' in any part of the body has its input on the origin of other tissues and subsequently influences the integrity of the original function/structure relationship.

One can subdivide the progression of the structure/function (S/F) relationship from early life expression to adult organism as follows:

- F1 (Embryological function), supported by S1 (Structure of integration for F1)

- F2 (Function belonging to imprinted structure), supported by S2 (structure that supports F2)

- F3 (Organogenetic function dependent on subsequent stages of organogenesis during fetal period), supported by S3 (Structure supporting and expressing F3)

- F4 (related to early postnatal function and influenced by gravity and atmospheric pressure), supported by S4 (Structure supporting and expressing F4)

- F5 (Function progressively adapted to different growth phases into adulthood), supported by S5 (Structure supporting and expressing F5)

- F6 (Function related to regression and ingression of organs and tissue, and inducting senescence), supported by S6 (Structure supporting and expressing F6) (Figure 9.8)

Where there is loss of function, the structure should be compressed in such a way that it can balance itself in its deteriorated pattern to 'pick up' the information stored in its unbalanced state. By doing so, it can alter its inner state, whether by passing directly to F2 (the operational function), or by going back to F1, the original function that stores embryological information. The structure should be treated in its compromised pattern for restoring its original potential of exchange and motion.

The functional state of a structure can be altered by traumas, for example those during early life. Such traumas, either pre- or postnatal, are known to be elicited by:

- compressive forces to the skull (the best known lesions to osteopaths)

- compressive forces acting on the vertebral column (torticollis capitis, torque)

- compression of the cervical spine or at the level of the sacrum

- the impact of compressive/de-compressive forces on soft tissues of the cardiovascular cavity or pleuro-peritoneal cavity (aspiration, birth by C-section)

- Infections and their incubation periods

   Most reproduction of pathogens occurs in the structuring tissue of the organs controlling homeostasis, such as in the meninges, pericardium, pleurae. A focal trigger point or tissue is established which by means of pro-inflammatory compounds disturbs and re-organizes the structure of other tissues (local irritation, fibrosis, and other structural disorganization)

- Surgical interventions also have to be considered a possible factor contributing to changes in the structure/function relationship of the body tissues

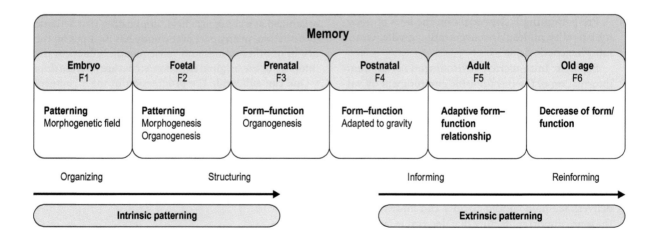

Figure 9.8
Life memory depends on intrinsic and extrinsic patterning

In conclusion, the therapeutic aim within the postnatal period can be defined by three objectives:

- conservation, support and restoring of the original life potency

- support of the 'imprinted' and functional pattern

- restoring the homeostatic equilibrium by balancing the traumatized tissue

Synchronicity: interdependence of developmental cycles and rhythms

Life is an expression of energy passing through matter

The energy management of a biological system generally aims to 'economize' its energy use or expenditure by functioning within the thermodynamic equilibrium. Some cycles function to retain or regain the spent energy, although a certain loss of energy (entropy) seems inevitable. Some economy is generated by the fact that the system tries to 'relate' different cycles of energy management by making them synchronous or by creating phases of energy interference and expansion. Cycles, such as respiratory and cardiac rhythms are evident in phases and are synchronous with the rhythms expressed at the brainstem by the oscillations of some cell groups that are responsible for the respiratory rhythm as well as cardiac tonicity and cardiac rhythms. The latter are themselves dependent on coherent fields of interaction within different brain areas.

Some physiological laws depend on thermodynamic laws, and some on hydrodynamic laws, but all are concerned with the development of the molecular frame of structure and function. These laws support electrodynamic, electromechanical and electrochemical exchange. The transition of energy (vibratory, electrical, magnetic) in an organism needs chemical, bioelectrical, and enzymatic reaction patterns which are not restricted to one specific functioning cycle but are involved in the whole of the developing organism in space and time. Hence, one type of cycle can be repeated almost infinitely in supporting different patterns of functioning. Furthermore, the developing organism structures itself by means of resonant energy patterns and coherency fields.

Function is integrated as a specific time-space unit in the developing tissue that integrates 'energy phases' into a structured pattern. The structure incorporates the energy phase as a space-time unit, which, in turn can be conceived as an integrated memory.

Each tissue, expressing a specialized function, is related to an important structuring process, which in itself is organized by a specific energy pattern. This pattern creates the integration of a certain time (frequency) into a well defined space. Both, time and space define a specific episode in the development, structuring and functioning of a type of tissue during developmental phases.

Dependent on the location where developing cycles are either synchronized or linear in their development, one can easily understand that for example the processes of liver structuring, heart building and brain maturation are functionally and structurally related. These processes are linked to some anatomical and functional space-time units which relate to function and structure development of each organ and original availability of energy.

In our example concerning the liver, this would mean that the venous-arterial left-right shifts organized by this organ in relation to a shift of a vitelline circulation to an omphalo-mesenteric one are equally important for the orientation of the cardiac cavities. Subsequently, the development of the brain, which is exposed to a major part of the cardiac output, is in itself functionally and structurally organized by the hydrodynamic information of the heart.

The brain develops not only based on genetic patterning but structures itself in a resonant way responding to the afferent information of the hemodynamic (hydrostatic) information related to the transitory stages of heart maturation and orientation. One could almost describe a common time-space unit for the development of the ductus venosus, the development of the septum primum of the heart and the mesencephalic flexure.

This example may be chronologically incorrect to a certain extent, but it indicates that a specific synchronicity could exist between the development of different anatomical areas and tissue-structure specifications.

The development of the brain is a function of the space-time building processes integrated into other organs (liver-heart) and its neuro-integrative function is built by space-time occupation, which is concerned with the structuring of specific organs and their subsequent function. The brain in itself is organized by the energetic patterns of liver and heart, before it can structure itself completely into a neuro-electric wire complex with its definitive integrative and organizing function.

For example, the development of the basal ganglia of the brain is not only the result of a compression phenomenon of this specific area by the expanding brain around the third ventricle. The structural organization of the area around the third ventricle is as much supported by the intrinsic hydrostatic pressure in the ventricle as it is dependent on the hydrodynamic information it receives by heart output and volume expansion of the liver.

Each nucleus in the brain could be described in a synchronous developmental pattern related to other patterns in the endodermal and mesodermal levels of organogenesis.

The brain in its entirety can be described as a space-time unit related to specific episodes of organ development and space-time building of the whole body. The neurological function is related to the specific 'wiring' and the development of a specific mapping, creating a memory chart that we call consciousness.

In conclusion, the brain function-structure transformation is determined by:

- Field interference (synchronicity, resonance, coherence between liver-heart-brain)

- Neurological patterning (genetic, epigenetic information)

- Neurological maturation (reproduction of embryological patterns in an adult neural circuit and functioning)

The interrelationship between the brain and the skull should in turn also be interpreted with the same point of view. Both are synchronous-coherent fields of patterns developing in a succession of resonant cycles of transforming function-structure relationship.

The development of the brain and the skull express:

- A genetically determined patterning

- A time dependent orchestrated migration of neural crest cells

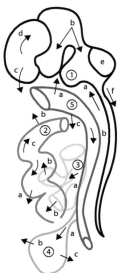

1 Development of cortex (a, b, c, d, e, f)

2 Development of heart bulge (a, b, c)

3 Development of lung buds (a, b)

4 Development of liver-pancreas (a, b, c)

5 Development of digestive tract (a, b, c)

Figure 9.9

Co-localization and co linearity of different morphological fields during embryological development[32,33]

- A spatial patterning dependent on maturation and mechanical interaction between brain-skull, skull-brain, brain vesicle and brain structure

Synchronous structuring and space/time units in body organization

A synchronous structuring with a whole body-organ organization and structuration during different space-time units of functioning is evident during all embryonic and fetal episodes. Each organ contains a full range of stored space/time related information in the centre of its own structure and function. The micro times of evolution and specialization of predetermined cells are not only valuable for brain development but also at all other levels of cell/tissue specification. Each organ has an actual function which is built on past micro times of cell determination/specification during morphogenesis and this information is still integrated in the organ and its function (Figure 9.9).

References

[1] P. Kaul., Motion moves sound, Ausgraph conference proceedings, Australia, 1990.

[2] E. Blechschmidt., The stages of human development before birth. S. Karger, NY., 1961.

[3] Heine H., Lehrbuch der biologischen Medizin. Hippokrates. Auflage 2, pp. 13-45, 1997.

[4] A.T. Still., The philosophicsal and mechanical principle of osteopathy. Osteopathic enterprise, Kirksville, 1986.

[5] A. Chila., Conferences on fascia. Namur (Belgium), 2000 & 2001.

[6] R. Becker., Life in motion. Stillness Press, 2001 & The stillness of Life, Stillness Press, 2000.

[7] S. F. Gilbert., Developmental biology. Sinauer, 7th ed., 2003.

[8] S. F. Gilbert., Developmental biology. p., 51, Sinauer, 7th ed., 2003.

[9] S. F. Gilbert., Developmental biology. p., 51, Sinauer, 7th ed., 2003.

[10] S. F. Gilbert., Developmental biology. p., 78, Sinauer, 7th ed., 2003.

[11] S. F. Gilbert., Developmental biology. p., 79, Sinauer, 7th ed., 2003.

[12] S. F. Gilbert., Developmental biology. p., 24, Sinauer, 7th ed., 2003.

[13] S. F. Gilbert., Developmental biology. p., 79, Sinauer, 7th ed., 2003.

[14] S. F. Gilbert., Developmental biology. p., 79, Sinauer, 7th ed., 2003.

[15] S. F. Gilbert., Developmental biology. p., 341, Sinauer, 7th ed., 2003.

[16] Le Douarin N.M. La crête neurale. Une structure pluripotente de l'embryon vertébré. Bull Ass Anat. 80(251), p.13, 1996.

[17] L. Wolpert., The development of pattern and form in animals. Carolina Biological, Burlington, 1977.

[18] E. Saliba et al., Médecine et biologie du développement. Masson, Paris, 2001.

[19] M. A. Seffinger & I.M. Korr, Osteopathic philosophy. pp. 3-14, AOA, Willams & Wilkins, 1997.

[20] E. Blechschmidt., Sein und Werden. Urachhaus, 1982.

[21] C. de Duve., Life evolving. Oxford university press, 2002.

[22] L.V. Beloussov., The dynamic architecture of a developing organism., Kluwer Academic Publishers, 1998.

[23] M-W. Ho., The rainbow and the worm., Utopia Press, 1998.

[24] D.A. Lovejoy., Neuroendocrinology., Wiley & sons, 2005.

[25] M.R. Edwards., From a soup or a seed? Trends Evol. Ecol. 13, 178-181, 1998.

[26] A. Deloof. The electrical dimension of Cells. Int Rev Cytol, (104); 251-352, 1986.

[27] S. F. Gilbert., Developmental biology. p., 24, Sinauer, 7th ed., 2003.

[28] S. F. Gilbert., Developmental biology. Sinauer, 7th ed., 2003.

[29] K.V. Hinrichsen., Human Embryology. Springer-Verlag, 1990.

[30] H. Heine., Lehrbuch der biologischen Medizin., Hippokrates Verlag, 1997.

[31] R.L. Birdwhistell., Kinesics and Context. Penguin books, 1970.

[32] P. Van Den Heede., International conference of osteopathic paediatric medicine, June 2000, Utrecht (NL).

[33] P. Van Den Heede., The Importance of Osteopathic Visceral Techniques for the Development of the young brain. De osteopaat, 1²; 18-23, 2000

10

The Incarnating Embryo – The Embryo in us
Human Embryonic Development in a Phenomenological Perspective

Jaap van der Wal in collaboration with Guus van der Bie

What I see is just the covering. The most important is invisible....
From: The Little Prince by A. de Saint-Exupéry

Introduction

When professionals refer to prenatal life or existence they most often implicitly refer to *fetal* existence. From a biological point of view prenatal existence includes the phase of embryonic life. The *fetus* is distinguished from the embryo by the fact that in the former the body plan has been completed, at least at the macroscopic level. Embryonic life is a matter of somatogenesis and organogenesis i.e. formation of the body and of organs. The transition from embryo to fetus is said to be at about 8 to 9 weeks after conception. This means that at about two and an half months of pregnancy the embryonic phase of human existence is considered to be completed and is followed by the next stages or steps in human life i.e. fetus, newborn, childhood and so on. One of the issues of this chapter it to show that embryonic 'way of life' is not a past episode but is psychosomatic actuality also in our later cycles of life including adulthood.

In terms of human biology and psychology the embryo functions in a way that differs essentially from the 'way of life' of an adult or a child (or even of a fetus). This in particular regards the functioning of the brain and senses. Nowadays it is widely believed that the nervous system in general and the human brain in particular have been proven to be the core of the human mind and human consciousness, of the human psyche or *soul* so to say. "Like a kidney produces urine, so the brain produces consciousness" is a widespread notion nowadays. In this typically *Cartesian* image of man the brain is considered as the origin, the *cause* of human behavior and psyche and therefore psyche, soul, mind and spirit are reduced to purely physiological i.e. material processes. Within the paradigm of natural science the view prevails that soul or psyche (belonging to the Cartesian realm of *res cogitans*) should be considered as nothing but a matter of brain action and therefore actually as belonging to the realm of *res extensa*. This view challenges the moral status of a human embryo: How could an embryo possess mind or soul if it does not even exhibit the shape of an actively functioning brain or nervous system? For most people therefore, the embryo has become a kind of half existence, a phase where man is not yet 'complete' or not yet entirely 'there'. As in the case of *brain death* the embryo is considered as *mindless*, which very often in the current moral and ethical debate is regarded as *not (yet) human*.

The questions at stake could be paraphrased as "What do we actually **do** when we are an embryo?" Or "Are we actually doing something?" Conventional definitions of human behavior are based upon the reductionistic image, that our nervous system in general and our brain in particular is the last *asylum* for what is called the human soul or mind. Soul has been reduced to consciousness, consciousness being reduced to brain activity. So, if you do not have a brain yet as is the case in our embryonic phase, how indeed could you act or behave? Within the frame of thinking of modern biological science no other domain (*locality*) and origin (*causality*) can be considered beyond that complex organ inside our skull. *Locality* and *causality* are pre-eminent *Cartesian* notions. But is *mind* to be located at all? It may also be experienced as something that 'happens' within our body so to speak. The reality of this realm can only be experienced by self-investigation and introspection, but that approach is no longer appreciated in conventional natural science.

Neurophysiologists nowadays study the **substrate** for soul and for consciousness. But finding an anatomical, physiological or genetic phenomenon ('body') apparently connected and associated with a certain mental activity ('soul') does not mean finding the phenomenon itself. Apparently brain activity can also be considered as a **necessary but not sufficient** condition for consciousness. Still, there is a risk of confusing the *condition* for a certain matter (body, brain, and gene) for the matter itself (soul, mind, and feature). Such reductionism prevails in genetics today. As a biologist, I however have never perceived that genes (here I mean the reductionistic concept of 'gene' as a formulated DNA-structure) are playing an active and causative role in a living organism. This is not to deny that genes play an important role in the phenotypic appearance of organisms. Yes, organisms have features and properties. Sometimes, they become ill. But I have never seen an "ill gene" or a gene with a certain property, like being able to move or to digest. But yet, seemingly without discussion, people seem to believe that genes are active principles and that they **cause** organisms. As a phenomenological embryologist, I reject that view completely. Only in pathologically abnormal or experimentally manipulated conditions (and of course in the evolutionary process of mutational changes in the genome) it appears to be the deviation of a given genomic pattern that causes the related different 'new' phenotype or phenomenon. In the normal integrated situation of the functioning organism, however, it is not the genes that cause the phenomenon. The organism itself is performing the biological activities and functions that characterize it (and for that it apparently needs genes).

What about an embryo? In the modern view of neuropsychology, the embryo does not have much chance to be accepted as a being with a mind, consciousness or soul. In an embryo, the least manifestation of a functional brain is completely absent. If one wants to define the moment at which a first brain 'activity' becomes discernible in the embryo, we must wait for the fetal phase in order to see some substrate for brain physiology like movements of limbs or a deducible EEG activity. In modern somatic philosophy – "you are not present there in that body, you are your brain" or "there is no Self

or soul living this body" - the body of the embryo also has been 'emptied' or 'ghosted.' Thus the embryo has become a brainless and therefore unconscious being. A body without a mind? How about all those organs in me of which there is not the slightest manifestation of awareness or consciousness? No mind there? But mind, awareness ('soul') produced by a specific organ? Does unawareness mean that mind is absent? The old philosophical dilemma of soul versus body is there. How do we exist in that so-called 'mindless' phase of our life? Just like we now function in our unconscious body and organs? Are we absent in those body domains? Or do we as sentient beings of soul and mind come into our body in some way: the concept of incarnation. Do we as 'souls' only live in our brains and is "the body" just serving the nutrition, locomotion and reproduction of that brain, as some diehard neuropsychologists nowadays state[1] ? What can the embryo teach us about a possible mind ('soul') living in our unconsciousness body? Is the 'embryo' still in us and therefore not only or simply a non-personal past in our life?

The performing of the body as behavior - existing in forms and shapes

A possible key to such dilemmas as presented here might be given by reconsidering the definition of **behavior**. One may also read behavior in living organisms from their *morphe* (form) and *Gestaltung* (shaping), i.e. from their continuously changing physical appearance. An organism always presents itself as a unity of shape, function and environment, continuously changing *in time*. The rose in the vase is not **the** rose. One has to include time into the image of the rose: from seed to plant, to bud and flower, to withering, etc. Far 'prior to that' the organism already shows behavior in a broader, morphological sense and exhibits behavior by means of its forms, its bodily organization and its shaping (*Gestalt*).

At first sight an embryo seems to be in a phase of life and development in which one cannot yet detect human behavior. Many people nowadays consider embryonic

[1]Apparently for philosophers that defend this stance, 'the body' begins somewhere at your neck. Below that level there is the 'body', on the one hand feeding, moving and reproducing the brain, on the other hand ruled by that organ. Above that level there is the brain ('the head') which apparently is on the one hand a regular part (organ) of the body, on the other hand not, but a special domain. This sounds like a vague and obscure re-introduction of outdated Cartesian dualism.

existence as 'purely' a matter of biological growth and differentiation, of metabolizing cells and tissues. The embryo is not yet functioning psychologically or 'being aware'. To answer the question "What is an embryo actually doing?" we first have to elucidate what actually goes on in an embryo. The embryo is a whole, a complete self-organizing being that seems to tend to 'fall apart' into its bodily components like organs, tissues and cells. The actual human embryo (human being) maintains its order within and through those processes and organizes them. During embryonic development one may describe a tree of cells, tissues, organs, which originate as a sequence *out of* each other and gradually differentiate in shape and function. This process, typical for embryonic development, is called *differentiation*.

The embryo therefore is neither the summation nor the result or consequence of its differentiating parts, its cells and organs. Organs and cells should be considered as secondary, the whole, the organism itself is primary. Biologically speaking one never observes that something is 'added'. At any one moment the human embryo may be seen as one entity that maintains a unity, a oneness. The 'whole' is not produced by building blocks; wholeness in living organisms is an activity, a lifelong process, performed, maintained against the resistance of 'falling apart' into separate body parts, cells and so on. This is how the German embryologist Erich Blechschmidt (1904-1992) characterized embryonic development. He proposed for the human embryo (as well as for every living being) the *Law of Conservation of Individuality*. By this is meant that the *shape of appearance* of an organism might change over the course of time but that *the essential being* itself remains unchanged, present and active within these outer shapes and forms. A human embryo is not *becoming* a human, it *is* a human being. The human organism (like every organism) is so to say not a being but a 'becoming', i.e. being in time. This means for example that a fertilized human egg (cell) the so-called *zygote* is not 'just' a cell, **it represents the human organism at that stage**. A human zygote is a complete manifestation of the organism *man* at that very moment, under the circumstances and environmental conditions that exist one day after conception.[2]

In *every* phase of its development the human embryo is a coherent whole, a unity of form, shape and function interacting with its environment. Every stage of the human embryo, in spite of homologies in form and shape with mammalian embryos, is a human manifestation (see Figure 10.1). We may look like a cell, or a fish (exhibiting homologies of gills) but *we* never are a cell or a fish! From the point of view considered here, there is no argument to regard any previous embryonic phase *less valuable* than a next one or to consider it as *not-yet-human*. The principle mentioned here is actually evident and perceivable for everyone. Have you ever met a person

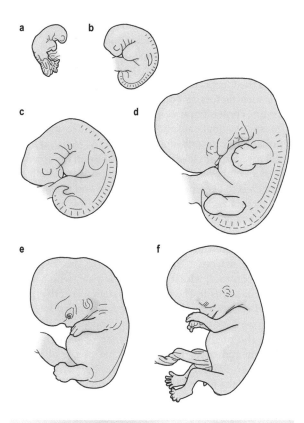

Figure 10.1

Stages of a human Embryo: 26 days (a), about 4 weeks (b), about 5 weeks (c), about 6 weeks (d), about 7 weeks (e) and 3 months (f). *From: The Human Embryo, E. Blechschmidt, Stuttgart, 1963*

[2]Actually the notion 'fertilized egg cell' is wrong. With conception the egg cell ceases to be a cell. Together with the fused sperm cell it transforms into a unicellular *organism*, called a *zygote*. A zygote might look like a cell (homology) but it is not a cell, it is a body, an (unicellular) organism, a whole!

who showed a photograph of themselves as a little child in the playpen (or, as a modern variant, a picture of a prenatal ultrasound when still in the womb) and stated: "Look! That was/is not me yet"? Like every living being we are appearances in time. From conception to birth, from birth to death, the human biography is an entity, a whole. *All* the appearances and expressions of a human organism, be they morphological, physiological, psychological or mental, are to be understood and interpreted as human expression, as human behavior.

The speech of the embryo

Describing and studying the shape of appearance gives us insight into the nature or essence of the living being or organism as it expresses itself by this behavior of growth and shape. It might help to *understand* a plant, an animal, but also the human embryo. Understanding is not the same as *explaining* the organism. The latter leads to the forms and shapes as causes, the former considers such factors as conditions. Like every scientific discipline contemporary embryology is mainly involved in questions about causality leading to the formulation of explanatory descriptions about HOW. What are the causal mechanisms leading to the shape and the appearance of an embryo? The ultimate perspective of such an approach is to become able to influence and manipulate those factors and processes. Understanding or perception of behavior however implies another approach, different from explaining the behavior. An example might elucidate this. The anatomist may explain how we make a fist, what 'causes' a fist so to speak: which muscles contract, which joints participate, which control mechanisms in the nervous system are active, and so on. However, to understand the fist as behavior, as a *gesture*, we have to apply a different approach. We have to take the phenomenological stance of participating in the phenomenon, rather than that of the observer or onlooker. For this one has to describe, perceive and understand the fist in the context of human action. How many feelings, meanings and gestures can be expressed by a human fist? The fist of restrained anger, the fist of triumph, of pain, of shame, of power. Placing myself assertively and empathetically into the gesture of the fist, it may be possible to trace the meaning and sense of that gesture. Forms as gestures, as intentions, as behavior. The hyphen between the domains of psychology, physiology and morphology is *motion*, understood and experienced as *gesture* or *intention*.

To understand the language of the embryo as meant here, it is a prerequisite to state that understanding the embryo means understanding the whole, the entity. Explaining – i.e. searching for causes of the shape, form, *Gestalt* of an embryo – brings one to the (body) parts, the cells, to DNA. It is the path of reduction and analysis. There is nothing wrong with that if one searches for the How and causes and explanations, but it doesn't enable the search for meaning or for answers about Why. Understanding leads to the whole, to the manifestation of the organism as a whole. The methodology needed for this approach of an organism may be found in *(Goethean) phenomenology* in general and in *dynamic morphology* in particular.

Dynamic Morphology – the Goethean approach

The approach of *dynamic morphology* is rooted in *Goethean* science and *phenomenology*. Like the phenomenologist the dynamic morphologist describes the form of an organism in its appearance in order to understand the dynamics of the underlying 'formative gesture'. Often the morphodynamic gesture of a biological shape can be recognized by the formative shaping gesture of the embryonic development and/or by the way the *definitive* form of an organ or body part is achieved in the adult organism. But such knowledge is not an absolutely necessary prerequisite for understanding the *gesture* that *speaks through* or is expressed by a form or shape.

The psychological internal restating of the underlying motion that is being expressed in the form, may recognize the gesture that, as it were, 'speaks' through a form. In this way the given form can be recognized as an internal motion or gesture, which means: psychologically understandable and imitable. This does not mean that the recognition of the morphodynamics of a given form has to be considered as a *subjective* action in the sense of *related to a personal and individual imagination that cannot be transmitted in an impersonal objective way.* The next example might elucidate this. Everybody will accept the containing character of the skull with which it protects and shields a given content from the outer environment, in contrast to the openness with which the limbs interact with that environment. One could therefore describe the skull as an antipathetic[3] (closing,

---

[3]Beware that the notions 'sympathetic' and 'antipathetic' are not applied here as 'good' or 'bad' or 'positive' or 'negative' but as two opposing qualities of behaving. Polarity, like the Yin-Yang principle, has nothing to do with good or bad, plus or minus.

separating) shape, the limbs as sympathetic (opening, connecting) gestures. The gesture of the form is evident in this case. The related mental act may have aspects of an *emotion* and feeling (sensing) rather than of a rational objective fact, but this does not mean it is only *subjective* and therefore nonscientific. We are dealing here with *intersubjective* objectivity. An essential component of the phenomenological approach is to consider organs, parts of a whole (a body, an organism) not in detail, isolated from the context to which they belong but to consider a form, a phenomenon in the context of the whole of the organism (the body) and to look next for the contrast in that same context so contrasting as a method of gaining insight. Comparative morphology is one of the manifestations of this approach. To understand a skull in its shape, its gesture, one should study it in contrast to the limbs or to the abdomen. This latter example is inspired by what will be introduced later on in this chapter as the craniocaudal gradient of development and organization in the human body. The craniocaudal gradient appears to express an essential polarity in form, function and behavior in the human body.[4] We term this approach *dynamic morphology*.

This implies that *dynamic morphology* does not apply an analytic process to describe shapes and forms. It tries to understand the gesture (*Gestalt*) and the form or shape in a more integrated and holistic way, it is a qualitative approach. Goethe referred to the perception and understanding of a so-called transcendental or *supersensible* quality in any form. By this expression he meant that the gesture or *forming language* of a form cannot be placed in the Cartesian category of an entity perceivable by our senses (*res extensa*)[5]. It is also important to be aware of the way the Goethean scientist approaches an object. In analytical science, the scientist has the attitude of '*onlooker*', in Goethean science, the scientist works with a *participative* attitude. He participates consciously in what is going on in morphological processes. This kind of consciousness enables the scientist to recognize movements and gestures (qualities) working in morphological processes.

---

[4]One of my teaching one-liners is: "To understand a brain, study a liver and compare".

[5] A good alternative for the Cartesian notions of *res extensa* and *res cogitans* could be *ponderable* and *imponderable* or *exact* versus *enact*. 'En-act' like ex-act 'is derived from the Latin word act or actum which means 'deed' and 'made'. 'Ex-act': what has been made, realized, 'en-act: that what makes or realizes (itself).

Morphology and Psychology: soul is being 'pre-exercised'

A human embryo does not 'function' in the sense that the latter term is used when applied to a body or an organ. The latter so to speak 'have' a function (or better: mechanism) as a prerequisite. The embryo still 'functions in forms'. Everywhere where one deals with living nature and with organisms, one is impressed by the perfect harmony that exists between form and function: the two categories always fit perfectly. The relationship between the two is close and subtle and refers to the well-known philosophical dilemma: What is first - the egg or the chicken? As to function and form there is really no solution for this dilemma: most of the time people consider the two as a kind of indivisible duality or twofoldness. One may study either the anatomy or the physiology but there is no one-directional causal relationship between the two. A similar dilemma is produced by the categories Mind (spirit, soul) and Body. For example: is a brain the cause or the (necessary but not sufficient) condition for a certain psychological activity. What is first? Mind or body? In several philosophical systems (including Osteopathy, Chinese Medicine, Anthroposophy) such dualities are considered as inseparable entities and therefore as polarities. Polarity is oneness, one cannot isolate or separate the two components of a polarity: two of a kind

In the view being developed here of human embryonic life and existence there seems to be an opportunity to overcome philosophically the supposed duality of form and function (or even more accurate: of form and mechanism). The embryo permanently changes its form(s) and shape(s) in a continuous process of metamorphosis. It is all a matter of motion and change of shapes. It could however also be considered as a very particular way of moving, a particular mode of 'behavior'. An example should elucidate this. When one takes a glass of water with one's hand, one performs an act, a performance by means of the hand and the arm as instruments to take a glass of water. An arm is an anatomical and physiological substrate that is perfectly fitted to take glasses of water and in this example functions as such. Considered in this way an embryo of about four or five weeks old does not yet 'have' (possess) an arm or a hand as an anatomical substrate. But in the weeks to come we may observe that a human embryo grows an arm and a hand out of its trunk as an act, a performance. The parts and elements that in the future will constitute an arm become discernible. This developing arm, as it were, 'performs' a movement of growth, an act of growing 'at the end' of which a structure will be formed, will be grown out, that is perfectly well fitted to grabbing glasses of water. This growing therefore represents a movement, a function of the arm. In general one is allowed to state that at the end of a long process of metamorphosis a very specialized and very special feature appears: an arm as 'result'. The form appears, comes forth out of the movement! The form, the shape may be interpreted as the final phase of a process of movement, come to 'rest'. Of course the process through which such an arm 'reaches' its final shape also 'determines', or at least constrains the forms of this structure and therefore its functional (i.e. mechanical) possibilities and constraints. The way in which the arm has been growing out, has been performed, is a very important defining (constraining) condition for the later 'function' of that arm. What connects the two is the principle of *gesture*: the gesture with which an arm grows and the gesture performed by that arm when it functions. A similar principle can be found in psychology. All our moving and locomotion can be considered as a continuous positioning and behaving in space. On the other hand do emotions move us in just the same way that our motives (i.e. what moves us) can bring us to motion. The concepts such as 'motive', 'e-motions', 'motion' and 'movement' are all derived from the Latin verb *movere*. Moving and gesture are *transdisciplinary* notions: gestures are both the 'language' of morphology and of physiology and … of psychology.

The summarizing and unifying formulation of the foregoing considerations might be that an embryo, unlike a so-called adult organism, does not yet 'have' forms or body shapes (that exhibit a function) but that an embryo 'still functions in forms and shapes'. In the adult and so-called full-grown organism form and function are considered as a kind of duality of two separate and discernible but strongly related and connected principles. One could state that in the embryonic organism those two principles are not yet 'separate' but still one and unified. The embryo functions, behaves (growing and changing) in its shapes and Gestalt. The embryo is motion in process. The embryo 'per-forms' gestures and movements. Its growth and metamorphosis, its continuous changing shapes, represent its performance and behavior. **The embryo behaves! The body is behavior!** These are the more or less one-liner conclusions to be drawn from considerations above.

This view could have interesting consequences for the mind-body dilemma. Is 'soul' something so to speak entering the body later, or is it produced later on by its major organ i.e. the brain? Or is it, to rephrase Erich Blechschmidt, that "soul is being pre-exercised in the body"? An adult human organism possesses a complete and principally different perspective and orientation to his/her world and environment. This perspective is completely opposed to the perspective of the embryonic way of being! This opposition between an adult and an embryo is schematically represented in Figure 10.2. For the adult organism the body represents an immediate 'instrument' for the expression of his/her essential being. In and by means of the body the human being is expressed so to speak 'centrifugally' into the world, the environment. For the adult, the world, the reality around is the aim of their existence: our body as an instrument of expression for the soul. In an embryo however the situation is absolutely the reverse. Realize that the method of contrasting and comparative morphology is applied now! In embryonic life the body itself is the centre of its existence; the human being is involved in the formation of the body itself. The latter is the centre of its existence and aim, goal of its functioning, not yet the 'world' around, not yet the environment in which we exist. In the embryo the spiritual-mental human being more or less sleeps itself unconsciously into the body in a 'centripetal' orientation. This means that *the gestures of growth* with which the embryo behaves, are expressions of human development, of becoming and being human. In a later phase the performance and *Gestaltung* in the development more or less comes 'to rest' (final forms) in the morphology and anatomy of the adult body (however not to the same extent for all various organs and body domains!). In the 'adult' state energies, forces, principles of growth and formation become available on other levels, serving the adult expressing and behaving. Considered in the way shown here, the adult human being and the human embryo appear as polarities in their mode of being. The first is a being of expression, finding its achievement and goal in the 'world', and the surrounding environment; the latter is more or less a being of 'im-pression', by which its spiritual essence is per-formed, 'expressed' in the formation of its body shape(s). If one considers a human newborn of about four months as a phase in

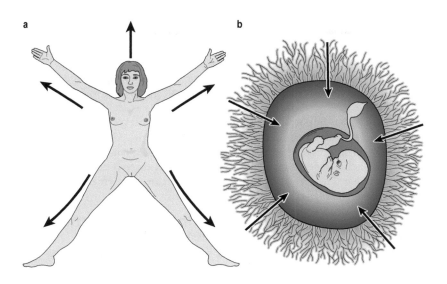

Figure 10.2

Revolution of Orientation in Existence between an Adult (a) and an Embryo (b). Centrifugality against centripetality. *From: Dynamische Morphologie, O.J. Hartmann, Frankfurt/M., 1959.*

between the described adult and embryonic orientation, then one could see that such a being still more or less follows an introverted pattern of existing ("it still only drinks and eats"). But already gradually something is emerging by means of this bodily organization, which will become more and more expressed and visible during human life.

Looking for movements and motions in human embryonic development we may find *growth gestures* and *developmental movements*. Those developmental movements are performances and therefore also to be considered as human behavior! An arm and a hand grow in the gesture of taking (and giving), the leg for instance grows in a gesture of supporting and walking upon. Breathing, taking, walking, going upright, these are not 'consequences' of a bodily organization. They are expressions of human nature, of human behavior that are first more or less pre-formed and pre-exercised during the embryonic phase, in order to 're-appear' later on at the physiological and psychological level.

The embryo 'pre-exercises its soul', with the physical body as resistance to perform. This resistance is a necessary condition for that performance; without it there would be no development possible, as Blechschmidt formulated as one of the major principles of embryonic development.

In fact Blechschmidt formulated three principles of embryonic development:

- "Soul is pre-exercised in the body".

- Developmental movements are performances.

- No performance without resistance.

Long before we take our first (physiological) breath, long before the first time we grab the finger of our mother, or make our first step, we have 'exercised' those movements as growth movements or developmental gestures, as so to say psychological performances. Breathing, grabbing, walking are not the result or consequence of a bodily physical organization, they are appearances of human behavior on the morpho-physiological i.e. functional level. And are breathing, grabbing, standing and walking not also psychological gestures? Also standing upright or going upright are both movements of the mind, i.e. movements of the soul or the I (am), as well as performances on the anatomical or physiological level. Also important in this context is the notion that a performance only can be undertaken against a resistance: no action without a re-action. Where we deal with re-action a performance has to be the primary act. It is motion that goes before everything. It is on the origin of every being and becoming, of every change, of every form. Movement (process) is the primary quality, not form or shape. In form a movement, a process comes to an end, comes to 'rest'. Another way to express this: for movement there is no cause, it is cause itself! "Am Anfang die Tat" (In the beginning the act) (Goethe). The ultimate consequence of considerations like this might be that the body is not producing us (or our soul or awareness) but rather that we from the very beginning function as a oneness of mind and body, of enact and exact, of soul and body and that it is as Rumi (1207 - 1273) said:

Wine got drunk with us, not the other way.
The body developed out of us not we from it.
We are bees and our body is a honeycomb.
We made the body, cell by cell we made it.

This approach helps us to understand the embryo at best, just because everything in the embryo has to do with becoming and shaping, with process. If we consider the movements and gestures that lead to the human body shape and *Gestalt*, it is evident that they are spiritual in nature. Take for example going upright. As we will see later, an embryo can already perform the act of coming to an upright position. It does so in an act of growing movement. Later on we will 'repeat' this act when we as a young child for the 'first' time become upright, in balance within ourselves. What a joy, what a performance, what "a small step for a man, but a giant leap for mankind". One or two years later the child may surprise its mother by no longer talking about him/herself in the third person but 'out of the blue' states: "I do want a piece of bread". A first psychological 'coming upright', perhaps? The force or power of becoming upright is not only present as the essential act of development and growing during the various phases

of embryonic development or early childhood, but it can also be recognized with admiration and wondering, when one meets a person who performs the act of 'going upright' on the spiritual level. For example like the professor during my student days, who exhibited an impressing power of walking upright as an individual although his so-called handicapped body was hardly capable of achieving a genuinely upright body position (M. Bechterew). Going upright as an act of strength of mind and spirit, not merely as a morphological or physiological act; becoming upright despite your bodily restraints or impairments; the 'body' as resistance for the 'soul'?

Birth as a the primeval gesture of development

So where do we come from? The question posed by the curious child philosophically relates to the issue of body and soul. Does our 'soul' emerge from our body, produced by an organ? Or are we a psychosomatic entity (polarity) and is our development also an act of incarnation, of embodiment? Or to state it more generally: do we live centrifugally from or centripetally towards the body? What is the gesture that might be considered as the essential gesture or prenatal development? Is it possible to 'read' such a gesture or principle from the phenomena that represent the 'speech' of the embryo, which is the 'language' of shaping and growing

During the first week of human embryonic development the so-called *zygote* starts to divide into two, four, eight, sixteen and so on smaller cells. After some three days the embryo looks like a spherical 'clod of cells', the so-called 8 to 64 cell *morula* stage. The *zygote* (which, it should be repeated here, is not a cell but represents the human body at that stage) differentiates into many smaller elements (cells). Each cell has its own nucleus and has its own cell membrane. All these events take place inside the whole of the zygote-sphere (*conceptus* or embryo). There is no physical growth yet; at the end of the first week the body still has the same shape (sphere) and size as the zygote. At the end of the first week when the whole system is subdivided into over a hundred cells, two differentiated types of cell appear. In the center an *inner cell mass* or *embryoblast*, representing what in a later phase will appear to be the so-called 'proper embryo' (or, a better notion in my view: the 'proper or actual body'); at the periphery a mantle of *trophoblast* (or *outer cell mass*) out of which in a later phase the placenta and membranes will develop. We may conclude that out of an entity (which is the zygote) via a stage of multitude (the *morula*) a duality or twofoldness (the so-called *blastula*) arises. 'The one divides into the two'. From now on we deal with a center (embryoblast), subdued to centripetal forces and tendencies (usually considered as the 'actual' or 'proper' body!) and an opposite pole with a centrifugal tendency, a periphery (trophoblast) that has a completely different relationship to the environment, because it interferes and connects with it and from now on will interact with the maternal environment in a metabolizing way.

One can see that during the first week, step by step, the zygote becomes more and more structured, more or less 'lifeless', and that it hardly interacts with its environment. The whole system more and more resembles a mineral-like structure: a spatial structure without growth, with hardly any metabolic interaction with the environment, i.e. still lacking features that are so typical for living organisms like time, growth and metabolism. This whole is nearly pure space and structure, constituted by particles (the cells), typical of inorganic nature. This first phase will end as soon as the embryo manages to nidate (or implant), which may happen after four, five or even seven or eight days. This so-called 'first week' is not a calendar week; it represents a way of being, of behavior, which through nidation becomes a completely different way of being in the second week. There exist animals where this first phase may last a few months, a so-called *embryo pause*. In such cases the blastula remains in the womb or Fallopian tube for months. When the conditions in the maternal organism have changed through seasonal factors in the environment and are ripe for it, the embryo nidates (implants) and in a revolutionary gesture a complete new and different way of existing and biological behavior brings the embryo to the next phase of development. This revolution is mainly characterized by an enormous 'peripherization' and expansion of the 'peripheral body', usually indicated as the *trophoblast*. It looks as if the first week of embryonic existence takes place 'outside' the biological time of the organism: "time[6] is not here yet". At least time is not 'incorporated' yet. The embryo still lives in the dimension of only 'space', as in 'eternity', as in mineral and inorganic nature.

[6]By 'time' we mean not cosmic time but the life time, so typical and characteristic of every living organism.

But development continues. At the center of the whole system that the embryo represents the embryoblast still exists as a kind of retaining center against the peripherizing tendencies of the trophoblast around it. It is in the periphery that the trophoblast exhibits the activities and tendencies related to growing, expanding, differentiation, metabolizing and interaction with the environment; in the center this is all more or less restrained or withheld. The principle of a duality/twofoldness still exists: the 'center body' now indicated as *entocyst* still opposes a 'periphery body' now described as *ectocyst* and still 'the two are one'. In the fourth week of development yet again names and structures of those two 'body parts' have changed. 'Periphery' is now called 'amniotic sac' and the 'center body' is now designated as the ('proper') embryo. Again however there exists this dual orientation to the environment: peripherizing and centrifugality against centering and centripetality. Even in the fetal period one might consider the two body parts or principles as opposed in '*fetus* versus *placenta* with *membranes*'. But it is the whole organism that we are dealing with here that represents the human embryo and the human body. In opposition to the 'regular' view in gynecology and embryology, the phenomenological approach which is applied here until so far did not give any clue or argument to distinguish between the 'actual' or 'proper' embryo (body) on the one hand with the placenta and membranes as a kind of secondarily added body dimension on the other hand. That is how they are usually interpreted and described in terms of *secundinae* and *adnexa*, added or auxiliary organs. It may be that there are good phylogenetic arguments to describe the development of placenta and membranes as a kind of secondary development – indeed one may observe that something like membranes and placenta are a later so-called 'invention' in evolution giving rise to a whole phylum of *placentalia* – but in the context of the human ontogeny there are no arguments for such a definition. The opposite might even be true: phenomenologically one could consider the periphery pole of the prenatal body as the rooting and primary dimension and the centre body, with the embryo (fetus) as the secondary one developing out the former (see below)

In prenatal life the physiological processes in the embryo are organized and oriented from 'outside' to 'inside', from 'periphery' to 'center', i.e. centripetally. It is in the outer 'envelopments' (first in trophoblast, next in the so-called ectocyst, next in amniotic sac and later in the placenta and membranes) that the embryo, the prenatal being finds it roots and 'origin'. There are the morphological and physiological necessary conditions for its biological existence, there it breathes, there it metabolizes, there it excretes, there so to say it roots and lives, there it exists!. In the third week of development, with the formation of first blood vessels and a heart, a stream of blood and nutrition is developed which brings the metabolic nutrients from the 'periphery body' to the 'centre body'. If this does not occur, the center with get lost from it periphery roots and the embryo (conceptus) will die off with a miscarriage as result.

Phenomenologically one could describe the relationship between periphery and center as a kind of En-velopment process as well as the gesture of a De-velopment. 'De' is Latin and means 'out of' or 'against'. Maybe this is what is made possible: a center can be De-veloped against the En-velope to which it is primarily related and connected? In the first week 'periphery body' (trophoblast) and 'center body' (embryoblast) are in immediate contact with each other. In the second and third week however there starts a kind of separation process in which the two entities tend to appear more and more as a duality: the two body domains start to grow and 'behave' in a very opposite way and direction. If not an intermediate system of mesoderm with blood and blood vessels and heart would be formed, the centre would die out the periphery and the whole system would perish. Consequently from the fourth week the center body (the so-called 'proper embryo' or, better, 'proper body') emancipates from its peripheral envelopments (the amniotic sac) by a space filled with clear water, the amniotic cavity. Now the embryo only survives thanks to the mediation of the umbilical cord. In the fetal phase this gesture of separation is also represented by shaping the poles of placenta and membranes within the 'periphery body'.

Summarizing one could describe the process morphodynamically as a gesture in which the centre step by step is De-veloped out of the periphery: a center is born out of a periphery. In this process the center gains autonomy, becomes more and more independent. What in the beginning was one, is step by step differentiated into a *duality* remaining an entity, so a twofoldness. The placenta and membranes also are in principle not a part of the maternal organism as is indicated in some languages using the term 'mothers' cake' (*Mutterkuchen* in German). In prenatal life they are part of the human body, of the human embryonic organism. If the placenta is a 'cake', it is at least a 'children's cake'.[7]

The essential and principal gesture of human embryonic development is the formation of a 'center body' *out of* a 'periphery body' with which and in which the embryo actually is rooting. This 'inner' or center dimension ('body') more and more emancipates from its rooting pole until at the end it completely separates from it. With the disconnection of the umbilical cord (birth!) this inner or center body develops out of its outer periphery and envelopment(s). This means that when we are born, we perform the act, the gesture of dying! During our prenatal existence our emancipating inner or center body - which we now in the postnatal stage consider to be THE body - was connected with, enveloped and sheltered by that periphery body in which we were oriented to and openly connected with the 'out there', with the environment. In German birth is called *Entbindung* which can be translated at best with de-composition, disconnection, untying, release. What was connected before, now is separated. The same can be applied to the process of dying, on one's deathbed. In Dutch the act of dying is described by the process of *ontbinding*: again a de-composition and untying! In prenatal development the gesture of De-veloping (literally) is predominant: something is De-veloped. In the dynamics of this emancipation gesture the center body comes forth out of the periphery pole. At birth a human being performs an act of dying: a human being is being born out of him/her self! The whole prenatal gesture is one of dying from your peripheral, isn't that your heavenly, celestial or spiritual roots and dimensions? How meaningful of the German language to describe birth as a process of *Ent-bindung*? As at a deathbed the process of dying could be interpreted as a disconnection, untying of the spirit from the body. At the same time one could state that a soul is born and that one is born out of a spiritual dimension. Where do we die from? We therefore do not come or originate from 'our mother's belly' - as so many times our children are being told nowadays - we come from our own roots, from our own (heavenly) origin. There seems to be a corpse at birth: the placenta and membranes as the periphery body that is left behind and that represents the peripheral

---

[7]That is why I do disagree with the usual notion in textbooks that there is a 'proper embryo' and something like *secundinae* or *adnexa*, secondary or added organs. No, the blastula as a whole, so also the later amniotic sac and placenta represent the embryo, our prenatal body! Apparently the body is suborganized into two domains.

dimensions where we have died from. Birth of the physical body may be seen as dying out of the periphery (spirit) while dying of our physical body may be interpreted as a birth of our spirit? So mother is not kicking us out of her womb or belly, we have to De-velop and die out of ourselves and mother is assisting us in that. She literally is our backup![8]

Is that gesture of enveloping and next developing not the principle gesture of human development during our whole life? Every time, again and again, we have to envelop ourselves so to say with an environment that supplies us with nutrition (physical or psychological), with stimuli. Next we root in that 'mantle', that nourishing environment and establish our roots there, we connect, we en-velop. But in order to reach a next stage or phase we have to de-velop, dismantle from that environment in order to find ourselves born in a new stage, a next phase of development. If we do not, retardation, staying behind is the consequence. The newborn human dies out of its prenatal way of living and existing. Certainly there is a risk in ending this way of being and existing, we will lose something, we even might literally die on it, but we may win new possibilities, new encounters, new impulses, and other nourishment. When we die out of that womb a complete new relationship with an up to then unknown dimension becomes an opportunity. In between the various stages and phases of development there are seldom smooth transitions of 'more of the same brings us to the next stage'. On the contrary, there are critical moments in between: disasters, discontinuities, let us say births, De-velopments. In our physiological birth we 'repeat' a morphological birth that was already performed in the fourth and fifth week leading to the morphological emancipation of the center body from the amniotic sac, the so-called delamination of the embryo. This gesture is again exercised at the moment of birth, this time physiologically. Could it all be a 'pre-exercising' of a primordial act of De-veloping that we also have to be capable of as psychological beings?

---

[8]Isn't it in this respect not very meaningful that at the end of the first 'week' when the embryo nests into the mucosa of the womb, we do that in the backward direction? At the moment of nidation there comes up in the embryo a body orientation (embryo pole and ab-embryonic pole) which only a few days later will manifest itself in the future dorsal and ventral body orientation.

Intermezzo

A tale about an unimaginable existence

Imagine you are (still) a fetus - *thinking* that the world is as you acknowledge and experience it at that time. How could you imagine another world, a different way of being? You just awoke in this world, in this reality. You awoke by opening and discovering your senses, but you are still dreaming. Slowly, step-by-step you are becoming aware of things, of the world around you. Your experience does not reach beyond a warm mantle of water. Dim warmth enfolds you, you know yourself carried in a rolling, softly giving cover. Awareness does not go beyond that. There is darkness, now and then a softly shining light. Vaguely soft rumors are heard. Voices and a murmuring sound of a heart. It is there, all around you. As yet things do not have names, there are no notions. You might 'think' (if one thinks at all when one is still a fetus): "This is it, this is the world, reality, so this is what my existence will be like." How could you know 'better' or otherwise?

And you become attached to this world. With complete surrender you build roots of confidence and being in this world, in this living mantle of membranes and placenta. That is your safety and surety. That is where you breathe and find nourishment, in there you exist, in there you root. A solid and safe base, *ground* under your feet. "Look at me, hanging on life-long cords" as the poet says. Imagine you are (still) a fetus and might 'think': "This is the way it is, this is the way it should be. This is life, existence; this is my reality, my world."

But then ....! Then comes a moment that the ground of membranes and covers under your feet starts to shake, starts to fail, to give way! Once reliable and safe connections are shaken. Blood vessels are torn, breath is nearly taken away! That reliable pouch that carried you starts to release you. The water that carried you all that time, that protected, fed and covered you, flows away. You are driven out, out of your paradise, your foundations are faltering. You are driven out! Out? What for? To where? Is there an *outside*? There is no such thing as an *outside*, there is no *there*, there is no other way of living, of being than this 'here' where you lived! It is UNIMAGINABLE that you could continue without that well-known world in which you awoke, that carried you and that you trusted! You are in pain, in distress, you are dying …!

But then....! The UNIMAGINABLE happens! At the end of a narrow, dark tunnel you live on! It is possible! Air singes your lungs, but you can breathe. It is a way of life hitherto unknown, unimaginable to you. There is light, there are loud noises, but also warm hands and arms that carry and comfort you. You can find nourishment: there is a warm breast you can come home to.

Is it not the same kind of notion that prevents us to look over the frontier of our death now? How UNIMAGINABLE it is that we could survive without everything that now represents our world, our current reality? To exist without this body, so familiar and a lifelong trusted house, without this world where I am safe and secure of my staying alive. Could there be a *somewhere else*, a *somehow else*? An existence *out there*? It surely cannot exist, it is unimaginable.

Imagine you are fetus again, in this reality, in this world! That one day you might be born through a tunnel into another way of being, living on at the other side? Existing in an unimaginable way. The unimaginable a possibility? Who knows, someone is waiting for you in that other reality? Are they aware of you during your pregnancy?

Being born: dying out of the coherence and wholeness of our prenatal existence, coming from a *there* to a *here*. Dying: going away from *here*, being born in a *there*, on *the other side*? Being born and dying, two sides, two aspects of a similar, of the same motion?

Conception, a gesture of incarnation?

Where do we come from? The child who nowadays asks his parents or school teacher the question will be taught that there is not a 'heretofore', a dimension 'where you may come from' but that "you are made, you are the product of the fusion of a sperm (cell) and an egg (cell)". No more, no less. However some children are told that they come from the stars, or from the same 'heaven' where granddaddy has gone to when he died. Who is right? What are the facts of human conception? In what various ways can we interpret the related facts? What are the gestures of the phenomena? Are we making or receiving children? In other words: Is there the gesture of either centripetality or of centrifugality again? Or both?

Gametogenesis (the formation of the so-called sex cells) starts with the primordial germ cell. From this stage on, differentiation into the oocyte in the female organism on the one hand, and into the sperm cell in the male organism on the other, is a process of increasing divergence and polarization. We may list a great number of properties of the primordial cells, which in subsequent differentiation develop in opposite directions into oocytes and sperm cells. (See Table 10.1). The approach of comparative and contrasting morphology reveals the two as a basic and fundamental polarity. Therefore, the context of a sperm is an egg and the reverse. They are not two, they are one, a polarity. Or, to state it more 'poetically': they belong to each other. When a sperm fuses with an egg, fulfillment takes place. They do not fuse and then become one; they fuse because they are One.

One may see immediately that a pronounced polarization is exhibited. The process of divergence includes germ cell differentiation in opposite directions. At the same time there is a reciprocal development in germ cell differentiation, typical for a polarization (see Figure 10.3).

The spherical shape of the egg cell is the shape that couples a minimum of contact with the outside environment to a maximum of volume and content (creates 'innerness' so to speak). The spherical shape of the egg cell represents the quality of being 'a world on its own'. The egg cell has a relatively large amount of *inner space* (content): it is the cell with the largest volume that may be found in the human body. The ripened egg cell is as big as a grain of sand and therefore **visible** with the naked eye, which is an extraordinary feature for a cell in the human body. For the dynamic morphologist it is important to realize that the egg cell is not only large in the sense of quantity and measures but that *she* exhibits the *gesture* of being *large*. During the ripening process the egg cell *gathers* a relatively large amount of cytoplasm, which is expressed in a relatively high (actually pathological) nucleus-cytoplasm ratio. This represents *the gesture of 'being large'*. The egg cell becomes so large that it becomes visible but also so large, so much cytoplasm so to say, that an egg cell can no longer live on her own: she needs to be incubated and taken care for by an ovary.

Compare that with a sperm cell; let us look at the sperm in contrast. There is a tendency to speak of sperm cells in the plural. Unlike the solitary egg cell a sperm is never by itself, only one sperm cell in the substance of a male ejaculation is pathology. The production of sperm cells (*spermatogenesis*) is characterized by the production of enormous numbers of cells while the process of *oogenesis* (production of egg cells) is characterized by a tendency of

	Oocyte (ovum)	Spermatozoon (sperm)
Shape	sphere	radius
Cell volume	++++ 'large'	- - - - 'small'
Nucleus-cytoplasm ratio	- - - - 'cytoplasmatic'	++++ 'nuclear'
Mobility (externally)	nil (being moved) so-called 'passive'	++++ (is mobile) so-called 'active'
Dynamics of the inner content	++++	- - - - (mere structure)
Total number of cells produced in a life time	400	billions
Total of cells released at fertilization	1 (seldom 2 or 3) 'one'[9]	millions 'many'
Localization of the gonad as to the body	inside body cavity (visceral)	'outside' body cavity (parietal)
Temperature quality needed for ripening	warm	cool
Shape of the gamete	ball, sphere	radius

TABLE 10.1: Some differences (contrasts) between gametocytes:

diminishing and reducing in number. The whole process of egg cell production and ripening might be described as a *converging* tendency (gesture). During the lifespan of a female the number of egg cells stored (not produced) in the ovary is reduced from millions via thousands to hardly any in the menopause. In contrast to this the male process exhibits a *diverging* tendency: continuously enormous numbers of sperm cells are produced (and recycled) in the testes. This numerousness is also functional. Very many sperm cells will be sacrificed in the process of overcoming a lot of anatomical, physiological and biochemical barriers, which a sperm has to face in order to be able to make contact with an egg cell in the end. The 'production' of egg cells from the ovary is a process of titration (one by one), the production of sperm cells in a testis is massive and explosive. These features cope with the polarity of *one* and *solitude ('oneness')* for the egg cell (see above) versus *many* and *community ('multitude')* for the sperm cells.

As to their shape there is also a very strong contrast between the two gametes. The egg cell could be described as purely spherical. In contrast the sperm cell should

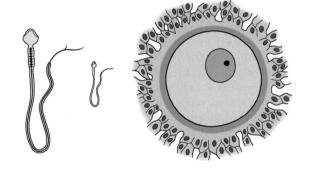

Figure 10.3

A sperm cell or spermatozoon (left) and a non-fertilized egg cell or oocyte (right). In the centre a sperm cell at the same magnitude as the egg cell.

be characterized as a radius-shaped cell. In the sense of morphodynamics the polarity is evident and impressive here. The egg cell is a ball. Is that not a shape with (endlessly) numerous *non-visible* radiuses? The sperm cell in contrast brings the principle of *radius* to appearance. A bunch of sperms may in a gesture of concentration constitute together a ('invisible') sphere. Moreover the sphere (of the egg cell) is also characterized as the shape of 'all-one-ness' or being alone, combining the minimum of contact with the outside environment with a maximum of volume and content (the gesture of creating 'innerness'). On the level of **extra**cellular mobility the sperm cell may be described as active and mobile. The egg cell should be characterized as 'passive' on this level. She can be moved, she listens to and follows the current of fluid she encounters, she yields to the environment so to speak. When we look at the **intra**cellular level however, the egg cell represents the active cell, the cell in its so-called interphase. This is in line with her characteristic as a metabolically active cell interacting with the extracellular environment. The cytoplasm of the egg cell should be regarded as relatively very dynamic, as such in strong contrast to the intracellular inactivity of a sperm cell! More than ninety percent of the content of the sperm cell consists of nucleus i.e. strictly organized and structuralized DNA-substance; there is some cytoplasm in its neck (mainly mitochondria) and the long tail is mainly constituted by structuralized fibrils. The sperm cell represents the gesture of a cell in its mitotic phase so to speak. In contrast to the egg cell, the sperm is not a metabolically interactive and 'open' principle. They 'shut themselves off' from the environment: it is traditionally the sperm cells that may overcome and survive drastic procedures such as freezing, centrifuging and acidification. Biologically speaking they are nearly invulnerable, certainly in contrast with the 'open and vulnerable egg cell!

The polar character of the two human gametes can also be discerned evidently by studying their behavior regarding cell division and ripening. Inherent to the phenomenon of bisexual reproduction the egg cell undergoes two reduction divisions (*meioses*) in order to reduce the number of chromosomes to half of the normal (i.e. *diploid*) number. As a rule the result of a cell division procedure is two so-called sister-cells and in the end both are about just the same size as the so-called mother cell they are derived from. This is not at all the case for the *meiosis* of the egg cell. She divides

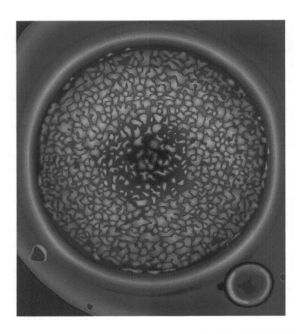

Figure 10.4

A human oocyte before conception. There is a clear zona pellucida and an so-called polar body

into one big voluminous sister cell which represents the actual *oocyte* and into an unusually small cell, the so-called *polar body*. The latter only contains the redundant half of the chromosomal substance and does not play a significant role anymore in the process of conception in humans as far as we know (See Figure 10.4). In the dynamic morphological view this **behavior** perfectly suits the dynamics of conservation of volume and content '(being-large'), which has been described as one of the most significant characteristics of the egg cell. In contrast the morphodynamic characteristics for spermatogenesis are fragmentation ('being-many'), division and reduction of volume ('being-small'). In such a context cell division seems an appropriate gesture. Sperm cells do not indeed 'resist' the reduction divisions occurring during spermatogenesis. The two *spermatocytes* that are the result of their meiosis are both equal in size. As noted before the sperm cell strives for reduction of its volume and for concentration. In the final stage of ripening from *spermatocyte* to the actual sperm cell (*spermatozoon*) it is biologically necessary that the sperm cell expels its superfluous cytoplasm. This process is completely in line with the signature and gesture of 'being-small'. It should be realized that in the phenomenological view 'large' and 'small' are not quantitative notions but qualities. How to measure the 'smallness' of a sperm? The head measures about 4 μ (micron) which is about half the regular size of 'a cell'. Compared to that the tail is relatively huge: about 60 – 80 μ (microns). But it is the **gesture** of making yourself small that apparently brings him to extrude nearly all the cytoplasm and to concentrate on the nucleus, even to the extent that the DNA inside the nucleus is almost completely dehydrated and condensed. In contrast to this the egg cell makes herself large, the gesture here is gathering so much cytoplasm that she becomes almost non-viable and becomes visible to the naked eye (*vide supra*).

Summarizing we can state that cell structures and properties that become more important, dominant or clearly expressed in the one cell become less important and less expressed in the other cell, and vice versa. In gesture and behavior both cells are a **polarities** of each other. Essential features of polarity are reversibility, being complementary and inversion. Developing in completely opposite directions, there is a strong inner **relationship** between the two processes, which is expressed by the reciprocal characteristics The polarization of the two gametes can be summarized as follows: the oocyte tends to express the features and qualities of the *cytoplasm* of the 'normal' ('regular') cell in a unidirectional way; the spermatozoon, on the other hand, exhibits the qualities and 'behavior' of the *nucleus* of the cell. In Figure 10.5 this is summarized by the two polar principles of the circle: on the left the morphological 'egg cell principle', on the right the morphological 'sperm cell principle'.

Conception or fertilization? – Where do we come from?

Most people nowadays consider conception as a kind of 'big bang', a moment of something starting. The popular notion is that a zygote (or so-called 'fertilized egg cell', also see Footnote 2) is the result of a kind of fusion of the two involved sex cells (gametes) and that during prenatal life the child develops out of that zygote. It

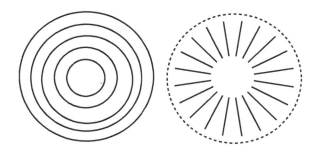

Figure 10.5

Circumferences and rays: the two polar principles of the circle. On the left the morphological "egg cell principle", on the right the morphological "sperm cell principle"

starts with conception; everything after that is a consequence or result of that primary or causal event. In this view children are more or less considered as a result of that conception or fertilization, children are 'made'. Our modern fertilization techniques are based on this view and on this principle.[9]

At conception the profound and intense polarity we have described eventuates in the formation of an interaction between the sperm cells and the involved egg cell. From observations made during *in vitro* fertilization procedures we know that in the non-manipulated situation for a few hours a subtle and labile complex is formed that may be described as a so-called *pre-conception attraction complex* (PCAC) (Figure 10.6). It is logical to consider the formation and presence of this biological complex as a necessary condition for the actual process of conception. We are dealing with a *state of activity* that is more than just a summation or spatial composition of two cellular elements. It is a process of encounter and interactivity: in this biological complex very specific biochemical interactions take place between the two cellular elements. During those few hours of interaction conception is a possibility not

---

[9]And they work and are successful! But "The result of the experiment does not prove that you **understood the phenomenon** in the right way"!

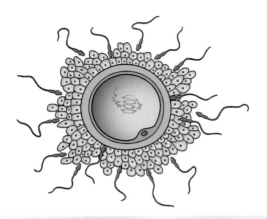

Figure 10.6

An egg cell (ovum) surrounded by sperm cells: a preconception attraction complex.

an inevitability. Whether it actually will come to a conception (which is the final process of fusion of the two gametes and their nuclei) is dependent on the outcome of various subtle reciprocal biochemical interactions and dependencies. Here it should be accentuated that at no time during the whole series of events (from the interactive encounter in the PCAC till the final fusion of the nuclei) any act of so-called penetration occurs. Nowhere and never is the continuity and integrity of the egg cell membrane ruptured, it is a matter of fusion of two membranes. [10]When this fusion of membranes is performed, the total content of the sperm cell may enter the egg cell cytoplasm. The popular image of one sperm cell actively and aggressively penetrating the passive and subdued egg cell is wide spread but not based upon proper observations. It is not correct: in the process of conception we deal neither with an active nor a passive partner, nor with a penetrating or penetrated one, nor with fertilizing and fertilized partner. Both cells, both elements are equivalent, it is all about the subtle equilibrium of interaction and exchange that takes place here between the two constituting equivalent but polar

elements. The egg cell, for example, is not a passive target; she is selective and receptive.

Important for the phenomenological approach applied here is the phenomenon of rotation. In IVF procedures we can observe that the PCAC starts to rotate. Not in a defined direction, not on a defined axle, but a global rotation. For the phenomenologist the question 'What causes this motion?' is not relevant. Rotation is more than a motion, it is also a gesture. Several hundred sperm cells attach themselves to the corona radiata of the egg cell and the whole complex starts to rotate, What is rotation? Radius-shaped ('limb-like') sperm cells move forward against a current of fluid in the Fallopian tube to find their target in this way (a typical 'sperm feature'). Egg cells are spheres. A sphere, a ball comes to rest, stays inert, centers so to speak, the ball is perfectly suited for **being** moved. Rotation is movement on the spot, it is neither forward motion nor standstill, a kind of movement without changing position neither rest nor movement but rest *and* movement. It is something else, something new. Rotation as it is performed by this polarity here, exhibits the gesture of encounter, of dialogue, of dancing with each other. In this respect the morphodynamics of conception is of the same quality as the mating encounters one so often can observe in the animal kingdom, for example during the mating 'dance' between male and female in all kinds of birds. Here also a whole complex of signals and interactions has to be exchanged and has to take place first between the mating male and female partners before the actual copulation ('fusion') can eventuate. This is the gesture of dance, encounter and dialogue. A completely different image than the one that nowadays usually is presented in fertilization biology and procedures exemplifying the sperm is an active, nearly aggressive principle out to penetrate and 'fertilize' the egg cell. An active principle fertilizing the 'passive' one, the 'fertilizer' and the 'fertilized'. In the gesture and image of a rotating PCAC it is a matter of the principle of encounter and dialogue between two equivalent qualities. Of course only for those who want to 'see' it, recognize it; the usually 'combative' mind of modern biology will never be able to see this. These two cells (we deal however with far broader principles than just two gametes) constitute a complex here for some hours to which they contribute equivalently. Does this exhibit 'zygote' quality. Is there 'zygote' in the air?

---

[10] The *zona pellucida* is the actual biochemical barrier that has to be 'taken' by the sperm. This is not the egg cell membrane, it is an enveloping spherical harness produced by the so-called theca cells of the ovary.

How could one interpret this biological complex of interaction phenomenologically (morphodynamically)? We are dealing with more than just two 'normal' cells that are going to fuse.[11] We deal here with the qualities of 'egg cellularity' and 'sperm cellularity'. The two contribute their polar qualities and potencies and so to speak sacrifice those qualities in order to accomplish ('perform') a biological reality ('complex'), a twofoldness that may raise the two constituting elements functionally to a higher level.[12] They perform something that could be interpreted as a kind of inversion or revolution of the 'normal' or 'regular' biological relationships. To understand what is meant here, the reader is invited to look at the first page of his/her biology book. There one may find a description and diagram of **The cell**. In regular biology 'The cell' is considered to be the principle or fundamental element of life and living nature, sometimes even as the 'building-block of life'. Where one deals with living organisms one deals with 'The cell'. The cell is an enveloped space of cytoplasm around a central nucleus, yes, surely, the fundament principle of life, of living nature.

But then look at what these sex cells are bringing about here. In a phenomenological sense one could correctly describe the sperm cell as 'a nucleus', a cell in which the nuclear component and principle of 'The cell' is more or less exaggerated (polarized). This culminates in a cell almost fully 'concentrated'(!) in regard to being a nuclear element (see Table 10.1). In this view the sperm cell is nearly pure nucleus, just structure, just centre, just formula (*formula* means 'little form'), hardly displaying any 'inner dynamics'. The sperm cell exhibits nuclear behavior, shows a gesture of 'nuclearity'. In contrast to this the egg cell lives in a gesture of 'cytoplasmity', it almost totally culminates in the quality and gesture of cytoplasm. It is an internally dynamic entity, with openness towards its environment (and therefore vulnerability); it lives in metabolic interaction with the environment in contrast to the sperm cells which biochemically spoken hardly

interact metabolically with their environment.[13] Both cells are very specialized to 'being active cytoplasm' on the one hand and 'being nucleus' on the other.

Contemplating this way one may see that a preconception attraction complex (PCAC) represents a kind of 'act of revolution or inversion': the regular relationships are almost literally turned inside out. As to the features of sperm cell and egg cell one may see here a complete inversion. What should normally be in the centre, is now in the periphery. What should bear the signature of rest and structure ('the nucleus'), is now actively in motion. What 'normally' is concentrated in the center (the 'nucleus') is now active in the periphery in a gesture of radiation and peripherization. What should be dynamically in the periphery or surrounding (the 'cytoplasm' usually functions as a dynamic mantle around a nucleus) is now in the center. What usually is a dynamic expansion ('egg cellularity') is now at rest forming the centre of a rotating complex. So, many sperm cells together with one egg cell create for some hours a situation that may be considered as a kind of complete (inside-out-)inversion of what is the fundamental principle and 'normal' relationship of life, i.e. 'The cell'. One could summarize the dynamics of the preconception attraction complex as a kind of 'de-biologicalisation', turning things inside out, upside down. It is a subtle balance of conditions in which something **might** happen, nothing **has to** happen. This subtle and labile equilibrium is not a matter of the dynamics of force or making, but instead a matter of the dynamics of a creative encounter, a reciprocal inviting and communicating activity. When the phenomena of this complex are experienced and understood in their formative dynamics and gesture - which is in fact the principle of the phenomenological approach and methodology -, the image, the impression, the quality of a 'receptive field' emerges. This represents the essence of the notion of 'conception' i.e. concerning and receiving, not making and constructing. Not (only) a 'horizontal' conception so to speak – which means a fusion of two gametes on the level of matter, of cells, of body, of biology and so on – is the essential process that takes place here, but here we might deal with the possibility at least of (also) a kind of 'vertical' connection or interaction

---

[11] Sex cells (gametocytes) even lack the capacity to express a biological identity. Somatic cells recognize the genetically similar partner and repel a 'foreign body' neighbor, sex cells lack this property of 'immunologic identity'. That is why they are so well fitted to fuse!

[12] Goethe could have considered this to be a *Steigerung* or 'functional elevation'. In his theory of colors (chromatics) the colors were the elevation (Steigerung) of the polarity encounter and interaction of dark and light, of day and night. Not the mixture of the two polar qualities but the active elevation on a higher level.

[13] This explains the properties of nearly invulnerability that are so typical for sperm. One can freeze them, centrifuge them, treat them with an acid solution, and no damage occurs. Do not even think of such procedures in the vicinity of a **mature** egg cell!

between a 'beyond' and a 'here', between mind (spirit) and matter. The matter dimension so to say is opened up here to become receptive and inviting as to the other dimension of 'en-actness' or spirit

It looks like a precious moment of keeping or taking a breath. From two sides the conditions for a conception (which at the end is the fusion of an egg cell nucleus with a sperm cell nucleus) are prepared in a process of reciprocal interaction and encounter, so it might **but does not have to** happen. This labile and dynamic balance enables the conditions for a possible encounter (connection) or 'non-encounter'. It is not only an egg cell and some sperm cells constituting a kind of enticing construct or complex but also two polar principles or forces: 'egg cellularity' and 'sperm cellularity' that cooperate here in an active encounter, functionally raising the level of the complex to a higher level. Regarded in this way conception is not just a passive fusion of an egg cell and a sperm cell but also an active process of so-called functional elevation or *Steigerung* in the Goetheanistic sense (see Figure 10.7).

Conception, which we successfully mimic and manipulate in our *in vitro* fertilization techniques, is not the actual or 'real' conception: the processes on the material, biological level are (at the risk of repeating the message again) necessary but not sufficient conditions for a conception on the other spiritual level. According to this view, not even *in vitro*, is a baby ever 'made' in the sense of 'constructed'. Conception rather is to be understood as a moment, a theme of connection and incarnation, of 'embodiment'. What is connected in conception, is disconnected ('untied', separated) in the moment of dying (excarnation). "Someone passes (away)", we say. What remains are the material remnants left behind, the dead body 'left' by the 'soul'. Conception may be seen as an event of inversion: what was separated before is connected and unites. If this connection is successful, the 'actual' conception (the fusion of the two gametes and so on) should rather be considered as a **result or consequence** than as a cause. In human conception we deal with three: a third person, entelechy comes to appearance by means of the physical and biological substrate offered by two other human beings, but not caused by the latter. In this view we are not involved in an act of reproduction as the principle of copying or reproducing, which is the successful act in the idea of survival of the fittest and evolution. A human being is not reproducible, at least not when one considers the

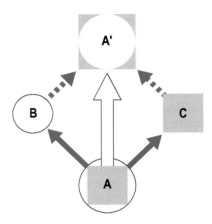

Figure 10.7

Diagram of a so-called "Steigerung" or 'Functional Elevation' (*Synergy*) in a Preconception Attraction Complex. A: Level of The Cell; B: Egg cell as 'Cytoplasm'; C: Sperm cells as 'Nucleus'; A' represents the 'inside out elevation' of situation A to an energetically higher level.

Grey square: 'Nucleus', White circle: 'Cytoplasm'.

biography as the true 'unit' or 'entity' of human life and existence. We do **not** reproduce ourselves in our children, that is a fundamental impossibility. Right in the setting free or releasing equilibrium of the preconception attraction complex the 'Other' (the 'Third')') may find the conditions to 'incarnate' and realize him(her) self. Not because of, but by means of conception. It is not a so-called fertilization that is taking place here but a 'real' conception.

Nidation – the gesture of pregnancy

Textbooks teach us that implantation (*nidation* or 'nesting') of the human embryo (*conceptus*) occurs at the end of the first week of development at about six days after conception. Actually this is not true. As mentioned before the formative processes in the first week are characterized by a relative lack of vitality. There is no growth, only a process of subdivision into cells. The *morula* and later the *blastula* does not have an intensive metabolic interaction with the environment. Though the young blastula represents a 'living' organism, there is evidence that it does not yet have an intrinsic biological clock. In some textbooks this is even acknowledged by regarding the first phase of embryonic development as the particular phase of blastulagenesis (blastula-phase), to be distinguished from the actual embryogen-esis; other authors even talk about a *pre-embryo* phase. That is related to the fact that the first phase ('week') of human development does not last a week, but should be considered as 'the phase that ends with the act of *nida-tion*'. This might happen after some four to five days but even at the seventh or eighth day after fertilization. The 'first week' of human development is also the period in which it is possible to manipulate the embryo techni-cally or preserve it by freezing without much harm for the organism (so far as we are currently aware). When we freeze an embryo, we preserve the substrate of what we may consider as the **physical condition for develop-ment**, a status that can 'wait' for implantation. In fact we artificially create a so-called *embryopause* that way, a phenomenon which is physiological for many mam-mals that are able to postpone the implantation for weeks or even months at a time. All these phenomena indicate that the first week is a kind of 'mineral' or 'non-viable' existence. It resembles the quality of a (plant) seed, also a very particular way of life with a physical material living 'outside of time' and with hardly active metabolism. The latter characteristics however may also be regarded as typical for inorganic 'life'.

The nidation (nesting) or implantation marks a com-plete and thorough revolution in the way of existence regarding the gesture and *Gestalt* of the human embryo. The *conceptus* and the maternal uterine mucous mem-brane start to establish an exchanging metabolic inter-action, the so-called phase of *adplantation*. As in the act of fertilization and conception there exists a situa-tion of equilibrium and dialogue in which something might happen but is not compelled to happen. It looks as if the phase of the first 'week' has reached its end and threatens to die off. Only a revolution, a new ges-ture might save the situation. Many embryos appear to fail in enduring this revolving activity of discontinuity. If the embryo is able to withstand it, the effect is dra-matic. From now on the outer or peripheral part of the embryo (the so-called *trophoblast*) starts to exhibit all the qualities and characteristics we usually attribute to living and growing organisms. In an extensive gesture

of peripherization it starts expanding and becoming metabolically very active. The embryo now shows a ges-ture completely opposite to the situation so typical for the young blastula before *adplantation*. The growth in the periphery with an increase of cells from about one hundred at the time of implantation to several thou-sand two days later has an almost explosive or cancer-ous character. Without respecting any boundaries the embryo grows into the tissue of the uterine mucous membrane, even breaking through the natural biologi-cal barriers of tissue. The cells of the trophoblast lose their boundary and fuse (*cytotrophoblast*), cell death occurs; phenomena also often seen in cancerous tissue!

Summarizing it may be stated that a revolution takes place from a centripetal to a centrifugal orientation, from 'mineral' ('dead') to 'living' ('vital'), from seed to plant, from closing off to being open. The embryo exhibits the gesture of a being without limits here. The fact that the trophoblast starts to produce substances now that influence the hormonal status of the entire maternal organism (in order to 'prevent' mother's next menstruation), is in agreement with this gesture. Nida-tion therefore represents a kind of discontinuity, a frac-ture. The prolongation of the gestures, the morphologi-cal behavior, characteristics of the first 'week' will never lead to (the gesture of) the second week. The embryo goes through a kind of crisis. This might 'explain' why a relatively high percentage of embryos fail to overcome this 'crisis' in development

Nidation is a kind of discontinuity, a fracture. Many biologists consider the act of the implanting embryo a kind of biological aggression. The embryo grows into the maternal organism, not respecting any biological boundaries. In the literature on biology one can even find the fetus described as 'the enemy inside', capable of making the mother ill from being pregnant! It looks like what happened with the act of 'penetration' by the sperm cell, which in fact also could be considered to be an act of dialogue and reception. Phenomenologically one may consider the relationship between mother and child during the process of nidation in a completely dif-ferent way! When a human being receives tissue (or an organ) from another human being, the first thing he/she will do, is to reject it. This is based on the principle of (biological) identity, at home in the immune system, which hardly ever fails in recognizing alien tissue. The embryo, the child, differs from the mother in genetic terms. If the mother were to be implanted ('transplanted') with tissue of her child, she would reject it, though not as strongly as in the case of a non-familial donor. In that case we would also have to help the transplantation by suppressing the immune system i.e. the identity of the receiver, in this case the mother. But at the moment of nidation the new (id)entity is implanting itself into the body of the mother and …….. (usually) the mother does not attempt to reject it at all! Does this not mean that actually the physiological mechanism of pregnancy phenomenologically might be characterized as a gesture of reception, but also of 'providing room' and of 'withdrawal'? The womb as a kind of biological asylum, where the mother's organism has withdrawn its identity! The status of pregnancy is not one of 'having' (or worse still 'possessing') a child, but one of receiving and hosting a child -the reverse of what usually is claimed to be the territory of the mother! The interaction so typical for ad- and implantation, the one of asking and responding, of literally inter-action, is continued during the whole duration of pregnancy till at the end either the motherly organism claims back its space, or the child 'decides' to 'withdraw'. As already mentioned, a trend exists in biology and gynecology nowadays of regarding pregnancy as a kind of war between mother and child. This seems to reflect rather the moral and social attitude and image of man of the researcher in question than it being a matter of biological factuality. In contrast the image of pregnancy as the primordial gesture of accepting and being accepted and hosted is presented here!

Centralization – the gesture of individuation

In an embryo of about two weeks old, we find the *endoderm* with the yolk sac on the (future) ventral side of the two-layered germinal disc and the *ectoderm* with the amniotic fluid in the amniotic cavity on the future dorsal side.[14] There already exists a dorsoventral (back to front) orientation. Following that, the craniocaudal (head to tail) body axis or orientation is formed with the appearance of the so-called *connection stalk*. At the

[14]In this script the terms 'endoderm' and 'ectoderm' are applied deliberately in spite of the contemporary habit in embryology textbooks of mentioning the involved germ layers as *hypoblast* and *epiblast* or (as a kind of compromise) *pre-endoderm* and *pre-ectoderm*. There are good (phenomenological) arguments however to maintain this terminology. Ectoderm and endoderm represent the later 'outer' or the later 'inner' 'skin–dimension' (body wall) of the human body.

location where the latter structure becomes attached to the germinal disc the caudal body pole is induced. In the germinal disc a preliminary head pole and pelvic pole are organized now with a trunk or thorax-abdomen-region (in this phase only slightly) developing in between. Just as the trunk is organized above (upon) the lower limb pole (pelvic pole) connecting it to the grounding surface of the earth, the germinal disc is connected by means of a connection stalk of mesodermal connective tissue to the ectocyst periphery, the rooting pole of the embryo system. Therefore the caudal pole may be regarded as the pole where we are oriented towards our cosmic periphery and origin, i.e. where the mediating connection stalk **connects** the 'terrestrial center body' to the 'celestial peripheral body'. In fact our pelvic pole which is part of our caudal pole is oriented more towards the periphery, to the cosmos ('celestial') while our head pole seems to be more emancipated and opposed to it ('terrestrial').

As soon as blood begins to flow through the small newly developed primordial capillary vessels, away from this enormous periphery (the ectocyst and trophoblast, our rooting pole), it concentrates, is gathered up and flows to that connection stalk. Subsequently, moved by peripheral forces of growth and metabolism, the blood flows in the cranial direction along the amniotic and yolk sac walls, along the flanks of the embryonic (germinal) disc to our head. As soon as the blood flow arrives at that cranial pole, it cannot flow on but has to 'congest' and 'flow back'. Very soon a specialized blood vessel is developed here, where the blood flow is redirected. This is what later will become the heart primordium. In a morphodynamical sense the heart primordium at the head pole of the embryo may be regarded as a place where the blood comes to **rest**. It is redirected and reimpulsed morphologically (heart loop) and later physiologically (primitive heart beat); it flows back along other capillaries to that connection stalk, 'disappearing' in the metabolic (extra- and intracellular) fluid of the ectocyst periphery. Then a 'fresh' flow of blood is directed toward the 'center' of the system which is now represented by the heart as the actual head pole of the embryo. Phenomenologically one can state that for the first time, a kind of 'Here' dimension arises in the embryo. Until that time the whole system seems to have been organized in a radiating direction away from the germinal disc as the axle of the system, but now with the heart, a real center **organ** has developed.

A center has developed opposite to, but also more or less originating from, the periphery. With the heart, a primordial 'Here' has developed in the embryonic organism. Very soon after the establishment of the primitive blood vessel loop (only at the fourth week will there be a closed circulation) the heart starts to beat on about the 21st day after conception.

After the critical moment of nidation a second critical moment of 'incarnation' occurs during the third week of human development. During the second week the gesture of peripherization remains the dominant feature of embryonic behavior. What is still lacking in the embryo, are two main principles: individualization and organization of an 'inner world', the latter morphologically as well as psychologically. The second week of embryonic development mainly exhibits the features, the gesture, of plantlike life. This happens to be in line with the phenomenon that the embryo does not seem completely individualized yet. In the second week a phenomenon that is also characteristic for the first week, might still occur: namely monozygotic twinship. The embryo is still '*dividual*' (divisible, 'dividable'), meaning it can still be divided into (or: shared by) two individuals. In the first week twinning will involve the complete embryo (later placentas as well as the 'proper bodies' become divided and separated). In the second week this involves the so-called 'proper body' (in this phase represented by the two-layered germinal disc) only; the identical twins now have to share their placenta and membranes. But at the end of the third week a human embryo has apparently individualized. Twin formation is no longer possible without complications. What is more significant however for the next phase which the human embryo is now approaching, is the fact that the embryo starts to exhibit the features that are characteristic for animalization. Until halfway through the third week the 'proper' embryo is a two-layered creature consisting of only two epithelia or 'skins'; in this case ectoderm and endoderm. There is nothing present yet that could be indicated as the substrate for innerness or for an 'inner world'. The whole being still lives in the periphery. In the middle of the third week the conditions within the embryo are turned upside down; a complete reversal of the bodily organization takes place. In the center of the organism the heart develops as the endpoint of a very delicate network of capillaries that start to connect the periphery i.e. the *trophoblast / ectocyst* with the nucleus i.e. the 'proper' body (see above). It is the heart that provides us with a center so that we can be present 'here', i.e. in or **within** our body. It means that with the formation of the heart a new gesture, a new orientation and a new phase of development and emancipation begins! Instead of the hitherto prevailing activity and gesture of peripherization and growing outward, the movement and the gesture of **growing inward** now begins. The first impulse for this action and re-direction is provided by the heart impulse. By means of the formation of the heart the act of incarnation can proceed more intensely. The heart represents the first organ that develops from out there to here and in this respect it is exemplary for all the other organ processes. If the heart has not formed properly, the embryo will die (or it may develop to become a so-called 'wind egg') and it is impossible for the human being to take root in a 'Here'. It are the dynamics and gestures of (animal) incarnation we are dealing with here.

In the slipstream of the formation of the heart, which represents the reorientation of the system bringing impulses and nutrients from the periphery to the center, the developmental processes of shape-giving and formation become more and more apparent **within** i.e. no longer **around** the germinal disc. How the forces of growing are actually involved, is not the issue in this text, but in any case, from about halfway through the third week a kind of '*gastrulation*'[15] takes place by means of which a middle layer of tissue, the inner germinal layer or *meso(derm)* is created. From the caudal pole of the embryonic disc onward, this 'inner dimension' is developed in the 'proper body'. The central inner axis of the body (*notochord*) is also part of this 'gastrulating' impulse. According to most textbooks it is the ectoderm that somehow starts to 'grow in' (or becomes positioned in between the two already existing layers) and differentiates into meso(derm). According to Blechschmidt's proposal we prefer the notion 'meso' instead of 'mesoderm' here because it represents a quality in the body organization which has no similarity to the limiting or body wall dimension of the ectoderm respectively the endoderm. That is why Blechschmidt proposed to abandon the terminology of 'derm' and talk about two limiting tissues ('skin layers' or body walls) and one in-between layer of the so-called 'inner tissue' (German *Innengewebe*) instead.

---

[15]In terms of developmental biology the term gastrulation is not applied correctly here, but as a description of the process of 'growing in' it satisfies.

Gastrulation (i.e. folding or growing in) can be seen as one of the archetypal phenomena of emancipation in animal morphology. In the fourth week of human development it is followed and intensified by the processes of delamination and body folding in which the anatomically individualized body becomes outlined by an outer body wall that represents the ectodermic parietal pole. Another aspect in animal organization is the development of a nervous system and a movement (locomotor) system. Animals develop sense organs, a nervous system and a locomotor apparatus, which all enable them to 'communicate' on a more or less conscious and autonomous level with the environment. Perception, awareness, and reaction are components of the interaction of the individual animal organism with its environment. From a phenomenological point of view, the external form induced by the folding process can be understood as a kind of gastrulation of the whole body form. Folding and gastrulation of the body are manifestations of animalization and individualization of the body and the organism. The outer world enters the organism by ingestion or perception, will be integrated by digestion or assimilation, and the organism interacts with the outer world by excretion or (re) action.

After the 'growing in' the 'growing beyond'

As stated before the process of 'gastrulation' is followed by the process of folding or *delamination*. By folding the so far more or less flat body, consisting of the three-layered germinal disc, the embryo attains the basic principle of the adult anatomical organization. It now becomes an organism with a body cavity, limited on the inside by a *visceral* body wall (the 'metabolic' boundary of digestion and secretion) and on the outside by a *parietal* body wall (the 'perception' boundary of skin and external sense organs and the dimension of locomotion and action). This folding does not only occur in the (ventro-)lateral direction leading to the closure of the body wall in the central ventral line (with the exception of the umbilical region), but also occurs in the craniocaudal direction. This leads to the organization of a body principle, which is a prerequisite for the already mentioned animalization of the organism, a process related to emancipation from the environment, individualization and autonomization. The beginning of the craniocaudal and the lateral folding (the so-called

delamination) marks the end of the third week. The embryonic body becomes maximally curved over the primitive umbilical cord. For most mammals and many other animal organisms, this external body shape more or less exists as a final morphological stage of the body. They will never reach the characteristic of the 'upright' body that human beings have. Apes too, regarded as the closest relatives of humans, show remnants of the craniocaudal folding in their external bodily form and vertebral column. Although primates can walk and stand upright for a few moments, they are not able to develop and maintain the upright posture of balancing of the human organism. This means that in the human embryonic development a further **different** phase is due to occur. From about the fifth or sixth week onward the folding process of the third week is partly unfolded to reach the typical human external bodily form: upright posture. Unfolding creates a morphological movement opposite to folding. This is superimposed on the folded bodily form of the preceding embryonic period.

Up to this phase the human embryo still looks more or less like a head-shaped form. The body shape is dominated by the gesture and formative movement of emancipation that represents the characteristic gesture of formative antipathy, a prerequisite for the *animal* possibility of gaining consciousness. It is also this formative principle that typically dominates the shape of the head pole in a human adult. Now however one could look for a subsequent gesture that might oppose the animal principle of delamination and flexion. With the latter we create ourselves an inner space with the possibilities of animal qualities linked with the capacity of consciousness and soul. An opposing gesture to this could lead to an inner center capable of 'centering the innerness' (self-consciousness). This opposition is presented on the outer bodily contour as the gesture of extension and coming upright, on the inside it is characterized by the ascensus of the head and the nervous system pole and the descending of the pelvis with the visceral (metabolic) pole. But it is also characterized by the gesture of de-flexion and un-folding. The embryo opens up its flexed and introverted body orientation on the ventral side by growing its limbs outwardly and at the same time by the de-flexion of the head pole out of the trunk, in opposition as to the de-flexion of the pelvic pole. Most markedly this extension or de-flexion can first be noticed in the cervical and the lumbar region. The human posture is characterized by the lordosis in the neck and the deepest lumbo-sacral angle of all primates. Described in another way: while head and pelvis are deflexed and unfolded, the neck and the waist appear. Now the extremities (limbs) grow outwardly in the dorso-ventral body axis (orientation) as well as in the orientation between the center (head) and the periphery (hands and feet). This body extension or erection is the start of the human gesture of coming upright: head, vertebral column and pelvis are organized on top of each other in the vertical axis, which is the very least prerequisite essential for the human upright position. However, balancing and centering are essential for staying upright. This unique position of the human body amidst that of related animals is due to the fact that the center of gravity of the body in the bipedal upright position is positioned **inside** the body contour. Balancing is something other than bipedalism which is a feature that we share with many bipedal animals. Going upright could therefore be interpreted as a human gesture. The gesture for achieving this balance, this equilibrium, this center in our body organization could be related to the mental gesture of self-consciousness, of centering and coming to oneself! Is self-consciousness not simply an enhancement of animal awareness and consciousness, but rather something opposing that gesture of the animal principle in us? Is that what we are performing and pre-exercising now as an embryo? The process of delamination and concentration of the former phase is maintained however. On the inner part of the organism it is preserved while the organs return to the body cavity of the trunk as it were. In the bodily organization the most explicit body axis i.e. the axis between head and tail (cranio-caudal) becomes expressed as the upper pole (head) and the lower pole (pelvis and lower limbs) again. But this time the latter body axis is not induced by outer and peripheral growing forces and conditions as it was in the second week of development, but it is now performed from a center **inside** the body contour itself. In the head pole the emancipating gestures of envelopment and concentration become more explicit: because of the skull (*neurocranium*), maintaining its closed roundness, the brain retains its spherical form while the facial skeleton (*viscerocranium*) more or less loses this with openings (including those for the eyes) oriented ventrally. Opposed to that the limbs (extremities) present the growing outwardly dimension of peripherization and decentration to the outside world (environment). It is important to recognize the

polarity between head and limbs: in the limbs (extremities) we open ourselves to the world and environment with our will pole of acting and locomotion in order to work 'out there' in the world; in the head we retain, we behold, in a morphological, physiological, and psychological gesture.

If one beholds the polar principles in bodily organization in composition with each other as described here, then one may discern the essential difference and polarity between the upper and lower limbs. Arms and legs are not only polar opposites of the head pole (skull) but in themselves are also polarized in the cranio-caudal axis. At their first appearance (fifth week) both pairs of limbs appear to have a finlike structure oriented towards each other like jaws in the head or skull (actually the whole embryo has a head shape during this phase of development). Subsequently by growing movements the limbs orient themselves toward the actual center of the embryonic folding and flexing body i.e. the navel. For the arms this leads to a kind of motion of turning inwardly (pronation) with flexion in the elbows which therefore point outwardly. In this way the hands come to 'rest' upon the heart or the heart region. The hand reveals a gesture of flexion in the wrist and the fingers like a grasping hand. It should be remembered here that all such gestures may be regarded as growing performances and functions. There are no functioning joints yet. A few days later the lower limb takes a position of slightly turning outwardly (exorotation) in relation to the umbilical cord which is relatively enormous at this stage of development and which is to be regarded as the pole opposite the heart in the systemic organization of the embryonic circulation. The knee also becomes flexed and oriented (pointing) outwardly, the foot is supinated and flexed dorsally and is pushed more or less against the body wall. It is a flat structure whilst no (growth) flexion of the toes exists yet. The orientation of the hands towards the heart and of the feet towards the umbilical cord is of significance: heart and hands are oriented 'here', while feet and umbilical cord are oriented 'there'. Regarded phenomenologically this is in agreement with the later functional position of the arms and the hands, being free from gravity and with a so-called open skeleton chain, suited to being an instrument 'for me' (taking, receiving, manipulating) while the legs with a so-called closed skeleton chain and involved with gravity and locomotion show rather an orientation open to the environment and periphery.

In the apes the unfolding in the brain, skull and pelvic region and in the pelvic organs is more or less exaggerated whereby the rounded off shape of the body ends gets lost. Therefore, the vertebral column never achieves the completely upright position. In humans, however, unfolding does not occur in the region of the head and the pelvic region. In humans, unfolding is important in the development of the cervical, thoracic and lumbar part of the vertebral column, therefore in the anatomical segmentation of head, trunk and pelvis. This means that in the apes the unfolding process is opposite to that of man: unfolding is prominent in the skull and pelvic region and does not persist in the vertebral column. In humans unfolding is prominent in the vertebral column and inhibited at the level of the pelvic region and the skull. In the human being, the upright posture is realized to completion by *unfolding*. The perfectly rectangular relationship between the frontal, sagittal and horizontal planes in the human body is due to the persistence in the unfolding process of the vertebral column. The unfolding process of the trunk therefore also induces the uprightness characteristic of the human being. Characteristic of this phenomenon is that as a result the atlanto-occipital joint, shoulder joint, hip joint, knee joint and ankle joint are situated in the same frontal plane. This represents the posture of equilibrium involved in walking upright. As already mentioned, the human body is the only body in which the center of gravity is 'situated' **inside** the anatomical body. In all the animals the forces of gravity distract the animal organization away from itself, away into the environment (gravitation field of the earth) as it were; in the human being the forces of gravity exerted on the body, bring him to **himself**!

Embryology of the Middle, of equilibrium and of freedom

Animal organisms are highly specialized as to their bodies as instruments. On the one hand, animals have unique and specialized skills for perception and reaction; on the other hand, the loss of developmental possibilities is evident. Being specialized also implies a 'condemnation' to only one particular way of functioning and living. A high level of specialization of an organism is paired with a loss of the possibility to use the body for multiple functions, a loss of plasticity. Perception

and reaction of an organism are strongly determined by morphological and physiological features, as well as being restricted in the sense of possibilities and faculties. The animal organism is a **perfect** entity of form, function and environment. Within the given framework of its instinct, the behavior of an animal is quite predictable. Instinct can be characterized as 'determinism of perception and reaction'. The human body however is not a tool for specialized instrumental functions. Sense organs, jaws, teeth, hands and feet are not fit for or limited to just a few particular functions. Human behavior is not necessarily predictable from the bodily instrumental organization. It is rather the unpredictable that makes human beings special. In humans it is their creativity that is most remarkable. Characteristic of this creativity is the freedom to act. Human beings 'can do whatever they want'. Animals 'must do what they can do'. Human beings can 'learn to observe what they want to observe', animals 'must observe what they are fit for'. In the words of the anthropologist Adolf Portman: "Animals are large in their small worlds, man is small in a large world".

The movements of flexion and enveloping, in this case delamination, provide an inner space (anatomically and psychologically) so to speak, which in its turn relates to and connects with the outer world of environment by means of the sense organs and the limbs. We recognize this 'inner world', this dimension of existence, in all behavior and expressions that we may observe in animals. The animal is animated ('souled').[16] The animal's structure and the anatomy are related intimately and immediately to their instinctive behavior. In a perfect (!) way the trinity of form, function and environment are interwoven in harmony in the animal, completely complementing each other. As an opposing tendency to those forces of closing off into an inner world one could place the gesture of opening up and unfolding, expressed in the forces of coming upright of the human body. Taking into account the qualitative expression that is performed in the embryonic growing gestures one could interpret the shaping gestures in their moral quality. Human embryology is the **embryology of freedom**. In this context freedom is considered to be the equilibrium and balance between 'too much' on the one hand and 'too little' on the other; freedom as it can be achieved and performed in the middle, the third level of being between the poles as it were, the level of balance and equilibrium.

---

[16]*anima* is Latin for 'soul'; The notion *animal* is derived from it.

Is there a gesture of, a form for freedom? In the morphology and physiology of the head we deal with antipathy as a gesture, here lives the freedom '**from**' so to speak, an extreme or polar form of freedom. In limbs and pelvis, where we open to and connect with the world, the gesture of sympathy, there is the domain of freedom '**to**'. Freedom to realize, to act, to accomplish. But is the 'real' freedom not the equilibrium of the two extremes, to be free '**with**'? With each other, with the world, with yourself? Freedom as the quality of the Middle, the in-between?

The trunk (with the arms) in general and the vertebral column in particular represents the mediating domain of the middle, of freedom so to speak. Here the polarities are balanced, as they present themselves as a pole of antipathy and being closed off in being 'Here' and a pole of sympathy and being open in being 'There'. In regard to this it might lead to a better understanding if one takes into consideration the notion of 'three heads' in the bodily organization. Three heads with three pairs of limbs: jaws, arms and legs? On the one hand the 'Head-head' in the skull with the most strongly introverted, 'antipathetic' and centripetal morphology, physiology and psychology; as an opposite there is the 'pelvis-head' in which the performances and activities of the viscera are expressed in a more open and centrifugal morphodynamics, organs of 'sympathy'. In the middle, in between there appears the 'mediating head' of the thorax. Every separate rib shows in its shape-giving 'behavior', every individual element on its own, the gesture of a radiating extremity (limb). But in context, in composition the ribs perform a functional elevation (*Steigerung*) and constitute the 'head of the thorax' as a whole, which enfolds and contains an inner space like a skull. The ribs in morphological collaboration achieve something that each individual rib is not capable of: they bring the two polar principles (limbs – head) in reciprocal interaction to a higher level which brings a third dimension into appearance, a new principle, the Middle or the 'in between'.

Something similar happens in the vertebral column composed of more than thirty elements. Each individual vertebra performs the enclosing gesture of the head (skull) with its closed vertebral arch (remaining open represents pathology here: spina bifida); but in composition and reciprocal interaction they constitute the so-called 'fifth limb', the vertebral column (the important domain for the physical therapist). Again the trunk is proclaimed as the domain of the Middle, of 'the three and the one', that everything comes forth from and to which everything leads. This might draw our attention to the entity of one vertebra and two ribs as the primordial unit of the skeleton. In this way we encounter the lemniscate in form, a primeval principle that could be regarded as a fundamental template of form and as a primeval gesture of metamorphosis for all other plans for the skeleton. In this way the shoulder blade (scapula) and the hip bone (coxal bone) for example could be considered metamorphoses of a vertebra, whilst in contrast to this and as a kind of inversion, the arms and legs can be understood as metamorphoses of ribs. Thus the polarity of the antipathy of the head versus the sympathy of the limbs can also be discerned in the dorsoventral orientation of the vertebrae versus the ribs, and even in the neurocranium (dorsocranial) and the viscerocranium (ventrocaudal).

In connection with the 'unfolding' extension and erection of the whole body of the embryo which is discernible by the development of the neck and the waist, the two pairs of limbs perform a kind of opposed rotation during their movement of growing out. While the arms rotate outwardly (*exorotation*), the legs rotate inwardly (*endorotation*), orienting themselves towards the 'earth' this way. This leads to the well-known opposition between the flexor and extensor side of the two limbs in the so-called 'anatomical position'. In the arms the so-called pre-axial zone is oriented outwardly, while in the legs it is oriented inwardly. The legs follow the backward 'rotation' or de-flexion of the pelvis in their growing gesture as it were and orient themselves towards the earth's surface, while the arms 'escape' this earthly orientation in an exorotating gesture so to speak by following the backward rotation of the head. As a consequence and as a general gesture for posture the embryo opens up into the typical upright posture of the human being. Humans balance their head on their vertebral column and above their trunk which in turn balances above (on top of) the pelvic girdle and the lower limbs.

It was Goethe who already recognized the strongly polarized organization of the upper and lower limbs as typical and essential for the human being. In our relatives the primates and mammals this polarity seems to have been 'lost' with the result that the lower pole (pelvic girdle and legs) has developed relatively too poorly to facilitate the upright posture. One could consider this an indication that within the organization of those animals the typical sympathetic openness of the lower pole has been lost and that the upper pole is dominated by the forces of gravitational and earthly orientation. The arms and hands of these species on the other hand do not reach (or retain?) the 'free of the earth' faculties and capacities which are so typical of the upper limbs of the human being. As in the head and the skull the arms open up again in those species to the influences of the environment and develop into specialized instruments capable of acting and performing with and in the environment. For example in the quadruped animal the exorotation of the arm is 'corrected' by a kind of movement of curving inwardly, which in fact is the continuation of the endorotational orientation that is the primary growing movement of an upper limb. In this way the limb is fixed in its position (as if the arms retain the function of a leg). In many primates the polarity in question is lost by an endorotational growing movement of the legs which is too weak, leading to the four-handedness of the animal. All this seems to evoke the idea that the erect and upright walking posture is a capacity that is performed and maintained in its explicit and essential manner only by the human being. This might open our eyes to the concept that the upright posture is the primary and that locomotion on four feet (or by means of four hands) is the secondary principle, quite in contrast to the usually and generally accepted notions in evolutionary biology. In this concept the human is not a being that has become upright out of a quadruped posture and locomotion, but a being primarily capable of walking upright and capable of maintaining this embryonic faculty and *talent (Anlage)*. This is recognized as the principle of so-called *retardation*, which was made explicit for the first time in the first decades of the 20th century by the Dutch morphologist Louis Bolk.

It was Louis Bolk who discovered that the human body seems to avoid the one sided tendency of instrumental specialization and therefore cannot be regarded as the subsequent example or effort of animal specialization. In human evolution something new, something different arises or becomes explicit. The human body has a shape and organization which represents the early phases of development. The human being seems to preserve or retain the embryonic relationships instead of abandoning them in a gesture of specialization and adaptation. For example our bipolar (digital) hand has

in fact a rudimentary form that goes back as far as the fishes and the early mammals. Only in humans is preserved this morphological property which results in an organization of hand and fingers that is suited well for instrumentalization.

In comparison to the hand of an ape or primate for example Bolk found that the human hand is quite retarded. But this original (take it literally) hand, this organization can be traced back to the oldest terrestrial vertebrates. The large mobility of the upper (cranial) or rostral limbs is a primordial feature that is already present in the so-called lower primates. The broad thorax, which is in line with the backward (dorsal) position of the scapula (which is a characteristic linked to the benefits of the upright posture), is an embryonic feature that is preserved (retained) by the human being, while it was more or less lost in the (so-called) higher mammals and primates. The human scapula for example lacks the longitudinal extension that is so typical of the mammalian scapula as a bone essential for support and locomotion. All this relates to the relatively great mobility of the shoulder girdle which is also a phenomenon of Bolkian retardation. The relatively strong outward rotation of the upper limb, shown among other things by the inwardly oriented head of the humeral bone which is strongly rotated in relation to the shaft of the bone also goes with the principle that the shoulder girdle and the arm refrain from locomotion and related specialization. Their embryonic appearance and features prevent this so to speak.

Retardation may also stand for a retarded and retained pattern and speed of growth. The limbs develop from their distal, peripheral parts onto the trunk; the growth of a limb follows a distoproximal gradient. A foot or a hand always follows the pattern of adult relationships (proportions) more (and therefore reaches the adult proportion earlier) than the lower leg (or arm) which in its turn exhibits a longer lasting growth pattern than the upper leg (or arm). In an organism with retarded growth this will lead to a relatively stronger and more pronounced development of the proximal limb parts (skeletal elements): a human being has relatively small hands and feet, relatively small toes and a relatively large heel, relatively short lower arms and so on. The legs of the human being are relatively long in comparison to the arms. This also may be explained as the result of strong retardation by means of a prolongation of the period of growing, an embryonic feature, in its turn resulting in the relatively long human legs. In general one could state that retardation also means 'avoiding' (or 'not giving in to') specialization which in fact is the typical feature of the animal organization. As if in evolution there is also the explicitation of the human Gestalt in question: "The more animal specialization there is, the less room there is for human explicitation". [20]

Walking upright is much more than a kind of movement or locomotion. As shown before in the gesture of retaining an upright posture against the forces of gravity, it is also a matter of maintaining an equilibrium or balance. Is this only a morphological Gestalt or is it also a physiological performance, or does it even represent a psychological faculty? A being capable of living in balance (at least having the faculty to do so), needs a morphological organization to act out this behavior, also in the sense of pre-exercising the embryonic principle as explained earlier in this chapter. Regarded as such, walking upright and the act of maintaining balance also represent an important gesture and therefore a faculty of the human soul. Comparative anatomy shows that the process of unfolding and coming upright, the process of development of the limbs as well as the development of the human brain are intimately related. The relatively large human brain is related to the development of an upright posture and is considered to be typical for the human being. The unfolding of the body organization (among other things, the de-flexion of the head) and the development of the characteristic human limbs also lead to the typical human brain development, resulting in a relatively disproportional quantity and quality of the brain. To a large extent those phenomena may be considered specific and unique to human development. Only the human being brings these originally embryonic relationships to an adult organization, the result of the retardation principle; and retains this morphology all through life. This potency leads to a 'multipotent or multipurpose organism', which is not possible for the animal organization. Consequently his biological status offers the human being the opportunity to be free from determinism, something a morphological specialization does involve. The human being acts out his quality against the resistance of the animal principle; he is not the simple extension of that latter principle; he has the possibility of overcoming it as it were. Freedom is something that has to be realized in our inner life; it is expressed in the self-consciousness

of man. Only humans possess a lifelong capacity and faculty of further development. Only humans are capable of overcoming the dictating forces of determinism and of entering the domain of freedom. In order to do so a certain bodily organization is required. To '**pre-exercise**' such an organization in form and function, is what embryonic development is all about.

The polarity body – the embryo still in you

In this text polarity appeared to be the central issue in all kinds of ways, in order to understand human forms and shapes. Is our whole body organization the manifestation of an essential polarity in our body formation, the fundamental polarity of mind and body, of spirit and matter? What about our consciousness and our soul; produced by the body or by a dialogue between spirit and matter within us? The last part of this chapter concerns itself with the 'morphology of consciousness'.

For this purpose we have to reconsider the manifestation of the so-called gradients of development in the human embryo with the so-called *craniocaudal gradient* as one of them and as the most well-known and appreciated one. The craniocaudal gradient of embryonic development is a term which in the first place signifies that the cranial pole or domain of the body development always runs ahead of the developmental processes in the caudal pole or domain of the body. This also relates to the fact that in the cranial pole the development of the organs tends to reach the more or less 'final adult' stage or organization earlier than in the caudal domain of the body. Your head becomes 'old' or 'adult' so to speak, whilst your viscera stay 'young' or 'embryonic'. In the growing embryo, one can observe that the development of the arm and the hand always runs ahead of the development of the foot and the leg for example, that the cranial nerves become manifest long before the lumbosacral spinal nerves, and so on. This phenomenon will also become manifest and 'repeated' in the physiological and psychological maturing of the limbs and the locomotion, for example from head to trunk, from arms and hand to legs and feet. Another body axis which displays such a gradient is the disto-proximal gradient in the limbs: the hands and the feet are 'older' than the shoulder and the pelvic region, the latter as the domain of the limbs for example, where indeed you continue with growing and formation far beyond your childhood.

One could however also describe the craniocaudal gradient as the polarity of movement and form, of embryo and adult, of **process** and **structure**. In the caudal pole of the body the processes actually tend to continue with the embryonic way of life as described here before, i.e. exhibiting morphological behavior with the physical body still in process, in metamorphosis. In contrast to this one may observe in more 'cranial' organs the tendency of more and more coming to structure and to 'anatomy' so to speak. So, the 'head pole' of the body as the structural form pole, the 'pelvic domain' of the body as the growing process pole. There (brain and nervous system, for example) function becomes more 'released' from morphological (growing and metamorphosing) activity. A good way of discerning this gradient or polarity is by comparing a liver ('caudal') with a typical 'cranial organ' like the brain. In the liver, function and form are still in motion, while in the brain, anatomy and structure become essential for the physiological function (See footnote 4); 'formlessness' of the liver and the liver cells in opposition to the tendency to structuralization of the brain and the nerve cells. Simplicity in form versus complexity in structure; the very complex biochemistry and physiology of the liver cell against the relatively simple nerve cell process of de- and repolarization. There is also the polarity of time (process) and space (structure). In the liver the embryonic phase, the 'en-act' dimension, still remains active in a morphological process, deeply involved and intertwined with matter. In the cranial area, in the possibility for mind, the 'en-act' is released from the material and bodily process and comes to function in a more body-free or intangible way. Think of the 'imponderable' mobility of our mind. This shows that the embryonic way of being is not in the past, is not a phase in our life we left behind. It is alive and active; in a large part of our body the interaction between body and mind is 'still' centripetal and 'embryonic'.

Could this be the expression of a polarity in our organism regarding 'interaction' between the en-act and ex-act dimensions of our psychosomatic being? In the 'caudal' ('visceral') dimension of our body, our mind seems to stay connected and intertwined with the body (matter) as is the general gesture in the embryonic phase. In the opposite pole, the body tends to become more structuralized, to become 'anatomy' so to speak. Is it that where mind and body are more or less disconnected and disconnecting, the mind is enabled to function in a more 'body-free' or purely 'conscious' way? Could it be that the embryonic way of being is the way of a sleeping consciousness enacting the body's life? And that when this process tends toward becoming a formalized and 'hardened' anatomical structure, the embryonic vitality and regenerative power is reduced and sometimes even disappears altogether ('death')? Or better still: is it this 'death' that enables awakening consciousness? What a fantastic idea: vitality and consciousness as oppositions: the more vitality, the more we sleep; the more death and structure, the more we are awake! In this view, mind is everywhere in the body as the acting principle, but levels of consciousness awaken to the degree in which the embryonic processes become subdued by the tendency to structure. In this view, the whole body is a psychosomatic manifestation with a great range of levels of consciousness. The will sleeps in the caudal pole, in the limbs and the muscles - the cognitive soul awakens in the head and the sense organs! Are psychological dimensions like thinking, feeling and willing related then to morphological dimensions of equivalent levels of consciousness and awareness: wakening, dreaming, and sleeping?

This may sound like a global concept. Nevertheless, the gradient we are describing may be observed in not only a craniocaudal 'direction' but in more than eight different bodily dimensions: dorsal-ventral, parietal-visceral, distal-proximal in the limbs, centripetal and centrifugal and so on. As a matter of fact, this gradient, this polarity is everywhere; and 'nowhere': it is a fundamental principle of polarity that rules the psychosomatic organization in all directions, levels and dimensions. For us, the holographic principle of the craniocaudal gradient overcomes the Cartesian error of **localizing** soul, psyche, awareness, and consciousness in a given organ or region. Not only or exclusively is the brain the domain of the soul, the mind or the psyche, but the several 'head organs' like the liver, the heart, and the kidneys exhibit a similar function to some degree. But the brain does represent the functional possibility of a high degree of awakening, that is, self-consciousness.

The phenomenological approach can yield great insight and renewal for the study of the human form and body. For it reveals that the body is not merely an appendage of the brain, but that it is an instrument of the soul from the very first day of life onwards. Consciousness is not synonymous or congruent with 'soul'; it is a function, an activity of the mind. The whole range and palette of consciousness shows that our soul is not a nebulous concept or illusionary 'something' but a 'soul body' just as complicated as our physical body. There is not one specialized organ for the psyche, but perhaps several - such as the brain, the sense organs, etc. - also function. But our mind is everywhere. The body is not a machine that functions; it is itself function, a function of the mind. Such an 'anatomy' would give us back the body that we are, that we live, where we do not have hippocampi in our heads at all, but where we think with our heads, also feel in our hearts and suffer pain in our toes. "We are awareness, consciousness and have a body".

Conclusion

In this chapter we have mapped the contours of a 'phenomenological embryology' that is searching for human expression and behavior in form and shape. The central issue in this approach is that a human being is a being of body and mind (soul), the fundamental polarities of spirit and matter, and that the morphogenesis of the bodily organization also represents human behavior and expression. From the very beginning we deal with soul and body; also during the embryo phase where (when) the body is being (per) formed. This process however is not exclusive for or restricted to the embryonic phase; during the following human life cycles this principle is continuously active, as the unconscious performance of the human mind or soul within the organs. This means that the conscious psychological life may be regarded as a kind of special psycho-somatic process, representing the actual or proper psyche of the human being, and not as restricted to only the physiological functioning of the brain, as the Cartesian paradigm would have us believe. Or paraphrasing the philosopher Delamettrie: "The human being does not **have** a soul, he **is** soul". Here we extend this view to the concept, that during embryonic development a human being is also not just a body but an animated and therefore experiencing being. The process of bodily organization and formation is also an expression of the human soul, of human behavior. In this regard it cannot be neglected that the human entelechy is active and present in the embryo and therefore may have experiences. Such experiences might be present as models and templates for the psychological functioning of the organism but may also lead to scars, pain or disturbances that may become consciously or subconsciously manifest in later life

cycles. If one considers that a human embryo is also an entity of body and soul (psyche), the whole embryonic phase represents **human** behavior as well. Our body is a human body that serves human consciousness; it is a human constitution and expression of human consciousness itself. In the formation of the human body morphology and psychology are a joined venture. It is the human mind, the human spirit that expresses the human body, not the reverse. The formation of our body is part of our biography.

References

Bie, G. van der, Embryology - Early development from a phenomenological point of view, Louis Bolk Instituut, Driebergen, Holland, Publication number GVO 01, http://www.louisbolk.org/nl/publicaties/bolk-s-companions; 2001.

Bie, G. van der, & Huber, M. (eds), Foundations of Anthroposophical Medicine - A training manual, Floris Books; 2003.

Blechschmidt E., The Beginning of Human Life, Science Library, Heidelberg; 1977.

Blechschmidt E., The Ontogenetic Basis of Human Anatomy – A Biodynamic Approach to Development from Conception to Birth – Edited and translated by Brian Freeman, North Atlantic Books; 2004.

Blechschmidt E. and Gasser RF., Biokinetics and Biodynamics of human differentiation, North Atlantic Books; 2012 (1978).

Blechschmidt E., Sein und Werden, Urachhaus; 1982.

Bolk L., Hersenen en cultuur, Scheltema & Holkema; 1932.

Bortoft H., Goethe's Scientific Consciousness, Institute for Cultural Research; 1986.

Bortoft H., The Wholeness of Nature, Lindisfarne Press; 1996

Drews U., Color Atlas of Embryology, Thieme Verlag; 1995.

Grossinger, R., Embryos, Galaxies and Sentient Beings – How the Universe Makes Life North Atlantic Books; 2003.

Hartmann O.J., Dynamische Morphologie, Vittorio Klostermann, Frankfurt/M; 1959.

Hartmann O.J., Die Gestaltstufen der Naturreiche, Verlag Die Kommenden, Freiburg; 1967.

Hinrichsen K.V. (Hrsg.), Humanembryologie, Springer-Verlag; 1990.

Langman J., Medical Embryology, Lippincot Williams & Wilkins; 1995.

Lipton, B., The Biology of Life, Cygnus Books; 2005

Odent M., The Scientification of Love, Free Association Books Ltd; 1999.

Poppelbaum H., Mensch und Tier, Rudolf Gering Verlag, Basel; 1933.

Portmann A., Biologische Fragmente zu einer Lehre vom Menschen, Basel; 1944.

Rohen, J.W., Functional Morphology – The Dynamics of Wholeness of the Human Organism Adonis Press; 2007.

Rohen, J.W., Lütjen-Drecoll E., Funktionelle Embryologie, Die Entwicklung der Funktionssysteme des menschliche Organismus, 3. Auflage, Verlag Schattauer; 2006

Rose, S., Lifelines., Penguin Books; 1997.

Seamon D. and Zajonc A. (eds.), Goethe's Way of Science, SUNY Press; 1998

Schad W., Die Vorgeburtlichkeit des Menschen, Urachhaus; 2005 (1982).

Schad, W. Die verlorene Hälfte des Menschen – Die Plazenta vor und nach der Geburt, 2. Auflage, Verlag Freies Geistesleben & Urachhaus; 2005

Verhulst, J., Developmental Dynamics in Humans and Other Primates: Discovering Evolutionary Principles through Comparative Morphology, Adonis Press; 2003.

Vögler H., Human Blastogenesis, Bibliotheca Anatomica 30; 1987.

Wilmar F., Vorgeburtliche Menschwerdung, J. Ch. Mellinger Verlag; 1979.

Wolpert L., The triumph of the embryo, Oxford University Press; 1991

11

Prenatal and perinatal worlds of experience

Ludwig Janus

A magic dwells in each beginning, that protects us and helps us to live.

H. Hesse, Lebensstufen (Steps of life)

Introduction

Humankind has always sensed that the experience of the mother has an influence on the developing child; expectant mothers, therefore, were always advised to avoid stress and experiences involving risk, and to nurture the development of the child with tenderness and loving care. It was feared that frightening experiences on the part of the mother could have negative effects on the child and cause it lasting damage. Only with the arrival of early psychoanalysis, however, did people begin to think of the child as a being able to experience in its own right, and with its own center of experience. Those early studies were of course concerned with suffering individuals, and for that reason the emphasis was on experiences of fear. Birth was understood as the first major fear situation, possibly linked to the experience of separation and abandonment.[1] Courageous as these observations and conclusions were, they did to an extent idealize the time preceding birth as one of freedom from troubles and disturbances.[2] The Hungarian psychoanalyst Nandor Fodor (1949)[3] was the first to describe the consequential effects of prenatal hazards in the form of fears and feelings of annihilation.

In the 1970s, research using psychoactive substances offered deeper insight into the subjective experience of birth and the prenatal period, making it possible to draw comparisons between the experiences of a number of subjects. A more precise understanding of the experience of the birth process became possible as a result, corresponding to the phases of the dilation of the cervix, expulsion, and emergence (Grof 1983).[4] The work with psychoactive substances also enabled researchers to capture frightening prenatal experiences, such as could be re-evoked in "horror trips."[5] One special dimension of prenatal experience concerned feelings relating to the umbilical cord, which might be felt to be nourishing and sustaining, or in contrast toxic and oppressive. This came to be known as "umbilical affect."[6]

Enlightening as these observations were, and as much as they expanded understanding, they did little to capture the physical dimensions of prenatal and perinatal experience. This was successfully addressed by the regression therapist William Emerson (2000)[7] whose approach concentrated on the experiencing of sensations of the body. His methodology looked at experiences before the development of language using physical techniques of regression and re-creation. These enacted the scene, recreating an experience for example by the physical simulation of the birth canal or uterine space, to help trace out spontaneous sensations or feelings of the body. Carrying out the regressions in groups enables group members to compare experiences and so prompt further insight. This methodology, which to some extent activates the right-brain, non-verbal side of experience, can render accessible very deep sensations and images going back to the embryonic period. It seems that earliest experiences are stored in the memory of our bodies and sensations, accessible to our experiential selves but not to our verbal selves. What is probably of importance here is that individuals are distanced a little from our human tendency to over-emphasize the centrality of language, so allowing entry to pre-verbal experience and memory.

Despite the accuracy of our understanding about the biological development that takes place during the embryonic and fetal period, our knowledge of the corresponding dimension of experience is fragmentary and incomplete; the more so the farther back we go. Our knowledge at the experiential level relating to the moment of birth and the preceding time is, on the other hand, much more complete. I shall therefore begin with an account of the later stages and then work backwards. This approach will also enable the reader to become gradually familiarized with the particular nature of these early experiences. I shall describe the milestones of early development in that reverse order. One important question here concerns how and by what means pre-verbal experiences are recalled. A few aspects are presented below.

In academic psychology, research into memory has mainly been concerned with linguistic memory and memories of matters that can be encapsulated in language. Study of the pathways of memory for feelings and for the body was mainly carried out in depth psychology and bodywork relating to individual cases only. It was only in the latter half of the 20th century that more systematic study of preverbal memory systems was carried out[8] and that this was recognized as an autonomous field. One characteristic of preverbal experiences is that they cannot be actively remembered, but only become accessible by re-evoking them in the present. Individuals re-immerse themselves in the early experience, and may also be able, in a second act, to assign an approximate time to it. In psychotherapy there are often external points of reference by which this can be assigned; for example fear of annihilation might be linked with a threat to the pregnancy. Of course, in dealing with such reconstructed "memories" there must remain some degree of question as to the reality of the content, since the only evidence is that of the individual case.

One important prerequisite lies in the fact that our capacity for empathetic understanding of the feelings and states of experience of childhood and infancy has grown enormously in the last 100 years. In the past, babies were allowed to "cry themselves out" and children were beaten without any sense of what the child might be experiencing. This has changed markedly in the second half of the 20th century. The experience and the sensitivity of infants and young children are now accepted as self-evident. The study of experiences before and during birth seeks to extend our empathetic understanding of the child's experience before and during birth. If this still seemed absurd only a few years ago, the predominant attitude now is quite different and ready to open up to this part of our biography. It is in this spirit that we try here to explore and understand early experience, by study and exercise, from within. Here, then, some ideas from the "film"

of early development, beginning with arrival in the world.

Arrival in the world – finding ourselves, or the painful sense of separation

Arrival in the world is a huge surprise, a moment of great astonishment. All that was inwardly, utterly familiar now looks and feels quite different. The very first act is as the child opens its mouth and draws its first breath, that existential act that gives life and banishes danger, as done formerly by the supply of oxygen from the umbilical cord. A new connection is forged through the agency of touch and the experience of being held, and through the familiarity of the voice. The child moves eagerly on its mother's abdomen, actively seeking the breast whose familiar scent it can smell. It is its arrival at this new source of nourishment that releases the umbilical cord. The child is now obtaining life and nourishment by its own actions, by breathing and sucking, where previously it obtained them passively from the placenta and umbilical cord. Ideally the child can make the link between the postnatal relationship and the prenatal one, deriving profound hope and comfort.

Nevertheless, at the beginning of its life the child is infinitely needy and dependent. Separation and times of abandonment are felt as a falling into nothingness; rejection and the experience of being unwanted lead to boundless pain and longing, which the child is totally unable to process. If the situation is unfavorable, the child can only try to shut off such painful experiences and protect itself from re-igniting them by avoiding close contact.

Birth – an adventure, or a trip to hell

Birth, according to the American Society for Obstetrics and Gynecology, is one of the most dramatic events in the life of any person. It is an irreversible, existential moment. The great task and change ahead is heralded by the increasing narrowness of space, decreasing provision of oxygen, and slow pangs of labor. The child has to engage in an unknown adventure in this first stage of birth, to seek and find an unknown path, and to endure an effort whose demands it cannot know, unknowing too whether it will have strength enough to cope. It is led in this by an instinctive knowledge, and ideally also aided and supported by its mother. She in turn will ideally have the help and support of others, the midwife and birth assistants. This situation of support is so important because the instinctive knowledge that enables the birth can only be effective in an environment of safety and emotional security.

Prenatal security is the basis for a successful birth; some might say faith and trust in God. This is a dimension of feeling that does also find expression in the religious sphere. It is only when such hopeful security and faith have been built up before birth that there is strength to endure the birth itself with confidence, and the sense that "the Lord is my shepherd, therefore can I lack nothing." Such a moment is when human individuals can truly take life's fate in their hands.

In the less favorable case when this undergirding of security is lacking, it can lead even in this first stage of birth to deep feelings of abandonment, anxiety about one's own existence, existential anger, depression, and fear of loss. The time when the cervix begins to dilate is associated with a sense of unavoidable change, which must be desired by both mother and child if it is not to be experienced as fateful or as endless, irreplaceable loss.

The strengthening labor gives the child a resistant surface against which to stem its feet, pushing itself forward, enabling the birth canal to open and enabling its head to press further into the lesser pelvis. This leads to the surprising discovery that there is a way forward, and that effort and decisiveness will be rewarded. In the opposite, unfavorable case, it can instead produce the sense that there is no way out, of being compressed and imprisoned, that all is in vain and a feeling of despair. All these feelings have a deep existential dimension; one that we find in representations of religious feelings of need and despair and of being a victim.

In the middle stage of birth, the child has to rotate. As it enters the lesser pelvis, its parietal suture is aligned transversely. Depending on position, the child has to turn 90° to left or right so as to be able to leave the birth canal by extending its neck. As it carries out this turn, the child once more faces the existential issue of finding and taking the right way. The child's instinctive knowledge and intuition and co-operation by the mother show the way. It may have the sense of being led by wondrous forces, and feel itself turning the corner and opening up a path for itself where there had seemed to be none, by actively turning and rotating.

The effort of opening up, head bent, turning in the middle stage of the birth process and stretching at the end of it are the first elemental actions by the child that change the world. This can be like the road to freedom, if the child's latter experience of its situation in the womb had seemed like a prison; or it may be an elemental battle, crowned by an elemental victory, if the child's passage into the world demanded all its reserves of strength. We encounter reflections of these different experiences of birth and the character imprinted by them in the tales of the birth of heroes. We learn, for example, how Hera prevented the birth of Hercules for eight days, causing him to make a superhuman struggle to come into the world and developing in him those qualities of a fighter that determined his whole life.[9]

In a case where conditions are unfavorable, this middle stage of the birth process brings a lack of orientation, panic, wrongly-directed activity, hopelessness, anxiety, anger, and the sense of not finding the solution, along with a feeling that there is no solution. If the stress is imposed mainly on the head during the dilation stage, in the middle stage the rotation also places the spinal column under pressure, or may often impose excessive stress. If the mother's pelvis is narrow, this could lead to existentially excessive demands being placed on the tissue and spraining.[10]

In the third stage of birth, the child must finally open the birth canal by extending its head, using its feet as the base from which to propel itself, to emerge into the light of the world. Its forehead and face press against the mother's sacrum and have to find their way downward. The sense here is of one final great effort and with diminishing resources: the absolute necessity of surmounting the last hurdle in order to reach the safety of the shore. This may be accompanied by a sense of triumph at the close of a battle well fought, as celebrated by every triumphal arch in history.

In the unfavorable case, the overwhelming feelings are those of exhaustion, fear of failure, mortal fear, or elemental fury and despair. There is no light at the end of the tunnel; instead there is eternal condemnation.

Birth is a great adventure and a heroic deed. Its varied reflection is therefore found time and again in the battles and adventures of heroes facing the great challenges of life.[11]

The fetal period – primal bonding or primal ambivalence

The period of gestation from the 3rd to the 9th month is one of growth, differentiation, and intensification of the prenatal relationship and bonding. The mother can feel the child moving and can establish a relationship through sensation and emotion. Today it is well known that prenatal relationship and reassurance are essential basic elements for later health, enabling the child to have experience of itself in a relationship and to "center itself" in that relationship. The process of bonding begins before birth and continues throughout life.[12-14]

Profound experiences of harmony and attachment are possible during this period, and similarly those of rhythm, harmonization, and difference. The child's experience of self takes place in a space in which it floats and which it explores; its first environment, a landscape reflected in images of paradise and the Elysian Fields. The writer Adalbert Stifter spoke of it in this way:

Far back in the empty nothingness is something like wonder and delight, powerfully seizing hold and flooding my being with an almost destructive force, like nothing in my future life. The features I registered were splendor, turmoil; it was somewhere below. This must have been very early on, for it seems to me as if a high, wide dark expanse of nothingness lay all about that thing. Then there was something else that permeated my inward self, softly and soothingly. The feature: these were sounds. Then I was swimming in something gently undulating. I swam now and again, within me the softness became greater and greater, then I became as if drunk; then there was nothing more.

Stifter, 1959[15]

The prenatal period also sees the first experiences of movement. Lux Flanegan's book (1984)[16] contains beautiful pictures showing how elegantly children move in this prenatal time. We can well imagine children's later pleasure in trampolining or dance as reflecting these early experiences of movement. This dimension of movement is aided by music, which is also fundamentally linked to the prenatal experience of sound.[17] Dance music, with its heartbeat rhythm, makes tangible the prenatal experience of sound and enlivens the prenatal sense of floating in the weightlessness of dance.

The experience of the umbilical cord and placenta is of major importance prenatally, and can be seen as reflected in the mythical tales of good serpents and venomous ones and of the tree of life. The child is dependent in an elemental way on its mother's body and the greater whole for its nourishment, supply of oxygen,

and removal of waste products. It can sense itself to be strengthened, invigorated, and sustained in constant plenty and satisfaction, as we find expressed in images of paradise and the land of milk and honey.

Dieter Lattmann's book *Jonas vor Potsdam* offers another poetic picture of the prenatal situation:

It was in the middle of my time (before birth) in the great fish, only then, that I was overcome by a feeling that never left me. I had been swimming in there, invisibly tiny, suffused by all those currents from the very beginning... I repeated the oscillations that it (the great fish) had engendered in me. One day I added my own, and hit against the boundaries. The fish paused, as if I had taken it by surprise, and suddenly performed a dance among the waves. Then I understood that it was pleased at that sign from me... I felt the incoming flow from the heartbeat of the great fish in which I stirred ... Like a miniature human in his biotope, I crouched in sloughed-off skin with my wizened head between my shoulders, legs flexed up toward me and hands entwined below ... And with this worried expression on my face as if I knew I had to make my way out... Maybe my mother was angry with everything that was around her, and just because she stayed too much in control to weep out loud I no longer felt as I was meant to inside her; I was bewildered. Later, I was never again so quadrupedal, so replete, so furious or contented, except when I was in love or ill.[18]

In the unfavorable case the child is faced with a situation of being unwanted or even threatened. Then the child can feel unworthy, extra to requirements, insignificant, or even under threat and fearful for its existence.[19, 20] If the mother is unhappy about the pregnancy or in social need, the child is directly exposed to the associated stress, with consequent damage to its vital consciousness. The child may withdraw into protective attitudes or maintain a constant irritated and disturbed mood. The uterine space becomes a prison or a lair, or the reverse may happen, with any prison or lair, together with the associated exposure and possible mistreatment, reflecting that primal imprisonment and exposure before birth. In that kind of situation, a child simply encounters too few positive experiences to be able to break out of the previous negative imprinting. The result can be lifelong dysphoric moods, irritability, sensitivity to stress, and pessimism.

LSD regression can render negative pre-birth experiences accessible in a very dramatic way. The Greek psychiatrist Athanassios Kafkalides gives a graphic description of the consequences that come from great unwantedness: the individual concerned was a 22-year-old single woman who had felt like a frightened animal ever since childhood. She was afraid of everyone and everything and was unable to find support anywhere. She had nothing but feelings of guilt and punished and tormented herself on account of them. Here is an extract from the notes recording the LSD experience of self-discovery:

As I saw my mother pregnant, I felt that I was in her belly, and she battered me terribly. I realized that she wanted to abort me and I felt frightened, because she was against me. And I felt very weak ... Mother's body is something dirty. It contains scraps of paper and splinters of glass. If anyone gets in there, they are nothing. It is like a grave; like a plastic bottle... because it is drowning me. I cannot see the sea, because it is drowning me. And if I drown I'll become a little baby, a fetus, and then... then the grave is there... And if I didn't exist in my mother's body, how could I think I would ever exist. I feel constantly dead and I'm constantly defending myself... When will I ever get out of this situation? It is black, I get out and I'm naked, and folk don't like naked people. I feel as if I'm burning... I see black ash... what is it? Mother's body is everything; I come into the world as if I'm burnt. When I come out of my mother's body I can't fight it, though, because, because everywhere I feel as if I'm in my mother's body. I have the feeling that I have something of my mother's body even when I am out of it. Now I'm the dirty little child they didn't want.[21]

The mother's body, then, is the place where we receive our first experiences of the world and ourselves, and where we learn the first lessons of life. It has been said that our mother's body is the first school we have all attended.

Implantation and the embryonic period

In contrast to the richness and diversity of our knowledge about the experience of birth and the fetal period, observations that could provide information about the preceding period are fragmentary and incomplete. One event that strikes our attention as a significant field of experience is the process of implantation. The experiences of that tiny being from which we develop, the blastocyst, during implantation are of the most elemental kind, as it begins to establish a relationship with the "other" being, its mother, to seek out a place that will be "home" and put down roots there. That can convey the sense that there is such a thing as home, nourishment, security and limitless support. Here it is possible to experience that sense of being at home and acceptable to express what we find in religious feelings.

In the opposite situation, implantation can be a battle for survival and an experience of homelessness, exposure, and nihilism. Words can only hint at the deep preverbal dissonances that can nevertheless leave their indelible mark on how it feels to us to be in the world.

There are remarkably few results from studies that look into the experience of self relating to the embryonic period, yet it is a time of fulminant, vital growth, differentiation of tissues, and the constitution of the infant body and self. It can be associated with exciting feelings of power and strength. On the other hand, there are some observations indicating that if anything prejudices the pregnancy at the given time when a particular organ system is developing, this can especially affect that system. For example, it may affect the cardiovascular system and predispose the individual to particular diseases in later life. One possible reason that there are so few observations deriving from regressions is that such threats posed an immediate risk to survival and led to the death of the fetus.

The initial cell stages – some speculative thoughts on the very first developmental processes

It is fair to assume that the origin of psychosomatic processes, rather than occurring at some time during prenatal development, in fact dates back to the very beginning, so that cells have an external life and an inner one (or internal competence) from the outset. There has always been speculation in the field of prenatal psychology that very early states of mind can predetermine the nature of later states, or that it is possible to arrive at intuitive insights in this respect by means of deep regressions. Although this area remains very speculative, an attempt can be made to make some statements about initial development, linking these to external developmental processes.

We develop from what are to outward appearances two very contrasting cell entities, the sperm and the ovum, the egg. The egg leads a very static existence in the ovary. At ovulation, when the follicle matures, one egg bursts out from its communal existence alongside its sister cells and, supplied by nutritive cells, undertakes a journey through the Fallopian tube. The sperm does not begin its existence until a few weeks before it matures, in the testicular tissue. Its journey is something of an extraordinary adventure, as the distance it has to travel is vast in comparison to its tiny size; it has to battle against adversities, faces the threat of exhaustion, and makes its journey in the company of a host of its fellow sperm. None but a few reach the egg cell, and only one sperm is allowed to enter. The event that follows in the egg cell itself is a highly dynamic process of encounter in which two haploid sets of chromosomes undergo complex ordering and unite to form a complete new cell. This process is the beginning of a new individual. The high drama of the event is like that mythological moment of the origin of the universe, which physicists believe happened in the "Big Bang." The new individual begins its journey to the uterus as a morula and blastocyst, and seeks out a place there for its implantation.

Some speculations suggest that the way the parents feel about their relationship to each other can exert an influence as marginal conditions of the conception, and may despite its marginality have deep effects.[22] Speculative as this may be, it may be instructive for individuals to ask what their parents' situation was at and after the time of their conception, and how ready they were to welcome a child, or how and in what way that preparedness might have been limited.

Closing remarks

It has become clear that the observations become more speculative and more sketchy the further back we go. However, this area will become a field of research in the years ahead. We need, as far as possible, to look inwardly at the beginnings of our own lives and forge a link with our beginnings in order to establish our identity and our authenticity more deeply. Just as it became clear in the field of depth psychology as it developed during the last century that we need to consider childhood feelings and experiences to be able to become truly adult and autonomous, so it has become clear in recent years that we also need to deal with the

preverbal period in order to establish the foundations of our own existence more deeply. The challenge to do so originated with patients who had lost the continuity of their own existence on account of unfavorable conditions and stresses. It became evident that this is not only true of stresses during the development of the child, but also of the preverbal period of the infant and the prenatal child. It can then become necessary in individual cases to concern ourselves with these stresses, if they had led to a loss of self. We can learn from such experiences with psychotherapy patients and experience of the self-stimulated by such therapy that even our inner competence and our spiritual experience have ultimately developed from the very beginning, and form part of our biography.

References

[1]Rank O: Das Trauma der Geburt. Gießen: Psychosozial; 1997.

[2]Graber GH: Die Ambivalenz des Kindes. Revised and expanded: Ursprung, Zwiespalt und Einheit der Seele. Collected works I. Obtainable from: Axel Bischoff, ISPPM Office/Sekretariat, Friedhofweg 52, 69118 Heidelberg; 1924.

[3]Fodor N: The Search for the Beloved. A Clinical Investigation of the Trauma of Birth and Prenatal Condition. New York: University Books; 1949.

[4]Grof S: Topographie des Unbewussten. Stuttgart: Klett-Cotta; 1983.

[5]Kafkalides A: The Knowledge of the Womb. Heidelberg: Mattes; 1995.

[6]Lake: Constricted Confusion. Obtainable from: Textstudio Gross, Brahmsstr. 1, 69 Heidelberg; 1980 (Unpublished).

[7]Emerson W: Treatment of Birth Trauma in Infants and Children, Collected Works of William Emerson, Vol. 1. Petaluma, CA 94952: Emerson Training Seminars; 1996.

[8]Schacter D: Searching for Memory. New York: Basic Books; 1996.

[9]Janus L: Zum Zusammenhang von Geburt und Lebensgestaltung im Märchen und Mythos. Kind und Umwelt. 1988;57:3–19.

[10]Biedermann: Manualtherapie bei Kindern. Stuttgart: Enke; 1999.

[11]Janus L: Wie die Seele entsteht. Heidelberg: Mattes; 1997. (Enduring Effects of Prenatal Life Time. Download from www.ludwig-janus.de).

[12]Krens I: Die erste Beziehung. Int J of Prenatal and Perinatal Psychology and Medicine. 200;13:127–153.

[13]Veldman F: Confirming Affectivity. The Dawn of Human Life. In J of Prenatal and Perinatal Psychology and Medicine. 1994;6:11–26.

[14]Veldman F: Haptonomie – amour et raison. Paris: puf; 2004.

[15]Stifter A: Nachgelassenes Blatt. In: Gesammelte Werke, vol.6. Gütersloh: Sigbert Mohn; 1959.

[16]Flanagan GL: Die ersten neun Monate des Lebens. Einbek bei Hamburg: Rowohlt; 1984.

[17]Parncutt R: Pränatale Erfahrung und Ursprünge der Musik. In: Janus L, Haibach S (ed.): Seelisches Erleben vor und während der Geburt. Neu-Isenburg: Lingua-Med; 1997.

[18]Lattman D: Reading from the book Jonas aus dem großen Fisch in the SDR broadcast of 7.6.1993.

[19]Häsing H, Janus L (ed.): Ungewollte Kinder. text-o-phon, Teutonenstr. 32b, Wiesbaden; 1999. Bindung beginnt vor der Geburt. Heidelberg: Mattes 2011.

[20]Levend H, Janus L: Drum hab ich kein Gesicht – Kinder aus unerwünschten Schwangerschaften. Würzburg: Echter; 2002.

[21]Janus L: Die frühe Ich-Entwicklung im Spiegel der LSD-Therapie von Athanassios Kafkalides. Zeitschrift für Individualpsychologie. 1991;16:111–124.

[22]Meistermann-Seeger E: Kurztherapie Fokaltraining. München: Verlag für angewandte Wissenschaften; 1986.

12

Evolution of the mind–body–spirit unit

James J. McGovern and Rene J. McGovern

Introduction

In this chapter we shall briefly outline the evolving scientific understanding of the mechanisms underlying how the mind and spirit communicate with the body. We shall explain how this suggests an interactive unity among the mind, body, and spirit. We shall also describe how these interactions evolve from infancy to old age and describe an osteopathic model to analyze problems involving mind–body–spirit interactions.

In order to describe these interactions, we need to establish common definitions. We adopted the word used by A.T. Still, and other osteopaths, namely *spirit*, since it indicated a relationship between emotions and autonomic functions.[1] Therefore, we define *spirit* as representing emotions that have semiconscious or unconscious origins and that are related to autonomic systems, while the *mind* is related to conscious thoughts that can control the non-autonomic systems of the body.

In ancient Greece people knew from experience that emotions (spirit) and bodily health were somehow related. They had asclepions, which were like modern spas or resorts, where there were baths, exercise routines, healthful diets, and good conversations to restore and augment health. Until recently, we had only limited research findings to support the physiological underpinnings linking the spirit (emotions) and the body. Through new technology, research evidence is now available to help us begin to understand the underlying mechanisms involved in the relationship between emotions and bodily health. The next section will describe some of the major contributors toward understanding this relationship.

Section 1: emotions

Recent research connecting the emotions to health has been summarized by Esther Sternberg, chief of the Neuroendocrine Immunology and Behavior Section at the Institute of Mental Health of the (U.S.) National Institutes of Health, and others. In her book, *The Balance Within*, Dr Sternberg discusses the connection between emotions and health, to show *how* stress produces physical responses in the body:

Rather than seeing the psyche as the source of such illness, we are discovering that while feelings don't directly cause or cure disease, the biological mechanisms underlying them may cause or contribute to disease.

Sternberg, 2000, p. 13[2]

Potential mechanisms, described by Sternberg, involve communication between the immune system and the central nervous system, or neuroimmunomodulation, as the field of mind–body communication is now being called. Additional work, described by LeDoux[3] in his book The *Synaptic Self*, articulates the physiologic impact of stress on brain structure and function. Antonio Damasio,[4] in his groundbreaking book *Descartes' Error* described the use of brain imaging techniques to demonstrate the importance of emotions (spirit) on rational thought. All three authors challenged the then accepted paradigm of mind–body dualism and helped establish the scientific credibility of mind–body interaction. The mechanisms underlying how the mind and spirit communicate with the body appear to specifically involve some brain centers, with several common central pathways activated, including the hypothalamic–pituitary–adrenal axis, peripheral nervous system, and autonomic nervous system. Neurohormones and neurotransmitters released into the blood or through nerve pathways then affect immune responses and disease expression.[5]

Esther Sternberg concludes a discussion of the above findings as follows:

Finally knowing all these different routes that connect the brain to the immune system helps us understand just how stress can make you sick and how believing can make you well.

Sternberg, 2000, p. 607[2]

On the last page of her book, Dr Sternberg ends with the following challenge for further research and for an overall understanding of the many fields involved:

But not all stress responses and diseases can be done away with solely by changing the environment. Part of the future in this field includes identifying which components of our physiological responses we can modify and which we can't; which can be changed by learning new ways of coping with stressful situations and which are unmodifiable except by medical intervention. Another important future task of this field will be to identify which of our behavioral and psychological responses to stressful situations are inherited, which are learned and how much is affected by early upbringing.

Sternberg, 2000, p. 210[2]

In the next two sections, we will see (Section 2) how the mind, body, and spirit evolved in animals and during our lifetimes and (Section 3) how modern healers can work with people to adjust natural structures not only in the body, but in the mind and spirit as well.

Section 2: evolution

In this section, we will illustrate how various stages of development of the mind and spirit have been "detected" (formulated) and how they have been applied to the evolution of different kinds of monkeys and early ancestors (hominids) of *Homo sapiens*. However, it is important to realize that scientists first studied developmental stages in human beings, then noticed some correspondence of their *lower stages* with the behavior of monkeys, and most recently suggested that *middle stages* of their development could be found in various hominids.

The following stages of human development, shown in Table 12.1, were proposed recently by Stanley Greenspan and Stuart Shanker.[6]

Development stage	Age of person
1. Self regulation and shared attention	From birth onwards
2. Engagement and relating	2–4 months onwards
3. Two-way intentional emotional signaling	4–8 months onwards
4. Co-regulated emotional signaling, social problem solving, presymbolic self	9–18 months onwards
5. Creating representations, symbols, or ideas	18 months onwards
6. Bridges between ideas and logical thinking	2.5 years onwards
7. Multicause, comparative, triangular thinking	Varies with individual
8. Reflective thinking with expanded sense of self	Varies with individual
9. Reflective thinking, considering the future	Varies with individual
10. Reflective thinking, philosophy	Varies with individual

TABLE 12.1: Stages of human development

Development stage (Numbers from Table 12.1)	Lowest animal involved
1 and parts of 2 and 3	Tamarins, marmosets, and selective others
2 and early 3	Rhesus monkeys and selective others
3 and early 4	Baboons and selective others
4	*Homo erectus, H. habilis*, australopithecines, ardepithecines, chimpanzees, bonobos
5	*Archaic H. sapiens* and early moderms (600,000 to 60,00 years age)
6	*H. sapiens* (130,000 years ago)
7 and 8	Magdalenian period (12,000 to 8000 BC)
8	Ancient civilizations (3500 to 720 BC)
9 and 10	Ancient Greece (700 to 300 BC)

TABLE 12.2: Stages of development in selected groups

The following stages of development (shown in Table 12.2 and using the numbers from Table 12.1) have been "seen" in the cognitive levels of various animals and historic human beings.[6]

While scientists from Charles Darwin to Richard Dawkins believed functional/emotional developments in hominids and modern man were the result of the somewhat passive, undirected process of natural selection, the authors of these last two tables, Stanley Greenspan and Stuart Shanker, believe that, while there are some biological developments that are *necessary* for this progression, the *sufficient* condition is due to "formative cultural practices that guide caregiver–infant interactions," and "were not genetically determined but rather, were passed down and thus learned anew by each generation."[6]

Greenspan and Shanker suggest that cognitive development is guided by *emotions* at every stage. Even just days after birth, a baby is coupling smells and textures (body) with feelings (mind and spirit) to begin their evolving, accumulating functional/emotional development.[6]

These baby–caregiver exchanges . . . can be quite extended. We refer to the long chains of emotional signaling as reciprocal, co-regulated, emotional interactions. . . The term "interaction". . . can be traced back to Lev Vygotsky and Jean Piaget, if not beyond. In Vygotsky's usage . . . the term primarily applies to social interactions.

Greenspan and Shanker, p. 30[6]

Vygotsky repeatedly used the terms *structure* and *function* to articulate development of cognitive processes and explained how we needed to construct new structures out of old structures to further develop them:

The first stage is followed by the first structure's destruction, reconstruction, and transition to structures of the higher type. Unlike the direct reactive processes, these latter structures are constructed on the basis of the use of signs. . .

Cole, 1978, p. 124[7]

Greenspan and Shanker go further and explain the key role of emotions (the spirit) in the formation of structures in cognition (mind):

...we will show, contrary to the views of Chomsky and Pinker on the genetic origin of language,

Scientist	Principle	Type of cause
1. Virchow	Interactive unity	Form(al)
2. Pasteur	Structure–function interdep.	Material
3. Darwin	Self-healing mechanism	Efficient
4. Bulger	Meaning–expectancy response	Final

TABLE 12.3: Sources of osteopathic principles

that language and cognition are embedded in the emotional processes that, in our hypothesis, led to symbols.

Greenspan and Shanker, pp. 7–8[6]

In Section 1: emotions, we saw that emotion or spirit interacts with the body to get things done. In the earlier text (Section 2: evolution), we noticed how the mind interacts with the spirit (emotion) to get things done. In summary, we have observed that the mind, body, and spirit need each other to get things done. That is, they are interdependent, i.e., an interactive unit.

Section 3: adjustment

The question for this section is: Can we adjust this mind–body–spirit interactive unit to help people? The adjustment or manipulation of units or structures sounds very osteopathic, even if it is on the mind, body, and spirit instead of just the body. Perhaps, we asked ourselves, osteopathic principles might work in the areas of the mind and spirit as well as on the body.

In 1892, Andrew Taylor Still founded the first osteopathic school (now A.T. Still University) and awarded the first D.O. degree in Kirksville, Missouri, USA. He developed several principles, the three most sustained being:

1 Interactive unity

2 Interdependency of structure and function

3 Self-healing mechanism.

Research on articles by contemporaries of A.T. Still revealed that his main inspirations for these principles were the works of Rudolf Virchow, Louis Pasteur/ Claude Bernard, and Charles Darwin/Herbert Spenser, respectively.[1]

It was recently noticed by us that these principles were related to the first three principles of perceiving reality (causality) of Aristotle: the formal cause, material cause, and efficient cause.[1] The fourth perspective, the final cause, did not have a corresponding osteopathic principle and so the meaning–expectancy response was proposed by us to summarize the osteopathic practice of explaining to patients what seems to be happening and thereby giving meaning and hence expectancy to the patient.[1]

The principles described in Table 12.3 can be quickly understood by realizing that they correspond to the four perspectives used by a manager running a business or used by a detective solving a crime (see Table 12.4).

In detective work, one starts with the perspective or dimension about which most is known, but invariably one needs to investigate the other dimensions (scene, suspects, etc.) to get the full picture, much as one shifts from vertical to horizontal clues in doing a crossword puzzle. So too in healthcare, we may have to shift perspectives to understand the underlying problems with patients. For instance, we may not be getting very far trying to understand a poor physical structure (e.g., poor posture) and so we might have to shift our investigation to the interactions or expectancies underway.

The discovery that the four osteopathic principles are just restatements of Aristotle's four perspectives on reality allows us to use them with the wide applicability of Aristotle's principles in analysis (as a detective) and in treatment (as a manager). The fact that Aristotle's four causes or perspectives have never been bettered in

Cause	Management	Detection
1. Form(al)	Plans	Plot
2. Material	Flow chart	Scene
3. Efficient	Organiz. chart	Culprit
4. Final	Objectives	Motive

TABLE 12.4: Applications of types of causes

2400 years suggests that we may be on solid ground in trusting their comprehensiveness.

There are also great implications in the recent hypothesis that the development of our cognitive stages were not evolved by the undirected process of natural selection but by the directed process of social interactions (training) in every new generation. One implication is that if parent–child interactions are helping individuals develop mental and spiritual structures, then perhaps health professionals can also help individuals form or adjust mental and spiritual structures.

We are, as Vygotsky suggested, continually destroying past structures and, using the old parts plus new-perspective parts, building new structures of our minds and spirits. Our bodies are doing similar reconstructions, and so it appears that we need a dynamic model of mind–body–spirit analysis and treatment to fully understand the interacting parts and evolving structures.

If the last paragraph is true, then the mind, body, and spirit are interconnected and changing as much as pressure, volume, and temperature are in thermodynamics. We would then need a unifying theory of the mind, body, and spirit as much as we needed the Gibb's equations to integrate our treatment of pressure, volume, and temperature.

Fortunately, Aristotle's perspectives, stated in Still's healthcare terms, are analytical and comprehensive enough to form a unified field theory for healthcare.

While the interconnectedness between the mind, body, and spirit sometimes has unfortunate consequences, as when diabetes increases the risk of getting depression, and going the other way, depression increases the risk of cardiovascular disease,[1] we should rejoice because the interconnectedness also means that we can sometimes treat problems stuck in one dimension by approaching them from another more accessible dimension. For instance, depression seems to be a

Healthcare Dimensions	Mind	Body	Spirit
1. Interactive unity	X	X	X
2. Structure–fn. interdependency	X	X	X
3. Self-healing mechanism	X	X	X
4. Meaning–expectancy response	X	X	X

TABLE 12.5: Outline of unified field theory for healthcare

systemic disorder, but that also means that treating it may lessen the severity of other (related) diseases.

The theory that the mind, body, and spirit are all parts of one system or unit suggests that healthcare professionals should at least understand some of the reactions at the interfaces of the mind, body, and spirit. A physical therapist or non-physician osteopath may not be able to treat serious mental disorders, but they should at least know that bad structures must be changed before we can function properly. For instance, a person with an attitude (spiritual structure) of guilt or low self-worth may continue to stoop or bend over while walking no matter how many physical treatments they receive. It is important to understand that the spirit expresses itself through the body and so bodily misalignments can be clues to misaligned mental or spiritual structures. Like a good detective, professionals can be alert to using other perspectives of the mind–body–spirit continuum to help solve problems in their work.

Besides realizing the possible interactions among the mind, body, and spirit (the principle of interactive unity), health professionals also need to recognize that people's structures, or "stories of how things happen" change during their lifetimes (the principle of structure–function interdependencies). Indeed, the hypothesis of a social evolution of cognitive development supports this principle and the possibility that health professionals can change people's mental and spiritual structures or "stories." Further, the social evolution of cognition also supports the application of the principle of self-healing mechanisms in the natural improvement of mental and spiritual functioning, as seen by natural tendencies among people towards developing rationalizations and other defense mechanisms to try to heal themselves.[8]

Lastly, the unity among the mind, body, and spirit and the social evolution of cognition gives strong support to the principle of meaning–expectancy response. That is, the emotions (spirit) allow our minds to develop better senses of meaning and this, in turn, provides clearer expectancy or sense of a final cause or objective behind naturally occurring events.

Even if a P.T., D.O., M.D., etc. is not interested in how their physical analyses and treatments might have mental or spiritual impacts, they should at least realize that the way they talk to patients has impact on their minds and spirits. For instance, research has found that when a patient makes a firm decision (perhaps with the help of a health professional), they activate their parasympathetic nervous system and burn the extra sugar in their blood stream, but when they fret undecided, they activate their sympathetic nervous system and may develop disturbance in their blood sugar regulation similar to that of a diabetic.[9] A health professional can help a patient activate (or deactivate) their autonomic system:

You cannot be stressed out and chilled out at the same time. While it's true that stress cranks up the sympathetic engine, the reverse also is true: Parasympathetic activity turns the sympathetic motor off and pulls the key out of the ignition.

Charnitski and Brennan, p. 67[9]

So, health professionals *can* help their patients mentally and spiritually. But how do they do it well? We believe that patients can be activated externally to the extent that professionals see their patients as "other selves," as people very like themselves and so very likeable. We believe that when the patient feels this "liking," they respond, as we learned children respond to their caregivers in cognitive growth. Likewise, the patient's own (internal) activation of parasympathetic mechanisms requires liking themselves, and their shortcomings.[1]

In summary, individuals evolve their bodily, mental, and spiritual structures throughout their lifespans and these structures and functions can and do affect each other. Because these structures interact, healthcare professionals cannot only activate the functioning and structures within one of these dimensions (mind, body, or spirit), but can deliberately cause adjustments between or among these structures and functions!

In this short article we have only hinted at the interactions, evolving natural adjustments, and malformations possible within and between the mind, body, and spirit. Whatever dimension health professionals primarily address, they should also try to see the other (mental, bodily, or spiritual) dimensions involved. In proactively trying to make adjustments, they may also be helped by realizing the *interactive unity, structure–function interdependencies, healing mechanisms,* and expectancy response perspectives as part of a unified field theory that can be used to formulate "causality" models for analysis and treatment. As the Dean of the Arizona School of Dentistry at A.T. Still University tells his students: "Remember that there is a complex human being attached to that tooth!"

References

[1]McGovern, J., McGovern, R. Your Healer Within: A Unified Field Theory for Healthcare. Tucson, AZ: Fenestra Books, 2003, pp. 33–39,65–66,76–79,130,142.

[2]Sternberg, E.M. The Balance Within: The Science Connecting Health and Emotions. New York: W.H. Freeman and Company, 2002, pp. 13,210,607.

[3]LeDoux, J. Synaptic Self. New York: Penguin Books, 2002.

[4]Damasio, A.B. Descartes' Error: Emotions, Reason, and the Human Brain. New York: Quill (Harper-Collins), 1994.

[5]Eskandari, F., Sternberg, E.M. "Neuroendocrine Mediators of Placebo Effects on Immunity", in: Suess, H., Kleinman, A., Kusek, J., Cengel, L. The Science of Placebo. London: BMJ Books, 2002.

[6]Greenspan, S.I., Shanker, S.G. The First Idea. Cambridge, MA: DeCapo Press (Perseus Book Group), 2004, pp. 7–8,30,56,88–95,101–102.

[7]Cole, M., John-Stiener, V., Scriberner, S., Souberman, E. Mind in Society. Cambridge, MA: Harvard University Press, 1978, p. 124.

[8]Brody, H. Stories of Sickness, (Second Edition). New York: Oxford University Press, 2003, pp. 66–67.

[9]Chartnetski, C., Brennan, F.X. Feeling Good is Good For You. New York: Rodale (St Martin's Press), 2001, pp. 60–78.

Further reading

Capra, F. The Hidden Connections. New York: Doubleday (Random House), 2002.

Capra, F. The Web of Life. New York: Anchor Books (Random House), 1996.

Cole, M., Cole, S. The Making of Mind. Cambridge, MA: Harvard University Press, 1979.

Dawkins, R. The Blind Watchmaker. New York: W.W. Norton Company, 1987.

Eccles, J.C. Evolution of the Brain, London: Routledge (Taylor and Fancis Group), 1989.

Konner, M. The Tangled Wing: Biological Constraints on the Human Spirit (Second Edition). New York: An Owl Book (Henry Hold and Company), 2002.

Kurzweil, R. The Age of Spiritual Machines. New York: Penguin Books, 1999.

Mayr, E. What Evolution Is. New York: Basic Books (Perseus Books Group), 2001.

Ridley, M. Nature Via Nurture: Genes, Experience, and What Makes Us Human. New York: Harper Collins, 2003.

13

Touch as a therapeutic intervention

Tsafi Lederman

Contribution from Eyal Lederman

Touch as a therapeutic intervention

I would like to invite you to think about what made you choose a profession where the main interaction with the patient would involve touch. You daily apply your hands to complete strangers with whom you may end up in a short or long-term therapeutic relationship. This tactile encounter is indeed an odd one: here is someone who hardly knows you, they are in pain and therefore vulnerable, they put themselves in 'your hands', and are most likely to be partially undressed while you are dressed. This daily routine, which may often be taken for granted, may be a profound experience for the patient. For some patients you may be the only person currently in their life who touches them.

The only knowledge that you have about your patient is their medical history; you do not know their emotional history. Their emotional history and their past physical, tactile experience, and their relationship to their body may affect the therapeutic interaction and therefore the treatment outcome.

Osteopathy is a manual therapy discipline where touch is extensively used. However insufficient attention is paid to the effects of touch itself, which is beyond the physical application of the techniques, i.e., the non-mechanical effects of touch. For example, when stretching a joint the therapeutic focus may be on the mechanics of stretching and the application of different manual forces. Yet the touch element and its effects beyond the local tissues may remain covert and its effects on other dimensions can often be missed. When we look at the effects of touch on the body we will recognize many of the physiological responses that are often attributed to different osteopathic techniques. As we shall later see these effects are not exclusive to any technique but are within the domain of its touch effects.

In this chapter we will examine the possible impact that the touch experience has on patients. The awareness of this impact may add another perspective to the way that touch can be used therapeutically. In order to understand why touch is such a potent therapeutic tool we need to look back to our early life experiences and the role that it has on our psychological and physical development.

Origins of touch healing

There was a time in our life when we couldn't survive without touch. Within six weeks of conception sensations arising from the skin are the first to appear [1-3] and are followed two weeks later by sensations arising from deeper within the body – proprioception. These early peripheral–central connections are not some random biological choice. Generally, structures that are important for the organism will be the earliest to appear and develop.

Indeed, touch, tactile, and skin-to-skin contacts have a nurturing effect on the psychological and physical development of the newborn. The nurturing effects of touch can be seen in premature infants, children, and adults. In the young, tactile contact has been equated with feeding in its level of importance for normal development. [4,5] Physical and tactile contacts are also important for reducing arousal and promoting emotional and self-regulation. [6-9] This will include the ability to handle stress, develop coping skills, mediate attention and learning processes, and achieve optimal functioning. Newborns are not able to self regulate. They "learn" this process through the experience of being soothed by their parent when they are distressed. This occurs largely by the physical contact of the baby with the parent and can be shown to influence different brain centers. Individuals who have inadequate holding and containing experiences in early life may fail to develop the related brain pathways/centers and may therefore have difficulties in self-regulating as adults. [10-16]

In recent years the profound effects of touch on psychological and physiological processes in the newborn, children and adults have been extensively studied. These effects are non-mechanical and are not associated with one single form of technique. For example in the newborn touch has been shown to improve weight gain,[60,61] behavioral development,[62] oxygen uptake,[63] red blood cell count,[63] sleeping patterns[65,66] and physical growth,[67,68] and reduce episodes of apnoea.[64] Some responses are quite remarkable. Massage given to adolescents and adults with HIV resulted in an increase in natural killer cells and their activity increased, suggesting positive effects on the immune system.[69,70]

Association between touch and healing can be traced back to the early infant-mother attachment behavior in which touch and tactile stimulation play an important part in bonding. This relationship begins in the womb in a primitive form, becoming a more complex attachment behavior from the moment of birth and over the first few years of life. In the womb, kinesthetic and tactile stimulation provides early sensations that are associated with security and support.[17] Following birth, when the baby is placed on its mother's body and suckling is initiated, the comfort and security of intrauterine life is extended into the outside world. During the first year of life the baby is totally reliant on the mother for all its needs. When the baby is in distress, be it emotional or physical, the mother will soothe it by holding, gentle stroking, or massage.[18] Some of this physical comforting behavior is continued throughout childhood. When the child falls or is physically hurt, the parent will stroke the skin over the injured area, kiss it better, or hold the child.[19] Most parents discover that, when their child is hurt, no measure of verbal comfort will stop the child crying unless physical contact is made and the child is hugged or kissed.

As adults our experience of comforting touch is mostly given by our partners or friends and occasionally a manual therapist. Although the need for comforting physical contact tends to reduce in adulthood, it still remains a powerful psychological and physiological regulator in times of danger, incapacity, anxiety, bereavement, and illness.[20,21] Furthermore, therapeutic touch in adult life can support healing and wellbeing.[20] Reite[6] states:

The strong belief that touch has healing powers may be related to the fact that, having once been a major component in the development of attachment bonds, it retains the ability to act as a releaser of certain physiological accompaniments of attachment – specifically, those associated with good feelings states and good health [brain chemicals].

Bowlby[5] points out that this behavior in adults is not regressive:

…in sickness and calamity, adults often become demanding of others; in conditions of sudden danger or disaster a person will almost certainly seek proximity to another known and trusted person. In such circumstances an increase in attachment behavior is recognized by all as natural. It is therefore extremely misleading for the epithet "regressive" to be applied to every manifestation of attachment behavior in adult life.

He further adds, "to dub attachment behavior in adult life regressive is indeed to overlook the vital role that it plays in the life of man from cradle to the grave."

Touch as therapy

Clinical experience and research into touch both support our belief that osteopathic manual events have non-mechanical influences associated with the physiological and psychological aspects of touch itself. This brings us to the next question – are all forms of touch therapeutic and what makes some forms of touch more therapeutic than others? In order to answer these questions we need to look at touch as the carrier of the therapist's intent. As will be seen later, the therapist's intent is the beginning of the tactile dialogue with the patient.

Different conditions require different therapeutic intents. Matching the therapeutic intent with the patient's condition is essential for a successful treatment outcome. Intent has physical manifestations that will affect the way in which the therapist touches the patient and the choice of technique. For the purpose of this article osteopathic technique can be classified into two main intention groups:[22]

1 Instrumental osteopathic technique: will aim to mechanically diagnose, "cure" or prevent the progression of the patient's physical condition.

2 Expressive osteopathic technique: will focus on accepting the patient as a whole – body and mind

– with the aim of supporting the process of healing with the awareness of the psychological and psychophysiological dimensions of their condition.

The aim of instrumental touch is to mechanically and by direct contact with the damaged tissues, cure, repair, or prevent progression of the condition.[23] The hands of the therapist are the therapeutic tools, just as a scalpel is for a surgeon. By the use of these tools, the therapist is attempting to "correct" a "mechanical failure" in the patient's structure or affect local tissue physiology and local repair. To stretch a shortened tissue mechanically or to increase blood flow through an ischemic muscle can be considered to be an instrumental approach. Instrumental osteopathic technique is also used in carrying out diagnostic procedures such as examining the range of movement of a joint. It can generally be said that instrumental osteopathic technique is biomechanical in its intent. The use of instrumental techniques is often associated with the view of the body as a mechanical entity separated from the self.[24]

The aim of expressive osteopathic technique is to support a wider healing and self-regulation processes. Expressive touch acknowledges the person as a whole – the multiple processes and dimensions associated with their condition. Expressive osteopathic technique involves awareness and empathy with the feelings and emotional state of the patient.[25] In expressive osteopathic technique, the technique becomes the vehicle for the therapist's intention. These intensions are integrated into a particular technique as a tactile, non-verbal and often subliminal message.

Differences between instrumental and expressive osteopathic technique can be illustrated by looking at two common clinical conditions: a patient suffering from a musculoskeletal injury such as an ankle sprain and a patient suffering from a painful neck due to emotional stress. Treatment of an ankle sprain will be largely instrumental, biomechanical in character, with an element of expressive touch (this is to acknowledge the fact that different areas of our body have different significance and personal meaning. For example, a

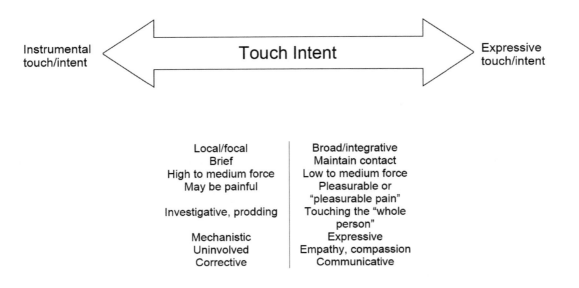

Figure 13.1
Contents of instrumental and expressive touch intensions. After E. Lederman, 1997, *Fundamentals of Manual Therapy*. Churchill Livingstone, Edinburgh.

dancer may experience an ankle injury differently to an office worker). In this case, instrumental osteopathic technique may consist of joint articulation to facilitate local repair of periarticular structures. In contrast, the patient who is suffering from neck pain due to emotional stress will require an expressive form of treatment, low on mechanical or instrumental elements. In this condition, a supportive, comforting, soothing and relaxing form of osteopathic technique may be more beneficial. In a psychosomatic condition such as this, using an instrumental intent may fail to meet the patient's emotional needs. Equally, treating a musculoskeletal injury solely using expressive osteopathic technique will fail to stimulate local tissue repair mechanisms. The differences between expressive and instrumental osteopathic technique are further summarized in Figure 13.1.

This classification of osteopathic technique into the two intention groups is somewhat artificial. These are not clear-cut groups. Each patient is unique and the balance using the two intentions should be applied according to the patient's needs and condition. It is advocated that a pragmatic approach should be used when matching the therapeutic intent with the patient's condition. If the diagnosis indicates a clear mechanical/structural condition, instrumental osteopathic technique will be the most effective approach. If the diagnosis indicates a psychosomatic condition, expressive osteopathic technique will be more suitable. This does not exclude the possibility that both forms of touch intent will be used simultaneously. For example, long-term stress may eventually lead to biomechanical changes in muscle. In this condition, instrumental osteopathic technique will can used to stretch the muscle physically, while expressive osteopathic technique can be used concomitantly to provide support and help the patient to relax.

The touch dialogue: touch as communication

Interestingly it is very difficult to "fake" therapeutic touch. Studies of the effects of touch on anxiety–stress level in patients in hospital settings demonstrates that when the patients are given therapeutic touch it is much more effective at reducing different markers of stress than a sham or procedural (instrumental) touch.[28,29]

This suggests that therapeutic touch may contain messages of intention that the patient can perceive. This may be either a conscious or subconscious process. In our Therapeutic Touch workshops we ask the participants

to list what message would be therapeutic and how they would convey it by touch. Some of the most frequently stated intentions were of acceptance, empathy, reassurance, comforting, trusting, providing safety, calming, and compassionate messages. Further to this we give the participants an exercise where they have to identify out of four intentions the one being communicated to them while they are receiving a mock treatment. Our experience from this exercise is that the recipients of touch are often successful in identifying the touch intent messages. However, the touch dialogue is no different to other forms of communication where messages can be misinterpreted. There is the possibility that the patient may misinterpret the therapist's intentions even when they are clearly conveyed.[26] Similar to other forms of dialogue, touch is also about listening to the messages from the patient's body. This feedback can be tactile. For example, is the patient relaxing or tensing their muscle as they are being touched? Further information can be gained from observing changes in breathing, facial expressions, and the patient's body language.

The interpretation of touch by the patient relies on different factors: their past experiences of touch, their social and cultural background, age, and gender, and their current emotional state. In addition to these a positive experience will be more likely to occur if touch is appropriate to the presenting condition, it does not intrude on the patient's personal boundary, does not communicate a negative message and its objectives and intentions are clear.[26,27]

Although expressive touch is non-mechanical the physical manifestations of it are important, i.e., how we physically convey these messages with our hands. When observing therapists using expressive touch several contact patterns can be identified. The speed of the technique is slowed down dramatically, the applied manual pressure tends to drop, and the duration the hands are kept in one area becomes longer. The applied hands tend to be in contact over broader areas, with sustained holding. Techniques are not applied in a mechanical succession but rather as a continuous flowing movement. There is more focusing on larger body areas, rather than specific tissues or joints, and the therapist's own stance and body expression seem to also play an overall role in the meaning of the message. Cranial osteopathy is a very good example where the technique incorporates many of the expressive touch elements and language, even if the main intention of the cranial therapist may be instrumental, i.e., to "manipulate" the cranial bones. Because the therapist is using the language of expressive touch the impact on the patient is similar to that of therapeutic touch intention. Indeed, many of the influences of cranial technique can be attributed to the positive effects of the touch interaction. (We know this because other manual therapy methods have been shown to have the psychological and psychophysiological effects that are often attributed to a cranial treatment.)

Broadly speaking different osteopathic techniques may contain covert psychological–emotional influences on the patient. For example, passive techniques are about letting go of control and trusting others, while active techniques (where the patient is using voluntary muscle contraction) are to do with trusting oneself and others (the therapist).[30] Active techniques[26] can highlight strengths and weaknesses. In areas of the body where the patient may feel weak, active techniques can be used to give a feeling of internal support, strength, and continuity.[31] This can be an empowering experience for the patient especially after injury where they may have lost confidence in their abilities and body.

Passive stretching can give a sense of opening and letting go and a general sense of outflow, whilst active techniques can support a sense of containment.[26] Deep work may give a feeling of being psychologically met; light work is less physically invasive (depending on the area being touched, its taboo value, and its symbolism). Light touch could be used as a reminder, directing the patient's attention to specific areas of the body; static touch could imply contact in the psychological sense and the supporting presence of another person.[32] This can be a profound and powerful experience for the patient. On the other hand passive technique may be regressive in nature where the patient is being cared for like an infant. Depending on the situation this form of touch may have either positive or negative effect. In one patient it may maintain their helpless passive stance as a recipient of care without ever taking charge. Yet in another anxious, hyperactive patient it may allow them to "let go." In contrast active techniques may encourage the "adult" in the patient and give a sense of being able to care for oneself.

Furthermore, techniques that stimulate skin receptors, such as massage, can be used to reinforce the sense of the body's envelope and being held as a whole within this envelope.[33] Passive technique can provide awareness of the internal space of the body and the quality and extent of movement.[31] Active techniques can also give a sense of the internal space of the body as well as the sense of the connectedness and relationship of different body parts to each other.

Psychological effects of touch

The positive psychological effects of touch have been shown in different settings (e.g., healthy or hospitalized individuals), different groups of individuals (e.g., different age groups) and with different manual techniques which are "carriers" of touch (massage, therapeutic touch, reiki, aromatherapy, reflexology, etc.).

Several studies have demonstrated the importance of touch in reducing stress and anxiety. Massage effects have been demonstrated to enhance alertness and reduce anxiety and stress levels of subjects at work.[34,35] In more clinical settings, the effects of touch have been shown to be psychologically important. Therapeutic touch has been shown to be useful during labor by helping to promote relaxation and reduce anxiety.[36,37] In different hospital settings touch was shown to reduce anxiety associated with the individuals illness or injury.[28,46] Burns patients,[38,39] patients recovering from cardiac surgery,[40] cancer patients,[41,42] HIV patients,[43,44] and patients undergoing surgery[45] were all shown to have reduced stress levels through different forms of touch (either in the form of therapeutic touch or different forms of manual therapy). Massage therapy was also shown to reduce anxiety and depression in teenage mothers.[47] Even in more complex psychological conditions where women had been sexually or physically abused massage therapy was shown to reduce aversion to touch and decrease anxiety and depression.[48]

In the elderly and dementia patients touch was shown to reduce anxiety and improve their immediate cognitive behavior.[49,50] Patients with chronic fatigue syndrome who received 10 days of massage therapy experienced fewer fatigue related symptoms, particularly anxiety and somatic symptoms as well as reduced depression and pain, and improved sleep. It was also found that the stress hormone (cortisol) levels were decreased whereas dopamine levels increased.[51]

Changes in emotion and mood will reflect in the individual's behavior. It is not unusual for patients to report dramatic changes in their behavior and in their experience of themselves after an osteopathic treatment. They may report feeling more confident, assertive, a better sense of boundaries and a positive feeling of wellbeing. This may be expressed outwardly in their posture and movement and even in their choice of activities following a treatment. Touch during treatment may also "touch on" traumatic memories and will be experienced as sadness, fear, and anger. The expression of these emotions and behavior will extend beyond the treatment session into their daily life.

The behavioral effect of touch has been shown in several studies. Touch has been introduced in school by a method called Massage in Schools where a group of children learned how to massage each other through play activity. The groups of children participating in the studies were shown to improve in various areas: their academic ability improved; there were reduced incidences of bullying; and the children were more respectful of each other and were less disruptive in class. Preschool children with behavior problems who received massage showed more on-task behavior, less solitary play, and were less aggressive.[52] Similarly adolescent children became less aggressive following weekly massage.[53]

Body image is another important area where the psychological effect of touch can be observed. Body image is the way we perceive our physical self.[54] Body image consists of the external envelope and the internal volume of the body. Body image develops in early life in parallel with sensory and motor development.[55] Early tactile and proprioceptive stimulation in the womb, infancy, and childhood provide stimulation and the basis for the development of body image and the sense of self.[56] Touch remains a potent stimulus for body image through life. Body image is dynamic and will change as a result of a variety of factors including injury, illness, and various psychological conditions. The positive effects of touch on body image have been observed in conditions where body image has been distorted such as in bulimia and anorexia.[57] Bulimic adolescent girls who received weekly massage therapy showed an improved relationship with their body image, and were less depressed and anxious.[58] Physiologically this change manifested in a decrease in cortisol levels and an increase in dopamine and serotonin levels. In anorexic patients massage therapy had a positive effect on body image resulting in decreased body dissatisfaction associated with this condition.[59]

Pain and injury can have a profound effect on body image. These experiences often bring into focus an area that before injury was a part of the whole. In these circumstances the patient's response is to segregate the injured part from the rest of the body. Segregation has perceptual forms. It is a process in which the damaged area is either being focused on and enlarged, diminished, or totally excluded from the body image. A treatment that is instrumental and local to the painful area may increase this perception of segregation. An expressive form of treatment that acknowledges the whole, using for example a broader/wider contact, could help the process of re-integration of the injured area into body image.

Summary

In this chapter we examined the power of touch beyond its mechanical effects, in particular in psychological and psychophysiological effects. The potency of touch as a therapeutic process is related to our early life experiences where tactile contacts formed an essential stimulus for our physical and psychological development. This therapeutic potency is also related to an instinctive need for touch that extends throughout our lives.

We looked at the way that touch is used as a form of non-verbal communication and how it can be used to convey therapeutic intention. Being aware of the extensive vocabulary of therapeutic touch will help the therapist utilize touch for a greater effect, providing a more effective clinical tool.

Acknowledgement

I would like to thank Dr Eyal Lederman for his osteopathic contribution to this chapter.

References

[1]Morris D 1971 Intimate behaviour. Corgi, London.

[2]Hooker D 1969 The prenatal origin of behavior. Hafner, London.

[3]Gottlieb G 1971 The oncogenesis of sensory function in birds and mammals. In: Tobach E, Aronson LR, Shaw E (eds) The biopsychology of development. Academic Press, New York.

[4]Burton A, Heller LG 1964 The touching of the body. Psychoanalytical Review 51:122–134.

[5]Bowlby J 1969 Attachment and loss. Hogarth Press, London.

[6]Reite ML 1984 Touch, attachment, and health – is there a relationship? In: Brown CC (ed) The many faces of touch. Johnson & Johnson Baby Products Company Pediatric Round Table Series, 10, pp. 58–65.

[7]Schanberg SM, Evoniuk G, Kuhn CM 1984 Tactile and nutritional aspects of maternal care: specific regulators of neuroendocrine function and cellular development. Proceedings of the Society for Experimental Biology and Medicine 175:135–146.

[8]Harlow HF 1959 Love in infant monkey. Science. In: Physiological Psychology. Thompson RF (ed) WH Freeman, San Francisco, pp. 78–84.

[9]Harlow HF 1961 The development of affectional patterns in infant monkeys. In: Foss BM (ed) Determinants of Infant Behaviour. Methuen, London.

[10]Feldman R, Eidelman AI 2003 Skin-to-skin contact (Kangaroo Care) accelerates autonomic and neurobehavioural maturation in preterm infants. Dev. Med. Child Neurol 45:274–281.

[11]Feldman R, Eidelman AI 2003 Direct and indirect effects of maternal milk on the neurobehavioral and cognitive development of premature infants. Dev. Psychobiol. 43.

[12]Hofer MA 1984 Relationships as regulators: a psychobiological perspective on bereavement. Psychosom. Med. 46:183–197.

[13]Schore AN 2000 The effects of a secure attachment relationship on right brain development, affect regulation and in infant mental health. Infant Mental Health 22:6–66.

[14]Schore AN 1994 Affect regulation and the origin of the self: the neurobiology of emotional development. Hillsdale, NJ, England: Lawrence Erlbaum.

[15]Weller A, Feldman R 2003 Emotion regulation and touch in infants: the role of cholecystokinin and opioids Peptides 24(5):779–788.

[16]Gunnar MR 1998 Quality of early care and buffering of neuroendocrine stress reactions: potential effects on the developing human brain. Preventative Medicine 27:208–211.

[17]Kulka A, Fry C, Goldstein FJ 1960 Kinesthetic needs in infancy. American Journal of Orthopsychiatry 33:562–571.

[18]Spitz R 1955 Childhood development phenomena: the influence of the mother–child relationship, and its disturbance. In: Soddy K (ed) Mental health and infant development. Routledge & Kegan Paul, London.

[19]Triplett JL, Arneson SW 1979 The use of verbal and tactile comfort to alleviate distress in young hospitalised children. Research in Nursing and Health 2(1):17–23.

[20]Dominian J 1971 The psychological significance of touch. Nursing Times

[21]Bowlby J 1958 The nature of the child's tie to his mother. International Journal of Psychoanalysis 39:350–373.

[22]Watson WH 1975 The meaning of touch: geriatric nursing. Journal of Communication 25(3):104–112.

[23]Weiss SJ 1986 Psychophysiological effects of caregiver touch on incidents of cardiac dysrhythmia. Heart and Lung 15(5):495–505.

[24]Nathan BT 1995 Philosophical notes on osteopathy theory. Part II. On persons and bodies, touching and inherent self-healing capacity. British Osteopathic Journal 15:15–19.

[25]Nathan B 1995 Philosophical notes on osteopathic theory. Part III. Non-procedural touching and the relationship between touch and emotion. British Osteopathic Journal 17:31–34.

[26]Lederman E 1997 Fundamentals of manual therapy. Churchill Livingstone, Edinburgh.

[27]Anderson D 1979 Touching: when is it caring and nurturing or when is it exploitative and damaging? Child Abuse and Neglect 3:793–794.

[28]Heidt P 1981 Effect of therapeutic touch on anxiety level of hospitalized patients. Nurs Res 30(1):32–37.

[29]Turner JG, Clark AJ, Gauthier DK, Williams M 1998 The effect of therapeutic touch on pain and anxiety in burn patients. J Adv Nurs 28(1):10–20.

[30]Bunkan BH, Thornquist E 1990 Psychomotor therapy: an approach to the evaluation and treatment of psychosomatic disorders. In: Hegna T, Sveram M (eds) Pychological and psychosomatic problems. Churchill Livingstone, London, pp. 45–74.

[31]Fisher S, Cleveland SE 1968 Body image and personality. Dover Publications, New York.

[32]Kepner JI 1993 Body process: working with the body in psychotherapy. Jossey-Bass, San Francisco.

[33]Bick E 1968 The experience of the skin in early object-relations. Int. J. Psycho-Anal. 49:484–486.

[34]Field T, Ironson G, Scafidi F, Nawrocki T, Goncalves A, Burman I, Pickens J, Fox N, Schanberg S, Kuhn C 1996 Massage therapy reduces anxiety and enhances EEG pattern of alertness and math computations. International Journal of Neuroscience 86:197–205.

[35]Field T, Quintino O, Henteleff T, Wells-Keife L, Delvecchio-Feinberg G 1997 Job stress reduction therapies. Alternative Therapies in Health and Medicine 3:54–56.

[36]Field T, Hernandez-Reif M, Taylor S, Quintino 0, Burman I 1997 Labor pain is reduced by massage therapy. Journal of Psychosomatic Obstetrics and Gynecology 18:286–291.

[37]Penny KS 1979 Postpartum perception of touch received during labour. Research in Nursing and Health 2(1): 9–16.

[38]Field T, Peck M, Krugman S, Tuchel T, Schanberg S, Kuhn C, Burman I 1997 Burn injuries benefit from massage therapy. Journal of Burn Care and Rehabilitation 19:241–244.

[39]Hernandez-Reif M, Field T, Largie S, Hart S, Redzepi M, Nierenberg B, Peck M 2001 Childrens' Distress During Burn Treatment is Reduced by Massage Therapy. Journal of Burn Care and Rehabilitation 22:191–195.

[40]Weiss SJ 1990 Effects of differential touch on nervous system arousal of patients recovering from cardiac disease. Heart Lung 19(5 Pt 1):474–480.

[41]Morales E 1994 Meaning of touch to hospitalized Puerto Ricans with cancer. Cancer Nursing 17(6):464–469.

[42]Stephenson NL, Weinrich SP, Tavakoli AS 2000 The effects of foot reflexology on anxiety and pain in patients with breast and lung cancer. Oncol Nurs Forum 27(1):67–72.

[43]Ireland M 1998 Therapeutic touch with HIV-infected children: a pilot study. J Assoc Nurses AIDS Care 9(4):68–77.

[44]Deigo MA, Hernandez-Reif M, Field T, Friedman L, Shaw K 2001 Massage therapy effects on immune function in adolescents with HIV. International Journal of Neuroscience 106:35–45.

[45]Moon JS, Cho KS . 2001 The effects of handholding on anxiety in cataract surgery patients under local anaesthesia. J Adv Nurs 35(3):407–415.

[46]McCorkle R 1974 Effects of touch on seriously ill patients. Nursing Research 23(2):125–132.

[47]Field T, Grizzle N, Scafidi F, Schanberg S 1996 Massage and relaxation therapies' effects on depressed adolescent mothers. Adolescence 31:903–911.

[48]Field T, Hernandez-Reif M, Hart S, Quintino O, Drose L, Field T, Kuhn C, Schanberg S 1997 Sexual abuse effects are lessened by massage therapy. Journal of Bodywork and Movement Therapies 1:65–69.

[49]Kim EJ, Buschmann MT 1999 The effect of expressive physical touch on patients with dementia. Int J Nurs Stud 36(3):235–243.

[50]Simington JA, Laing GP 1993 Effects of therapeutic touch on anxiety in the institutionalized elderly. Clin Nurs Res 2(4):438–450.

[51]Field T, Sunshine W, Hernandez-Reif M, Quintino O, Schanberg S, Kuhn C, Burman I 1997 Chronic fatigue syndrome: Massage therapy effects on depression and somatic symptoms in chronic fatigue syndrome. Journal of Chronic Fatigue Syndrome 3:43–51.

[52]Escalona A, Field T, Cullen C, Hartshorn K, Cruz C (In Review). Behavior problem preschool children benefit from massage therapy. Early Child Development and Care.

[53]Diego M, Field T, Hernandez-Reif M, Shaw J, Rothe E, Castellanos D, Mesner L 2002 Aggressive adolescents benefit from massage therapy. Adolescence 37:597–607.

[54]Gorman W 1969 Body image and the image of the brain. Warren H Green, Missouri.

[55]Schilder P 1964 The image and appearance of the human body. John Wiley, Chichester

[56]Krueger DW 1989 Body self & psychological self: a developmental and clinical integration of disorders of the self. Brunner/Mazel, NY.

[57]Stark A, Aronow S, McGeehan T 1989 Dance/movement therapy with bulimic patients. In: Hornyak LM, Baker EK (eds) Experiential therapies for eating disorders. Guildford Press, New York.

[58]Field T, Shanberg S, Kuhn C, Fierro K, Henteleff T, Mueller C, Yando R, Burman I 1997 Bulimic adolescents benefit from massage therapy. Adolescence 131:555–563.

[59]Hart S, Field T, Hernandez-Reif M, Nearing G, Shaw S, Schanberg S, Kuhn C 2001 Anorexia symptoms are reduced by massage therapy. Eating Disorders 9:289–299.

[60]Field et al 1986 Tactile/kinesthetic stimulation effect on preterm neonates. Pediatrics 77(5):654–658.

[61]White JL, Labarba RC 1976 The effects of tactile and kinesthetic stimulation on neonatal development in the premature infant. Developmental Psychology 9(6):569–577.

[62]Solkoff N, Matuszak D 1975 Tactile stimulation and behavioral development among low-birth weight infants. Child Psychiatry and Human Development 6(1):33–37.

[63]Schaeffer JS 1982 The effect of gentle human touch on mechanically ventilated very-short-gestation infants. Maternal Child Nursing Journal, Monograph 12, 11: 4.

[64]Kattwinkel J, Nearman HS, Fanaroff AA, Katona PG, Klaus MH 1975 Apnea of prematurity: comparative therapeutic effects of cutaneous stimulation and nasal continuous positive airway pressure. Journal of Pediatrics 86:588–592.

[65]Scafidi F, Field T, Schanberg S, Bauer C, Vega-Lahr N, Garcia R 1986 Effects of tactile/kinesthetic stimulation on the clinical course and sleep/wake behavior of preterm neonates. Infant Behavior and Development, 9:91–105.

[66]Field T, Hernandez-Reif M 2001 Sleep problems in infants decrease following massage therapy. Early Child Development and Care 168:95–104.

[67]Scafidi F, Field T, Schanberg S, Bauer C, Tucci K, Roberts J, Morrow C, Kuhn CM 1990 Massage stimulates growth in preterm infants: A replication. Infant Behavior and Development 13:167–188.

[68]Field T, Scafidi F, Schanberg S 1987 Massage of preterm newborns to improve growth and development. Pediatric Nursing 13:385–387.

[69]Deigo MA, Hernandez-Reif M, Field T, Friedman L, Shaw K 2000 Massage therapy effects on immune function in adolescents with HIV. International Journal of Neuroscience 106: 35–45.

[70]Ironson G, Field T, Scafidi F, Hashimoto M, Kumar M, Kumar A, Price A, Goncalves A, Burman I, Tetenman C, Patarca R, Fletcher MA 1996 Massage therapy is associated with enhancement of the immune system's cytotoxic capacity. International Journal of Neuroscience 84, 205–218.

14

What is health? What is disease? Thoughts on a complex issue

Torsten Liem and Matthias Flatscher

Although health is the greatest of all goods relating to the body, it is nevertheless the one that we consider and enjoy least: when we have health we do not think of it.

R. Descartes (Descartes, 2004, p. 54)[1]

Difficulties with regard to method: the hiddenness of health

This is a subject that affects us all – not just health professionals. Nevertheless, health is usually something that is hidden, only coming to the fore when it is not an automatic "given." When we are sick, the loss of health is evident. But what is health? Is it simply the absence of disease?

The question "What is disease?" seems easier to answer than the question of health. Disease manifests itself as disorder and announces its presence in the form of symptoms. Disease phenomena, cases of disease, the clinical picture, and the course of a disease; all these can be described, objectified, and classified. Can the same be said of health? We face problems if we simply see each as the reverse of the other – disease as the negative counterpart of health, its opposite – and it hardly helps us arrive at a positive definition.

The 1948 WHO definition of health

The World Health Organization defined health as follows:

Health is a state of complete physical, mental, and social well-being and not merely the absence of disease or infirmity.

Constitution of the World Health Organization of 1948[2]

The following aspects of this definition are very helpful:

- Health goes beyond physical considerations.

- Health is viewed in its psychosomatic entirety.

- Health is not limited to the person as an individual, but is also expressed in the person's relationship with the world around.

- Health is more than the absence of disease.

- Health is understood in terms of (subjectively experienced) wellbeing.

The following aspects of this definition however present problems:

- Health is described as an ideal, static state (how many people can claim to enjoy "complete" (physical, mental/spiritual, and social) wellbeing?).

- Health is equated with the highest good, but in doing so the definition fails to present it as a means of enabling a successful personal life plan (it follows, surely, that the entire responsibility for a person's whole life plan would then become the concern of healthcare, instead of the person's own concern?).

Definition of health as given in the *Lexikon für Ethik*[3]

In the *Lexikon für Ethik* the entry for "health" revealingly refers the user to that for "disease." The WHO definition is criticized as idealistic and subjective:

A helpful middle course seems to be, on the one hand, to interpret disease as functional disorder, i.e., the disturbance of a functional balance, and on the other hand to let the criterion by which we define disease be, not the failure to achieve the ideal state, but rather the deviation from statistical normal values. (Horn, 2002, p. 142)[3]

According to this definition disease is understood as functional disturbance and health as functional efficiency. The understanding of health is thus derived from disease – to be more exact it is seen as the absence of disease. The achievement of health is interpreted as the removal of these functional disturbances. The measurement of (dys-) functionality is based on statistically determined controlled variables, and health consequently understood as a biologically programed set point.

The functional concept of disease and health is a descriptive one. Statistical, scientific analysis can identify a deviation from mean values, but is quite incapable of identifying states of health or disease. Physical, chemical, or biological data are inadequate as prerequisites for understanding disease. This method of approach describes facts, but cannot say what should be the norm. It is a mistake (a naturalistic one) to proceed from statements of fact to normative statements of what ought to be. "Ought" does not follow from is." Descriptive medicine finds itself in a "normative vacuum" (Waldenfels, p. 116).[4]

Health is what is "normal," but not in the sense of the statistical meaning. If (almost) all are blind, that is not "normal" (take as an example of this idea José Saramago's *Blindness*). There is nothing normative in a statistical statement of fact. It is precipitate to equate the "mean" with "standard," and to be avoided.

A functional understanding of disease leads to the practice of medicine as repair. Repair medicine assumes a statistical mean value that has to be restored. The achievement of health is understood simply as a matter of restitution, in the sense of establishing the old order of set values.

In contrast to this, in the context of osteopathy, the author uses a resource concept in which healing is not necessarily oriented towards a previous state of health, but is based on a concept of health as an evolutionary process, and embraces a higher-order dynamic balance of the person as a whole.

Disease and health link back to the psychosomatic wellbeing of the particular individual. This must definitively involve reference to the individual biography (history of disease and attainment of health) and the socio-cultural context of the individual. (See pp. 22ff.)

Health from a living systems perspective

Health comprises a set of resources necessary to achieve goals, adapt to environmental changes, satisfy needs, and sustain life. Health is generally perceived to possess instrumental value, enabling the individual to pursue his or her life goals, which can be variably defined as individual or biological in nature. Philosophically, health is rarely regarded as an end in itself but rather a prerequisite to a desirable life.

Health has been regarded as a mere adaptation to environmental challenges. This notion may be limited in that it is purely reactive, thus neglecting the active properties of health that enable the individual to grow and to thrive.

According to Forrest,[5] previous definitions of health failed to examine the constituent parts of health itself. What are the individual aspects of health and how do they interact to produce the features generally attributed to health? Adopting a living systems perspective, Forrest[5] includes such "assets" in an examination of health. This conceptualization rests upon fundamental notions of living systems theory: living systems are energetically open systems that are in dynamic interaction with their environments, constantly working to reduce internal entropy. They comprise individual parts that, in interaction with each other, assume a complex systems character, delineating the organism from the environment and maintaining structure of the unit as an autopoietic entity. Hierarchical arrangements are characteristic of complex systems.[6]

Human beings are a prime example of complex systems, with health being a potential attribute of these systems; systems theory justifies an investigation into the hierarchically subservient parts, or "assets," of health. Accordingly, these "assets" would dynamically interact with each other and the environment to produce emergent properties of health.[5]

Forrest[5] proposes to organize the assets of health along five dimensions: energetics, restoration, mind, reproduction, and capabilities (see Table 14.1). Properties of each asset depend on a multitude of processes at cell, tissue, and organ level. For example, an individual's capacity to recover from tissue injury can be classified as a restoration asset. Amongst others,

Dimension	Definition	Theoretical basis	Explanation
Energetics	Managing energy to maintain self-organization, enable self-transcendence, and support the energetic requirements of essential functions of a living system	Living beings are dissipative systems that continuously exchange energy with the environment to support system functions, such as growth, maintenance, reproduction, and action	Comprises physiological processes concerned with the overall energy metabolism and more specifically electrolyte balance, water, gas, and nutrient metabolism. Can generally be seen to make up the person's physical fitness level
Restoration	Maintaining the integrity of self via a set of processes that prevent, overcome, and heal damage from system perturbations inflicted by the internal and external milieus	Continuous interaction with the environment requires that living systems prevent, withstand, and repair damage from environmental challenges that threaten the integrity and development of self	For example, radiation, chemical, and mechanical factors are potentially harmful and so are psychological stressors or pathogens. The skin is just one example of tissues designed to defend the body against those insults
Mind	The capacity to sense, interpret, and act on data available from the parts of the whole (i.e., organs, tissues, and cells) and the environment, and learn from those experiences	Living systems process information from their internal and external environments in order to formulate action plans, learn, and experience life	The process of "knowing." Provides the ability to sense data in the environment through sensory systems. Also, perception of emotions, understanding the meaning of sensory and emotional data to create information that can be interpreted individually. Experience thus accumulated eventually informs actions when re-exposed to similar information: learning
Reproduction	Creation of offspring	To sustain the species, living systems reproduce	Defining factor for any species. For human beings this health asset also includes their sexuality and the ability to pursue sexually oriented needs and goals
Capabilities	Functional capacities that enable an organism to execute tasks, engage in activities, and, for social beings, interact with others and the social environment	Depending on stage of development, living systems have functional capacities that enable action related to satisfaction of needs and attainment of goals	Highly individualized: depending on individual history, life experience, values and beliefs; also on overall cultural, political, and economic context. Processes supporting communication, mobility and social interaction fall within this dimension

TABLE 14.1: Health asset dimensions*

*Living systems theory suggests that "health" as a property of a complex system needs to be examined for both its constituent parts and for the emergent properties resulting from interaction between them and the environment. Individual dimensions of health interact to produce emergent properties of health. Individually, they depend upon cell, tissue, and organ properties and on each other. Adapted from Forrest, 2014.[5]

it would depend on current immune function, blood clotting properties, and previous tissue state, etc. The restoration asset will then, for example, also depend on the organism's oxygen metabolism, part of the energetics dimension.

Complex systems, and human beings in particular, are special in that they not only possess adaptive mechanisms allowing interaction with their environment, they also possess a mind, which enables them to experience and learn from experience. Any examination of health and its assets will thus have to include such biography-dependent features. This notion ties in with the resource concept previously discussed in an osteopathic context, where health can only be understood as a dynamic and evolutionary process. The personal experience of health is itself an emergent property of the lived experience of individual health assets, past and present and always in an environmental context.

Based upon the above complex systems analysis, Forrest (2014, p. 212)[5] proposes a new definition of health:

Health enables individuals to adapt to their physical and social environments, satisfy their needs, attain their goals, and live long lives free from distress and suffering.

Here, health is regarded philosophically as a means to other individual and biological ends. A passive adaptation component of health is acknowledged, but is not exclusive of active aspects, which enable individuals to grow, develop, and reproduce. Adopting a complex systems perspective allows for a more appropriate examination of the constituent parts comprising health, thus enabling the osteopathic practitioner to appreciate both the role of parts and the non-linear emergence of system properties.

An attempt at a fresh definition of disease and health

There is a difference between disease and being ill. Being ill is not something that can be reduced to the clinical picture of the disease or to the somatic dysfunction/lesion (etc.). The functional, scientific perspective forgets that diseases link back to the individual *experience of being ill*. Diseases cannot be separated from the person who is ill. How far, we may ask, does osteopathy, as a system of manipulative treatment, take account of these perspectives in its historic course of development

– other than in terms of metaphysical speculation? (Gevitz, pp. 180–181.)[7]

The WHO took up the problem of a static concept of health as against the dynamic and process-based, and formulated a blueprint for health policy in its Ottawa Charter. This is underlain by certain "resource" prerequisites for the promotion of health.[8] The Ottawa Charter represents an integration model, in terms of both content and method, the aim of which is to apply and develop various strategies to inform, educate, train, and advise on matters of health, encourage self-help, and promote preventative medicine.

According to Hörmann[9] the main influencing factors on the maintenance and restoration of health are lifestyle and the treatment of diseases. The spiritual dimension of health (WHO 1998) should also, according to Raithel et al.,[8] be taken into greater account.

Antonovsky's *Salutogenese*[10] takes a similar direction by investigating the means by which individuals develop towards health and help to unlock the resources of healthy capacities. Common to both Salutogenese and the Ottawa Charter is the aim of enabling healthy development, the centrality of prevention and health promotion, and the fact of addressing several context dimensions (system levels).[11] Whereas *Salutogenese* ("health genesis") asks about options for healthy development, gives a central place to self-regulation in treatment, and adopts a dynamic understanding that sees sickness and health as a continuum, pathogenesis asks about the causes of disease, applies analytical approaches and objective findings and combats disease, based on a dichotomy between healthy and sick.[11] Many approaches of complementary and alternative medicine, as well as approaches within osteopathy, correspond to "salutogenic" views, for example in seeing health and disease as a continuum and in the view that disease can to some extent also be seen as part of physiology. This also includes the self-healing powers of the human body essential to the osteopathic concept of 'health'. In this sense osteopathy focuses on supporting these self-healing powers in the human organism.* A.T. Still's much quoted statement[12] "To find health should be the object of the doctor. Anyone can find disease."

---

*This embraces the cornerstones of Still's osteopathy, which state that all cures are already present in the patient and treatment therefore centers around activating the former.[12a]

It is the doctor's responsibility to support his patient in finding health. According to Petzold[12b] a salutogenic approach considers 'attractive' aims, that motivate the patient to find solutions and resources.

This is rooted in early osteopathy. Nevertheless, parts of osteopathic diagnostics are oriented towards pathogenetics, and therefore more of a diagnosis of disease. In Petzold's view holistic diagnostics should be further complemented by health goals and include resources, as well as establishing a connection to the patient's motivation for health, for instance by asking, "Why do you want to regain your health?" The latter would be consistent with a health diagnosis.

Therefore, on the one hand, osteopathy does exhibit signs typical of a 'salutogenic' approach. However, on the other, the interpretation of human and interpersonal phenomena in exclusive terms of anatomical and physiological processes – which often characterizes actual, current osteopathic methods – risks the reduction of the person, especially when inner experiences are reduced to the energetic or physical level. We can of course regard structural and physiological dynamics as a precondition, but not as an adequate cause of human phenomena. If we wish to treat the *wholeness* of the patient, it does not suffice to treat only the correlate represented in the tissue.

It is also not uncommon to find in practice that patients take the approach of simply handing over their bodies for treatment to the osteopath, as they might hand over a car to a garage for repair. An osteopath who unquestioningly accepts this role misses the opportunity of enabling the patient to take a conscious decision to participate actively in the healing process. This also increases the likelihood that the patient will suppress psychological associations.[13] A further problem is that the language in which a great proportion of osteopathic approaches are expressed is bio-reductionist.

These last two points make it difficult for patients to recognize the connections between the circumstances of life, their own experience, and behavior on the one hand, and the associated dysfunctions and disturbances of their state of health on the other, enabling them to take personal responsibility for their physical and psychological state of health.

Further, in osteopathy there is an almost complete lack of methods that could provide a basis to promote the development of subjective experience in the practitioner (or indeed the patient), apart from techniques to experience the tissue by palpation, taught in osteopathic training. Osteopaths are therefore usually little prepared to consider subjective realms of experience in their patients (or indeed in themselves).[14] In this respect, phenomenology teaches that it is especially the act of dealing with the space–time character of existence, and dealing with the physicality of existence, co-existence in a common world, attunement of mood, memory, and existence in history, mortality, openness of existence and, beyond this, the unfolding of these supportive possibilities, that lead to freedom of existence (Boss, pp. 237–314).[15]

The medical finding should be understood from the experience of being ill, and not the other way around. To be ill means to have a disturbed relationship with oneself, one's fellow beings and environment. Applied to osteopathy, this means that against the objective reality of the tissue structures and associated energies there stands the subjective reality of inner consciousness or subjective experience (both that of the patient and that of the practitioner). This is embedded in interobjective realities (sociobiological environment) and intersubjective ones (culture/family) as previously discussed (see pp. 22ff.)).

It is sick people rather than diseases that are healed, persons in their psychosomatic–social wholeness. The dimension of experience of the sick person who complains of symptoms cannot be straightforwardly equated with the objective level. What is meant by the achievement of health (in terms of the healing process) is not determined from the outside (e.g., by the use of statistical mean values), but from the direction of patients themselves.

Standard values cannot establish what it is to be healthy, nor can this be measured technologically. Rather than this, health appears to be a state of "inner adequacy and agreement with oneself" (Gadamer, p. 138).[16]

Sick patients each bring with them an individual history, bound up with the person's particular biography and relationship with the world and people around. The aim of therapy cannot be to bring about a statistical mean value, but to find a fresh balance, matched to the individual. Being ill is not something that can be reduced to a biological, social, or psychological dimension; it must take into account all related concerns in their entirety from the point of view of the patients.

Achieving health does not therefore mean a return to a pristine biological state. Rather, what is past is treated as something that has indeed existed and whose consequences in the present and future must always be taken into consideration. Therapeutic methods must therefore be innovative and not just restitutive. There is no preset "what" or universal "how" in being healthy:

Not everything is equally healthy for every individual. There are no definitions of being healthy or being ill that apply infallibly to every single case. (Pöltner, 2002, p. 82).[17]

Being ill and being healthy link back to the particular person's individual experience. Medicine has therefore been viewed since ancient times from more than just the scientific point of view, and has been seen rather as the art of healing. This art lies in the ability to appreciate the suffering and specific characteristics of the individual person. In sickness, the requirement inherent in this specific individual experience is this: change is required when individual suffering needs to be alleviated. Taking this normative and practical basis of the particular individual and that person's life experience as a starting point, we can then look at socio-cultural, descriptive scientific aspects.

Osteopathy therefore has to give recognition to individuals as they are, and it is in this sense that it offers the potential to be able to act – to give treatment. Examples of possible approaches can be found in *Morphodynamik in der Osteopathie*.[18]

Being healthy is the essential capacity to be open towards oneself and others and enter into communication. Healthy individuals are neither at the mercy of what they encounter, nor are they slave to it (as in addiction or compulsion), nor do they shut themselves off from their own selves or others. Being healthy is the fundamental experience of the person's own ability to be:

Hidden as it is, health becomes apparent in a kind of wellbeing; more than this, in that this very sense of wellbeing makes us eager to be active, open to discover, and forgetful of self, so that we hardly even notice stresses and strains… .

Gadamer, 1993, p. 143f.[16]

In the process of achieving health, according to Liem, an increase in health finds expression in increasing coherence, for example in increasing understanding for the meaningfulness of the entire world in which the person lives; individuals grow in understanding for their life history as a whole, including their state of health, suffering, and associations of meaning, and there is an increase in trust.[19]

Summary and conclusion

Health – unlike disease – is hard to put into objective terms. Attempts at a definition rest on certain reductionist ideas (health cannot be defined as an ideal state). Most current attempts to conceptualize health adopt a living systems perspective, seemingly beginning to do justice to the complex nature of the human organism and its properties.

Health/disease cannot be understood simply from a functional perspective or objectifiable values. A norm cannot be derived from a description (false reasoning on naturalist premises).

The achievement of health does not rest upon restorative methodology (repair medicine). Health/disease should be seen from the perspective of the individual's experience. Therefore, in addition to the localization of dysfunctions, osteopathic diagnostics could contain health goals as well as resources and should establish a connection to the patient's motivation.

The determining factor in the achievement of health is not by way of objective mean values but patients' inner agreement, with consideration being given to the individual, along with the personal history and the contexts surrounding that individual.

Normative requirements can only be arrived at when working from the perspective that relates to experience, and these norms are always individual. Medicine and osteopathy as healing art must conform to this individuality.

To be ill is to have a disturbed relationship with self and one's fellows and with the world around. To be healthy is the essential capacity to be open to self and others and to enter into communicative exchange.

References

[1]Descartes, R. (1649/2004): Brief an Chanut vom 31. März 1649. In: Canguilhem, G.: Gesundheit – eine Frage der Philosophie. Berlin.

[2]Constitution of the World Health Organisation (WHO). In: http://www.admin.ch/ch/d/sr/i8/0.810.1.de.pdf

[3]Horn, C. (2002): Krankheit, in: Höffe, Otfried (ed.): Lexikon der Ethik. München.

[4]Waldenfels, B. (1998): Der Kranke als Fremder. In: Grenzen der Normalisierung. Frankfurt am Main.

[5]Forrest, C.B. (2014). A living systems perspective on health. Medical Hypotheses. 82: 209–214.

[6]Kaneko, K. (2006): Life: An Introduction to Complex Systems Biology (Understanding Complex Systems). New York: Springer.

[7]Gevitz, N. (2004): The D.O.'s: Osteopathic Medicine in America. Baltimore.

[8]Raithel, J.; Dollinger, B.; Hörmann, G. (2007): Gesundheitspädagogik. In: Einführung Pädagogik. Wiesbaden, 232–249.

[9]Hörmann, G. (2002): Die Krise des Gesundheitssystems: eine verkannte Bildungskrise. In: Bildung, 1, 1, 24–30.

[10]Antonovsky, A. (1997): Salutogenese. Zur Entmystifizierung der Gesundheit. Tübingen.

[11]Petzold, T.D. (2007): Salutogenese und 20 Jahre Ottawa – Charta. In: Gesundheit Berlin (ed.): Dokumentation 12. Bundesweiter Kongress Armut und Gesundheit, Berlin (www.gesundheitberlin.de).

[12]Still, A.T. (1986): The Philosophy and Mechanical Principles of Osteopathy. Kirksville, p. 58.

[12a]Still, A.T. (1908): Autobiography of A. T. Still. Revised edition. Kirksville, Montana: Published by the author.

[12b]Petzold, T.D. (2012) Interview mit Theodor Dierk Petzold über Salutogenese und Osteopathie. Osteopathische Medizin. 13(4), 20-21

[13]Nathan, B. (1999): Touch and emotion in manual therapy. Edinburgh/New York.

[14]Liem, T. (2011a): Osteopathy and (hatha) yoga. In: Journal of Bodywork & Movement Therapies. No. 15, 92–102.

[15]Boss M. (1999): Grundriss der Medizin und Psychologie. 3rd Ed. Bern.

[16]Gadamer, H.-G. (1993): Über die Verborgenheit der Gesundheit. Frankfurt am Main.

[17]Pöltner, G. (2002): Grundkurs Medizin-Ethik. Wien.

[18]Liem, T. (2006): Morphodynamik in der Osteopathie. Stuttgart: Hippokrates

[19]Liem, T. (2011b) Wechselseitige Beziehungsdynamiken und subjektive Ansätze in der Osteopathie. In: Osteopathische Medizin. 12. Jg., H. 2/2011, 4–7.

15

Somatic dysfunction and compensation

Torsten Liem, Michael Patterson and Jochen Frühwein

Introduction

The concept of the somatic dysfunction has been central to the osteopathic profession since its inception. Views concerning the interaction of form and function and vitalism have set their mark on osteopathy from its beginnings, and have influenced the different definitions of the osteopathic lesion, osteopathic dysfunction, and somatic dysfunction. Today, views deriving from neurophysiology, information theory, systems theory, phenomenology, and other approaches can also help us to a more comprehensive understanding, or more integrated view, of the somatic dysfunction.

The somatic dysfunction is not simply an altered state of a somatic or visceral structure, but can be seen as a type of altered functional pattern, a dysfunction complex, made up of various components and complex multiple associated interactions that increase the probability of functional breakdown.

A further characteristic feature of osteopathy is that treatment does not necessarily involve the symptomatic region to the exclusion of all else. On the contrary, in line with the osteopathic model, somatic dysfunctions possibly related to the symptoms may also be located at some considerable remove from the site of the symptomatic disorder itself.

Form, from the standpoint of osteopathy, means the physical aspect in its various guises, i.e., that which is external and objective (see pp. 22ff.). Function, in the context of osteopathy, means the functions or physiological aspects associated with the particular structure. This includes not only such physiological parameters as range of motion when flexing the arm, heart rate, EEG, hormonal and enzyme activities, neurotransmitter metabolism and other neurophysiological aspects (i.e., the external and objective), but also processes of the consciousness, and consciousness as an inner subjective phenomenon. Function thus encompasses both objective and subjective dimensions. These views will be discussed later in the chapter.

While the somatic dysfunction as an important osteopathic concept is currently still some distance away from being comprehensively elucidated,[1-8] it is supported by a wealth of scientific evidence from many fields. By using emerging information from various scientific disciplines related to the full range of human function, the concept of the somatic dysfunction is enriched and can properly be viewed as a central player in the loss of optimal health that leads to disease.

This chapter will outline and discuss the historical development of the concept of the somatic dysfunction, together with current concepts and definitions of somatic dysfunction, hypotheses concerning the underlying mechanisms of its effects and its origins, and finally approaches to its diagnosis.

Historical development

Historical definitions of the osteopathic lesion

The founder of osteopathy, Andrew Taylor Still, viewed the human body as a whole and did not differentiate any "osteopathic lesion" such as we recognize today. A.T. Still referred to strains, sprains, twisted vertebrae, osseous lesions, and hypermobility.[9,10]

In his teaching he also did not demonstrate any special techniques; instead he simply treated the whole system, e.g., he stimulated healthy tissue in order to improve a particular function. It was left to Still's pupils to introduce further differentiations in order to be better able to analyze the individual parts.[11]

In subsequent osteopathic teachings the concept of the somatic dysfunction achieved elemental significance for osteopaths and evolved to become a central concept of the osteopathic profession. The somatic dysfunction was initially known as the "osteopathic lesion." Under this name, the profession built a rich clinical and modest scientific tradition that ascribed fairly specific meaning to the term.

The early concept of the osteopathic lesion was that of functional disturbance caused by pressure. Writing in 1903, Hulett defined the osteopathic lesion as the "osteopathic concept that is any structural perversion which by pressure produces or maintains functional disorder."[12] He further clarified that while a bone may be commonly thought of as the genesis of the lesion, a muscle, ligament or viscus may act as the lesion agent. In addition, the concept included the notion that the structure may not be normal (perverted), but that it must also, and fundamentally, have altered function. An organ or tissue may be abnormal structurally, but be functioning normally. Thus the concept of the osteopathic lesion and by extension, the somatic dysfunction, is based on the idea of functional disturbance in any part of the body.[13]

At that time the "osteopathic spinal lesion" came to assume particular importance in the etiological consideration of disease. Early osteopaths such as McConnell explained both local and distant tissue disorders as resulting directly from the anatomical malalignment/malpositioning of the spinal column and ribs which causes a blockage of the "vital channels", thus inhibiting the free flow of all fluids (arteries, veins, lymph, cerebrospinal fluid) and free conduction along the nerve pathways.[14] The early osteopaths adopted a critical stance vis-à-vis the germ theory of Pasteur, according to which micro-organisms were the cause of disease.[15–17]

Downing, writing in 1923, broadened the concept of the lesion to include its secondary adaptive consequences on the nervous system, circulation, and secretory and excretory systems. He called this the "greater osteopathic lesion complex."[18]

McCole started from the assumption that all organs, membranes, bones, muscles, and nerves, all blood and lymph vessels must stand in harmonious balance ("adjustment"). By contrast, he understood the osteopathic lesion to be the imbalance ("maladjustment") of any tissue in the body that, by feedback to specific centers in the spinal cord, produces a reflex disturbance of function in this part or in another part of the body.

According to McCole, the osteopathic spinal lesion represents any change in the normal function of a spinal articulation. In his view, this leads to posture-related stress and joint disorders or to a disorder of the tissues of a joint (also including the spinal cord segment and the associated sympathetic ganglia). In addition, it is said to cause local or distant tissue disorders. The disorder in the joint does not comprise any definitive pathology, e.g., severe contusions or malformations. The movement restriction is within or outside the physiological limit of movement, but always within the anatomical limit and is susceptible to osteopathic correction.

As a result, pathologies such as infections, tumors, tissue tears, severe sprains, bone fractures, dislocations, malformations, and ankyloses are automatically excluded.[19]

However, even within the osteopathic camp, there were from the very outset dissenting opinions as to whether the osteopathic lesion is a structural anatomical[20, 21] or functional physiological disorder.[22] Downing described the lesion as a pathology and structural disorder.[23] Littlejohn considered the abnormal arrangement of the tissues from the viewpoints of immobility and disordered function which leads to pathological changes only after a prolonged period.

Historical classifications of the osteopathic lesion

One of the earliest classifications was that proposed by Hulett (1906). He distinguished three types of osteopathic lesions characterized by the change in the positional relationship of the bone/joint partners and organs:

1 Dislocation (complete separation of the articular surfaces)

2 Subluxation (incomplete separation of the articular surfaces)

3 Displacement.

Already with these subcategories he was drawing a distinction between severities of dysfunctions. The first two he related primarily to bony tissue and distinguished between complete (dislocation) and incomplete (subluxation) separation of the articular surfaces; he related displacement in particular to yielding structures such as the viscera, e.g., a displaced uterus.[24]

McCole in his classification distinguishes principally between four types of lesion[25] (see Table 15.1). Although McCole subdivides lesions into these four main classes they are in his opinion all composite lesions to a certain degree and all lead to the same pathology, regardless of their etiology or the time when they arise.

Lesion type	Cause	Symptoms/acting on
Traumatic	Accident/trauma	Due to impulses from the associated spinal cord centers; reflex symptoms
Reflex	Abnormal impulses arriving from distant regions	Stimuli are processed in corresponding spinal cord centers of the segment: acting on muscles and blood vessels of the joint
Acute	Traumatic or reflex	Able to develop chronic attributes such as fibrous infiltrations
Chronic	Traumatic or reflex; frequently from untreated acute lesions, so-called fibrous contracture	Able to repeatedly cause acute symptoms; no clear boundary between acute and chronic lesions

TABLE 15.1: Four lesion types (after McCole)

MacDonald made a distinction between the primary lesion and secondary lesion, based in particular on causal aspects.

1 The primary lesion. From MacDonald's perspective the primary lesion is necessarily a joint lesion. It arises as a result of either an acute strain/acute trauma or chronic tension. According to MacDonald these factors may produce an osteopathic lesion that primarily affects the weak points in the vertebral column, e.g., L5/S1, T11/12,1/2, C2/3, and C0/C1. Not infrequently these become symptomatic as a response to chronic strain or poor posture.

2 The secondary lesion. MacDonald described secondary lesions as reflex lesions in which the primary cause is not located in the joint in question. Clinically primary and secondary lesions are very similar to each other and in MacDonald's opinion they are triggered secondarily to organic disorders, but also by thermal or mental causes. Secondary lesions are thought to be caused by either a reflex arc or by irritation at a distance from the spinal cord segment (viscerosomatic reflex), e.g., due to irritation of the gastric muscosa.

Afferent nerve connections give rise to muscular or ligamentous tension, leading to a joint disorder in the supplying segment that consequently does not have a primary joint lesion.[26] A similar classification was propounded by Littlejohn. He drew the distinction between a primary and a secondary reflex lesion, in which a close connection is assumed between somatic problems and the associated viscera. These are approximately consistent with a reflex viscerosomatic/somatovisceral lesion. Littlejohn defined osteopathic centers in the vertebral column in relation to visceral function. Dysfunctions occurring are termed "reflex lesions."

According to Littlejohn, the primary reflex lesion refers to an original dysfunction in the locomotor apparatus that exerts a reflex action on an internal organ; in contrast, the secondary reflex lesion refers to the dysfunction of an internal organ that exerts an effect on somatic structures.

The spread of the impulses from a dysfunctional vertebra to an organ, a primary reflex lesion, is now termed a somatovisceral reflex. The opposite phenomenon of a secondary reflex lesion, in which an internal organ facilitates the corresponding spinal segment, would today be called a viscerosomatic reflex.[27]

Terminology relating to the osteopathic lesion/somatic dysfunction

However, by the mid-1960s the term osteopathic lesion had become a flashpoint for animosities between osteopathic and allopathic professions that threatened continued payment for treatment from insurance carriers and governmental agencies for osteopathic care. In addition, with growing awareness of the osteopathic profession by the general public, it became obvious that the older term meant little and conveyed almost no meaning to the lay audience. Ira Rumney, D.O., coined the term "somatic dysfunction" to replace the name but not the concept of the "osteopathic lesion." During the ensuing several years, the term somatic dysfunction became widespread and accepted in the osteopathic profession and was officially adopted as the term of choice by the Educational Council on Osteopathic Principles (ECOP) who refined its definition to its present form.

In addition, re-naming as "somatic dysfunction" takes account of the demands made by many osteopaths who emphasize the functional and physiological aspects of the dysfunction. This runs counter to the understanding of the term "lesion" in the world of allopathic medicine. Here it is used to refer to a pathology/tissue disorder – a fact that possibly hampers communication between osteopaths and allopathic physicians/other healthcare professionals.[28]

While the term "somatic dysfunction" may not carry the accumulated rich meanings given to the term "osteopathic lesion" over the years, it is more descriptive of the most common characteristics of the dysfunctional complex diagnosed by the palpating osteopath.

Over the years, the profession has produced a general understanding of the usual palpatory diagnostic signs for recognizing the presence of a somatic dysfunction, such as tissue texture abnormality, asymmetry, restriction of motion, and tenderness (TART), but these are palpatory manifestations and not functional alterations.

In contrast, the term "subluxation" is used in the chiropractic treatment model, although the use of that term is usually limited to the altered position of joints, traditionally for the most part those of the spinal column.

Early osteopathic research

Research over the first half of the twentieth century, notably by Louisa Burns, D.O., J.S. Denslow, D.O., and I.M. Korr, Ph.D., looked at the functional implications of an osteopathic lesion. Burns's work provides a compelling vision of the, often dramatic, effects of ligamentous strains of vertebral structures on both short- and long-term function of associated somatic and visceral organs. Thus, for example, attempts were made to induce osteopathic lesions under laboratory conditions.

In the course of these experiments it was found that acute stress applied to bone leads to congestion and edema formation, that chronic stress leads to ischemia, fibrosis, and tissue contracture[29-31] and that vertebral dysfunctions induced experimentally by stretching the ligaments of the small vertebral joints lead to short- and long-term functional disorders in associated organs.[32]

Denslow and Korr began to look at correlations of palpatory signs with function[33,34] and to develop a neurophysiological model of these interactions.[35] Due to the nature of their studies, Denslow and Korr placed greatest emphasis on the intervening actions of the nervous system for many of the deleterious actions of the structurally disturbed site on local and distant functions. Denslow discovered that even very small amounts of pressure on the spinous process of the dysfunctional segment stimulated muscle activity in the same segment; in contrast, even fairly heavy pressure did not produce any stimulation in the neighboring segments. On the other hand, even light pressure on the neighboring segments led to reflex contraction at the level of the lesion. Korr also investigated the change in tissue quality and texture over the vertebrae of a dysfunctional segment. In experimental studies Denslow established that the degree of tissue changes correlated closely with the degree of lowering of the motor stimulus threshold. When palpating a subject Denslow was able to predict relatively accurately the stimulus threshold of each segment.

Korr conducted experiments to measure the irritation of the sympathetic nervous system. He proceeded on the assumption that the change in sweat gland activity could be determined by measuring the electrical conductance of the skin over dysfunctional and non-dysfunctional segments. The change in activity of the sympathetic vasomotor fibers, which regulate vascular smooth muscle tone, was measured by Korr on the basis of skin and deep-muscle temperature.

Korr also made reference to initial study results that pointed to altered sympathetic activity in the skin of dysfunctional regions. Korr further proposed that the lateral horn cells, which influence the specific visceral functions, behave exactly like those that control the sweat glands. Korr drew attention to the changes in various visceral functions experimentally induced in animals by acute spinal lesions.[36]

Later on in the discussion below we will outline the contemporary neurophysiological findings related to the effects of somatic dysfunction on total body dynamics and suggest additional possibilities for the dysfunctional aspects of a somatic dysfunction.

Somatic dysfunction: prevention and predisposition

A.T. Still hypothesized that the existence of osteopathic spinal lesions was a causal factor in the development of disease. Disordered structure gives rise to altered function. His manual concept involved the restoration of health using appropriate manual techniques.[37] He believed that the chronic occurrence of such a lesion leads to autonomic, visceral, and immunological disturbances, i.e., to the occurrence of disease. As early as 1902 Still had the visionary idea of practicing prevention. By eliminating physical movement restrictions, irritations, and pain, osteopathic treatment improves the state of health even before the onset of disease.[38]

George G. Conley wrote in 1934 about the relationship between the disturbance of the osteopathic lesion and the resultant clinical disease that could appear very much later. Conley recognized that many physical disorders for which surgery was seen as the treatment had their functional "cause" in osteopathic lesions. Conley regarded the functional disturbance provoked by the osteopathic lesion as the "hidden cause" of the resultant disease process. Conley considered the early diagnosis and treatment of the somatic dysfunction to be one of the most important elements in the daily practice of every osteopathic physician.[39]

According to the neurophysiologist Irvin Korr, the osteopathic lesion is characteristic of a predisposing location that is thought to increase the probability of disease. To begin with the body is able to compensate. A disease process develops only after a certain degree of decompensation and depletion of physiological reserves has been reached. The osteopathic lesion causes local hyperactivity of sympathetic innervation and is the "silent" herald of chronic disease.[40] However, the severity of this pattern is decisively influenced by the descending pathways from the brain, with the result that the same structural disorder may cause massive symptoms in one individual but no symptoms in another. Even apparently healthy individuals have segments characterized by reduced electrical skin resistance. These seem to point to disease occurring at a later stage or else the segments were susceptible to disorders under conditions of stress.[41] Korr does not regard the lesion

as necessarily being the cause of disease, but rather as a "channeling" factor. Since the lesion may sometimes produce no symptoms, he considered its elimination to be the chief preventive role of osteopathy.[42]

Current definition of somatic dysfunction

According to Parsons and Marcer (2006), definitions and descriptions of somatic dysfunction are still bedeviled by much confusion even today. They have proposed the following logical outline:[43]

1 Etiological considerations (e.g., traumatic, compensatory, postural)

2 Temporal considerations (e.g., acute, chronic)

3 Hierarchical concepts (e.g., primary, secondary, compensatory)

4 Physiological aspects (e.g., neuromusculoskeletal, fascial, viscerosomatic, somatovisceral).

The current definition of somatic dysfunction is that of the Educational Council on Osteopathic Principles (ECOP)[44] of the American Association of Colleges of Osteopathic Medicine (AACOM):

Impaired or altered function of related components of the somatic (body framework) system: skeletal, arthrodial, and myofascial structures, and their related vascular, lymphatic, and neural elements. Somatic dysfunction is treatable using osteopathic manipulative treatment. The positional and motion aspects of somatic dysfunction are best described using at least one of three parameters:

1 *The position of a body part as determined by palpation and referenced to its adjacent defined structure.*

2 *The directions in which motion is freer.*

3 *The directions in which motion is restricted.*

An acute somatic dysfunction (according to the 2009 ECOP glossary) is an immediate or short-term impairment or altered function of related components of the somatic (body framework) system and is characterized in the early stages by vasodilation, edema, tenderness, pain, and tissue contraction.

A chronic somatic dysfunction (according to the 2009 ECOP glossary) is impairment or altered function of related components of the somatic (body framework) system and is characterized by tenderness, itching, fibrosis, paresthesias, and tissue contraction. A somatic dysfunction is identified by TART (see page 244) and other palpable tissue qualities.

As "somatic dysfunction" relates particularly to osseous articular complexes and their associated structures, the 2002 edition of the ECOP glossary also featured visceral dysfunction for the first time, alongside somatic dysfunction. A visceral dysfunction is the impaired or altered mobility or motility of the visceral system and related fascial, neurological, vascular, skeletal, and lymphatic elements.

Discussion of the current definition of somatic dysfunction

Somatic dysfunction was regarded as either the cause of or a contributing factor in the development or maintenance of symptoms or diseases. Neurophysiological processes and impairment of the function of fluids were among the causes held to be responsible for this.

According to Klein and Sommerfeld, it is not only range of motion that needs to be restricted to qualify as a dysfunction. The displacement of the fulcrum or axis in three-dimensional space is another kinematic criterion that can be put forward.[45]

Chauffour and Prat use the term "osteopathic lesion" with similar meaning to "somatic dysfunction." For them, however, the quality of tissue resistance is more important in osteopathic diagnosis than the amplitude of the movement.[46] For them, the examination of the various parameters of an osteopathic lesion is essential to its successful treatment.[47]

According to Fossum, if we relate our concept of the soma or the somatic system back to the stage of embryological development, then most osteopathic approaches, including those treating the visceral and cranial systems, can be integrated into the concept of the somatic dysfunction. The mesodermal germ layer develops in the third week of gestation (the gastrulation stage). In view of the symbiotic connection between the mesodermal structures, i.e., bones, muscles, ligaments, fasciae, and fluids, it must therefore also include the ligamentous and fascial structures of the visceral system and most of the structures of the "craniosacral system." The motility of the visceral organs and that of the brain represent an exception. Motility, seen as a component of the structure itself, is defined as the capacity to change form or morphology. The motility of the visceral organs thus relates to the endoderm and the motility of the brain to the ectoderm.[48]

Somatic dysfunctions can be very evident, e.g., when a person has turned over an ankle, resulting in marked movement restriction, inflammation, and tissue swelling. Often, however, all that is evident is a very slight change in movement, mobility, elasticity, density, bioenergetic expression of the tissue and other tissue qualities.

Somatic dysfunctions must be palpable, or they cannot be treated. The diagnosis of somatic dysfunction by palpation appears to be commonplace in osteopathy/manual medicine. In particular, the studies conducted by Denslow and Korr provide a starting point to examine the evidence for a somatic dysfunction.[49] Recent years have witnessed a flurry of further studies devoted to the palpation of somatic dysfunctions.

For instance, in the case of tender or trigger points, palpation for sensitivity and palpation for pain have been shown to be apparently reliable.[50,51] Likewise, a study by Fryer et al. indicates that abnormal segments can be identified by palpation, confirmed as sensitive by the patient, and objectively demonstrated using a palpometer (pressure algometer).[52] Furthermore, interobserver reliability of osteopathic palpatory tests of the lumbar spine has been found to be acceptable following consensus training.[53]

Highly functional and gentle approaches have also achieved good intra- and inter-examiner reliability, e.g., for detecting the partial total lesion in spinal findings,[54] and substantial intraobserver reliability has been obtained when diagnosing cranial strain patterns in healthy subjects as well as in those with asthma or headache.[55] As part of the diagnostic process the patient's pain gestures also show acceptable inter-examiner reliability.[56]

Yet more research is needed, for example, to identify the components of a somatic dysfunction and their detection/palpation, to verify the nature and existence of an intervertebral dysfunction, and to investigate the many factors influencing palpatory diagnosis.[57-59] In palpatory diagnosis, not only the interpretation of palpatory sensations, but also the perception process itself can be affected by multiple factors, most of which act on the subconscious of the palpating individual. Palpation is a complex process and is influenced, for instance, by previous experiences, the type of information being sought, as well as the context in which palpation takes place. The various influences that shape the perception and interpretation of palpatory findings may create challenges when treating a patient.[60] Awareness of these factors, coupled with consensus training, may lead to more adequate palpation procedures and to enhanced competence in palpation practice, as demonstrated by the improved reliability of osteopathic palpatory diagnostic tests following consensus training.[61,62]

The model of the primary and secondary somatic dysfunction

Dysfunctions are subdivided into primary and secondary dysfunctions (ECOP Glossary 2009), and compensation:

1 A primary somatic dysfunction is the somatic dysfunction that maintains a total pattern of dysfunction (ECOP Glossary 2009). It is the dysfunction that is either the most significant or the one that has been present in the body for the longest time. A primary dysfunction is usually of the traumatic type, remains monosegmental, and is produced by exogenous (external) influences. According to Chauffour and Prat, the "primary lesion" (their term for the primary dysfunction) is at the center of all other dysfunctions. They define it as "the individual osteopathic lesion, which during the examination of a given patient at a given moment, and in comparison with all other lesions present, has the greatest degree of tissular resistance."[63] Again according to Chauffour and Prat, it is not the original dysfunction; the original dysfunction may be likened to the foundation stone of the building, whereas the primary dysfunction is the keystone in a classical tectonic architectural structure. The dysfunctional chain develops in various ways, depending on the morphology of the individual, and on other dysfunctions present, etc. While the patient history can disclose the triggering factor and the symptoms, it cannot localize the primary dysfunction. The total dysfunction and the primary dysfunction depend to some extent on time and circumstances. The primary dysfunction can undergo change, and can vary over time. Osteopathic examination of the

patient by palpation is the only way to localize this as a specific space–time phenomenon.[64]

2 A secondary somatic dysfunction is one that has arisen either as a mechanical or neurophysiological response subsequent to or as a consequence of other etiologies (ECOP Glossary 2009). It can follow a primary dysfunction – usually insidiously and passively, can represent an adaptation to or compensation for primary dysfunctions or anomalies, or represent a situation en route to correction of primary dysfunctions. In the spinal column they are usually plurisegmental, i.e., several segments are usually affected. Secondary dysfunctions can be seen as endogenous (due to internal causes). Secondary dysfunctions may also be followed by tertiary dysfunctions.

3 Compensation is the adaptation of the body to abnormal function or pathogenic influences. Compensation does not yet involve any loss of mobility, although it may bring a tendency to dysfunction. Unlike primary und secondary dysfunctions, it is reversible. In the case of inherited or anatomical malformations, however, it is irreversible.

Discussion of the model of the primary and secondary somatic dysfunction

Total osteopathic lesion

Chauffour and Prat also describe the total osteopathic lesion. This they define as the sum of all "individual osteopathic lesions" found during a general osteopathic examination.[65]

The individual osteopathic lesions are interrelated, and they affect each other while differing in their individual potential to affect the body as a whole. The sum of all individual "osteopathic lesions" (the "total osteopathic lesion") significantly impairs the body as a whole. The osteopathic diagnosis proceeds from the general to the specific, thereby ensuring that it includes the total osteopathic lesion and also the primary lesion.

The center of the total osteopathic lesion is the primary lesion; at the time of the examination this should exhibit the greatest tissue resistance by comparison with all other lesions.[66]

According to Chauffour and Prat, elimination of the primary lesion should be the goal of any osteopathic treatment because its correction will also eliminate the other secondary lesions.[67]

Key lesion

Mitchell also proceeds on the assumption that once the "key lesion" has been resolved, most secondary segmental dysfunctions will resolve spontaneously.[68] However, Parsons and Marcer have criticized this approach, claiming that it ignores the temporal aspect of a somatic dysfunction. While a recently established compensatory pattern can probably be resolved in this way, this is not the case with long-standing problems. The longer a dysfunction is present, the more marked will be the fibrotic changes in the connective tissue. In such a situation it is unlikely that elimination of the primary lesion will also be followed by resolution of the secondary lesion. Instead, as argued by Parsons and Marcer, the "old secondary lesion" could potentially become the "new primary lesion," thus reinstating the "old primary" as the "new secondary." This process can be extended via reflex arcs to all the structures of the body.[69]

Zink's model

According to the law that "The rule of the artery is supreme," Zink's circulatory model is based on the failure of the circulation of lymph and blood and the consequences of this on musculoskeletal and fascial mobility. In Zink's theory, musculoskeletal movement restrictions can give rise to organ dysfunctions because the supply of oxygen and nutrients and the removal of toxic waste products are disturbed.

According to Zink, a somatic dysfunction always leads also to localized inflammation and edema, due to the disturbance of circulation in terms of arterial restriction or disturbed venolymphatic drainage. It is his belief that the restoration of adequate circulation ushers in a correction of the musculoskeletal system and all affected organ systems.[70]

Complicated lesion

Webster described a complicated series of lesions. The typical clinical finding was that a first-degree lesion becomes superimposed on a pre-existing second-degree lesion.[71]

Hoover had noted that there are lesions that do not function in accordance with the typical lesional mechanisms that are generally taught. He observed the development of lesional patterns on top of pre-existing lesional patterns and assumed that careful clinical examination would uncover these lesions. Hoover's thesis was that a lesion of this type is superimposed on top of another pre-existing lesion of a known lesional type. In other words, a second lesion is placed on a pre-existing original lesion, and for this reason he used the name "complicated lesion."

According to Hoover, "complicated lesions" represent severe functional disorders because the tissues have a markedly reduced capacity for adaptation due to their pre-existing dysfunction. The irritation caused by the very pronounced tensions also gives rise to severe reflex segmental disorders. Examples of "complicated lesions" include heart problems and a complex lesion at TH3, asthma and TH4, gastric ulcer and TH5, and so on.

Careful diagnosis must precede accurate and complete correction, otherwise the lesion will deteriorate and the results will be disappointing. According to Hoover, correction is ensured best by eliminating the "superimposed lesion." Only then can the original lesional pattern be treated and eliminated using appropriate techniques. Hoover's work also suggested the existence of further complications of complicated lesions (complicated lesions superimposed on pre-existing superimposed lesions).

Total structural lesion/total lesion

In the 1920s Arthur Becker introduced the idea of the total structural lesion. This included the primary structural lesion and all resulting mechanical sequelae. Overall he viewed it as "one" mechanical lesion and treated it as a whole. In 1954 this idea was further developed by Fryette, who broadened the concept of the total lesion beyond mechanical considerations to also include psychological, emotional, and spiritual factors as well as physiological, dietetic, and environmental factors.[72]

Further distinctions can be drawn:

- Somatosomatic dysfunction. A primary somatic dysfunction (of the bony skeleton or skeletal muscle) leads to further somatic dysfunctions via fascial, ligamentous, muscular, or neural connections.

- Somatovisceral dysfunction. A primary somatic dysfunction can lead to disturbances affecting visceral structures, via fascial, ligamentous, or vascular connections. This especially involves vertebral dysfunctions, via neural segmental connections. Somatic dysfunctions can develop a visceral aspect via the sympathetic ganglia that originate from these segments and also supply sensory and motor innervation to the joints or muscles.[73]

- Viscerosomatic dysfunction. Disturbances of the internal organs can lead to disturbances in the musculoskeletal system.[74]

- Viscerovisceral dysfunction. Via fascial, ligamentous, neural, or vascular connections.

- Psychosomatic or psychovisceral dysfunction. Psychological stress factors or situations that affect the individual either powerfully over a short period of time (death of parents, rape, etc.) or less intensely over a long time period (conflict, anxieties about one's existence, etc.) can overwhelm the homeostatic capacities of the individual. The body reacts to this both globally and locally. Examples of local reactions would be by contraction of particular muscles or muscle groups. Examples of a global reaction are:
  - via the nervous system, causing a reduction in lymphocyte function;
  - via the neuroendocrine system, causing increased secretion of cortisol;
  - via the limbic system and autonomic nervous system, bringing about certain involuntary reactions of the body.

- Somatopsychological or visceropsychological dysfunction. These may occur, for example, as a result of increased sympathetic tonus, pain, motion restrictions, or neuroendocrine changes, all of which can lead to psychological disturbances. A somatic dysfunction may also reflect mental–spiritual overload, fear avoidance strategies, unresolved conflicts, or unconscious patterns of life. The tensions caused by these in the body may result in somatic dysfunction, depending on the strength and duration of their occurrence. More precise studies are required to examine the extent to which emotional factors might need to be

simultaneously addressed in order to achieve the release of somatic dysfunctions.

Cranial somatic dysfunctions can be further subdivided into the following categories, based on subjective palpatory experience: osseous, membranous, neural, fluid, and electrodynamic dysfunctions:

- Osseous dysfunctions include all dysfunctional change in the structure, physiological movement, and position of the cranial bones. An extension of this category would be changes in the other bony articulations.

- Membranous/fascial dysfunctions: these consist of dysfunctional changes in the membranous/fascial structures of the craniosacral system, such as the structure and function of the meninges of the brain and spinal cord, the connective tissue sheaths of the cranial and spinal cord nerves, etc. This corresponds to palpatory findings relating to the other fasciae of the body.

- Neural tissue dysfunctions: the neural structures too may exhibit dysfunctional changes and they are possibly accessible to a palpatory approach.

- Fluid dysfunctions: this refers to dysfunctional changes in the cerebrospinal fluid (CSF) – for example, in the subjective perception of rhythmic activity or volume of the CSF. This palpatory concept is also by extension applied correspondingly to the other body fluids.

- Electrodynamic dysfunctions: electrical and magnetic forces influence physiological processes in the body, such as those of growth and healing. Some osteopaths claim to be able to sense some portion of these forces.

Every somatic dysfunction is highly individual and depends, for example, on the type and intensity of the cause, the duration of the forces and noxious agents involved, the activity, the age and emotional state of the person concerned, their constitutional character and posture/attitude, structural and physiological predispositions, anomalies and pathologies, as well as the individual's current state and the position of the tissue or joints at the moment when the forces exerted their effect.

Mechanisms underlying the development and effects of somatic dysfunction

Somatic dysfunction can be seen as representative of a mechanical or physiological reaction to internal and external influences. Some factors that potentially predispose to or participate in the development of a somatic dysfunction include:

1 Genetic influences

2 Intrauterine, perinatal, or postnatal influences

3 Trauma, such as accidents, birth trauma, whiplash injury, falls, wrong movements, or repeated incidences of microtrauma

4 Results of infection (brought about by inflammation reactions) and other severe diseases such as encephalitis, meningitis, or otitis media

5 Sequelae of surgery, lumbar puncture, medications, vaccinations, or scars

6 Sequelae of dental extractions or other dental procedures such as a bridge or brace

7 Mechanical influences such as work-associated abnormal stresses or posture

8 Visceral influences such as organ dysfunctions or diseases

9 Psychological influences/emotional trauma

10 Influences relating to nutrition, lifestyle, and rhythms of life on the body tissue

11 Influences from the external world, such as environmental pollution, climate, and hygiene conditions.

A somatic dysfunction can arise if exposure to the above-listed influences is short-term and too strong or too protracted for the local or systemic regulatory forces to be able to resolve, remove, or compensate for them or their effects.

Many functional systems may be involved in the development of a somatic dysfunction and in its effects. A somatic dysfunction can be seen as a kind of abnormal functional pattern, a dysfunction complex, made up of various components and multiple associated interactions. Theories and models that may offer possible explanations include:

- Nociceptive model: peripheral and central neural changes with special reference to the sympathetic nervous system

- Allostasis model with impairment of neuro-endocrino-immunology

- Progressive dysfunctional development

- Tensegrity model

- Changes in connective tissue, matrix, or continuum consciousness as proposed by Oschman

- Psycho-neuro-immunology

- Somatic dysfunction as a region of restricted vitality and consciousness

- Model of dissipative systems

- Holon concept

- Holarchic qualities of somatic dysfunction

- Somatic dysfunction and new physics (see also Chapters 1 and 4)

- Biodynamic and biokinetic forces according to Becker

- Changes in biophoton, electromagnetic fields, and liquid crystalline structures (see Chapter 4)

- Changes and mechanical impairments in inter- and intraosseous, muscular, fascial, and other connective tissue and visceral structures, e.g., restrictions, spasm, shortening, etc.

- Hydraulic impairments/multiple effects on fluids in the body, e.g., poor lubrication, restricted drainage and circulation

- Polyrhythmic interactions and resonance phenomena (see Chapters 18-20)

- Emotional, mental, and spiritual interactions (see Chapters 18, 20 and 38).

Some of these models are more speculative than others. Some of these theories and models will be described and discussed in the following text.

Nociceptive model

At present the effects of somatic dysfunction seem to be best researched through nociceptive mechanisms.[75–78]

In their model of the somatic dysfunction, Korr and Denslow suggested that the basis for the deleterious effects of the somatic (or visceral) structural disturbance was the production of altered outflows from spinal areas receiving neural inputs from the disturbed structure. These altered outflows to neurally associated somatic or visceral structures would disturb their function and hence reduce the total functional capacity of the body to maintain health.[79–81] Korr and Denslow placed great importance on the interactions between somatic and autonomic components of the spinal cord and on the influence of the sympathetic nervous system in overall body function.

Korr and Denslow's emphasis on the interactions between the somatic and visceral structures was influenced by their work on the effects of somatic stressors on visceral function.[82] Indeed, early in the profession, there had been a strong recognition that sensory impulses from somatic structures would influence visceral function and vice versa.[83] In fact, the interaction between somatic and visceral structures was one of the primary reasons given for the effectiveness of manipulative treatments of somatic structures; such treatments would affect visceral function. Burns[84] provided evidence of strong somatic and visceral interactions, but it was not until many years later that the scientific community began to conduct research on the mechanism of viscerosomatic and somatovisceral reflexes.[85] Now it has become evident that most sensory inputs from somatic structures connect not only to spinal or brainstem circuits that convey information to the brain or back to somatic structures, but also to circuits that end on autonomic circuits that influence visceral function. Even more dramatically, sensory inputs from visceral structures almost always send collaterals to circuits that influence somatic structures.[86,87] Hence, disturbances in visceral tissues would be reflected in somatic structures and vice versa. Thus,

the importance that Korr and Denslow placed on the interactions between visceral and somatic structures seems well placed.

Due to the state of knowledge about nervous function, Korr suggested that the hyperactive state of spinal reflexes, and hence overactive muscle activity in dysfunctional areas seen in their studies, was due to continued inputs from disturbed proprioceptors.[88] He termed these areas of hyperexcitable spinal tissue as "facilitated segments" which were responsible for disrupted function of both local and distant visceral and somatic structures.

In 1990, van Buskirk[89] proposed that proprioceptive inputs could not cause the strong effects that accompanied somatic dysfunction and suggested that nociceptive inputs would be much more likely candidates for long-lasting changes seen in most somatic dysfunctions. The mechanisms responsible for such changes were still in question.

By the early 1980s evidence was accumulating that spinal reflex arcs were not static entities, relaying information from input to output, but were subject to alterations in their functional characteristics.[90–94] Increasingly, work on spinal reflex function in both learning and pain fields was showing that various sensory inputs, but especially pain inputs, could alter both peripheral and spinal information flow for long time periods and perhaps permanently.[95]

Peripheral and central neural plasticity

Peripheral changes

Mechanisms of long-term alterations in peripheral receptor and nerve fiber excitability are now being elucidated. When tissue injury occurs, cellular damage results in release of various substances, such as substance-P, peptides, and others, that alter the chemical milieu of sensory receptors in the area. Nociceptors, usually high-threshold organs, are sensitized, that is, their firing thresholds are lowered. In addition, neural impulses traveling toward the spinal cord (orthodromic flow) branch out to other nociceptors on the same neuron and travel outwards (antidromic flow) to invade the receptor area of the nerve. This causes release of substance-P and further sensitizes the nociceptor endings in the area. The acute sensitivity of the skin around a wound is the result of this type of nociceptor sensitization. This is an adaptive process in that it causes the person to avoid further damage to the area. In addition, however, this causes increased levels of nociceptor inputs to the spinal circuits. Usually, this type of sensitization is short-lived.

If, however, an injury results in peripheral nerve damage, the resulting release of nerve growth factor can cause functional changes in local mechanoreceptor sensory neurons, resulting in the stimulation of central pain pathways with mechanoreceptor inputs.[96] Thus, in some instances, sensitization of peripheral sensory inputs can result in altered inputs to the central nervous system, thus disrupting the normal functional relationships between input and outflow. This type of sensitization may be long-lasting and results in an abnormal and nonadaptive situation that can be part of a somatic dysfunction syndrome.

Spinal circuit changes

Over the past 20 years, it has become increasingly apparent that the spinal cord is not merely a transmitter of information from the body to the higher nervous system and back, but that the cord's gray matter itself is an information processor. While spinal reflexes are well known and some have even been studied extensively, what is now becoming apparent is that sensory inputs as well as descending inputs from higher brain structures can alter the information processing capabilities of spinal neural circuits.

Four overlapping, but distinct changes in spinal circuit excitability have been identified.[97] The first type is termed spinal "sensitization." Sensitization occurs very rapidly in response to many types of stimuli, but particularly to painful stimuli. In a single burst of input lasting less than a second, the spinal circuit can be shown to increase its activity to subsequent stimuli and with several stimulus inputs over several seconds, may increase to 200% or more of the original responsiveness. Thus, a short-lived burst of input can cause an alteration of spinal excitability that lasts for up to two minutes. Once the stimulus is stopped, the spinal excitability returns to normal over 90–120 seconds.[98]

If, however, the stimulus burst lasts for several minutes, the spinal circuit level may not return to its baseline excitability. If an increased excitability remains, it may last for hours and is termed "long-term sensitization" (the second type of change).[99]

If the stimulus lasts even longer, the spinal excitability may not return to normal for weeks, a phenomenon known as "fixation."[100] In this third type of change,

sensory inputs into the affected area can cause larger-than-normal outputs to both somatic and visceral areas for a significant time, which is an abnormal and nonadaptive situation.

If sufficiently intense or long-lasting sensory inputs impinge on spinal circuits, the results can be the seemingly permanent changes in spinal circuit function (the fourth type of change). In this case, spinal inhibitory neurons die and there is evidence of the sprouting from remaining excitatory neurons onto the areas left vacant by the dying axons. In this case, the excitability of the affected circuit would be seemingly permanently increased, resulting in perhaps permanent increased outflows from the area to related somatic and visceral structures and to the higher brain centers.[101]

The four levels of spinal alterations described here are apparently mediated by separate mechanisms ranging from simple increased neurotransmitter release for sensitization, to altered genetic expression for fixation and rampant abnormal cellular repair mechanisms resulting in cell death (permanent change). However, all these processes result in increased spinal circuit excitability.

While many of the effects seen in the studies of spinal excitability have been the result of nociceptive inputs to the spinal circuits, an increasing number of studies are showing that spinal excitability alterations can occur with mechanoreceptor inputs or inputs descending from brain centers.[102] The alterations from non-nociceptive inputs do not alter the excitability as rapidly as nociceptive inputs, but may in fact be more like inputs acting over a long term from altered motion patterns that are often associated with osteopathic palpatory findings.

Such a long-term or permanently increased excitability of spinal areas was exactly what was described by Korr and Denslow from their work[103,104] and what Korr described as the facilitated segment, although they had no idea that the alterations in spinal excitability they observed were occurring within the spinal neurons themselves.

The sympathetic nervous system plays an essential role in nociceptive mechanisms. The controversially debated centerpiece of the models behind all descriptions of the putative role of the sympathetic nervous system in the generation of pain involve positive feedback pathways from the spinal cord to the periphery of the body via the sympathoneural or sympathoadrenal system.[105,106]

Central changes

While alterations in spinal circuits are now observed in many circumstances, there are increasing indications of somewhat similar alterations in the circuits devoted to processing sensory inputs in the brain, from subcortical to cortical levels. These changes occur in many brain areas, and range from the simple sensitization to possible inhibitory cell death in areas of the frontal cortex involved in the highest levels of personality function.[107] If such brain changes are found to indeed occur with nociceptive inputs, and even with non-nociceptive inputs, the concept of "facilitation" could extend from the spinal cord to the brain itself.

Peripheral inflammation leads to nociceptor sensitization, followed by central sensitization of second-order neurons (e.g., in the spinal or trigeminal dorsal horn), with an amplification of the transmission of nociceptive impulses (Figure. 15.1). A peripheral nerve lesion, e.g., induced mechanically in the case of a somatic dysfunction, is followed by generation of ectopic impulses in nociceptive and non-nociceptive primary afferent neurons, leading to central hyperexcitability.

Following nerve lesion, e.g., induced mechanically in the case of a somatic dysfunction, the lesioned primary afferent neurons and corresponding central representations (e.g., in the dorsal horn, thalamus, and cortex) may undergo dramatic biochemical, morphological, and physiological changes. Sympathetic coupling to afferent neurons with large-diameter axons may now be important, since activity in these neurons could generate central hyperexcitability and feed into central circuits that have changed as a consequence of the peripheral nerve lesion.[108,109]

Autonomic changes observed under the condition of ongoing pain are dependent on the integrated activity of many centers in the central nervous system (Figure. 15.2).[110,111]

Fryer's (1999) hypothetical model of somatic dysfunction points in a similar direction: strain to the zygapophysial joint capsule creates inflammation (synovitis) and synovial effusion and activates the nociceptors. Axon reflexes produce vasodilation and inflammation at the terminal nerve endings, producing typical segmental tissue texture changes, i.e., tension in the tissue, which can be caused by segmental muscle inflammation and engorgement/blood congestion. Range of movement and end feel are altered due to tissue engorgement and joint effusion. Nociceptor activation sends action potentials to the dorsal horn and stimulates sympathetic activation, which in turn produces visceral and immunological sequelae. Segmental "stabilizing" muscles, such as multifidus, are reflexly inhibited, while the excitability of long, polysegmental muscles (such as the erector spinae) is increased, making the joint vulnerable to further strain. Over time connective tissue changes occur in the strained capsule, producing typical range of movement impairment. The multifidus atrophies, causing loss of functional stability and control and exposing the joint to continuing strain. Ongoing nociceptor activation provokes further segmental tissue inflammation and continued sympathetic stimulation, causing the cycle to become self-sustaining. Although pain perception need not be involved, nociceptive processing in the dorsal horn may become disturbed. The resultant "central sensitization" leads to hyperalgesia and chronic pain.[112]

Homeostasis and allostasis

The concept of the somatic dysfunction is also tied to the idea of total economy of the individual. In the mid-1800s, Bernard wrote of the concept of the defense or stability of the internal milieu.[113] This was further discussed and developed by Cannon in 1915 with his concept of homeostasis, or the stability of the internal milieu.[114] Cannon amplified his ideas into the concept that the body had internal set points for various internal functions, such as temperature, Na^+ concentration, and so forth, and that these set points were maintained by feedback mechanisms and regulatory functions, influenced by emotions as well as non-voluntary regulatory physiology. He described the "fright or flight" response as a part of this mechanism, all part of the need of the organism to maintain its internal state.[115]

Hans Selye[116] built upon these ideas as he incorporated the general adaptation syndrome (GAS) that suggested a greater role for stress, both psychological and physiological, in the internal regulatory systems. He postulated that chronic stress, activating the hypothalamic/pituitary/adrenal (HPA) axis that produced body responses vital to meeting stressful situations, was a potential vital component of functional breakdowns. With episodic stress, the HPA

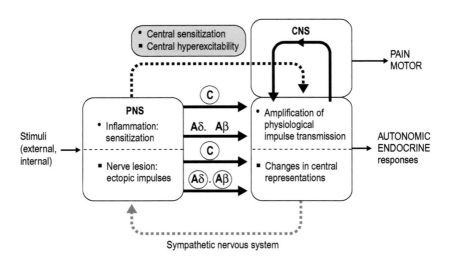

Figure 15.1

Concept of the generation of peripheral and central hyperexcitability during inflammatory pain or neuropathic pain involving the sympathetic nervous system (CNS, central nervous system; PNS, peripheral nervous system). The pain is always associated with motor, autonomic, and endocrine responses. The upper dashed arrow indicates that the central changes are generated (and possibly maintained) by persistent activation of nociceptors with unmyelinated (C) fibers (e.g., during chronic inflammation), called here "central sensitization," or after trauma with nerve lesion by ectopic activity in myelinated (Aδ, Aβ) and C-afferents and other changes in the lesioned afferent neurons, called here "central hyperexcitability." The lower dashed arrow indicates the efferent feedback via the sympathetic nervous system (including the sympathoadrenal system) to the primary afferent neurons. The transmission of nociceptive impulses is under multiple control of the brain (bold arrows, upper right). Primary afferent nociceptive neurons (in particular those with C-fibers) are sensitized during inflammation. After nerve lesion, all lesioned primary afferent neurons (unmyelinated as well as myelinated ones) undergo biochemical, physiological, and morphological changes, which become irreversible with time. These peripheral changes entail changes of the central representations (of the somatosensory system), which become irreversible if no regeneration of primary afferent neurons to their target tissue occurs. The central changes, induced by persistent activity in afferent nociceptive neurons or after nerve lesion, are also reflected in the sympathetic efferent feedback system that may establish positive feedback loops to the primary afferent neurons.

axis would activate appropriately and ensure that the body could meet the threat, a "heterostatic state." With chronic stressors, however, the long-term activation of the HPA axis would lead to overactivation of the axis and chronic heterostasis, and soon to functional collapse.

However, in 1981, Sterling and Eyer[117] proposed that homeostatic and heterostatic concepts were insufficient to explain observed function. They proposed the term "allostasis" to denote the concept

not of static internal states (homeostasis) or heightened internal response (heterostasis), but of changing internal and mental states designed to meet the demands of the environment. Thus, allostasis denotes the process by which an organism achieves internal viability through bodily changes of state, including both behavioral and physiological processes. Allostasis implies that the physiological and psychological states can in fact change in order to maintain total functional integrity.

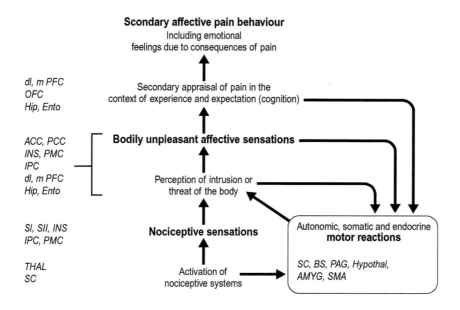

dl, m PFC
OFC
Hip, Ento

ACC, PCC
INS, PMC
IPC
dl, m PFC
Hip, Ento

SI, SII, INS
IPC, PMC

THAL
SC

Scondary affective pain behaviour
Including emotional
feelings due to consequences of pain

Secondary appraisal of pain in the
context of experience and expectation (cognition)

Bodily unpleasant affective sensations

Perception of intrusion or
threat of the body

Nociceptive sensations

Activation of
nociceptive systems

Autonomic, somatic and endocrine
motor reactions

SC, BS, PAG, Hypothal,
AMYG, SMA

Figure 15.2

The interaction between nociceptive sensations, bodily unpleasant affective sensations, and secondary affective pain behavior and the brain centers possibly involved. Activation of autonomic, endocrine, and somatic motor systems occurs on all integrative levels during activation of the centers representing nociception and pain. The mechanisms of activation of these motor systems by higher centers (see interrupted arrows) have been little studied. Simplified scheme. ACC, anterior cingulate cortex; AMYG, amygdala; BS, brain stem; Ento, entorhinal cortex; Hip, hippocampus; Hypothal, hypothalamus; INS, insular cortex; IPC, inferior parietal cortex; PAG, periaqueductal gray; PCC, posterior cingulate cortex; PFC, prefrontal cortex (dl, dorsolateral; m, medial); PMC, premotor cortex; SC, spinal cord; SI, SII, primary and secondary somatosensory cortex; SMA, supplementary motor area; THAL, Thalamus. Designed after Jänig.

These reactions are transmitted by the hypothalamic–pituitary–adrenal (HPA) axis, the sympathetic nervous system, and the immune system (cytokines).

The hypothalamic–pituitary–adrenal axis involves corticotropin-releasing hormone (CRH) from the hypothalamus that causes the pituitary to release adrenocorticotropic hormone (ACTH), which in its turn causes the release of cortisol from the adrenal glands. This axis, and also "allostatic load," is maintained by the following factors, according to Willard:

- Diurnal rhythm (see Chapter 3)

- Nociceptive somatic stimuli

- Nociceptive visceral stimuli

- Emotional stimuli.

Sterling and Eyer further defined an "allostatic state" as a chronic overactivation of regulatory systems and the subsequent alterations of physiological set points, and an "allostatic overload" as the expression of pathophysiology by the chronic overactivation of regulatory systems. Thus allostasis and its related pathological states encompass much more than the concepts of homeostasis encompassed. However, all these concepts include the idea that stressors can come from inside as well as outside the body.[118]

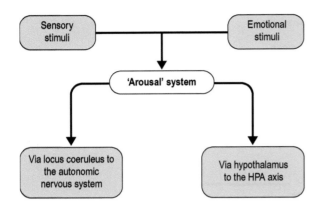

Figure 15.3
The arousal system according to Willard.

An important arousal system (Figures 15.3 and 15.4) is the HPA–locus–coeruleus–noradrenalin axis (HPA–LC–NA axis):[119] the hypothalamus activates the locus coeruleus by means of corticotropin releasing factor (CRF). The locus coeruleus in turn activates the hypothalamus by releasing noradrenalin. This "feedback–forward system" is activated rapidly and has a profound effect on homeostasis. The hippocampus has an inhibiting effect on CRF release, and the amygdala a stimulating effect.

Whereas acute adaptations are useful for the functioning of the body, long-lasting adaptations are damaging. Long-lasting, uncontrolled compensatory responses are referred to as "allostatic load." The four factors listed above are responsible for the inability to switch off the allostatic reactions.

Pathological processes brought about by the allostatic load are associated with the effect of cortisols, catecholamines, and cytokines. Some of these effects are listed below (according to Willard: AAO Convocation 2004 in Colorado Springs):

- In the cardiovascular system: hypertension, arteriosclerosis, left heart hypertrophy, disinhibition of the fibrinogen system, and increased risk of myocardial infarction.

- In the nervous system: depression, anxiety together with memory loss, reduced cognitive capacities, changes in behavior.

- In the endocrine system: increase in insulin resistance.

- In the metabolic system: rise in blood pressure, hyperlipidemia, and hyperglycemia.

- In the immune system: immune suppression of T-cell activity, etc.

- In the adrenergic steroid system: disturbances of bone metabolism, fat and glucose metabolism, tissue oxidation, and the immune system; increased insulin resistance.

The correction of somatic dysfunctions reduces the uncontrolled feedback mechanisms and improves homeostasis and hence the state of health of the patient. Osteopathic theory must therefore encompass both the concept of physiological regulation on the segmental level and that of central regulation of autonomic activity and nociception. Only in this way can the wide-ranging results that follow osteopathic manipulation be understood.

The concepts embodied in allostasis, reflecting both a physiological and a mental state change designed to maintain the viability of the organism, are predicated on the ability of the organism to successfully carry out such alterations. The imposition of a somatic dysfunction of any sort within the homeostatic/allostatic mechanism would produce a barrier to full operation of the regulatory processes. Thus, the somatic dysfunction would necessitate a greater response to achieve continued viability, or would not allow full adaptation to the impinging stress, and thus downgrade the ability to maintain viability, creating an allostatic overload. Commonly, this leads to loss of health, or disease or clinical symptoms (see below for a model of allostatic function).

The evidence presented here suggests that the somatic dysfunction, whether primarily in a somatic or visceral structure, with the concurrent alterations in spinal reflex function and possibly brain function, can have far-reaching consequences for far-flung body areas through both the neural and tensegrity systems and by interfering with allostatic mechanisms.

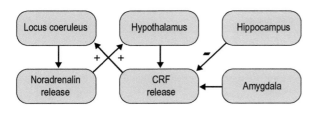

Figure 15.4
Noradrenaline and CRF release.

Further perspectives on the development and ramifications of somatic dysfunction

Progressive dysfunctional development using the example of Dolet, Chauffour and Prat

For Dolet, a structural imbalance represents in effect the last stage of a progressive dysfunctional development (see Figure. 15.5). This theoretical progression can stop at any level and need not necessarily proceed through to the final stage.

According to Chauffour and Prat[120b] an "osteopathic lesion" is primarily expressed in the mesodermal tissue. Usually the scarring reaction of connective tissue following inflammatory processes is responsible for the development of "osteopathic lesions": inflammation → fibrosis → sclerosis. The acute inflammation (tumor, dolor, calor, rubor) leads to edema and spasm of muscle tissue. This is normally fully reversible and, depending on the extent and duration of the inflammatory reaction, can initiate repair processes in the tissue. However, this phase can also be the first stage of an "osteopathic lesion" and transition into fibrosis. If the inflammatory reaction has been too important, too prolonged, or too frequently recurring, tissue reorganization occurs. This is associated with an increase in the number of collagen fibers and a change in their orientation. This phase is not spontaneously reversible. Osteopathic treatment can enable the fibrosis to revert to the inflammatory stage and lead to better reorganization of the tissue and to partial or total normalization of tissue mobility.

Sclerosis is the final stage of a pathological scarring process; it is irreversible and is accompanied by ligamentous and tendinous calcification, exostosis, arterial sclerosis, etc. Osteopathic treatment can improve the body's adaptation capacity in relation to this dysfunction. The linear development presented here is not necessarily the process encountered in reality. The fibrosis stage can be associated with phases of inflammation, or different stages may co-exist in a single tissue.

Tensegrity model[††]

While much emphasis has been placed on the neural mechanisms underlying somatic dysfunction, there are features of the syndrome that cannot readily be explained by neural effects. One of the observations often made by osteopaths and others working with manual medicine is that treating a local area for somatic dysfunction can cause dramatic and seemingly instantaneous changes in somatic and visceral mobility in areas far removed from the treatment site.

One of the underlying constructs of osteopathy is that the body is a functional unit. The great unifying systems certainly tie the body into such a functional whole; the circulatory, endocrine, and nervous systems are thought of as great unifiers. However, another construct is now emerging as another great mechanical unifying system: the concept of "tensegrity."

Andrew Taylor Still's focus on the inter-connectedness of structure and function has been carried forward by Fryer with reference to the now well-known process of mechanotransduction. This is the name given to the possibility that mechanical stress brings about alterations in cell physiology in such a way that fibroblasts react to mechanical forces. Not only are their physiological processes altered, but so too is their gene expression. This process lends support to the principle of the inter-connectedness of structure and function and points up possible clinical implications.[121] Mechanotransduction potentially provides pathophysiological justification for the tensegrity concept. For example, it might explain how mechanical tensions in connective tissue disturb the function of every individual cell right down to its nucleus. This phenomenon might lead to the development of disturbances of cell function leading to the onset of disease. It might even provide a hypothetical explanation for a gene mutation or a tumor.

*see also p. 60

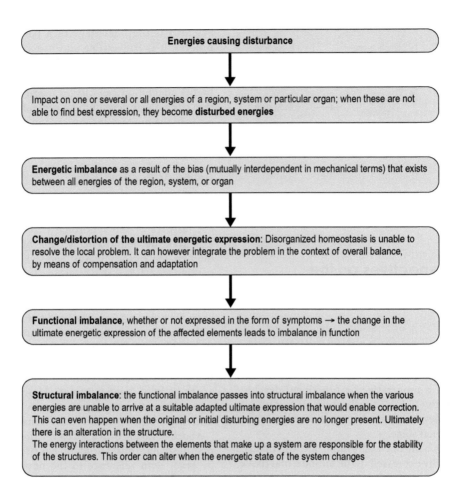

Figure 15.5
Progressive evolution of dysfunction (after Dolet).[120a]

The tensegrity principle is commonly used in buildings and art forms. Interestingly, it seems to be the basic principle underlying cellular architecture at both the whole cell and intracellular levels. At the larger level, the bones, ligaments, and muscles make up tensegrity structures in the body. In fact, the tensegrity principle is used at all levels of the body.

Buckminster Fuller developed the concept of tensegrity and the word is a portmanteau formation derived from a combination of "tension" and "integrity." The tensegrity model is a structural system of rigid, discontinuous parts, linked by continuous tension cables. Stresses are distributed discontinuously, while strains within the system are distributed continuously. Tensegrity structures are characterized not only by great stability, but also by their capacity to transmit mechanical energy or information within the system as a whole. In this way tensions are distributed continuously across all the structural elements, so that an increase in tension in one element always leads to an increase in tension in other elements of the system. This increase in tension is compensated for by an increase in compression in certain components of the system, and by this means the system itself is stabilized.

Interpreted in the same light, the bony skeleton can be seen as representing the rigid parts of the system and the muscles, tendons, and fasciae as the continuous tension cables.

Ingber has described this reciprocal tension system on the cellular level. A network of contractile microfilaments operates as tension cables, exerting a tensile force on the cell membrane and components in the direction of the cell nucleus. The intracellular microtubules or large bundles of interwoven microfilaments and the extracellular matrix counteract this force. Intermediate filaments in the cell function as integration elements between microtubules and contractile microfilaments and between the cell membrane and nucleus.

The significance of cell form for the functioning of adherent cells has been repeatedly demonstrated.[122–127] Stamenovic and Coughlin studied the underlying mechanisms regulating cell form and cell deformation in more detail.[128] The cytoskeleton plays an important role in this regulation,[129–138] so that the stretching of a cell can activate particular genes. Genes in turn, by producing proteins, are able to alter the mechanical properties of a cell.

Stamenovic and Coughlin describe three models: tensegrity structures, prestressed cable nets, and open cell foam networks. They concluded that prestress and the architecture of the cytoskeleton are the key features for the elastic cell response.

Tensegrity structures

These are prestressed cable nets in which the cable tension is completely balanced by the local compression of the supporting struts. Stamenovic and Coughlin demonstrated that the mechanical properties of simple tensegrity models of cytoskeletons match the mechanical behavior observed in adherent cells.[139–141]

Prestressed cable nets

Prestressed cable nets describe a balance of the response of adherent cells under low mechanical tension. They provide an explanatory model for the mechanical roles possibly played by important molecular structures of the cytoskeleton in resisting cell deformations.

The actin framework of the cytoskeleton carries prestress, giving stability of form to the cell. When minor deformations of the cell occur, the rigid actin filaments do not bend, nor does their length change to any noticeable extent. Instead they rotate and alter the size of the intervening space to create balance in the configuration. The prestress of the actin of the cytoskeleton is to a certain extent counterbalanced by compression of the microtubules. When the compression reaches a critical point, the microtubules bend and distort. (For this bending to occur, the tension in the actin filaments must significantly exceed the peak force that can be generated by a single actomyosin unit.)

Open cell foam networks

If major compression stress acts on the cell, the filaments of the cytoskeleton can bend and distort. In this case, the open cell foam model becomes the more appropriate description of the mechanical response by the cell.

Tensegrity from the perspective of osteopathy

The extracellular matrix allows the creation of a continuum in our bodies that corresponds to the principles of tensegrity and also links all organs, systems, and structures. Tensegrity provides some endorsement of the osteopathic approach in diagnosis and treatment, for example, as regards the importance of the fasciae as a communication network in the body.[142] In fact it seems very possible that the fasciae of the body are part of this tensegrity construction, distributing imposed and intrinsic forces at any one area to the total structure. Thus, a change in body mechanics allowing normalized motion at one area could be immediately transferred to other areas of the body, allowing them to return to normal tensions and functional characteristics. The possibilities of the tensegrity model for somatic dysfunction appear to be difficult to overstate.

The tensegrity model extends far beyond such considerations, however. For Buckminster Fuller, there are in the first instance no objects or rigid substances but simply "events operating in pure principle"; even the Universe itself is only coordinated, formed, transformed, and held together by tension, repulsion, electromagnetic, and gravitational forces.[143] Even interpersonal relations can be interpreted from the point of view of tensegrity. They develop in a fine tension network of attraction and resistance: "push" and "pull." The individuals concerned represent the discontinuous compression elements, and the existing patterns of relationship form the continuous tension network.[144] From the point of view of tensegrity, a somatic dysfunction comes about when either the compression elements (bones) or the tension elements (soft tissues), or the balance between the two, change. Inflammatory processes can alter tissue, for example, in this way. Increased accommodation or compensation then occurs in the tensegrity system. Ultimately the extent of the compensation in the tensegrity system is a decisive factor in whether disease symptoms appear. This compensatory play is mainly provided by the tonus/tension of the soft tissues. The complete collapse of the tensegrity system could only come about through the destruction of the elements involved.

Applied tensegrity is when an osteopath takes up contact with tensions in the body, and with forces of attraction and repulsion; likewise, the release or normalization of tensions that have been therapeutically induced according to the pattern of the dysfunction to enable a state of higher order to be achieved.

Dysfunction from the perspective of matrix consciousness as defined by Oschman[145]

Oschman distinguishes two kinds of consciousness:

- Neurological consciousness. We form a picture of our world and our place in it through the impressions received from our senses and processed selectively or by logical, rational analysis. Our sensors are continuously monitoring our internal and external environment.

- Connective tissue, matrix, or continuum consciousness. This kind of consciousness appears only at the fluid boundaries of perception, and as a realm of experience directly preceding the formation of a mental image of the world. It arises before we initiate any movement in response to this mental image. Oschman speaks of this realm of experience as being the unconscious, and understands it as indwelling not only the nervous system, but also – or indeed primarily – the living matrix. He sees this kind of

(unconscious?) "consciousness" as forming within the continuous living matrix system that contains the connective tissue types and nuclear matrices of the cells in the entire body. According to his hypothesis, a continuum consciousness comes about in the connective tissue because the living matrix is a high-speed semiconducting communication network. The living matrix represents an information and energy system in the following ways:

- As an excitable medium and whole-body, integrated conduction system, it is able to generate and transmit signals.
- As an energy system, it is able to take up information and energy from the environment, store it, and release it at any particular point (or at all points) in space or time.

Oschman bases his hypothesis on the discoveries of Mae-Wan Ho regarding the liquid crystalline properties of tissue. The continuum route proposed in this hypothesis is understood to operate by conduction through the excitable medium of the living matrix far more rapidly than via classical nerve conduction. The matrix perceives the environment by sensory means and can initiate processes long before the neurological consciousness has formed a conscious perception.

According to Oschman, the signal is transmitted by the cytoskeleton of the sensory cell, directly through the connective tissue to the myofasciae, and on to the cytoskeleton of the muscle cells. The arrival of energy and information from sensory input at the myofilaments of the muscle cell triggers a contraction.

Oschman's view once more points to the great importance of the state of the matrix for the homeostasis of the body. Osteopathy has always attributed great importance to the connective tissue in treatment. The essential functions of the connective tissue for higher development reveal the way in which disturbances arise.

Dysfunctions of the connective tissue or dysfunctions in the functional unit consisting of the sensory cell–connective tissue–myofasciae–cytoskeleton of the muscle cells lead to disturbances in energy and information in the body as a whole, and also, according to Oschman, in the body's "subconscious."

From the evolutionary point of view, the nervous system is thought to have developed from specialized cells as an extension of pre-existing matrix communication. According to the holonic view, the systems that are older (in evolutionary terms) are encompassed by those that are younger. This means that the matrix system, if it does exist, would have been relegated, transcended, and integrated by systems that developed later. Otherwise more recent developments would be reduced in their holonic quality to stages that are earlier in evolutionary terms, which would surely be wrong. From this point of view the matrix system appears to be more fundamental, since it serves as a component for subsequent developmental stages; however, the development of the brain would be more significant because it enables a deeper and more comprehensive consciousness to emerge and stands higher in the holarchical order. There is some contradiction here to the ideas presented by Oschman.

Psychoneuroimmunology

Some interactions in osteopathy which support higher-order stages of integration in the body – for example, those that involve differentiation and integration of somatopsychological consequences of trauma by accessing these via the tissue – can be explained in terms of psychoneuroimmunology. Insights from psycho-neuroimmunology suggest that emotions have a key function as they travel between the two realms of body and mind.[146] Biochemical substrates deriving from emotions transport information to and fro between brain structures and endocrine, gastrointestinal, and immunological systems. Scattered throughout the entire digestive tract are neuropeptides and their receptors.[147] The ligands that act on immune cells do not only consist – as was long assumed – of particular neurotransmitters and neurohormones, but also numerous other hormones and neuropeptide transmitter substances. It has also been demonstrated, for example, that on contact with a pathogen, a number of cytokines and nerve cells can be synthesized; conversely, that immune defense cells generate neuropeptides. Neuropeptides are not only found in the brain, but also in non-neuronal structures; together with their corresponding receptors on the cells they supply cognitive and emotional information to the whole body. On the other hand the subjective experience of self is formed through a dynamic interaction of ligands and receptors (formerly seen as belonging to the physical category). It became very clear that psychological factors affect the immune system and vice versa. Stress of long duration (H. Selye's "distress") such as

hopelessness, despair, and chronic suppression of strong emotions weakens the immune system and even affects the gene expression of immunological cells. Therefore, the immune system by no means only operates as a defense system; according to Booth and Ashbridge, it also participates – as part of the psychoneuroimmunological network – in distinguishing "self" and "non-self," the creation and maintenance of self-identity and the integrity of the organism.[148]

Somatic dysfunctions as regions of restricted vitality and consciousness

The body is a kind of feedback system for access to vitality. Somatic dysfunctions are in this sense regions of restricted vitality and consciousness. Somatic dysfunctions can be likened to local zones of non-admittance and control, to an extent shut off from the vital force and from rhythmic regulation – a kind of conditioned state of the tissue with reduced vitality or local limitation of potential vitality. In a certain sense they are a kind of filter between an individual and the direct experience of life. At the same time there is inherent in them the potential to open up to what is hidden within, to a greater order, and to become whole or healthy.

The extent to which exogenous or endogenous forces affect the interaction between tissue and consciousness, and body physiology, also depends on the extent to which the individual in question is able to be "present" in and permeable to these forces. It is hypothesized that this will directly determine the quality and pattern of the dysfunction.

Changes can therefore arise even before any other palpable or visible changes in tissue or mobility become apparent. There are those in the osteopathic community who claim to be able to detect some of these changes. More evident motion restrictions and changes in the tissue develop subsequently (e.g., loss of elasticity, swelling, hardening, fibroses, etc.).

It is assumed that somatic dysfunctions that develop before the second or third year of life can exert a much stronger effect on the unity of body, mind/spirit, and soul than those that arise later. This could be in part associated with the fact that they can negatively affect subsequent development/maturation, and that a young child has not yet developed an episodic memory and cannot relate the experience in any way in space and time. In the case of this kind of dysfunction, the processes of release during osteopathic treatment will therefore be less a matter of accompanying the patient using verbal means, and far more experience-oriented.

Dysfunction from the perspective of dissipative systems

Dissipative, self-organizing systems are continually active in order to produce entropy, which forms part of a continuous exchange of energy with the environment. These systems are characterized by the fact that their order is destroyed when close to an equilibrium state, whereas in a state far from equilibrium, order is maintained, or new order can emerge via instabilities.[149] Thus humans, in the course of their physical, emotional, mental, and spiritual developmental dynamic, pass from an ordered state into a disordered one and spontaneously back to a higher-order state. There is a tendency to order and stability with phases of disorder – these can also be expressed through the appearance of certain disease symptoms and acute somatic dysfunctions – that are necessary to the development of a new order.

The patient passes through a stage of instability, so that patterns of order that are no longer adequate can disintegrate and a new structure or higher-order integration can develop. A certain necessary disorder precedes the new order.

Superficially, this process can sometimes look like one of disintegration on the part of the patient. The practitioner must not make the mistake of remaining on the surface or perhaps even supporting the patient in reorganizing and stabilizing the old or dysfunctional pattern of order. Instead, the practitioner can take up contact with the inner movements and homeodynamic forces, and accompany the spontaneous processes of reorganization. From time to time, of course, and from case to case, the decision needs to be made as to whether translative measures are necessary (see Ch. 1, pp 18,19; Ch. 20) to achieve some stabilization.

Somatic dysfunction as a holon (Wilber's AQAL model)

Every form of appearance of every kind exists as a holon. Disease and somatic dysfunction are therefore not completely independent entities; each is a whole in its own right, as well as a part of something else, of other wholes/parts (for example, tissue, functions, consciousness, sociobiological and cultural environment). Somatic dysfunctions are temporary phenomena. Our objective as osteopaths is not to treat symptoms, and certainly not simply to get rid of the symptoms. Manipulation carried out with the aim of simply eliminating a symptom, without taking account of the diverse patterns of relationship in the patient, comes across on the contrary as invasive and becomes a problem itself.

As osteopaths, we try to detect the pattern of relationships and discover their significance and information both in themselves (as a "whole") and as part of other wholes/parts, and by palpation to make them capable of being discovered by the patient.

Every somatic dysfunction manifests itself in a number of ways; not only does it appear as a particular tissue quality, but at the same time it exists in at least four aspects:

- As an external, palpable tissue dysfunction with functional parameters that are to some extent measurable.

- As an inner, subjective perception of the self, or "intention," in the patient.

- As an inner, intersubjective component/cultural aspect/familial constellation.

- As an external, collective, interobjective aspect of biosocial systems.

Each of these aspects or quadrants also appears on different levels, e.g., on the physical, mental, or spiritual level, increasing at each stage in its significance for the health or ill-health of the patient; meanwhile the stages that emerged first are more fundamental for all the following stages (see also Ch. 1, p. 13ff and Ch. 18).

Osteopathy diagnoses and treats mainly on the basis of understanding the way in which structure and function are interrelated, the prime focus being on the external tissue expression.

This treatment approach becomes reductionist and inadequate if we try to understand and treat the person and ill health of our patients purely from the point of view of their tissue pattern (Wilber's upper right-hand quadrant), leaving the other aspects out of consideration. The other aspects must therefore be incorporated into osteopathic methodology of diagnosis and treatment. Table 15.2 makes clear that exclusive consideration of

Inside–individual	Outside–individual
- Spiritual level: resonance of being, communication (5th chakra) - Anxiety and hysteria states - Mental level: stress due to work or relationships - Belief systems: "no-one will understand me" - Emotional level: communication problems - Emotional trauma in adolescence and childhood - Early childhood, e.g., being left alone, verbal utterances (crying) eliciting no response, not being understood - Pre-, peri-, and post-natal trauma - Physical level: emotional stress → tension of the geniohyoid muscle → sensation of tightness of the larynx - Lump in the throat	- Imbalance of body posture, of the anterior and posterior muscle chains, of the hyoid muscles (continued caudally as the infrahyoid muscles and cranially as the suprahyoid muscles), etc. with multiple consequences, e.g., compression of the carotid body and carotid sinus, narrowing of the jugular vein, disturbance of the thyroid gland, sensation of tightness, etc. - Cervical fascia, hyoid ligaments - Shoulder girdle dysfunction (via the omohyoid muscle) - Dysfunction of C1 (→ hypoglossal nerve → geniohyoid muscle) - Dysfunction of CN V/3, CN VII - Functional swallowing disorder - Functional tongue disorder - Underlying pathologies in the cervical region - Ineffective behavioral patterns in communication with others
- Destructive and dissociated world views - Dysfunctional cultural behavior and perception - Cultural isolation - Dysfunctional family dynamics, e.g., due to alcohol-dependent parents, etc. - Lack of intimacy and contact with others	- Social isolation - Socially low income class with economic and financial problems - Poor economic climate - Structural violence in society (social injustice) - Unhealthy environmental conditions - Poor working conditions

TABLE 15.2: Etiology of somatic dysfunction of the hyoid bone (after George)[150a]

tissue–energy patterns does not fully exploit the potential for prevention and healing, because every case of ill health is reflected in at least these four aspects (adapted from George).[150]

According to the AQAL model, the main focus in treatment is less on analytical and reductionist diagnosis of the disease, and more on recognizing the holonic character of every somatic dysfunction. It also becomes clear that it would be impossible to separate the examiner (or practitioner) from the object of examination (or patient). Recognition of the holonic and holarchic pattern of relationship and dynamics is fundamental in the treatment.

Human bodies as well as physiological phenomena or symptoms are linked one with another in a non-local, non-causal way and are facets of a multi-dimensional, holarchical order. A change occurring during therapeutic interaction therefore permeates all aspects of human existence, not only the physical or psychological.

Every pattern is characterized by a specific motion in space and time and by a particular oscillating infolding and unfolding. It reflects the relationship between different, apparently separate phenomena. Recognition of patterns of relationship (of different interacting tissues and patterns of motion in space and time, and also the interrelationship of different patterns, their rhythms and their significance for the patient) is important. This approach makes it clear (depending on breadth of perspective) how one pattern is contained within another, etc. For example, a particular interrelationship of function and structure such as abdominal pain can be contained within an energy pattern; this in turn within a pattern of consciousness; and that within a familial pattern or a particular social pattern, and so on. The whole is expressed in the patterns of interacting networks of relationship, so that the patterns enable us to discover the whole.

The aim of our therapeutic procedure is not necessarily to change the patterns, but to allow the information that arises from the whole to appear, so that it becomes possible for the patient to perceive the relationship to the whole. A certain dynamic emerges in this process, together with a field in which a change and transmutation of the somatic dysfunction can occur. The practitioner cannot foresee what specific form the change will actually take.

The aim is not primarily to achieve a symptom-free state, but to bring about health or wholeness in the form of a greater order or higher complexity. The idea of health as wholeness and being at one with oneself is contained in the fact that both words (health and wholeness) derive from the same Anglo-Saxon word "haelan."

Dysfunction from the perspective of the holarchic organization of regulation

The organization of regulation is structured in a holarchic way. Each level of regulation maintains integrity in its own specific way. Each higher level encompasses and integrates the lower one. An example that makes this plain is the capacity of higher neural levels to inhibit lower ones.

Example: the phylogenetic shift in the neural regulation of the autonomic nervous system passes through three stages, each associated with a specific behavioral strategy. The higher and more recent centers inhibit the lower, older centers:[151]

1 Primitive, unmyelinated visceral vagus: fosters digestion and responds to threat by depressing metabolic activity.

2 Sympathetic nervous system: capable of increasing metabolic output and inhibiting the primitive visceral vagus to foster mobilization behaviors necessary for "fight or flight."

3 The third stage, unique to mammals and to humans in particular, is characterized by a myelinated vagus. The sympathetic structures are inhibited. The myeli-

nated vagus is able to rapidly regulate cardiac output to foster engagement with or disengagement from the environment. The mammalian vagus is neuroanatomically linked to the cranial nerves (CN V, VII, IX, X, XI) that regulate facial expression and vocalization.

In the normal situation, when individuals feel sufficiently safe, they respond to stress via the myelinated vagus. In cases where this response is not successful (or in traumatized patients, for example) there is progressive disinhibition of the lower structures, first in the form of sympathetic response and finally in a stage of immobility.

The lower levels then define the framework of possibilities for the higher. The lower levels are contained in, and present in, higher or later stages of development. This means that even when mammals and humans go beyond the exclusively sympathetic response state, it nevertheless remains fundamentally important to their well-being and their survival. Even if the human body goes beyond simple physics, it is still subject to physical laws.

The higher developmental levels are not contained in the lower, however, and so cannot be defined in terms of them. For example, neocortical organization cannot be reduced to the biological regulatory mechanisms of the reptilian brain, cells, or the laws of physics. Although it is true that the laws of physics and those that govern cells and the reptilian brain still apply in neocortical organization, the properties of the neocortex go far beyond them (see below). This means that therapeutic approaches that take their direction only from lower evolutionary stages such as quantum physics, for example, are not necessarily appropriate for higher stages of development, since they only comprehend part (in this case the quantum physics part) of the higher developmental stages. (The laws of quantum physics apply equally when we are dealing with atoms, molecules, stones, coffee cups, plants, animals, and human beings, but human beings possess other qualities that stones and coffee cups do not have.) Likewise, approaches that claim to be holistic, but make no hierarchical distinction in the developmentally determined manifestation of certain organizational principles, are not really working holistically, because they cannot do justice to the various significant issues that have resulted from that development.

The following categories are mainly based on those differentiated by Zweedijk, and in part on the triune brain as described by MacLean:[152]

- The cellular level.[153] Cells require nutrition, and need to dispose of metabolites, etc. They communicate with their environment; for example, the cell membrane reacts to the slightest changes in its surroundings (pH, tension, temperature, etc.). The cell possesses autocrine regulation, meaning that it regulates itself by means of self-produced cytokines, and is influenced by growth factors, enzymes, prostaglandins, and neurotransmitters. It is a form of regulation retained in single-cell organisms to this day, but this stage is also present in humans. If something goes wrong at this level in mammals, it can find expression in the form of cancer, for example. When osteopaths palpate tissue, then (along with much else) they exert an influence on this level.

- The tissue level. As cells differentiate and become ordered in characteristic spatial patterns, this enables increased cooperation by cells and increasing complexity through evolution.[154] Multicellular assemblies of cells such as connective and epithelial tissue, etc. are regulated by similar substances to those that operate on the cellular level, e.g., cytokinins, interleukins, histamines, prostaglandins, etc. Tissue organization, cell growth, and cell differentiation are also regulated by direct interactions with the cytoskeleton by means of integrins (heterodimeric transmembrane proteins). This tissue organization is also found in primitive life forms such as molluscs. Despite lacking a nervous system, they are able to communicate with each other, by producing chemical substances transported via intercellular fluid and vascular systems or by means of tensegrity structures. This level is also present in humans and may exhibit dysfunction. Here, too, pathologies can arise, e.g., in the form of certain kinds of cancer, bone tumors, leukemias, etc. From the functional point of view, it is possible for example to correct local regulatory functions of tissue regions. Imbalances, e.g., in skin metabolism, can be improved by changes in diet, sport, fresh air, water, and sunshine; increased

tension, and loss of elasticity or mobility in soft tissues can be normalized by total body adjustment or general osteopathic treatment, etc.

- The intrinsic plexus. In the animal kingdom, for example in starfish and sea urchins, we find a nervous system with afferent and efferent nerves but no central nervous system. In humans we find these in such places as the urogenital system and myenteric plexus of the gastrointestinal tract. Marked pathology on this level is expressed for example as achalasia, pylorospasm, or megacolon. The osteopath will work on this level by taking up palpatory contact with the intestine, for example, and releasing abnormal endodermal tensions, to enable the reestablishment of relative autonomy and improvement of the functional dysregulation between the intramural nervous plexus and, for example, the tissue in the digestive tract. In some cases therapy will also need to be given on a higher level, such as the celiac ganglion or inferior mesenteric ganglion, or possibly on a still higher level in the paleocortical part of the conditioned reflexes, etc.

- The extrinsic nervous system; archicortex, or reptilian brain. In humans this comprises the spinal cord, the brainstem, and a small part of the mesencephalon and cerebellum. Their function is primarily reflex and instinctive in nature, and includes visceral or glandular regulation and that of sleeping and waking. The capacity for conditioned learning is not yet present at this level, although awareness of species would appear to be. In humans too, this level is still effective in the form of regulation of essential functions through the connection between the brainstem and spinal cord, etc. with the periphery (e.g., in the form of the organs). The extrinsic nervous system regulates organ functions and integrates them with other body functions, and through the production of neurotransmitters it also influences the intrinsic nervous system. This is the level of somatic dysfunctions in the narrower sense (models according to Korr). Dysfunction of a vertebra, for example, can impair organ function.

- The oldest mammalian brain/limbic system. In humans, this comprises the limbic system arranged around the third ventricle (the thalamus, hypothalamus, etc.). This level of organization introduces feelings/emotions into the regulation of the body as a whole. Basic needs such as hunger, thirst, sexuality, fear and aggression are regulated in the limbic system. This level encompasses and integrates the extrinsic nervous system. On this level, learning in the sense of conditioning is possible for animals and humans. The processing of information is much more primitive than in the case of the neocortex, but more rapid and better suited for survival reactions. Emotions in this sense are the conscious experience of a greater interplay of physiological reactions, and serve to monitor the activity of the body's biological systems and adapt them to the necessities of the internal and external environment.[155] According to Servan-Schreiber, the limbic system is far more easily accessible through the body than by means of language. Fear is not learned through the neocortex, but through the limbic system. These fear patterns can be temporarily blocked by the prefrontal cortex, but persist in the limbic system.[156] Diseases such as anorexia nervosa may have their roots here. On this level, the osteopath can promote integration by such means as compression of the third ventricle; however, this is a mechanical method and so is limited and reductionist, because this level of organization goes far beyond an exclusively tissue level. There is again a very close connection between somatic dysfunction and this level (see also p. 231ff.).

- The more recent mammalian brain/neocortex. This developmental level has taken place only in certain mammals and above all in humans. The complexity of organization has increased massively, and has the potential to integrate and inhibit or partially suppress all other levels of organization. Symbols of language and logic, self-reflection, associative cognitive thought, belief, knowledge, art and cognitive thought are aspects of this developmental stage. In humans, the prefrontal cortex in particular is greatly enlarged as compared with all other mammals, and controls attention, concentration, inhibition, and suppression of impulses and instincts, governs social relations and moral behavior and is capable of symbolic thought. In the mental sphere, the neocortex brings the possibility for a person to "think themselves into being ill." When we think that we are becoming ill, these thoughts foster a weakening of the immune system. These processes are initiated by consciously or (usually) unconsciously operating systems of belief, which may be subjective or intersubjective and cultural. Health can also be adversely affected by the neocortex through exaggerated control or suppression of the emotional life, since minor indications and alarm signals from the limbic system are no longer consciously perceived. Dissociations on this level are difficult to correct by purely osteopathic treatment; however, recognition of this level is of essential importance for all treatment. The more practitioners are able to recognize their own inner world, the more they will be able to establish contact with the patient on this level in an empathetic, conscious, and competent way.

Somatic dysfunction and the new physics

The new physics has forced a revision of many dogmas stemming from Newtonian paradigms in physics, and has dispersed the reductionism of Newtonian linearity and revolutionized our understanding of the physical world. Quantum physics gives expression to a coherence, unity, and wholeness on the physical level. We can to some extent see it as representing the unitary deep structure of the physical level that underlies the explicate surface structure of the elementary particles.[157]

Models from quantum physics can make pronouncements about quantum reality and non-living matter/energy, that is, about the mutual influence and the wholeness of subatomic levels of existence. Quantum reality is also fundamental for all subsequent evolutionary stages of development; it underlies them. As a result not only non-living natural objects, but also plants, animals, and humans are subject to its laws. It therefore seems necessary to take quantum reality into account in osteopathic treatment.

Chapter 3 presents the insights of quantum physics and their possible consequences and interactions with regard to biological life in a clear and comprehensive way linked to practice, together with their implications for integrative treatment of human patients.

However, we should avoid treating realities of quantum physics as an absolute and reducing all existence, along with the whole of human experience and therapeutic interaction to this level; being human is not just limited to the laws of quantum physics, but is also confronted with phenomena belonging to many fields: biological life, emotional and mental levels, and spiritual experience. This means that, although as human beings we are also subject to the laws of quantum physics, at the same time we go far beyond simple quantum reality, so that in osteopathic treatment we must likewise take account of particular physiologies, sensations, feelings, and thoughts, as well as the links that bind the person into a cultural life and social or biosocial systems and correlations of matter, energy, and consciousness on all levels.

Indeterminism, non-locality, observer effect, and interbeing in quantum physics

Quantum physics explains the fundamental workings of things in the everyday world and the elemental components of that world. Some of these aspects also reveal important ideas from an osteopathic perspective, and these will be discussed here.

At a subatomic level the position and momentum of a subatomic particle can never be measured simultaneously (indeterminism). Like this uncertainty relation, therapeutic test methods can also only ever measure partial aspects and, depending on what is being tested, other aspects are relegated to the background.

In quantum physics it is possible that correlations between particles are not bound/linked to fields and do not diminish with increasing distance (non-locality). Sheldrake conducted a number of experiments which indicate that, by morphic resonance, activity patterns are able to operate non-locally in a way that is not attenuated by spatial or temporal distance.[158,159]

Particularly given the imprecise nature of unobserved quantum particles, these are not isolated units; instead, in this dynamic process of interactions, each point in a system is always informed about the whole. Any elementary particles that have mass or energy contact with each other in any way whatsoever are connected or quantum entangled with each other in informational and energetic terms (interbeing). Interbeing and interconnectedness also exist on the structural–physiological level and between patient and interacting surroundings.

In the subatomic realm there are no isolated "particles"; instead there exists a complicated network of energetic inter-relationships in which everything is connected to everything and – in quantum physics terms – that which we customarily think of as solid matter consists of light, vibration, information, resonance, etc. (relativization of the concept of matter).

Depending on experimental design, light can be measured in quantum physics either as particles or waves. This means that the researcher and the observation/experimental design convert possibilities into reality (observer effect). In the therapeutic interaction too the way in which osteopathy is "observed," i.e., its conscious and unconscious perspectives and patterns of belief, influences the examination as well as the therapeutic interaction and the healing process in the patient.

One example of quantum physics influences on biological systems can be illustrated by the experiment conducted by Kaznacheyev and Mikhailova in which a viral disease was transferred from one cell culture to another cell culture in a separate glass flask by electromagnetic waves or biophotons.[160] Information and energy transfer phenomena familiar from quantum physics also operate simultaneously in primarily neural and humoral function circuits.

Biodynamic and biokinetic forces according to Becker

Becker's model of biodynamic and biokinetic forces emerged from reflection on his therapeutic experience and represents a rather personal perspective on somatic dysfunction.

A "total rhythmic balanced interchange" relating to the system as a whole is taking place: between body physiology, life (motion in space and time relationships), and environmental processes (genetic factors, trauma, diseases of all kinds, physical and psychological stress, and nutritional factors).[161]

Biodynamic energy describes health or the bioenergy of health. This comes into being at conception and ends at death.[162] During a traumatic event, vectors of force or biokinetic energy (K) enter the bioenergetic systems (D) of the body. Becker expresses this as: $D + K = DK$. The concept of "biokinetic energy" covers the forces that exert an effect on the body and act as pathogenic/disturbing factors: physical traumas, psychological traumas, infections, poisoning, faulty nutrition, etc.[163]

The incoming environmental energy induces a change in the patterns of the body's fluid matrix (with effects down to the cellular level), a new functional pattern in the body and the development of tissue tensions, which may still be present in the tissue years later. It produces the following consequences: imprinting of the nervous system (by afferent stimulation as a result of changed fluid patterns), a change in arterial supply and venolymphatic drainage of the affected tissue and the development of a somatic dysfunction.[164,165] There is an environmental energy field, which forms part of the tension pattern, and a compensatory mechanism on the part of the body, which forms the somatic dysfunction in its anatomical and physiological aspects and which is the body's own energy field.[166] The somatic dysfunction is a kind of response to these forces; together with the environmental energy it forms a complex. Account needs to be taken of both the somatic dysfunction and the environmental energy in order to release this complex, in diagnosis and in treatment.[167]

The "potency" is continually working to direct these biokinetic forces back into the external world, in a process that Becker himself sees as mysterious, and which he describes as "something happens," with the aim of achieving a better state of health. The degree to which it achieves this depends on the strength of the biokinetic forces. This process unfolds during the hours to weeks following the trauma.

In patients in whom the process was not successful, or in acute cases, biokinetic forces are active. The osteopath examines the bioenergetic factors. The treatment assists the "potency" in its work of releasing excessive biokinetic energy to the external world.

Findings in somatic dysfunctions

According to Fryette, the good practitioner should be able to identify and normalize the majority of adverse factors by appropriate assessment and treatments,[168] even though every practitioner is preconditioned in terms of assessment, meaning that a bias toward favorite dysfunctions can never be ruled out entirely.

The most important assessment findings in the osteopathic model of somatic dysfunction are today characterized by the following abbreviations/acronyms:

TART[169] (first described by Denslow in 1947 as ART[170]): "T" – tenderness; "A" – asymmetry of

motion and relative position; "R" – restriction of motion; "T" – tissue texture change.

STAR:[171] "S" – sensitivity (abnormal tenderness); "T" – tissue texture change such as altered tone, laxity; "A" – asymmetry (malalignment); "R" – range of motion and pliability reduction.

The TART or STAR designation does not constitute a diagnosis but merely reflects observed phenomena. Further assessments would be necessary from an osteopathic perspective in order to clarify causal, temporal, hierarchical, and physiological inter-relationships.

According to Chauffour and Prat, the individual osteopathic lesion is the smallest identifiable osteopathic lesion found during the general examination. In particular it characterizes a disturbed tissue quality that leads to a palpatory diagnosis. For Chauffour and Prat, restriction of mobility plays a secondary role in diagnosis. In their view, testing for mobility is a major source of error and positional imbalances are often an adaptation.[172]

The somatic dysfunction also involves sliding and gliding functions in the assessment of fascial structures.[173]

Additional possible palpatory parameters of relevance in the assessment of somatic dysfunction may include: temperature, pliability restriction/tissue elasticity (resistence/resilience), density, hardness, rigidity, laxity, instability, ability to slide, glide, and accommodate to the movements of adjacent structures, viscosity, tension, adherence, vibrational frequency, alignment, positional displacement, shifting of the fulcrum/axis in three-dimensional space, tissue hernias, compressive/decompressive forces.

Observation of posture,[174] and even gestures of the patient [175] may be used for the assessment of somatic dysfunctions.

In osteopathic treatment, the foremost concern is not the naming of the disease, but rather an understanding of the organization of the body and person in its unity of form and function, in relation to the whole and to the social, familial, and cultural environment; of the importance of somatic dysfunctions in the emergence of disturbances in an individual's state of health and the development of disease symptoms.[176]

References

[1]Licciardone JC. Osteopathic research: elephants, enigmas, and evidence. Osteopath Med Prim Care 2007;1:7.

[2]Fryer G. Somatic dysfunction: updating the concept. Australian Journal of Osteopathy 1999;10:14–19.

[3]Fryer G. Paraspinal muscles and intervertebral dysfunction: part one. J Manipulative Physiol Ther 2004;27:267–74.

[4]Fryer G. Paraspinal muscles and intervertebral dysfunction: part two. J Manipulative Physiol Ther 2004;27:348–57.

[5]Fryer G, Gibbons P, Morris T. The relation between thoracic paraspinal tissues and pressure sensitivity measured by a digital algometer. J Osteopath Med 2004;7:64–69.

[6]Lederman E. The fall of the postural–structural–biomechanical model in manual and physical therapies: exemplified by lower back pain. J Bodyw Move Ther 2011;15:131–38.

[7]Fryer G. Research and osteopathy: an interview with Dr. Gary Fryer by Helge Franke. J Bodyw Move Ther 2010;14:304–08.

[8]Korr IM. The emerging concept of the osteopathic lesion. J Am Osteopath Assoc 1948;48:127–38 (reprinted in J Am Osteopath Assoc 2000;100:449–60).

[9]Still AT. Osteopathy Research and Practice. Kirksville: The Journal Printing Company; 1910.

[10]Still AT. The Philosophy and Mechanical Principles of Osteopathy. Kirksville: Journal Printing Company; 1902.

[11]Parsons J, Marcer N. Osteopathy: Models for Diagnosis, Treatment and Practice. Edinburgh: Churchill Livingstone/Elsevier; 2006.

[12]Hulett G. A Textbook of the Principles of Osteopathy. Kirksville: Journal Printing Company; 1903:76.

[13]Hulett G. A Textbook of the Principles of Osteopathy. Kirksville: Journal Printing Company; 1903:76.

[14]McConnell CP. The Practice of Osteopathy. Kirksville: Journal Printing Company; 1906.

[15]Still AT. The Philosophy and Mechanical Principles of Osteopathy. Kirksville: Journal Printing Company; 1902.

[16]Korr IM. The emerging concept of the osteopathic lesion. J Am Osteopath Assoc 1948;48:127–38 (reprinted in J Am Osteopath Assoc 2000;100:449–60).

[17]McConnell CP. The Practice of Osteopathy. Kirksville: Journal Printing Company; 1906.

[18]Downing CH. Principles and Practice of Osteopathy. Kansas City: Williams Publishing Company; 1923.

[19]McCole GM. An Analysis of the Osteopathic Lesion. Great Falls, Montana: GM McCole; 1935.

[20]Still AT. Osteopathy Research and Practice. Kirksville: The Journal Printing Company; 1910.

[21]Downing CH. Osteopathic Principles in Disease. San Francisco: Orozco; 1935.

[22]Littlejohn JM. The Science of Osteopathy: Its Value in Preventing and Curing Disease. Boston: Crosby; 1900.

[23]Downing CH. Osteopathic Principles in Disease. San Francisco: Orozco; 1935.

[24]Hulett G. A Textbook of the Principles of Osteopathy. Kirksville: Journal Printing Company; 1903:76–77.

[25]McCole GM. An Analysis of the Osteopathic Lesion. Great Falls, Montana: GM McCole; 1935.

[26]MacDonald G.The Osteopathic Lesion. Kirksville: USA Medical Books; 1935.

[27]Parsons J, Marcer N. Osteopathy: Models for Diagnosis, Treatment and Practice. Edinburgh: Churchill Livingstone/Elsevier; 2006.

[28]Parsons J, Marcer N. Osteopathy: Models for Diagnosis, Treatment and Practice. Edinburgh: Churchill Livingstone/Elsevier; 2006.

[29]Burns L. A Contribution to the Study of The Pathology of the Vertebral Lesion. Bulletin no. 4. Chicago: AT Still Research Institute; 1917.

[30]Burns L. Further Contributions to the Study of The Effects of Lumbar Lesions. Bulletin no. 5. Chicago: AT Still Research Institute; 1917.

[31]Burns L, Chandler L, Rice R. Pathogenesis of Visceral Disease Following Vertebral Lesions. Chicago: American Osteopathic Association; 1948:347.

[32]Burns L, Chandler L, Rice R. Pathogenesis of Visceral Disease Following Vertebral Lesions. Chicago: American Osteopathic Association; 1948:347.

[33]Denslow JS. An analysis of the variability of spinal reflex thresholds. J Neurophysiol 1944;7:207–15.

[34]Korr IM. The emerging concept of the osteopathic lesion. J Am Osteopath Assoc 1948;48:127–38 (reprinted in J Am Osteopath Assoc 2000;100:449–60).

[35]Korr IM. The neural basis of the osteopathic lesion. J Am Osteopath Assoc 1947;47:191–98.

[36]Korr IM. The neural basis of the osteopathic lesion. J Am Osteopath Assoc 1947;47:191–98.

[37]Still AT. Osteopathy Research and Practice. Kirksville: The Journal Printing Company; 1910.

[38]Still AT. The Philosophy and Mechanical Principles of Osteopathy. Kirksville: Journal Printing Company; 1902.

[39]Patterson MM. The osteopathic lesion as a factor in disease. J Am Osteopath Assoc 2001;101:456.

[40]Korr IM. Clinical significance of the facilitated state. J Am Osteopath Assoc 1955;54:277–82.

[41]Korr IM. Clinical significance of the facilitated state. J Am Osteopath Assoc 1955;54:277–82.

[42]Korr IM. The neural basis of the osteopathic lesion. J Am Osteopath Assoc 1947;47:191–98.

[43]Parsons J, Marcer N. Osteopathy: Models for Diagnosis, Treatment and Practice. Edinburgh: Churchill Livingstone/Elsevier; 2006.

[44]Educational Council on Osteopathic Principles (ECOP). Glossary of Osteopathic Terminology. AACOM; 2009. http://www.aacom.org/resources/bookstore/Documents/GOT2009ed.pdf

[45]Sommerfeld P. Personal communication. 2002.

[46]Chauffour P, Prat E. Mechanical Link: Fundamental Principles, Theory and Practice Following an Osteopathic Approach. Berkeley/CA: North Atlantic Books; 2002:23.

[47]Chauffour P, Prat E. Mechanical Link: Fundamental Principles, Theory and Practice Following an Osteopathic Approach. Berkeley/CA: North Atlantic Books; 2002:27.

[48]Fossum C. Osteopathische Sicht des viszeralen Systems. In: Liem T, Dobler T, Puylaert M: Leitfaden viszerale Osteopathie. Munich: Elsevier; 2014.

[49]Fryer G. Research and osteopathy: an interview with Dr. Gary Fryer by Helge Franke. J Bodyw Move Ther 2010;14:304–08.

[50]Fryer G, Gibbons P, Morris T. The relation between thoracic paraspinal tissues and pressure sensitivity measured by a digital algometer. J Osteopath Med 2004;7:64–69.

[51]Degenhardt BF, Snider KT, Snider EJ, Johnson JC. Interobserver reliability of osteopathic palpatory diagnostic tests of the lumbar spine: improvements from consensus training. J Am Osteopath Assoc 2010;110:579–86.

[52]Fryer G, Gibbons P, Morris T. The relation between thoracic paraspinal tissues and pressure sensitivity measured by a digital algometer. J Osteopath Med 2004;7:64–69.

[53]Degenhardt BF, Johnson JC, Snider KT, Snider EJ. Maintenance and improvement of interobserver reliability of osteopathic palpatory tests over a 4-month period. J Am Osteopath Assoc 2010;110: 465–73.

[54]Hafen-Bardella C. Reliabilitätsstudie über die Befunderhebung der Wirbelsäule nach der Methode der Lien Mécanique Ostéopathique. Master's thesis: Donau Universität Krems; 2009.

[55]Halma KD, Degenhardt BF, Snider KT, Johnson JC, Flaim MS, Bradshaw D. Intraobserver reliability of cranial strain patterns as evaluated by osteopathic physicians: a pilot tudy. J Am Osteopath Assoc 2008;108:493–502.

[56]Anker S. Interrater-Reliabilität bei der Beurteilung der Körpersprache nach dem Fasziendistorsionsmodell (FDM). Donau Universität Krems; 2011.

[57]Fryer G. Paraspinal muscles and intervertebral dysfunction: part one. J Manipulative Physiol Ther 2004;27:267–74.

[58]Fryer G. Paraspinal muscles and intervertebral dysfunction: part two. J Manipulative Physiol Ther 2004;27:348–57.

[59]Liem T. Pitfalls and challenges involved in the process of perception and interpretation of palpatory findings. Int J Osteopath Med 2014 (accepted for publication).

[60]Liem T. Pitfalls and challenges involved in the process of perception and interpretation of palpatory findings. Int J Osteopath Med 2014 (accepted for publication).

[61]Degenhardt BF, Johnson JC, Snider KT, Snider EJ. Maintenance and improvement of interobserver reliability of osteopathic palpatory tests over a 4-month period. J Am Osteopath Assoc 2010;110: 465–73.

[62]Degenhardt BF, Snider KT, Snider EJ, Johnson JC. Interobserver reliability of osteopathic palpatory diagnostic tests of the lumbar spine: improvements from consensus training. J Am Osteopath Assoc 2010;110:579–86.

[63]Chauffour P, Prat E. Mechanical Link: Fundamental Principles, Theory and Practice Following an Osteopathic Approach. Berkeley/CA: North Atlantic Books; 2002:29.

[64]Chauffour P, Prat E. Mechanical Link: Fundamental Principles, Theory and Practice Following an Osteopathic Approach. Berkeley/CA: North Atlantic Books; 2002:29–30.

[65]Chauffour P, Prat E. Mechanical Link: Fundamental Principles, Theory and Practice Following an Osteopathic Approach. Berkeley/CA: North Atlantic Books; 2002:28.

[66]Chauffour P, Prat E. Mechanical Link: Fundamental Principles, Theory and Practice Following an Osteopathic Approach. Berkeley/CA: North Atlantic Books; 2002:28.

[67]Chauffour P, Prat E. Mechanical Link: Fundamental Principles, Theory and Practice Following an Osteopathic Approach. Berkeley/CA: North Atlantic Books; 2002:28.

[68]Mitchell FL. Muscle Energy Manual. Volume I. East Lansing, MI: MET Press; 1995.

[69]Parsons J, Marcer N. Osteopathy: Models for Diagnosis, Treatment and Practice. Edinburgh: Churchill Livingstone/Elsevier; 2006:30.

[70]Zink JG, Lawson W. An osteopathic structural examination and functional interpretation of the soma. Osteopathic Annals 1979;7:12–19.

[71]Hoover HV. Diagnosis and treatment of lesion patterns and complicated lesions. J Am Osteopath Assoc 1953;52:553–55.

[72]Fryette HH. Principles of Osteopathic Technic. Carmel, CA: Academy of Applied Osteopathy; 1954.

[73]Fossum C. Osteopathische Sicht des viszeralen Systems. In: Liem T, Dobler T, Puylaert M: Leitfaden viszerale Osteopathie. Munich: Elsevier; 2014.

[74]Fossum C. Osteopathische Sicht des viszeralen Systems. In: Liem T, Dobler T, Puylaert M: Leitfaden viszerale Osteopathie. Munich: Elsevier; 2014.

[75]Jänig W.Sympathetic nervous system and inflammation: A conceptual view. Auton Neurosci 2014;182:4–14.

[76]King HH, Jänig W, Patterson MM (eds.). The Science and Clinical Application of Manual Therapy. Edinburgh: Churchill Livingstone/Elsevier; 2011.

[77]Patterson M, Wurster RD. Somatic dysfunction, spinal facilitation, and viscerosomatic integration. In: Chila AG (ed). Foundations of Osteopathic Medicine. Philadelphia: Lippincott Williams & Wilkins; 2011.

[78]Willard FH, Jerome JA, Elkiss ML. Nociception and pain: the essence of pain lies mainly in the brain. In: Chila AG (ed). Foundations of Osteopathic Medicine. Philadelphia: Lippincott Williams & Wilkins; 2011.

[79]Korr IM. The spinal cord as organizer of disease processes: some preliminary perspectives. J Am Osteopath Assoc 1976;76:35–45.

[80]Korr IM. The spinal cord as organizer of disease processes: III. Hyperactivity of sympathetic innervation as a common factor in disease. J Am Osteopath Assoc 1979;79:232–37.

[81]Korr IM. The spinal cord as organizer of disease processes: II. The peripheral autonomic nervous system. J Am Osteopath Assoc 1979;79:82–90.

[82]Korr IM. Abstract: Skin resistance patterns associated with visceral disease. Federation Proceedings 1949;8:87.

[83]Page LE. Osteopathic Fundamentals. Kirksville: Journal Printing Company; 1927.

[84]Burns L.Viscero-somatic and somato-visceral spinal reflexes. 1907 . Reprinted in J Am Osteopath Assoc 2000;100:249–58.

[85]Patterson MM, Howell JN (eds.). The Central Connection: Somatovisceral/Viscerosomatic Interaction. Athens, OH: University Classics; 1992.

[86]Patterson MM, Howell JN (eds.). The Central Connection: Somatovisceral/Viscerosomatic Interaction. Athens, OH: University Classics; 1992.

[87]Patterson MM, Wurster RD. Neurophysiologic mechanisms of integration and disintegration. In: Ward RC (ed.). Foundations for Osteopathic Medicine. Philadelphia: Lippincott, Williams & Wilkins; 2003:120–36.

[88]Korr IM. The neural basis of the osteopathic lesion. J Am Osteopath Assoc 1947;47:191–98.

[89]Van Buskirk RL. Nociceptive reflexes and the somatic dysfunction: a model. J Am Osteopath Assoc 1990;90:792–94.

[90]Patterson MM. Spinal responses: static or dynamic? J Am Osteopath Assoc 1972;72:156–62.

[91]Patterson MM. A model mechanism for spinal segmental facilitation. J Am Osteopath Assoc 1976;76:62–72.

[92]Patterson MM. Louisa Burns Memorial Lecture 1980: The spinal cord – active processor not passive transmitter. J Am Osteopath Assoc 1980;80:210–16.

[93]Patterson MM, Grau JW (eds.). Spinal Cord Plasticity: Alterations in Reflex Function. Boston: Kluwer Academic Publishers; 2011.

[94]Patterson MM, Steinmetz JE. Long-lasting alterations of spinal reflexes: a potential basis for somatic dysfunction. Manual Medicine 1986;2:38–42.

[95]Patterson MM, Wurster RD. Neurophysiologic mechanisms of integration and disintegration. In: Ward RC (ed.). Foundations for Osteopathic Medicine. Philadelphia: Lippincott, Williams & Wilkins; 2003:120–36.

[96]Woolf CJ, Salter MW. Neuronal plasticity: increasing the gain in pain. Science 2000;288:1765–68.

[97]Patterson MM, Wurster RD. Neurophysiologic mechanisms of integration and disintegration. In: Ward RC (ed.). Foundations for Osteopathic Medicine. Philadelphia: Lippincott, Williams & Wilkins; 2003:120–36.

[98]Groves PM, DeMarco R, Thompson RF. Habituation and sensitization of spinal interneuron activity in acute spinal cat. Brain Research 1969;14:521–55.

[99]Pinsker HM, Hening WA, Carew TJ, Kandel ER. Long-term sensitization of a defensive withdrawal reflex in Aplysia. Science 1973;182:1039–42.

[100]Patterson MM. Spinal fixation: long-term alterations in spinal reflex excitability. In: Patterson MM, Grau JW. Spinal Cord Plasticity: Alterations in Reflex Function. Boston: Kluwer Academic Publishers; 2011:77–100.

[101]Patterson MM, Wurster RD. Neurophysiologic mechanisms of integration and disintegration. In: Ward RC (ed.). Foundations for Osteopathic Medicine. Philadelphia: Lippincott, Williams & Wilkins; 2003:120–36.

[102]Wolpaw JR. Spinal cord plasticity in the acquisition of a simple motor skill. In: Patterson MM, Grau JW. Spinal Cord Plasticity: Alterations in Reflex Function. Boston: Kluwer Academic Publishers; 2011:101–26.

[103]Korr IM. The neural basis of the osteopathic lesion. J Am Osteopath Assoc 1947;47:191–98.

[104]Denslow JS, Korr IM, Krems AD. Quantitative studies of chronic facilitation in human motoneuron pools. Am J Physiol 1947;150:229–38.

[105]Jänig W. Pain and the sympathetic nervous system: pathophysiological mechanisms. In: Mathias CJ, Bannister R. Autonomic Failure: A Textbook of Clinical Disorders of the Autonomic Nervous System. Oxford: Oxford University Press; 2013:236–46.

[106]Jänig W. Autonomic nervous system and pain. In: Basbaum AI, Bushnell MC (eds.). Science of Pain. San Diego, CA: Academic Press; 2009:193–225.

[107]Grachev I, Fredrickson B, Apkarian A. Abnormal brain chemistry in chronic back pain: an in vivo proton magnetic resonance spectroscopy study. Pain 2000;89:7–18.

[108]Jänig W. Pain and the sympathetic nervous system. In: Squire LR (ed.). Encyclopedia of Neuroscience. Volume 7. Oxford: Academic Press; 2009:371–83.

[109]Jänig W. Pain and the sympathetic nervous system: pathophysiological mechanisms. In: Mathias CJ, Bannister R. Autonomic Failure: A Textbook of Clinical Disorders of the Autonomic Nervous System. Oxford: Oxford University Press; 2013:236–46.

[110]Jänig W. Pain and the sympathetic nervous system: pathophysiological mechanisms. In: Mathias CJ, Bannister R. Autonomic Failure: A Textbook of Clinical Disorders of the Autonomic Nervous System. Oxford: Oxford University Press; 2013:236–46.

[111]Jänig W. Author comment: Autonomic reactions in pain. Pain 2012;153:733–35.

[112]Fryer G. Somatic dysfunction: updating the concept. Australian Journal of Osteopathy 1999;10:14–19.

[113]Bernard C. Memoir on the Pancreas. New York: Academic Press; 1974 (translation of 1856 original).

[114]Cannon WB. Bodily Changes in Pain, Hunger, Fear, and Rage. New York: Appleton; 1915.

[115]Cannon WB. Organization for physiological homeostasis. Physiological Reviews 1929;9:399–431.

[116]Selye H. The Stress of Life. New York: McGraw-Hill; 1956/1976.

[117]Sterling P, Eyer J. Biological basis of stress-related mortality. Soc Sci Med E 1981;15:3–42.

[118]Schulkin J. Rethinking Homeostasis: Allostatic Regulation in Physiology and Pathophysiology. Cambridge, MA: MIT Press; 2003.

[119]Chrousos GP. The hypothalamic–pituitary–adrenal axis and immune-mediated inflammation. N Engl J Med 1995;332:1351–62.

[120a]Dolet JP. Biomécanique et Bioénergetique comprendre et corriger. Aix en Provence: Editions de Verlaque; 2000:125.

[120b]Chauffour P, Prat E. Mechanical Link: Fundamental Principles, Theory and Practice Following an Osteopathic Approach. Berkeley/CA: North Atlantic Books; 2002:24–26.

[121]Fryer G. Research and osteopathy: an interview with Dr. Gary Fryer by Helge Franke. J Bodyw Move Ther 2010;14:304–08.

[122]Folkman J, Moscona A. Role of cell shape in growth control. Nature 1978;273:345–49.

[123]Ingber DE, Jamieson JD. Cells as tensegrity structures: architectural regulation of histodifferentiation by physical forces transduced over basement membrane. In: Anderson LC, Gahmberg CG, Ekblom P (eds.). Gene Expression during Normal and Malignant Differentiation. St Louis, Missouri/New York: Academic Press; 1985:13–32.

[124]Ingber DE, Folkman J. Tension and compression as basic determinants of cell form and function: utilization of cellular tensegrity mechanism. In: Stein WD (ed.). Cell Shape: Determinants, Regulation and Regulatory Role. New York: Academic Press; 1989.

[125]Heidemann SR, Buxbaum RE. Mechanical tension as a regulator of axonal development. Neurotoxicology 1994;15:95–107.

[126]Singhvi R, Kumar A, Lopez G, Stephanopoulos GN, Wang DI, Whitesides GM, Ingber DE. Engineering cell shape and function. Science 1994;264:696–98.

[127]Chen CS, Mrksich M, Huang S, Whitesides GM, Ingber DE. Geometric control of cell life and death. Science 1997;276:1425–28.

[128]Stamenovic D, Coughlin MF. The role of prestress and architecture of the cytoskeleton and deformability of cytoskeletal filaments in mechanics of adherent cells: a quantitative analysis. J Theor Biol 1999;201:63–74.

[129]Harris AK, Wild P, Stopak D. Silicone rubber substrata: a new wrinkle in the study of cell locomotion. Science 1980;208:177–79.

[130]Dembo M. Mechanics and control of the cytoskeleton in Amoeba proteus. Biophys J 1989;55:1054–80.

[131]Sims JR, Karp S, Ingber DE. Altering the cellular mechanical force balance results in integrated changes in cell, cytoskeletal and nuclear shape. J Cell Sci 1992;103:1215–22.

[132]Ingber DE. Cellular tensegrity: defining new rules of biological design that govern the cytoskeleton. J Cell Sci 1993;104:613–27.

[133]Davies PF, Tripathi C. Mechanical stress mechanisms and the cell: an endothelial paradigm. Circ Res 1993;72:239–45.

[134]Wang N, Butler JP, Ingber DE. Mechanotransduction across the cell surface and through the cytoskeleton. Science 1993;260:1124–27.

[135]Wang N, Ingber DE. Control of the cytoskeletal mechanics by extracellular matrix, cell shape, and mechanical tension. Biophys J 1994;66:2181–89.

[136]Thoumine O. Control of cellular morphology by mechanical factors. J Phys III France 1996;6:1555–66.

[137]Janmey PA. The cytoskeleton and cell signalling: component localization and mechanical coupling. Physiol Rev 1998;78:763–81.

[138]Chicurel ME, Chen S, Ingber DE. Cellular control lies in the balance of forces. Curr Opin Cell Biol 1998;10:232–39.

[139]Stamenovic D, Fredberg JJ, Wang N, Butler JP, Ingber DE. A microstructural approach to cytoskeletal mechanics based on tensegrity. J Theor Biol 1996;181:125–36.

[140]Coughlin MF, Stamenovic D. A tensegrity structure with buckling compression elements: application to cell mechanics. J Appl Mech 1997;64:480–86.

[141]Coughlin MF, Stamenovic D. A tensegrity model of the cytoskeleton in spread and round cells. J Biomech Eng 1998;120:770–77.

[142]Raab C. Tensegrity. In: Liem T, Dobler T: Leitfaden Osteopathie. 2nd edn. Munich: Elsevier; 2005.

[143]Letter on Tensegrity from Buckminster Fuller, Section 1. Copyright Estate of Buckminster Fuller.

[144]Raab C: Tensegrity. In: Liem T, Dobler T: Leitfaden Osteopathie. 2nd edn. Munich: Elsevier; 2005.

[145]Oschman JL. Connective tissue as an energetic and information continuum. Structural Integration: The Journal of the Rolf Institute. August 2003.

[146]Pert CB. Molecules of Emotion. New York: Touchstone; 1999.

[147]Gershon M. The Second Brain. New York: Harper Collins; 1999.

[148]Booth RJ, Ashbridge KR. Teleological coherence: exploring the dimensions of the immune system. Scand J Immunol 1992;36:751–59.

[149]Jantsch E. The Self-Organizing Universe: Scientific and Human Implications of the Emerging Paradigm of Evolution. Oxford/New York: Pergamon Press; 1980.

[150]George LE. Integral medicine: an AQAL-based approach. AQAL Journal of Integral Theory and Practice 2006;1 (2): 38–59.

[150a]George LE: Integral Medicine. AQAL-Journal 2005;1(2):1–22

[151]Porges SW. The polyvagal theory: phylogenetic substrates of a social nervous system. Int J Psychophysiol 2001;42:123–46.

[152]Zweedijk R. Viszerale Manipulation bei Kindern. In Liem T, Schleupen A, Altmeyer P, Zweedijk, R. Osteopathische Behandlung von Kindern. Stuttgart, Haug; 2012.

[153]De Duve C. Die Zelle. Heidelberg: Spektrum der Wissenschaft; 1986.

[154]Servan-Schreiber D. Die neue Medizin der Emotionen. Munich: Verlag Antje Kunstmann; 2004:36f.

[155]LeDoux JE. The Emotional Brain: The Mysterious Underpinnings of Emotional Life. New York: Simon & Schuster; 1996.

[156]Bohm D. Wholeness and the Implicate Order. London: Routledge; 1980.

[157]Wilber K. Eye to Eye: The Quest for the New Paradigm. In: The Collected Works of Ken Wilber – vol. 3. Boston: Shambhala; 1999:275.

[158]Sheldrake R. Seven Experiments that Could Change the World. Rochester, Vermont: Park Street Press; 2002.

[159]Sheldrake R. The Presence of the Past. London: Collins; 1988.

[160]Kaznacheyev VP, Mikhailova LP. Ultraweak radiation in intercellular interactions [in Russian]. Novosibirsk: Nauka; 1981.

[161]Becker RE: Force factors with body physiology. Academy of Applied Osteopathy Yearbook 1959:89–97.

[162]Brooks RE (ed.). The Stillness of Life: The Osteopathic Philosophy of Rollin E Becker, D.O. Portland: Stillness Press; 2000;75,114–18.

[163]Brooks RE (ed.). The Stillness of Life: The Osteopathic Philosophy of Rollin E Becker, D.O. Portland: Stillness Press; 2000;75,114–18.

[164]Brooks RE (ed.). The Stillness of Life: The Osteopathic Philosophy of Rollin E Becker, D.O. Portland: Stillness Press; 2000:114.

[165]Brooks RE (ed.). The Stillness of Life: The Osteopathic Philosophy of Rollin E Becker, D.O. Portland: Stillness Press; 2000:115,118.

[166]Brooks RE (ed.). The Stillness of Life: The Osteopathic Philosophy of Rollin E Becker, D.O. Portland: Stillness Press; 2000:115,118.

[167]Wilber K. Eye to Eye: The Quest for the New Paradigm. In: The Collected Works of Ken Wilber – vol. 3. Boston: Shambhala; 1999:275.

[168]Fryette HH. Principles of Osteopathic Technic. Carmel, CA: Academy of Applied Osteopathy; 1954.

[169]Educational Council on Osteopathic Principles (ECOP). Glossary of Osteopathic Terminology. AACOM; 2009. http://www.aacom.org/resources/bookstore/Documents/GOT2009ed.pdf

[170]Denslow JS, Korr IM, Krems AD. Quantitative studies of chronic facilitation in human motoneuron pools. Am J Physiol 1947;150:229–38.

[171]Dowling DJ. STAR: a more viable alternative descriptor system of somatic dysfunction. AAOJ 1998;8:34–37.

[172]Chauffour P, Prat E. Mechanical Link: Fundamental Principles, Theory and Practice Following an Osteopathic Approach. Berkeley/CA: North Atlantic Books; 2002:23.

[173]Chaitow L. Somatic dysfunction and fascia's gliding-potential. J Bodyw Move Ther 2014;18:1–3.

[174]Myers TW. Anatomy Trains: Myofascial Meridians for Manual and Movement Therapists. 3rd edition. Edinburgh; Churchill Livingstone/Elsevier; 2013.

[175]Typaldos, Stephen. Clinical and Theoretical Application of the Fascial Distortion Model Within the Practice of Medicine and Surgery. Brewer, ME: Orthopathic Global Health Publications; 2002.

[176]Fossum C: Die somatische Dysfunktion. In: Liem T, Dobler T (eds.). Leitfaden Osteopathie. Munich: Urban und Fischer; 2002:57.

16

Thoughts on the significance of systems theory* for osteopathic diagnosis and therapy

Peter Sommerfeld

Supposing that we should carry our empirical intuition even to the very highest degree of clearness, we should not thereby advance one step nearer to a knowledge of the constitution of objects as things in themselves. For we could only, at best, arrive at a complete cognition of our own mode of intuition, that is, of our sensibility, and this under the conditions originally attaching to the subject, namely the conditions of space and time; while the question – "what are objects considered as things in themselves?" remains unanswerable even after the most thorough examination of the phenomenal world.

I. Kant, *Critique of Pure Reason*[1]

Introduction

Osteopathy is generally understood as a system of diagnostic and therapeutic methods based on the one hand on specific theoretical foundations,[†] and on the other, on various empirical findings. If we observe practicing osteopaths at work, we find it increasingly difficult to separate their actions into those performed for diagnosis and those actions carried out for therapy. From a certain point on, they seem indistinguishable; both visibly merge into a single homogeneous interventional act that we might interpret as a communicative process between osteopath and patient. Hardly a word is said in this process, however; rather, it seems to be maintained by the constant interchange of three elements: the investigative, diagnostic act, the therapeutic act and the response (reaction) of the patient. If the procedure is successful, two problems are avoided: on the one hand, an attitude of therapeutic nihilism (a description inspired by W. Wieland),[4] which would be a purely intellectual labor of understanding that completely separates diagnosis from therapy; on the other hand, the trap of diagnostic nihilism, which would separate therapeutic decisions from any labor of understanding. This leads on to the following understanding: that osteopaths investigate and treat in a single process, which appears as a continuum. This can be understood as a communicative process, and the relationship between osteopath and patient can thus be described as a system, as understood by systems theory. The tension between diagnostic and therapeutic nihilism forces the osteopath to adopt an ever-repeating but constantly changing circular process of sensing and perceiving, establishment (and assessment) of the facts, decisions and actions.

This means that for anyone involved in the practice of osteopathy it is unavoidably necessary to take both theory of knowledge and theory of action into consideration. Only by doing this can we bring the two polar opposites of perception and action into relationship in a way that might be termed therapeutically appropriate. At this point it is also worth mentioning two further basic assumptions that clear the way toward a connection between a problem of understanding and an approach to a solution by means of systems theory.

*The concept of systems theory was introduced by Bertalanffy (1950),[2] and applied and developed as an interdisciplinary approach in research in the second half of the twentieth century (also under the names of constructivism and cybernetics). Those who have worked in this field include biologists (Humberto Maturana, Francesco Varela), linguists (Ernst von Glasersfeld), sociologists (Thomas Luckmann, Niklas Luhmann), those engaged in research in neurology, cognition, and communication (Heinz von Foerster, Gregory Bateson), in the disciplines of mathematics (Norbert Wiener, John von Neumann) and information theory (Claude Shannon and Warren Weaver) for the analysis of complex situations.

†Although these are known as "osteopathic philosophy" (see, e.g., Seffinger[3]), there is some question as to whether the principles of osteopathy, or indeed osteopathy as a whole, should (as is sometimes maintained) be understood as philosophy in the academic sense. Rather, they involve paradigms that depend in many respects on the way in which osteopathy developed in the America of the late nineteenth century. This was as much historical, cultural, and geographical. It is not our concern here to examine this in detail.

Firstly, in the empirical sciences, each piece of knowledge acquired is linked in to a process that is normally based on the following four factors:[5]

1 The data, the experience itself.

2 Construction of a database.

3 Formation of a hypothesis or assumption arrived at by inductive reasoning.

4 Development, by means of a deductive procedure, of a mathematically consistent theory that will finally need to be tested again with reference to the experience(s) by applying reduction.

Setting out the process in this form clearly shows that what generally applies in the empirical sciences need not necessarily apply in medicine and its related fields. We gather the clinical data, construct a database by means of diagnostic and investigative procedures of varying specificity, and on the basis of these we build up one or more suppositions (findings, diagnoses), which direct the therapeutic intervention. There is certainly some attempt to carry out the fourth element, the deductive stage (by which a theory is constructed by conclusive mathematical deduction and formal logic)[‡] but deduction often tails off into the realm of probability theory (statistics); attempts in this direction are often less than satisfying and lag far behind the apparently stable theories of the hard sciences. Precisely the element that might guarantee the clinician a degree of certainty in making decisions is lacking.

Secondly, the manner in which perception is focused, in which links are made between the acquired experience data, and knowledge is derived from this, is dependent on the practitioner's subjective experience in the context of therapy and/or experiment, as well as on the (intersubjective) exchange of experience with colleagues. Drawing on Husserl's concept of life-world, we might speak here of a world of osteopathic experience, or life-world experience, as opposed to scientific experience with its emphasis on objectivity. We cannot take as our basis a "world out there" that is capable of objective description and independent of us. (Even for the physicist objectivity is an ideal state). What we perceive at the moment of the intervention (functional deficit; primary dysfunction, etc.) cannot be separated from the world of experience of the osteopathic community and the life-world experience of the practitioner

in that moment. In the context of a communication process with the patient that refers back to itself (i.e., is recursive), and on the basis of the current state of knowledge, we "constitute"[§] what we perceived, so as to create a basis of action or treatment. This, however, raises the question: How and why do we "constitute" this basis, or how does it become constituted?

Complexity, system and contingency

The question as to "why?" is central to the osteopathic approach. It would be possible, in principle, to take a catalogue of symptoms encountered as problems to be addressed in therapeutic practice and match them to a suitable catalogue of specific treatment techniques. This kind of "treatment by numbers" is based on a behaviorist model, in which the person carrying out the treatment performs preset procedures on an "input–output" basis, and assumes that the application of a particular therapeutic stimulus will always produce the same reaction in every patient. Here we have an entirely practical, easy-to-negotiate world in which unpredictability plays hardly any role. In such a world, clinical action could be decided by mathematical deduction. This would do away with the deficiency with regard to the four-stage procedure used in the empirical sciences, described above. However, daily experience with patients teaches us that the therapeutic reality we are usually dealing with is quite different. This is true not only in the case of therapeutic or clinical reality, but also for reality as such. There is a quite straightforward parallel here; the situation that Niklas Luhmann outlines in the preface to *Soziale Systeme* (Social Systems) as a problem for a theory of sociology can be applied to our own daily experience: "The issue, then, is the relation between complexity and transparency. One could also say, a relation between opaque and transparent complexity."[7]

[‡]Conclusions established by deductive means, such as those arrived at in mathematics or formal logic (e.g., $2+2=4$), are based on the underlying assumption of an axiomatic system (e.g., the number system).[5]

[§]I prefer to say "constitute" rather than "construct" here, in order to draw more closely on Edmund Husserl's conception of what is involved. Constructivism, a variety of systems theory, would tend to prefer the meaning of "construct," emphasizing the idea that the brain constructs reality. However, this suggests a certain one-sidedness in the way that reality comes about, which does not adequately describe the problem. Reality would then be causally dependent on our brain activity. The process implied by "constitute," on the other hand, involves a permeation of subject and world.[6]

Although unpredictability and complexity play a major role in medicine as a whole – one that is often denied – this is true in a very special sense in osteopathy. Over the past century, osteopathy has increasingly developed in a direction that is widely concerned with what are generally called "functional disturbances." The particular problem with this field that is labeled "functional" is that it is concerned with disturbances or symptom complexes for which there are often no traditional medical findings, or, when they do exist, they are hazy. Consequently they yield no clear diagnoses to indicate what the therapeutic intervention should involve. This is connected with what medicine accepts as "findings"; these are normally computable, and so quantifiable, observations (measurements) and those that are visually accessible. Some of these visual observations can be described in quantitative terms, and others in qualitative terms. The role of tactile findings, for example, if they have one, is very subordinate. Osteopathy therefore deals with a "gray area" situated between medically relevant symptom complexes and the associated diagnoses, and the resulting given treatment, and the "normal" or "healthy." I suggest that in industrialized societies this gray area appears to be growing.

I should now like to look in a little more detail at the background of system, complexity, and unpredictability. This will help to make a clearer case for the usefulness of an approach based on systems theory, or indeed "systems practice." The work of Niklas Luhmann certainly offers one of the most consistent theoretical examinations of matters relating to systems theory. I shall therefore draw on his structure and concepts in the following accounts.

System

In Luhmann's work, system is understood using a difference theory approach; a system is not a "thing" (which would be ontological), but "a system "is" the difference between system and environment."[8] That is a very formal approach, but one whose formal clarity is able to cast light on very complex matters. "System" occurs twice in this statement; once as the difference, and once within this difference, as part of the two-sided formulation of system/environment. Even on this quite formal level, then, there is a system within the system. Although this may seem paradoxical, paradoxes are one of the characteristics of systems theory arguments, and

this is particularly the case in Luhmann. Difference can also mean differentiation: making distinctions. So, what is specified is part of the two-sided formulation: in our present context (for example) what is dysfunction, and what is not. (The complete two-sided formulation would be spelled out as: dysfunction/everything else that is not this dysfunction.) This concept of system thus contains an operational component. It involves a process of distinguishing and decision making that requires time. One side is decided on (e.g., dysfunction on the left) and the other, which in the language of systems theory is called the "unmarked space," remains outside and not precisely defined. "The system [then] takes shape as a chain of operations. The difference between system and environment arises solely from the fact that an operation generates a further operation of the same type."[9] What happens, therefore, is not a once-and-for-all event that places a system in an environment, but a process that – and this is an essential aspect – is maintained by a single type of operation. This process creates differences and hence systems. Luhmann, drawing on Maturana and Varela,[10] characterizes such a process as autopoietic: one of circular self-reproduction. For Luhmann, in the case of social systems, this type of operation is communication.[11]

Contingency

Contingency is another central concept in Luhmann's thoughts on system. Here, however, it appears in an extended form as double contingency. Contingency, which is often treated together with concepts such as chance or unpredictability, can be traced (among other sources) to Aristotle, who uses the word endechó-menon[12] to describe something encompassing the tension between the impossible and the necessary. Luhmann's definition is the following:[13]

This concept results from excluding necessity and impossibility. Something is contingent insofar as it is neither necessary nor impossible; it is just what it is (or was or will be), though it could also be otherwise.

If we understand the world as being neither some deterministically operating clockwork nor uncontrollable chaos, then the appropriate expression to describe this would be contingency. If two people encounter one another, double contingency comes into play. Both parties, in our case the osteopath and the patient, are mutually subject to unpredictability; both are to a high degree contingent. A very few of the immeasurable range of possibilities for the creation of a connection are selected, in order to establish communication. Against this background it is quite remarkable that anything resembling communication does come into being. Differences, then, are set up (as discussed under the previous point) and decisions made in favor of one side of the system/environment formulations. The problem in this connection is to establish the balance between self-reference and "hetero-reference." (Self-reference involves referring to one's own states of condition, thoughts, etc. while hetero-reference attempts to react to, or to anticipate, changes in the states of the other.) This means that there are expectations relating to each side, one's own and the other, which it is necessary to work with. Tackling a problem area of that kind in terms of systems theory may be described as system formation. System formation re-establishes:

...transparency despite opaque complexity... The system is first set in motion and orients itself by the question Will the partner accept or reject a communication? or, in terms of action, will an action hurt or harm him?[14]

In the case of failure communication will not come about, hence any system formation. Considering this, any clinical context is very special because the expert has to decide and act under a high degree of uncertainty dominated by double contingency. "The behavior of others," Luhmann states:

...is indeterminable only in the situation of double contingency and specifically for the person who tries to predict it in order to use this prediction to determine his own behavior.[15]

We might say that this is the dilemma facing therapy professions. For osteopaths, the situation is a challenge to the extent that they consciously take into account the possibility that matters could always be otherwise. However, the dilemma lies in the constant threat of being overwhelmed by the demands or lapsing into a random approach to therapy, in which contingency dissolves into indifference.

Complexity

Complexity is usually understood today as a measure of the options for relationship between the elements of a system.[16,17] If, in this respect, a system is understood

as a number of elements and the relationships existing between them,[18] problems arise regarding the concept of complexity. The more elements a system contains, the more potential connections are possible, i.e., the complexity increases. Maximum complexity would then mean that every element could relate to every other element (complete interdependence). Complete interdependence implies that change on the part of one element will always affect all other elements; a situation to some extent described in popular accounts of chaos research as the butterfly effect.[19] Changes in one element would force the entire system to change. Some aspects of the discussions specific to osteopathy concerning the concept of dysfunction appear to assume such a state of affairs.

Two points in essence show the problem of the concept of complexity outlined above: the variations in complexity between environment and system, and the impossibility of complete interdependence. No system is able to construct a point-for-point relationship with its environment. It is impossible for the system to master perfectly all the potential factors of disturbance. The complexity of the "environment" element of the two-sided formulation is always greater than the complexity of its "system" element. Additional time is required for possible reaction. It has become clear in this context that, when the number of elements increases beyond a certain point, the possibility of complete interdependence becomes less and less likely. This is because it becomes impossible, even in terms of sheer time, for the system to react adequately to disturbances, because of the constant necessity of reacting to changes in the condition of all the elements involved, and time is needed for this reaction.[20] No system can realize the logical possibility of connecting every element to every other one. This is the point of departure for any reduction of complexity.[21] Systems therefore serve to reduce complexity, or are products of a reduction of complexity and thus of a selection process.[22] However, complexity so understood produces the paradox that the reduction of complexity in its turn produces complexity: the inherent complexity of the system itself. Systems therefore increase their complexity by interruptions of interdependence (termed "loose coupling"). Loose coupling means that irritation of one element no longer forces the entire system to adapt: just one specific region. From the point of view of difference theory, the complexity/simplicity distinction is replaced by the following distinction: complexity without/complexity with interruptions of interdependence (or simple/complex complexity).

Simple complexity, if we may formulate it in such paradoxical terms, is complexity that still allows everything to be linked to everything. Complex complexity is the case in which patterns of selection are necessary.[23]

According to the concept of contingency Luhmann describes the following process: "[c]omplexity […] means being forced to select; being forced to select means contingency; and contingency means risk."[24]

Summary

We might express these ideas, if they seem somewhat cumbersome, in simpler terms by saying that we live in a contingent, complex world to which we react by creating systems. In doing so, we reduce complexity, but at the same time we build up a complexity that is inherent in the system. This process creates a foundation for knowledge and action, although the world has remained the same, i.e., it is still contingent and complex in relation to our descriptions.

I should like to take this deliberately a stage further by pointing the way from theory toward practice. Relating this to the therapy situation, from what has already been said (and even if we look at the issues in an entirely ironic way) we can see three dilemmas emerging:

1 The great complexity of biological, psychological, and social systems; whose susceptibility to disturbance means that no conceptual therapeutic approach (understood as ultimately founded) can do justice to them.

2 The unavoidability of selection in creating a system; the contingency of the world (which is axiomatic) means that the risk of failure is immanent within it; it could also be said from the strict scientific viewpoint that any experience is tainted by subjectivity. However, a particular characteristic of systems theory involves the fact that the concept of "subject" is resolved through the concept of "system" (which is also used as a point of criticism).

3 Double contingency in therapeutic communication; this places an enormous pressure of expectation on the person performing the therapeutic activity, in that the patient expects the practitioner to know. The dilemma that arises from this is that the person performing the therapeutic activity is tempted to deny contingency.

In this situation, and seen in simple terms, three negative routes are open, in the sense that they either deny the dilemmas or seek some trick to circumvent them:

1 Therapeutic nihilism: the risk being known, the person performing the therapeutic activity avoids actions of a therapeutic nature and retreats to a purely observer position: "I know what is wrong with you, but it is very complicated, so I cannot help you. You will have to live with the problem."

2 Diagnostic nihilism: the person performing the therapeutic activity decides that attack is the best form of defense and rejects the process of cognition as such, on the grounds that all knowledge is inadequate in principle. This approach makes intuition, or some other deciding authority, the basis for therapeutic actions: "I do not know what is wrong with you, but an inner voice tells me that I can help you."

3 "Treatment by numbers": the person performing the therapeutic activity denies complexity and contingency, regards the human individual as a simple machine, able to be determined, and sees the disturbances affecting that individual as capable of being addressed using a precisely laid out procedure. In this process it is possible to find final causes (perfect diagnoses) and to deduce from them clearly indicated therapeutic actions (perfect treatments): "I know exactly what is wrong with you. What has to be done in this case is this and that, in order to solve your problem."

I believe that osteopathy has a variety of very interesting solutions to offer with regard to this dilemma, particularly in its field of competence dealing with "functional disturbances," and that these solutions can be worked out in terms of systems theory. I should however like to emphasize that systems theory is only one of a great variety of ways of reacting to the problems outlined here. The decision to use it is more a personal matter than one related to the nature of osteopathy itself. The ideas set out below have essentially a practical focus and so also tend away from formal consideration of "systems theory" in the sense of pure theory.

Constitution of a system

Contingency can become a recurrent theme and creative element in the osteopathic interaction. In view of the high degree of contingency of biological organisms and the complexity inherent in the system, we need to analyze them into subsystems in order to gain any clear perspective. Complexity is reduced, and the facets of the individual systems rendered knowable for the observer (the osteopath) and so capable of treatment.** In the light of this, osteopaths can be said to form an environment such as can be perceived, by constituting a system, in order to be able to act. This happens in several overlapping and even repeating phases:[26]

- Differentiation

- Creating relationships

- Synthesis and preparation of a treatment approach.

I should like to stress here that, in an osteopathic intervention, the constitution of a system (the investigative, diagnostic act) and treatment (the therapeutic act) merge one into another with no clear boundary between, and that each influences the other. The division into sequential, separately operating stages presented in the text does not correspond to what actually happens in therapeutic practice.

Differentiation

The concept of differentiation is, as already stated, fundamental to Luhmann's systems theory approach. This theory, in contrast to an ontological description of the world, chooses to take the route of difference theory.[27,28] Maturana gives a definition related to biology.[29] The process of proceeding from complex, supraordinate levels to less complex, subordinate levels is reflected in the process of focusing during osteopathic examination. From the point of view of systems theory, the first stage is to establish global differences (e.g., in fascial screening), and it is only when this is done that subsystems emerge for the observer.

These differences are expressed for the observer as anomalies, differences or disturbances within the system level in question (e.g., tensions tending to pull the tissue in a particular direction).

Osteopaths are constantly making such decisions, in the form of: left/not right, anterior/not posterior, etc. As they do so, a subsystem is built up (for the sake of simplicity let us say "spatial differentiation," e.g., the left half of the body. However, osteopaths also work with other kinds of differentiation: temporal, e.g., rhythm, or qualitative). They can then proceed to work within this complexity, as for example: it is the left foot/not the left hip, the left knee, etc.; it is the liver/not the duodenum, etc. On a further level of differentiation, it would then be possible to establish differences such as: it is the left anterior talus/not some other possible dysfunction; it is the right triangular ligament/not something else, etc. So Luhmann's difference theory, dry as it may at first seem, can be seen here to have great pragmatic advantages, helping us to reflect on this very complex process and to begin to understand it.

Subsystems such as those that come about by the process of differentiation within these differentiations are always part of higher, overarching system levels, with boundaries that are in principle open, both in the upward and the downward direction. Here it is important to interpret the significance of the differences in this investigative step only within the level in question, with no interpolation into other levels, since the end result of doing that would be the problem of complete interdependence. This would also leave sufficient room that could then be more precisely or freshly defined in subsequent sub-levels. This approach respects contingency on every level and does not regard the body and person as a trivial machine[30] and this in turn avoids treading the route of "treatment by numbers."

**This may sound reductionist. However, this reductionist element is resolved when we realize that, in systems theory, the system also features as a unit of difference. Another solution is the one proposed by Wilber[25] that uses the concept of the holon: "Reality is not composed of things or processes; it is not composed of atoms or quarks; it is not composed of wholes, nor does it have any parts. Rather, it is composed of whole/parts, or holons."

It is also essential to employ the same type of operation in developing and exploiting the system. I began by pointing out that the interaction between osteopath and patient can be described as a social system, and that the type of operation in social systems is communication. To make this point more specifically and forcefully, what gives an intervention its particular osteopathic character is that it is communicative in nature. Whereas the process of examination in traditional (allopathic) medicine increasingly acquires the character of a monologue, in which the observer looks broadly, in as detached and distant a way as possible, at the body of a patient delivered in unawareness for the practitioner's attention, the process of examination in osteopathy relies on each and every response of the body, however slight, that the practitioner thinks might answer the questions being put. This dependence fundamentally rests on the immediate proximity, which finds expression in touch.[††] A dialogue takes place in this touch; it operates in both directions and produces changes on both sides. One system (a person practicing osteopathy) affects the other (the patient), and for each "other" system, its own operates as an environment. This is precisely what must be avoided at all costs in the traditional (allopathic) examination procedure, which seeks to operate on the lines of the empirical sciences as its ideal; there it is axiomatic that the patient, as the object of observation, must not influence the "measurement apparatus." That is impossible in osteopathic intervention; not even required, and, I should like to add, not desired. The patient is called upon to influence the observer so that such a thing as communication can come about. It is only this specific form of communication that makes a selection process possible, and, with it, the constitution of systems.

Creating relationships

Communication can only create links when it makes sense to both parties. If no meaning is conveyed, all that is perceived is a kind of "white noise" of interference not open to interpretation and offering no access point for action. For the osteopathic practitioner it is therefore essential to distil meaning from the verbal and the non-verbal communication process.

In creating relationships, the systems arrived at through the communicative activity are placed in relationship one to another. Now, a kind of therapeutically useful sense needs to be produced. Without a reflexive process, all that happens in the patient/osteopath system is a meaningless collection of disturbances that have been sensed; this is a problem that many students of osteopathy are faced with at first. They have sensed a number of things during the examination process, but do not know what to do with the information they have collected. On the other hand, they must act in order to gain experience. This is a particularly clear demonstration of the circular connection between knowledge and action.

So it is not the elements that constitute a particular system level that are fundamental to the construction of the system and the therapeutic interaction, but the relationships between them. The essence of the system is expressed in the relationships between the elements, and not in the elements themselves. Creating relationships enables an understanding of individual subsystems, and their possible significance for problems of the patient, which is necessary in the moment of the therapeutic interaction. In this way, re-presentation (i.e., presenting again) of what has already been discovered ("we've seen something like this before") and assimilating it into the plan of action in the way envisaged by Jean Piaget, creates a constant process of learning and development carried out by the osteopath during the work with the patient. Piaget says:[32]

To my way of thinking, knowing an object does not mean copying it – it means acting upon it. It means constructing systems of transformations that can be carried out on or with this object [...] Knowledge, then, is a system of transformations that become progressively adequate.

The synthesis and establishment of a treatment approach

The risk of diagnostic nihilism is present here, since ultimately it is the meaning provided by the point above that produces the plan for the therapeutic act. We can understand "meaning" as being the comprehension of a practically complete picture of certain functional aspects, together with their significance for actual and potential decompensation in the patient. It creates the starting point and provides the elements of planning for the therapeutic action. Depending on the complexity of

---

[††]A particularly detailed analysis of this from the point of view of phenomenology can be found in Waldenfels.[31]

the case, it is possible to begin afresh, time and again, and, from this point, to restart an attempt at communication that may have floundered. This also helps us see that we should not take simple cases as a basis for the construction of complex ones, because the contexts – and so the appropriate degree of complexity – are determined by the particular problem at hand.

Constitution of the system makes it possible to arrive at a viable[‡‡] treatment approach within the currently applicable, individual patient/osteopath system. "Viable" here does not mean the best of all possibilities, but simply one that is selected and is adequate to meet the current context. Other possibilities, which might have been equally adequate, were simply not considered in the differentiation process. That was how it became possible to reduce complexity. We might say, following Foerster,[34] that observers do not perceive that they miss what is beyond their perception. However, the risk of misunderstandings and of failed attempts at making the connection is ever-present here.

Two things are achieved here: firstly, the decision as to where the focus of treatment should be, and the sequence of steps in the treatment. (This stage includes such concepts as the "dominant dysfunction" and "priority.") Secondly, the overall view that this stage tries to build up then provides patients with a rough picture of the options as regards osteopathic treatment in their current situation.

The therapeutic act

The triad of assessment/diagnosis, therapeutic act, and response of the patient have already been mentioned at the opening of this chapter, where the point was made that these three elements run right through the osteopathic intervention. Consequently, the therapeutic act does not follow on from the end of the stage when the system is constituted, as the second movement of a symphony follows on from the first; rather it is constantly taking its turn and is interrupted in turn by the other. Operationally, this interchanging activity is maintained by "osteopathic communication."

It follows on from our theory that treatment according to osteopathic principles must take its direction from relationships and not from individual elements of a system. The line of approach is therefore quite different. It is not the structure itself but its relationship to other structures; more than that, how it relates to other relationships (second-order relationships), which provide the fundamental direction. Here we see a striking difference between the osteopathic approach and other kinds of manual therapy, where attention is directed purely to the structure. Systems, as has already been mentioned, are defined by the relationships between their constituting elements, not by the elements as such. It is this that makes it helpful and necessary to treat the person in terms of connections. The synthesis of processes, consisting of making distinctions and establishing relationships, consequently enables decisions to be made regarding the choice of which relationships and connections to treat, and not which structures to treat.

There is a positive solution to the dilemma outlined at the outset, because in the context of the interaction with the patient, there was no need for any of the three escape strategies mentioned. Instead it has been shown that osteopathic action can consciously bring in both contingency and complexity. This is achieved by constituting a system that enables treatment. The kind of operation that maintains this is like a dialogue, something that is characteristic of the osteopathic approach. Constitution of a system is carried out in awareness of the fact that successful treatment cannot be guaranteed. This is entirely acceptable. The idea of humans as simple machines capable of precise determination, being objects that can be manipulated, would be a depressing prospect, and in no way one that corresponds to the fundamental idea of osteopathy.

Reflection on what we do is an important factor in osteopathic work with the patient. In the field of therapy, both extremes – unfounded action as well as action founded on first principles – represent ethical problems. Constructive reflection can serve as a regulatory factor. Hence this suggestion should neither be underestimated nor overestimated.

References

[1]Kant I: Critique of Pure Reason. Translated by JMD Meiklejohn, London: Henry G Bohn; 1855. Everyman's Library, London: Dent and New York: Dutton; 1974: 54f.

---

‡‡This concept has developed from evolution theory. To be "viable" is essentially to "fit," although this does not (as presented in some theories) necessarily imply that it is the best fit. Glasersfeld says in this connection[33]: "Both in the theory of evolution and in constructivism, "to fit" means no more than to have passed through whatever constraints there may have been."

[2]Bertalanffy L: General System Theory. Foundations, Development, Applications. 13th edn. New York: George Braziller; 2001.

[3]Seffinger MA: Osteopathic Philosophy. In: Ward RC (ed.) Foundations for Osteopathic Medicine. Baltimore: Williams and Wilkins; 1997: 3–12

[4]Wieland W: Strukturwandel der Medizin und ärztliche Ethik: Philosophische Überlegungen zu Grundfragen einer Praktischen Wissenschaft; lecture given 17th Nov 1984. Heidelberg; 1986.

[5]Zeidler KW: Prolegomena zur Wissenschaftstheorie. Würzburg: Könighausen & Neumann; 2000:114ff. a) 127ff.

[6]Zahavi D: Husserl's Phenomenology. Stanford/Ca: Stanford University Press; 2003: 72–77.

[7]Luhmann N: Social Systems. Transl.: J Bednarz, D Baecker. Stanford University Press. Stanford, Cal.; 1995: xlvii

[8]Luhmann N: Einführung in die Systemtheorie. Heidelberg: Carl-Auer-Systeme-Verlag; 2002: 66.

[9]Luhmann N: Einführung in die Systemtheorie. Heidelberg: Carl-Auer-Systeme-Verlag; 2002: a) 66, b) 77, c) 174.

[10]Maturana HR, Varela FG: Autopoiesis: the Organization of the Living. In: Autopoiesis and Cognition. Dordrecht: Reidel 1980

[11]Horster D: Niklas Luhmann. Munich: C.H. Beck; 1997.

[12]Smith R. 2011. Aristotle's Logic. In: EN Zalta (ed.). The Stanford Encyclopedia of Philosophy. Fall 2011. edn. URL = <http://plato.stanford.edu/archives/fall2011/entries/aristotle-logic/>. [30.1.2012].

[13]Luhmann N: Social Systems. Transl.: J Bednarz, D Baecker. Stanford University Press. Stanford, Cal.; 1995: 106.

[14]Luhmann N: Social Systems. Transl.: J Bednarz, D Baecker. Stanford University Press. Stanford, Cal.; 1995: 111, 112.

[15]Luhmann N: Social Systems. Transl.: J Bednarz, D Baecker. Stanford University Press. Stanford, Cal.; 1995; 121.

[16]Luhmann N: Komplexität. In: Ritter J, Gründer K (ed.): Historisches Wörterbuch der Philosophie. Basel: Schwabe; 1976; 4: 1027–1038.

[17] Luhmann N: Einführung in die Systemtheorie. Heidelberg: Carl-Auer-Systeme-Verlag; 2002.

[18]Steinbacher K: System/Systemtheorie. In: Sandkühler HJ (ed): Enzyklopädie Philosophie. 2 vols. Hamburg: Felix Meiner; 1999; 2: 1579–1581.

[19]Kriz J: Systemtheorie für Psychotherapeuten, Psychologen und Mediziner. Eine Einführung. 1st edn. Vienna: Facultas; 1999.

[20]Luhmann N: Einführung in die Systemtheorie. Heidelberg: Carl-Auer-Systeme-Verlag; 2002: a) 66, b) 77, c) 174.

[21]Luhmann N: Social Systems. Transl.: J Bednarz, D Baecker. Stanford University Press. Stanford, Cal.; 1995: 44.

[22]Krieger DJ; Einführung in die allgemeine Systemtheorie. 2nd edn. Munich: Wilhelm Fink Verlag; 1998: 11ff.

[23]Luhmann N: Einführung in die Systemtheorie. Heidelberg: Carl-Auer-Systeme-Verlag; 2002: 174.

[24]Luhmann N: Social Systems. Transl.: J Bednarz, D Baecker. Stanford University Press. Stanford, Cal.; 1995: 25.

[25]Wilber K: Sex, Ecology and Spirituality: the Spirit of Evolution. Shambhala; 2000: 45.

[26]Krieger DJ; Einführung in die Allgemeine Systemtheorie. 2nd edn. Munich: Wilhelm Fink Verlag; 1998: 11ff.

[27]Krieger DJ; Einführung in die Allgemeine Systemtheorie. 2nd edn. Munich: Wilhelm Fink Verlag; 1998: 11ff.

[28]Luhmann N: Die Gesellschaft der Gesellschaft. 2nd edn. Frankfurt am Main: Suhrkamp; 1999: 60ff.

[29]Maturana HR: The Organisation of the Living: a Theory of the Living Organisation. In: Int. J. Man-Machine Studies vol. 7: 313–332.

[30] Foerster H v: Wissen und Gewissen. Versuch einer Brücke. 4th edn. Frankfurt am Main: Suhrkamp; 1997: 357–363.

[31]Waldenfels B: Bruchlinien der Erfahrung. Phänomenologie, Psychoanalyse, Phänomenotechnik. Frankfurt a. M.: Suhrkamp; 2002.

[32]Piaget J: Genetic Epistemology. Transl. Duckworth E. New York, The Norton Library. New York: WW Norton & Co Inc. and Toronto: George J McLeod; 1971. [First published 1950 in French].

[33]Glasersfeld E: Radical Constructivism: A Way of Knowing and Learning. London: Routledge Falmer; New York: Routledge Falmer; 1995: 41.

[34]Foerster H v: Wissen und Gewissen. Versuch einer Brücke. 4th edn. Frankfurt am Main: Suhrkamp; 1997: 357–363.

17

The osteopathic experience of fulcrums and the emergence of stillness

Stephen F. Paulus

Introduction

Fulcrums, as applied in an osteopathic context, originated with the work of William Garner Sutherland, DO. Sutherland took the essential principles of osteopathy, as presented by Andrew Taylor Still, and expanded them into areas not previously thought to be readily accessible to the average osteopath. Sutherland told us:

Dr Still could not speak of all the things he understood about the living human body. We were not ready to hear him.[1]

I believe that one of the many abstract or non-material concepts that Still could not speak of or was not able to articulate well to the early osteopathic profession was the practical application of fulcrums. The majority of early and mid-twentieth century DOs were primarily interested in biomechanical, material, objective, and linear methods of applying osteopathic principles and were not ready to hear Still's whole message. Fortunately for us, a few of Still's students received what today's scientifically oriented DOs would call an esoteric osteopathic education.

Etymologic origins of fulcrums in an osteopathic context

If we dig deeper into the etymologic origins of the osteopathic meaning of fulcrums we find that the non-mechanical classification comes from a non-osteopathic source. If we want to honestly understand the groundbreaking work of William Garner Sutherland, we must study not only the writings of Andrew Taylor Still but also Sutherland's influential friend and teacher Walter Russell. It was Walter Russell (1871–1963) who originated an expanded, metaphysical, and non-material meaning to the word Fulcrum. Russell was an architect, sculptor, writer, and self-taught scientist. Most of all, he was a mystic who received spiritual teachings that he

transcribed into a series of books. He was an American spiritual master who co-founded the University of Science and Philosophy in Virginia. Both William Sutherland and his wife Adah were deeply influenced by the spiritual teachings of Russell. It is surprising how much of what we call osteopathy in the cranial field has its origins in the teachings of Russell.

It sounds unexpectedly osteopathic when Russell writes:

There is no motion in a fulcrum. All motion is in the moving lever, which extends from the fulcrum. Likewise there is no power in the moving lever, which extends from the fulcrum. The power which is manifested by the lever is in the fulcrum upon which the lever oscillates.[2]

Or when he says, "The power is in the still fulcrum and not in the moving lever nor in the expression of power extended from the fulcrum."[3] However, when Russell says, "The fulcrum is always in balance with the universe,"[4] we get our first glimpse at the expanded significance of a fulcrum and begin to understand where Sutherland got his more esoteric osteopathic understanding of fulcrums.

When most Cranial osteopaths think of fulcrums, the conventional association is with the anatomic/functional unit known as the Sutherland Fulcrum named by Harold Magoun, DO. Magoun specifically defines a fulcrum as:

The descriptive name given to that point of rest, located in the area of the straight sinus, around which the entire membranous articular mechanism of the cranium moves. Its precise location is shifted by the motivating force transferred to it, the influence of the shift moves all the component parts of the mechanism accordingly and simultaneously.

Thus the two-phase cycle of position of the cranial bones is directly related to the respiratory cycle of the motility of the neural tube and the fluctuation of the cerebrospinal fluid.[5]

This definition of a fulcrum offers a biomechanical perspective that takes the basic laws of Newtonian physics and applies them to a biologic model. In biomechanical osteopathy and cranial geometric teachings, the utility of a mechanical fulcrum is important. Every mechanical osteopathic treatment uses concepts from classical physics that include simple machines, mechanical advantage, levers, pulleys, shear forces, creep, nut and bolt dynamics, ball and socket joints, tongue and groove joints, etc.

The other common osteopathic application of fulcrum biomechanics occurs when we describe an osteopathic lesion, or what is now called a somatic dysfunction. The localized physical region of a somatic dysfunction, more often than not, has relative inertia when contrasted with the surrounding tissues. We commonly utilize the term inertia to describe a focal area of dysfunction that does not physically move or does not manifest inherent motion. The confined area of restriction acts as a fulcrum relative to the levers of the surrounding tissues. During the diagnostic portion of a treatment session, we identify areas of restriction, i.e., inertia, and then apply a specific osteopathic treatment to help motivate therapeutic change or motion. These fulcrums of dysfunction, on the surface, have no obvious link to stillness. However, concealed below the surface, fulcrums of dysfunction can have direct links to still points. Fulcrums of dysfunction can act as windows, allowing access to stillness.

The purpose of this article is not to have a detailed discussion of classic or Newtonian physics and its application to a biologic model. That has been, and continues to be, the dominant teaching model in the osteopathic profession and has been well documented elsewhere. The explicit intent of this article is to discuss some of Sutherland's, and by association Still's, non-mechanical and non-material teachings and discover their practical application. Sutherland expressed his frustration at the lack of appreciation the early osteopathic profession demonstrated for the old doctor's out of the ordinary spiritual pursuits and he wrote:

I have often said that we lost something in osteopathy that Dr Still tried to get across. That was the spiritual that he included in the science of osteopathy.[6]

Sutherland was, and remains, a deep resource of applied spirituality for the osteopathic profession. He did not lose the "spiritual that [Dr Still] tried to get across", he interwove it seamlessly around and into the standard mechanical osteopathic principles.

Categories of fulcrums

I believe that Sutherland taught at least four different categories of fulcrums. The first category is a physical and mechanical fulcrum (as demonstrated in the confluence of the falx and the tent known as the Sutherland Fulcrum and the membranous/bony fulcrum located at the second sacral segment). The second variety relates to the inertial fulcrum of a dysfunction. The third type is a non-material fulcrum utilizing potency (or what Sutherland called "the fluid within the fluid"). A fourth version includes the perception of a non-mechanical and non-material fulcrum and the awareness of a spiritual Fulcrum from a Russellian perspective, where "the fulcrum is always in balance with the universe." When Sutherland said:

You, as one of the mechanics of the cranium, become a pharmacist in your art of knowing this mechanism – not merely the articular mechanism and that little fulcrum of the falx and the tent, but the fulcrum in the fluctuation of the cerebrospinal fluid, its still point.[7]

[The] balance point is the fulcrum around which the action occurs, that shifts automatically from point to point. Even so, the fulcrum remains still – the fulcrum wherein you get the balanced vision.[8]

Sutherland was asking us not to look at the material "little fulcrum" of the falx and the tent, rather he was revealing to us that it is from the fulcrum, or the still point of the mechanism in the cerebrospinal fluid (CSF) that we are able to have a balanced and even greater osteopathic vision than that afforded by mere palpation. He also was asking for us not to focus on the temporal event of a still point but to honor the stillness as a dynamic process. Sutherland made sure that Andrew Taylor Still's applied spiritual teachings were intimately interwoven with status quo osteopathic biomechanical instruction.

Metaphysical Fulcrum

Sutherland accessed the metaphysical fulcrum primarily (but not exclusively) via the function of the cerebrospinal fluid. It was Still who said, "that the cerebrospinal fluid is the highest known element in the human body . . ."[9] Sutherland expanded upon this axiom and said, "The arterial stream is supreme but the cerebrospinal fluid is in command . . ."[10] He also recognized the vital importance of the CSF as a rarefied access portal for engaging the "something other" or "the lost something in osteopathy" or what he called the "fluid within the fluid" or the "stillness of the tide." Sutherland astutely said, "There is something within the cerebrospinal fluid that nourishes that no scientific laboratory will ever find."[11] Within the discipline of osteopathy in the cranial field, the function of the CSF is recognized as the primary way to access the "stillness of the tide"; however, Sutherland's approach can be applied anywhere in the body, not just the cranial–spinal–sacral mechanism where CSF is present. When we expand the cranial concept beyond the material fluid of the CSF and extend a non-material concept of fluid below foramen magnum to include the entire body, we pose a vital question, "Is what we call the fluid material and mechanical or is it non-material and thus unrelated to the laws of Newtonian physics?" In other words, is cerebrospinal fluid an osteopathic euphemism for a metaphysical perceptual field? Or, is it a category of subtle material motions or biologic processes that have not yet been measured and named?

Both Sutherland and Russell could be quite mysterious and oblique in their teachings. It can be difficult understanding abstract explanations of personal experiences and they can leave the average osteopath reeling in the stormy waves of intellectual perplexity. It was Rollin Becker, DO, one of Sutherland's closest students, who was able to put into more accessible words how we can understand and utilize fulcrums. Becker said:

A fulcrum is a still point, a source of power. Fulcrums aren't levers; fulcrums are still points. Out of the fulcrum flow levers. The tissues that you've got a hold of are the levers that are going to be doing the moving around for you.[12]

More specifically he tells us:

At the fulcrum point – at the point where this tide changes from one direction to the other – is the point at which the breath of life interchanges with the cerebrospinal fluid.[13]

Becker also studied with Walter Russell and incorporated many Russellian concepts into his osteopathic

way of life. It becomes interesting to sort out who said what when discussing fulcrums, still points, and stillness. When Russell says, ". . . the power is not in the motion. It is in the stillness of the fulcrum,"[14] it sounds a lot like Sutherland or Becker!

Like Sutherland, Rollin Becker recognized the profound significance of the CSF. Becker revealed that:

At the fulcrum point – at the point where this tide changes from one direction to the other – is the point at which the Breath of Life interchanges with the cerebrospinal fluid. It then, in turn, is transmitted into the lower energies that the body needs.[15]

When we engage the CSF, it is the fulcrum or the balance point of interchange with the Breath of Life where stillness finds us. Once we understand what Becker means by "The fulcrum is the source of power. It's the point of reference . . . ,"[16] then we can offer an osteopathic treatment based on the "lost something" in osteopathy that Still tried to get across rather than on an exclusive biomechanical approach. This is the spiritual manifestation of osteopathy that transcends theology or religion.

The fulcrum as a reference point

When we use the power manifested in a fulcrum as our reference point for an osteopathic treatment, we are accessing the forces of nature to do the work of healing. Still said, "Osteopathy is to me a very sacred science. It is sacred because it is a healing power through all nature."[17] On the surface, we can employ a biomechanical osteopathic treatment and at the same time keep our awareness oriented toward stillness manifested in a non-material fulcrum.

Following closely in the footsteps of Sutherland and Becker is James Jealous, DO. His expansive osteopathic biodynamics curriculum discusses fulcrums in a nonmechanical way and has given osteopaths the opportunity and ability to experience for themselves what a fulcrum is and how to utilize this knowledge in everyday practice. Jealous and Eliott Blackman, DO, introduced to the osteopathy community the concept of midlines originating from an embryologic field. Midlines are not just embryologic energetic remnants: they are fulcrums. Midlines are linear fulcrums. Midlines are a function located within structure. Midlines are perceived as localized quiet lines that reference stillness. The non-material fulcrum of the posterior midline, which originated from the embryologic field of the primitive streak, is the reference point for all other midlines in the body. Midlines are orienting embryologic axes that are perceivable as a non-material field in any physical location within the body.

We can historically give the scholarly references and subsequent expanded applications of fulcrums, but deeper understanding is not based upon information received from a lecture or a book but from the real world of experience. True knowledge is only gained from having our own personal experience of fulcrums when working within the sacred confines of an osteopathic treatment. While the expanded metaphysical experience of fulcrums is fundamentally simple and always accessible, it takes, as Becker says, "... skill, time, and patience to learn to feel this functioning."[18] Having an experience of stillness in a fulcrum is not foreign territory, unavailable, and inaccessible, but is our birthright. Experiencing the stillness in a fulcrum is not exclusively an osteopathic birthright; it is the inheritance we receive as human beings. Stillness is essential and elemental to what it means to be a human being.

Expanding the concept of fulcrums beyond a mechanical perspective

When we speak of the expanded metaphysical Fulcrum, it is important that we utilize accurate language. The functions of abstract, non-material Fulcrums are different from that of physical fulcrums used in simple machines or Newtonian physics applied to a biologic model. Just as Becker capitalized the "H" in health in this famous quote:

It is extremely difficult to find words to express health. Health is a word with an unknown meaning ... However, health in the broadest sense, "Health" with a capital "H," is something. It's the very reason, we are all here ... I mean on earth. We are here because we have Health.[19]

He gave the word health an expanded spiritual meaning beyond the ordinary, totally in accordance with the teachings of A.T. Still. *The Chicago Manual of Style*, the definitive reference on writing rules and guidelines, explains that capitalizing words elevates the selection to a transcendent idea or it makes reference, directly or indirectly, to one supreme God.[20] To more accurately distinguish between a mechanical fulcrum and a "Fulcrum" based upon non-material stillness, I have capitalized the

"F" in the latter. The word Fulcrum (with a capital "F") refers to the source of power, the reference point for all levers/motion. It is the still point where the tide changes from one phase to the other. Stillness is not a lifeless experience; it is vital, living, and dynamic and has a feeling of power, potency, and creativity. Motion is an extension of stillness. Motion is an effect of stillness. All levers are in motion. All tissues, somatic elements, and fluids are levers. A lever (tissue) gets its power from a Fulcrum (stillness). The inherent force driving the cranial mechanism and all the mechanisms in the body emerges from the dynamics of a Fulcrum.

The grammar of fulcrums

When we refer to a "fulcrum on" or a "fulcrum over which a lever moves" we are describing a mechanical fulcrum that uses the physical laws of simple machines. We use this mechanical fulcrum when applying a biomechanical osteopathic treatment. When we mistakenly refer to the metaphysical "Fulcrum on" the CSF as a "lever over a Fulcrum" or a "Fulcrum between" we are implying the presence of a barrier or a separation between stillness and the CSF or other structures. When we speak of a Fulcrum, it is more accurate to speak of the "Fulcrum in" the CSF or of the "Fulcrum emerging" when treating any physical location anywhere in the body. Commonly, osteopaths refer to the "Fulcrum of" a particular region, or globally to represent a more generalized emergence of stillness. Speaking of a "Fulcrum of" makes reference to stillness contained within, or better said, of being in relationship to our living patient.

The perception of a "Fulcrum in," a "Fulcrum of," or a "Fulcrum emerging" is an event. It is not a point on a map. During an osteopathic treatment, we generally perceive stillness contained within the body of our patient. We can also have an experience of stillness being in relationship not only with our patients but also with ourselves. Our experience of a Fulcrum sometimes appears to be localized anatomically, and at other times it emerges throughout the entire body. When our consciousness is not localized, the awareness of stillness occurs beyond the confines of our physical bodies.

The Fulcrum of stillness in osteopathic treatment

The language involving Fulcrums and stillness can get confusing, but personal experience will clarify the cognitive dissonance. Ultimately, there is no barrier between stillness and levers; they are in a continuous dynamic relationship. They are seamless in function. One goal of an osteopathic treatment is to remove the barriers between Fulcrums and levers, thus allowing the inherent therapeutic processes to heal via the laws of nature. Becker advised us that during an osteopathic treatment to:

Moment by moment . . . attune to the stillness and reattune to it. And there's no point in time where it just happens – you just go along and that's the way it is – because this is something dynamic. This dynamic is intrinsic [to stillness] . . .[21]

And Russell says, "Wherever stillness is, there is God – and God is everywhere."[22] In osteopathy, what we call stillness is always available. Our task is to use osteopathy to discover or experience the Fulcrum in the CSF or any location in the body. The Fulcrum of stillness is not exclusive to the CSF, but can be found or revealed anywhere and in any tissue or fluid in the living human being we call "the patient." It is also within us as osteopaths. We, as the person giving the treatment, also have the presence of stillness. Becker tells us:

You contact your stillness, you contact the patient's stillness, and from that time on, you're feeling. That's all there is to it. But you're not a passive machine.[23]

This is similar to what Anne Wales, DO instructed us to do in an osteopathic treatment. Wales asked for us to "unlearn the principle of the doctor being the active force which operates upon the passive patient . . ."[24] and instead create a situation in which the doctor allows for a process of "an active agent applying itself to an active body."[25] Becker and Wales are directing us, and giving us permission, to become a part of the osteopathic treatment – to also receive and experience the stillness that manifests during a change in the tide.

False fulcrums

We can also discuss the notion of false fulcrums. The inappropriate or unconscious application of force by the osteopath during treatment may create a type of fulcrum that is dysfunctional and has no link with stillness. False fulcrums can be created in situations whereby the overly active osteopath perceives the patient to be inactive. In this situation, the osteopath is not fully engaged with the dynamic interchange between the

material and non-material fields. Simply put, the osteopath is not paying attention. False fulcrums can cause the inherent tidal forces to shutdown, creating a lack of localized or global motion that appears to be a still point. False fulcrums are in fact, footprints left by the osteopath. False fulcrums are iatrogenic dysfunctions. When we treat, we must not leave remnants of our personal presence in the tissues.

Stillness emerging

I have found that it is easier and more effective to speak of stillness emerging, rather than us bringing forth stillness. We don't direct stillness, as some might direct the tide (as a fluid force) in a cranial osteopathic treatment or as we might if using a direct action approach in an osteopathic biomechanical procedure. We don't control the arrival of stillness. We, as the osteopath, hold or create a container or an environment for stillness to emerge. In my experience, stillness only emerges when I am humble and receptive, while at the same time recognizing that neither the patient nor I are passive – we are both active agents imbued with stillness. The only difference between me and the patient is that "most of the time" I am actively aware of the opportunity for stillness to emerge at any moment and I can assist the process with conscious awareness and make sure that I am not just willing to receive stillness, but I am also ready to utilize the effects of stillness to help the patient achieve healing. We hold the space for stillness to emerge and at the same time maintain the awareness of the patient's necessity. In a generic sense, necessity is the reason why a patient seeks our help. Necessity can be a localized osteopathic somatic dysfunction; it can be a non-specific alteration in function; it can be a non-material obstruction or separation from structural elements; or it can be a lack of expression of health; etc. When stillness merges with necessity, healing begins.

Spiritual Fulcrum

Stillness is not exclusive to somatic elements of a living human being. Sutherland spoke mystically of the cerebrospinal fluid as being everywhere, as a "sea around us."[26] He said:

Where is that cerebrospinal fluid? Is it only in my body? No. It is in each and every one of your bodies. There is an ocean of cerebrospinal fluid in this room. Here is a fluid within a fluid. There is a fluid within a fluid. The Breath of Life is within each.[27]

Becker tells the story of feeling the stillness come into the room where William Sutherland was teaching:

Those of us who were privileged to be in his classes while he lectured on this subject have observed and shared in the experience of feeling the whole classroom becoming still. He would call it to our attention and would tell us that it was something that frequently occurred when the Potency of the Tide was being discussed. It occurred spontaneously and was not something that was planned or predetermined. Those who experienced this could feel the stillness, and his comment would be, "Can you feel the change in the Tide?"[28]

Becker also spoke of the spiritual Fulcrum in the room during an osteopathic treatment.[29] It is a common occurrence in my practice to experience a change in the tide taking place outside of the patient, in the treatment room. It feels as though stillness is enfolding the patient and me in an embrace of love. In those moments, I am also being "treated." I don't begin my treatment invoking some God of stillness or ritualizing a separate spiritual aspect of osteopathy. I am simply open in every instance for the opportunity for stillness to find us. I remain receptive and patient. Anne Wales was fond of reminding her students that, when being with the intricate living mechanism of a human being, "we must be patient and then wait some more."[30] We cannot manipulate stillness to be delivered when and where we want.

Perceiving the change in the tide

We can feel "the change in the tide" and stillness emerging during an osteopathic treatment or at nearly any time in our lives when we are in a state of acceptance and humility. The emergence of stillness occurs far from the demands of the ego. In other words, we must also drop our ego's need to do something in order to receive stillness in our lives. During an osteopathic treatment, to realize the emergence of stillness, we must release our grip upon the need to fix something. Once you begin to recognize the power of stillness to be a source of healing, then you are free to experience the many textures of stillness. There are innumerable expressions of stillness. Stillness emerges partially or completely. The time frame for stillness may be instantaneous, as a flash of beauty, or more prolonged and pervasive. It is not the osteopath who determines the length, breadth, or quality

of stillness. However, it is the osteopath, by virtue of his or her skill, attention, patience, awareness, and serenity that helps create the context for Stillness to emerge during an osteopathic treatment.

Stillness: local and non-local

We have two possible means of identifying stillness when we experience it as a reference point. Stillness is appreciated by some as a non-local phenomenon without a distinct position in time or space. For others stillness is local and distinct, either within or outside of the body. Each osteopath must be open for either experience and not feel constrained by thinking they should feel one or the other. Sometimes the inertial dysfunctional fulcrum of a lesion will be the doorway to the beauty of stillness. The access portals, timings, and types of Fulcrums coming into a treatment are myriad.

Motion vs stillness and still point vs stillness

While we cannot command stillness to emerge, we can understand the processes that help to enhance its manifestation. Becker once said, "Motion is not life. Motion is a manifestation of life."[31] To have an opportunity to experience stillness we must ultimately drop our sensation of bone, membrane, and fluid. We can appreciate one of the many tides, or rhythmic effects of stillness; but we must know that the power is not in the motion of the tides – even the subtle tides. The power is in the pause–rest or the stillness manifested in the still point. We must not confuse the still point with stillness. The balance point in the to-and-fro movement of the tide is where the interchange occurs. There are many different kinds of still points, both induced and spontaneous. Still points are not the end of a treatment as some assume, but are often the beginning. As I mature in this work, I have found that the process of creating or finding still points is not the goal of an osteopathic treatment. The therapeutic process does not originate from the generation of a still point or from the chronological recognition of its presence. It emanates from what creates a still point – from what Russell, Sutherland, and Becker call the rhythmic balanced interchange. I have found that being open to the moment-to-moment opportunity for stillness to emerge is a more effective approach; however, it in itself must not become a goal. Stillness is basic to an osteopathic treatment. Becker said, "Stillness is to me, the very key to what Dr Will was trying to give us."[32] And he revealed that, "I definitely utilize stillness, as the motive force for securing changes in the patients."[33] I understand that Andrew Taylor Still "could not speak of all the things he understood about the living human body," he did not have a clear reproducible vocabulary to verbalize what he experienced.

When I read in between the lines of Still's writings, I am convinced that he utilized stillness as the motivating force for healing. He may have publicly taught the biomechanical principles of osteopathic manipulation, but he consciously and privately worked with metaphysical Fulcrums and stillness.

The lost something in osteopathy

As we expand beyond the box of biomechanics and open our consciousness to the metaphysical in osteopathy we can personally discover the "lost something in osteopathy that Dr Still tried to get across." We can discover for ourselves "the spiritual that he included in the science of osteopathy." We can, in every moment, "be ready to hear . . . of all the things he understood about the living human body." As we try to sort through the confusing language and attempt to understand complicated concepts we must remember to get back to "Be still and know" within our consciousness.[34] Finally, we must follow one of Sutherland's most essential gifts of wisdom: "It matters not what interpretation one may apply, providing one's mental trolley is on the *Wire*."[35]

I interpret Sutherland's comment to mean that we must maintain a conscious engagement with the stillness manifested in a Fulcrum during our work as osteopaths. Ultimately, it doesn't matter how we interpret or name the forces of nature that do the work of healing. We only need to maintain our conscious spiritual link via the "Wire" of what A.T. Still called, "connected oneness."[36] Having a conscious spiritual connection was, I believe, the essence of what "Dr Still could not speak of." What he could not speak of is our true reference point as osteopaths.

References

[1]Sutherland, W.G. Contributions of Thought, Second Edition, Edited by Adah Sutherland and Anne L. Wales. Rudra Press, Portland, Oregon, 1998. p. 293.

[2]Russell, W. The Message of the Divine Iliad, Volume One, University of Science and Philosophy, Virginia, 1971, p. 160.

[3]Russell, W. The Message of the Divine Iliad, Volume One, University of Science and Philosophy, Virginia, 1971, pp. 173–174.

[4]Russell, W. The Message of the Divine Iliad, Volume One, University of Science and Philosophy, Virginia, 1971, p. 243.

[5]Magoun, H.I. Osteopathy in the Cranial Field, Third Edition, Edited by Harold I. Magoun, DO, Sutherland Cranial Teaching Foundation, 1976, p. 339.

[6]Sutherland, W.G. Contributions of Thought, Second Edition, Edited by Adah Sutherland and Anne L. Wales. Rudra Press, Portland, Oregon, 1998, p. 351.

[7]Sutherland, W.G. Contributions of Thought, Second Edition, Edited by Adah Sutherland and Anne L. Wales. Rudra Press, Portland, Oregon, 1998, p. 342.

[8]Sutherland, W.G. Teachings in the Science of Osteopathy. Edited by Anne L. Wales. Rudra Press, Portland Oregon, 1990, p. 44.

[9]Still, A.T. (1899) Philosophy of Osteopathy, Self-Published by A.T. Still, Kirksville, Missouri. (Reprinted by The American Academy of Osteopathy, Colorado Springs, Colorado, 1977). p. 39.

[10]Sutherland, W.G. Contributions of Thought, Second Edition, Edited by Adah Sutherland and Anne L. Wales. Rudra Press, Portland, Oregon, 1998, p. 231.

[11]Sutherland, W.G. Quoted in: Journal of the Osteopathic Cranial Association, 1948–1949, 1954, 1957–1958, Edited by Keith Swan, DO. The Cranial Academy, 1988, p. 57.

[12]Becker, R.E. Stillness in Life. Edited by Rachel Brooks, MD. Stillness Press, 2000, p. 51–52.

[13]Becker, R.E. Stillness in Life. Edited by Rachel Brooks, MD. Stillness Press, 2000 Life. Rudra Press, 1998, p. 6.

[14]Russell, W. The Message of the Divine Iliad, Volume Two, University of Science and Philosophy, Virginia, 1971, p. 204.

[15]Becker, R.E. Stillness in Life. Edited by Rachel Brooks, MD. Stillness Press, 2000, p. 6.

[16]Becker, R.E. Life in Motion: The Osteopathic Vision of Rollin E. Becker, DO. Edited by Rachel Brooks, MD. Rudra Press, 1998, p. 51.

[17]Still, A.T. (1910) Osteopathy Research and Practice, Self-Published by A.T. Still, Kirksville, Missouri (Reprinted and reformatted by Eastland Press, Seattle, 1992). p. 7.

[18]Still, A. T. (1910) Osteopathy Research and Practice, Self-Published by A. T. Still, Kirksville, Missouri (Reprinted and reformatted by Eastland Press, Seattle, 1992). p. 178.

[19]Still, A.T. (1910) Osteopathy Research and Practice, Self-Published by A.T. Still, Kirksville, Missouri (Reprinted and reformatted by Eastland Press, Seattle, 1992). p. 219.

[20]The Chicago Manual of Style, 14th Edition The University of Chicago Press 1993, p. 265.

[21]Becker, R.E. Stillness in Life. Edited by Rachel Brooks, MD. Stillness Press, 2000, p. 31.

[22]Russell, W. The Message of the Divine Iliad, Volume One, University of Science and Philosophy, Virginia, 1971, p. 139.

[23]Becker, R.E. Stillness in Life. Edited by Rachel Brooks, MD. Stillness Press, 2000, p. 54.

[24]Wales, A.L. Osteopathic Dynamics, Academy of Applied Osteopathy Yearbook 1946, The Academy of Applied Osteopathy, 1946, p. 38.

[25]Wales, A.L. Osteopathic Dynamics, Academy of Applied Osteopathy Yearbook 1946, The Academy of Applied Osteopathy, 1946, p. 38.

[26]Sutherland, W.G. Contributions of Thought, Second Edition, Edited by Adah Sutherland and Anne L. Wales. Rudra Press, Portland, Oregon, 1998. pp. 254–255.

[27]Sutherland, W.G. Teachings in the Science of Osteopathy. Edited by Anne L. Wales. Rudra Press, Portland Oregon, 1990, p.139.

[28]Becker, R.E. Life in Motion: The Osteopathic Vision of Rollin E. Becker, DO. Edited by Rachel Brooks, MD. Rudra Press, 1998, p. 30.

[29]Becker, R.E. Life in Motion: The Osteopathic Vision of Rollin E. Becker, DO. Edited by Rachel Brooks, MD. Rudra Press, 1998, p. 31.

[30]Wales, A.L. Personal Communication, July 1997.

[31]Becker, R.E. Stillness in Life. Edited by Rachel Brooks, MD. Stillness Press, 2000, p. 159.

[32]Becker, R.E. Stillness in Life. Edited by Rachel Brooks, MD. Stillness Press, 2000, p. 33.

[33]Becker, R.E. Stillness in Life. Edited by Rachel Brooks, MD. Stillness Press, 2000, p. 67.

[34]Sutherland, W.G. Contributions of Thought, Second Edition, Edited by Adah Sutherland and Anne L. Wales. Rudra Press, Portland, Oregon, 1998. p. 146.

[35]Sutherland, W.G. Quoted in: Becker, R.E. Life in Motion: The Osteopathic Vision of Rollin E. Becker, DO. Edited by Rachel Brooks, MD. Rudra Press, 1998, p. 38.

[36]Still, A.T. (1892) Philosophy and Mechanical Principles of Osteopathy, Hudson-Kimberly Publishing Co., Kansas City, Missouri. (Reprinted by Osteopathic Enterprises, Kirksville, Missouri, 1986). p. 73.

18

Principles of diagnosis

Torsten Liem

Inspection: To look, see and perceive
History: to listen, hear and understand.
Palpation: to perceive, understand and know.

A.G. Chila[1a]

Introduction

Diagnosis aims to establish correlations between the osteopath's findings (both objective and subjective) and the patient's subjective experience, cultural and biosocial environment, and to make them capable of being discovered.

Diagnosis in osteopathy should consist of taking the case history, inspection and examination of the patient, and, most particularly, palpation. Following the taking of an accurate history, the process firstly involves the eyes, in accurate observation and inspection. (For example, the osteopath will consider the characteristics of movement of a newborn that has been subjected to trauma, looking at details such as whether the legs are bent or extended, whether the feet are tense or relaxed, whether the hands are clenched or open, and whether the child has assumed a resigned attitude or one of resistance, etc.) It involves the ears, listening intently, and performing careful auscultation and percussion.

The osteopathic "touch"

Osteopaths can train themselves in the observation of patients' general behavior, gestures, posture or mannerisms, way of making contact, voice and what they say, and these are enough to provide an initial understanding of the person and the patterns of tissue and consciousness that may be exerting a restrictive effect. However, for the osteopath it is touch that communicates most information about function and dysfunction of individual tissues and the way they interact. It is the fingers that have the most direct contact with the tissue dynamics in the patient.

Achieving competence in palpation

Anne Wales[1] makes clear the need for continual practice to train all our senses – especially that of touch – in observation, in order to develop the capacity to read the full story that the body has to tell. In order to develop competence, Esteves and Spence propose that students should be encouraged to use available opportunities to experience normal and altered patterns of structure and function; and reflect on the validity and reliability of their diagnostic judgements.[2] Aubin et al. present for instance a seven-step palpation model that promotes the development of palpation skills by gradually mastering the complexity of the palpation process.[3]

Influences that shape the perception and interpretation of palpatory findings

Palpation is seen as the cornerstone of osteopathic diagnosis and treatment and considered the major building block of clinical decision making within osteopathy. Palpation is generally a complex process and is influenced by previous experiences, the type of information to collect as well as the context in which it takes place, influencing the perception and interpretation of palpatory findings and thereby creating challenges when treating a patient.[4]

Diagnostic palpation is experienced and interpreted on the basis of multisensory integration of vision and haptics, but other influences may also play a role, such as habitual and context-related influences, as well as cultural and social imprinting.[4] Knowing about the challenges, becoming aware of them and dealing with them consciously may result in more adequate palpation procedures and enhance competence in palpation practice.[4]

Intersubjective relationship between osteopath and patient

Our heart, with its love, sympathetic insight, and understanding, also has its part to play in each approach to the patient. The results of imaging and laboratory tests, etc. can provide further information as necessary, but the characteristic that distinguishes the osteopath lies in the findings and the treatment given on the basis of an intersubjective relationship between osteopath and patient. In particular this involves osteopaths' abilities to support, to open themselves to the patient with as much empathy and freedom from conditions as possible, and to focus their intuition and whole spectrum of consciousness in relation to the patient, so as to be able to discover the varied and often disparate aspects of the patient.

Methodology of diagnosis

The methodologies of diagnosis and treatment presented here (see also Chapter 20) can be seen against the background of two viewpoints in particular, which are complementary and can be applied in parallel:

1 AQAL diagnosis. Each of the approaches developed in medicine to date (see Chapter 1) has significantly broadened our understanding of health and disease. (This has come, for example, through their recognition of genetic influences, and those of the environment, morphogenetic fields, biochemical processes, biomechanical processes, vitalist concepts, previous personal experiences, present stimuli, unconscious processes, conscious decisions, etc.) The therapeutic interaction, however, is limited by two main factors: the treatment methods being used by the practitioner (based on the particular approach being applied), and the view of the wholeness of the body and person of an individual, which arises from this. Disease, seen as something that affects the whole person, is not just limited locally to the occurrence of a particular dysfunction: it extends to all aspects of human existence. At present, the approach that especially deserves mention as a means of developing an integral diagnosis that is as inclusive or comprehensive as possible is, in my view, Wilber's AQAL model. This diagnostic model seeks to achieve an awareness of the following aspects in the patient:

a Levels of existence: form/function or material/energetic levels.
b States of consciousness (as part of the subjective functional aspects in the interaction between the structural and the functional).
c Intersubjective cultural/family levels.
d Interobjective levels: social, biosphere.
e Types (e.g., masculine/feminine).
f Lines of development (especially of values).
g Levels of development (e.g., gross, subtle, causal or physical, biological, emotional, cognitive, spiritual (Figure. 18.1) or levels of spiral dynamics (see later in this chapter)).

2 Whenever one of these factors is either ignored or treated as absolute, this risks reducing the person and diminishing the healing potential. When taking the history, the aim is to elicit as comprehensive a picture as possible about the interacting dynamic levels of existence and to establish the link between them and the other examination findings (especially those from palpation). In palpation, very different and specific methods are used to differentiate tissue/energies associated with particular inner states of consciousness, and also with certain kinds of cultural/familial experiences and sociobiological structures.

3 Tissue–energy–consciousness complex (Figure. 18.1). Rather than being made up of soma and psyche, human beings are a psychosomatic unity. The tissue, as the external aspect, is present through to the very top of Wilber's system of quadrants, to the highest level of the internal aspect (i.e., the highest consciousness) (see also Chapter 1). The increasing complexity of material form that emerges in the course of evolution is associated with an increase in the sophistication of energies and an increase in inner consciousness. Therefore, the more complex the gross forms, the more subtle are the accompanying energy patterns or fields, and the greater the inner consciousness. In this phylogenetic and ontogenetic dynamic, the material element (including the energy fields linked to the material) can be seen as the external, objective aspect or external form. As such it is constantly present throughout, and its presence extends upward to the highest level of the inner, subjective aspect, the highest possible consciousness. Tissue dysfunctions in

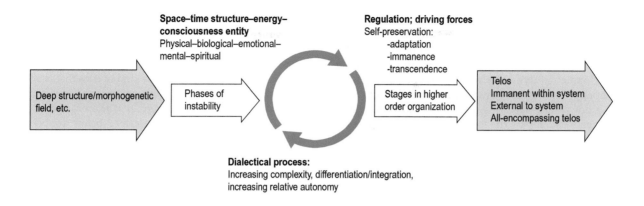

Figure 18.1
Developmental dynamics of the person.

certain stages of development of the tissue can often be associated with certain conditioned dysfunctional patterns of consciousness. Therefore there is generally an association between regressive palpation (and the palpation of developmental dynamics in the tissue), and certain inner dynamics of consciousness.

It would be a mistake, however, to reduce inner experiences to the energetic level or to the physical. If our aim is to treat the "wholeness" of the patient, we need to do more than just treat the tissue correlate. Osteopaths also need the ability to discover those components that arise from the inner consciousness, and to take due account of them. The degree of consciousness that osteopaths are able to exercise towards the inner emotional, mental, and spiritual elements in themselves and in their patients will determine how able they are to recognize tissue–consciousness patterns in their patients; in other words, to make the link between the patterns found in the tissue and the inner dimension in the patient, and to take due account of it. Further, the more they are able to do this, the more likely it is that the treatment they provide will not give rise to fresh dissociative patterns. In deciding the treatment approach, it is necessary to distinguish between the different osteopathic viewpoints as appropriate, and also to distinguish

the interaction of structure and function. This offers a solid methodology for the treatment of tissue dysfunction complexes and the associated subjective patterns of consciousness.

The following will assist with interpretation of Figure 18.1. The entity composed of structure–function–consciousness exists on the physical, biological, mental, and spiritual level (see, for example, Table 25.3). In osteopathy, the idea that the body possesses its own self-regulatory powers has usually only been stated in relation to the biological level. In fact it extends to every level of the structure–function–consciousness entity. Characteristic features of this entity are the maintenance and assertion of the self, and self-adaptation. The wholeness, autonomy, and identity of the person have to be maintained against environmental constraints; otherwise its existence is threatened. On the biological level, this principle similarly applies to each cell, tissue, organ, and organ system. It applies equally on other levels, such as emotional and mental.

At the same time, there is a need for self-adaptation. If the person, cell, or tissue, e.g., the liver, is no longer able to adapt as a part to the whole or to another system, then its existence is likewise threatened. In diagnosis we look for findings that underlie the "horizontal capacity" or balance of self-preservation and self-adaptation of the person as a whole, of individual tissues/organs to each other, and also emotions, etc. We also seek those that underlie the "vertical capacity" of immanence and transcendence, which plays a determining part in the developmental dynamics of the person. Findings that may appear in terms of immanence would, for example, be a downward-operating process in which the higher elements encompass the lower and place them in their relative context. An example of this might be the way that the limbic system subsumes the reptilian brain, or the cerebral cortex the limbic system. Dysfunctional findings in this kind of process might appear as dissociation of the higher element relative to the lower (e.g., in the form of anorexia, see Chapters 1 and 15) or as a diminution or dissolution of the higher element. Self-transcendence as an evolutionary drive toward a higher level, which reaches out beyond what is, is by no means something that only exists in phylogenetics or embryonic development; it is part of being human and of all phenomena. The developmental dynamics of the person follow a course that proceeds through phases of instability. These may be expressed as disturbances in wellbeing, life crises, or diseases. We need to find out the extent to which these present a danger, for example of dissolution of the self.

Transcendence is part of a dialectical process leading to greater complexity. Differentiation from something multiform and partial leads to the creation of something new, by a process of integration that leads to a higher state of unity.

This step-by-step evolutionary process of increasing differentiation and integration takes place in each of the levels mentioned above, so that there is a process of development within each of the various levels (emotional, mental, etc.). In addition, development is taking place – characterized by breaks in symmetry – from one level to another. This ultimately leads to an increase in coherent heterogeneity. The result of this, as explained later in this text, is the formation of wholes/parts organized in a holarchical way, and an increase in relative autonomy. Within the particular system, the deep structure (the morphogenetic field) acts as a driving force, representing a kind of pattern of higher probability, a blueprint of characteristics for that system. Forces of attraction direct the dynamics operating in the particular system. These are attractors immanent within the system (i.e., endpoints that exist within it).

The system is also affected by a telos outside itself, since it is in turn part of another, "higher" system. The process recurs ad infinitum.

Another possible explanation is that the force operating might be a chaotic attractor, a kind of telos that is all-permeating and all-encompassing, or immanent in all that exists, which Teilhard de Chardin calls the omega point.

The investigation methods described below are possible approaches designed to turn these viewpoints to practical application. It is not necessary to adopt all the methods presented; quite the contrary in fact, as they can be adapted and replaced by others that work better for the particular osteopath.

Factors that influence the body shape

Many factors influence the way in which the body takes shape: they include those present in the physical, biological, social, and cultural environment (from the prenatal stage to the end of life), the subjective consciousness that emerges in the particular individual, the hereditary and constitutional tendencies that are expressed, the way in which the body is used, moved, or nourished, the accustomed posture, and the breathing pattern. The way in which the body takes shape is also influenced by the emotional patterns or systems of belief with which individuals identify and the mannerisms by which they express themselves; by how they experience their bodies themselves or as a result of the sociocultural environment or the teaching of their parents, those parts of the self that they come to value more, and which less, and the way in which they as individuals interpret certain experiences, states, and disease symptoms. All these decisions and experiences, some conscious, others quite unconscious, exert their formative effect on the body and person and on the tissue. They also find expression by means of the body, and the osteopath can discover them by taking the history, by inspection, examination, palpation, and specific tests.

Subjectivity in diagnosis

However, there are limits to the objectivity of the findings made in the course of diagnosis, since these are also affected by the subjective influence of the osteopath's range of experience, knowledge, and consciousness, and by the interpretation consequently placed on the findings. The subjective influence can be all the more marked depending on the degree of validity of the diagnostic procedures. This becomes increasingly evident, the more the procedures relate to functional matters.*

Osteopaths can, however, develop greater neutrality in their empathetic assessment by working to train their consciousness. It is not helpful to treat subjective findings as irrefutable truths when presenting them to the patient, and sensitivity should be exercised when judging which subjective findings in the tissue should be communicated to them. Firstly, there is no benefit to patients if these findings are not related to their own experience; secondly, the very nature of the therapeutic situation means that everything a practitioner says has enormous influence on the patient. What should be encouraged, however, is patients' awareness, their ability to experience their own bodies and recognize the interdependence of their internal and external worlds.

Diagnosis does not simply mean a list of symptoms

In osteopathy, a diagnosis that seeks to do no more than compile a list of symptoms, from which to give a name to the particular disturbance or disorder, is of limited therapeutic value. There is no harm in doing so, but an exclusive focus on describing the disease or its symptoms is to be avoided. It brings the risk of giving the symptoms a significance that is not justified by their actual importance in terms of ontogenesis, and may then lead to treatment that is directed at suppressing the symptoms. It makes the patient dependent on the disease description. As a general rule the symptoms can be seen as an indicator light signaling the fact that something is wrong. They are the outward manifestation of inner processes. The pattern of symptoms enables the osteopath to assess whether the disease course is chronic or acute, and to distinguish degenerative, inflammatory or necrotizing processes. When interpreting the findings, the point is not to reduce the diagnostic process to a linear, mechanistic procedure (for example, looking for the primary dysfunction) but to integrate this into a complete, holistic view of the patient.

*Quite apart from the fact that strict scientific objectivity, such as is applied in the examination of non-living matter, is inappropriate when examining living things, i.e., chaotic and open systems; indeed, this is impossible in practice. Nevertheless, the additional use of objective procedures, such as laboratory tests or medical imaging, is of course entirely appropriate in given cases as an aid to diagnosis.

For a diagnosis to be particularly helpful, it should always give a clear idea of the changes that have taken place in the person and the type of restrictions present in the tissue:

- The way that the patient's body as a whole functions in relation to past events: how did the patient's body function in the past and what influences have led to its present way of functioning?

- The way that the patient's body as a whole is organized and functions in the present: what types of coordination and organization maintain its present homeostasis? What imbalances are reflected in particular dysfunctions? Where is the imbalance brought into balance (and is that place of balance within or external to the body)?

- The way that the patient's body as a whole will function, if the situation is projected into the future: how will it function with the organization it has at present? In what direction does the imbalance tend; toward what potential state of balance does it seem to be oriented? What potential challenge does this present and what risks might it pose?

A good diagnosis also always involves a search for the possible causes of the disturbance, those things that elicit symptoms, and conditions that tend to give rise to pathology.

The history should seek to establish whether the patient has suffered any accidents or physical trauma, even if these appear to be trivial or insignificant. Even if long forgotten, they may nevertheless have played an important role in the development of the dysfunction: the patient's tissue may not have forgotten. Even a post-operation scar, or one left by a past accident, can be associated with the patient's present problem.

Particular attention should be paid to prenatal, perinatal, or postnatal trauma. This often only produces symptoms years or even decades later, when the patient's capacities of compensation are exhausted. It is also often the case that such subtle disturbances and changes in tension only become apparent some time later, as the body grows and takes shape. The osteopath, however, may be able to sense them long before the symptoms appear.

Another influence is (conditioned) belief systems, or the state of emotional, mental, or spiritual development of the patient; the effect that these belief systems exert on the patient's life is very important for treatment. (For example, they will determine whether the treatment given should be translative or transformative.) They influence the kind of communication that takes place between osteopath and patient, the options that are open and the ways in which they are able to work together in the healing process.

An essential point when looking at disease causation is that the osteopath should not regard the patient's emotional life, cultural and social environment as a separate issue from the physical disturbances. All form part of an interconnected complex. Subjective, intersubjective, interobjective, and objective dimensions are all partial aspects that together influence health, disease, or dysfunction. Recognition of this fact will prevent treatment from becoming too one-sided in its approach.

Further, good diagnosis offers the possibility of preventive application of osteopathy, averting unnecessary suffering. Other courses of action, besides the manual treatment, can also help: such things as a change of diet, workplace or occupation may also be needed so that the patient does not continue to suffer the effects of one-sided physical or psychological stresses.

Finally, the body's state of homeostatic balance also enables us to assess the extent to which the patient's body and person will be able to integrate particular therapeutic impulses: whether they can do so at all, or whether the demands would be too great for their resources. Is the body system so altered and impaired that it is no longer able to "listen" or react to other systems?

Diagnosis begins as soon as the patient enters the room, with the very first handshake. Even such details as the patient's gait and the quality and strength of hand pressure can provide an indication that will help you decide where to look in the course of further examination (how the patient's head is held, the position of the shoulders and the pelvis, curvatures of the spine, etc.).

It is very important to give the patient a sense of being valued and taken seriously, from the very first moment of meeting. The more patients are able to feel this, the more willing they are to cooperate. As in all kinds of therapy, a good rapport between practitioner and patient is fundamental to success. In this case rapport refers to an immediacy in the contact that is established,

good communication, and being "on the same wavelength." Conscious ways that practitioners can use to establish this are by adapting their volume and tone of voice, speed and rhythm of speech, and choice of words to match the patient, similarly their breathing rate and body posture, gestures and facial expressions. In sheer spatial terms, the practitioner can adopt a position at roughly the same height as the patient, so that the patient does not have to look up or look down to make eye contact when giving the history.

Sometimes, in the professional situation, we find it difficult to do things that come so easily and automatically in everyday life when dealing with people and relating to friends, and in the therapeutic process we imagine these normally simple things to be beyond us, demanding impossible intellectual effort. It is very helpful if we can allow ourselves in professional practice to apply all the resources that we use without a moment's thought in normal life.

The whole and the part

In assessing the patient, the person needs to be seen both as a whole (consisting of subholons, see also pp. 13ff.) and as a part of other wholes. The findings to be noted will take the subjective, intersubjective, and objective levels of the patient (physical, biological, emotional, mental, and spiritual) equally into account. They must at the same time be seen in relation to the interactive unity of the person as a whole and the dynamic interactions between function and structure. The patient's evolutionary and holarchical development should also be discovered and noted, observing with empathy and sympathetic insight. To observe in this way will immediately cure us of objective absolutism, and enable us instead to see the deep intermeshing of ourselves and others, both subjectively and objectively.

- What physical and biological components are not fully integrated in the patient? What emotional, mental, and spiritual aspects, situations, or experiences is the patient refusing to accept? These need to be differentiated, integrated and experienced. Whatever the person refuses to accept must be re-experienced: the patient will have to live through it again.

- What are the underlying physical and biological patterns of dysfunction and the emotional, mental, and spiritual belief patterns? Patients constantly reinforce and express these patterns in the situations of their lives.

- What are the conscious and unconscious decisions and intentions that are present in a patient's various levels of experience? These determine and produce the individual's future experiences, since every intention (and even every thought) has its consequences. Every action produces a reaction. This is where opportunity and freedom and the potential growth of patients are to be found. As patients learn, not only to become aware of their intentions but also to place them consciously at the outset of their actions, they assume responsibility for their lives.

- How does the body as a whole maintain its order and intactness in the face of the given circumstances? It is here that we can find out the tendencies that exercise a homeodynamic and regulatory effect. It is vital to resource-oriented therapy to establish a connection and synchronization with these. (This is therapy that utilizes the patient's own resources for the purpose of healing.) The right approach is generally to establish this connection before resolving dysfunctions. (However, important as it is, this rule is not absolute.)

An essential part of the diagnostic process is to enquire about the relationship between the "wholes" aspect and the "parts" aspect of the patient, to find out what balance exists between the two. The relationship of the particular part (e.g., particular tissue) to the whole changes during the development of dysfunctions and the disease processes. This is found both in palpation and in history taking where we try to discover what patients' relationships are to their inner and external worlds. In essence, two basic tendencies are found:

- Patients' relative autonomy or self-assertion may be dysfunctionally exaggerated with respect to the external world. There may be a kind of egocentric bolstering of the person over other persons, nature as a whole, and other kinds of being. In this case, the increase in relative autonomy is not based on internalizing and embracing more levels of being, as in healthy development, but rather in separating and distancing oneself from them. This strengthens the separation between the self and the world outside in favor of the egocentric importance of the person.

There has been a dysfunctional shift that displaces the "parts" aspect of the person to the benefit of the "wholes" part. The typical finding in terms of energy is that the person's body and being absorbs more energy than it gives out.

- There may be a loss of relative autonomy, in that the natural boundaries of the individual are weakened. In this situation, relative autonomy is lessened in that the "wholes" aspect of the person declines and there is a dysfunctional increase in the "parts" aspect or in the person's receptiveness. The boundaries of the self relative to the world outside are diminished, weakened with respect to the external world. In this case, the diminution of boundaries is not a lessening of egocentricity, as it would be in healthy development (where in fact it would be a sign of greater relative autonomy), but a reduction in the capacity to maintain the self over the external world. There has been a shift that displaces the "wholes" aspect of the person to the benefit of the "parts" aspect. The typical finding in terms of energy is that the person's body and being gives out more energy than it absorbs.

A similar method is used to establish the vertical capacity that the patient has (see also p. 16). This means that we look for the relationship between self-immanence and self-transcendence, or between the dysfunctional dissolution and dissociation of the self:

- Dissolution of the self: regression occurs if it is no longer possible, for whatever reason, to maintain either individuality or any form of relatedness, for both are necessary to existence. The higher resolves into the lower element: the holon into its subholons. This would mean, for example, that certain somatic or psychological parts of the patient are no longer as well integrated as they could be, and instead disintegrate. (For example, the function of a limb or organ is restricted, or hormonal regulation becomes disturbed.) The dissolution of a holon happens in the reverse direction to the process of its formation. (In the opposite scenario, features characteristic of regression often make their appearance during the healing process. What this means in practice is that previously repressed disturbances or emotions can reappear, and chronic states can change back into acute ones.)

- Dissociation:[†] on the intellectual level there can be a pathological dissolution of the link with the biological level (e.g., in the form of anorexia) or with the person's surroundings in the biosphere (e.g., environmental destruction).This points to the fact that autonomy can only ever be relative, since on the one hand it reflects the "wholes" aspect of a holon, but on the other it is always part of some other context.

- Dissociations can also become evident in the form of subjective or objective changes. (For example, there may be a change in the patient's behavior, or a disorder such as anorexia.)

In clinical practice in osteopathy, these tensions are not only observable through palpation, despite the fact that this forms the major part of osteopathic treatment (e.g., palpation of tissue that has lost some degree of its autonomy and is being compensated by other tissues). In taking the history and in the observation of the patient, the osteopath tries to discover which tendency predominates.

This stage of diagnosis also proceeds from the general to the specific. The first step is to observe the patient as a whole entity. Attention then passes to particular regions, following the leads to the dynamics of particular aspects of tissues and organs (which can be seen as the objective correlate of subpersonalities).

The osteopath palpates the patient. The relationship between the particular part (e.g., a given tissue) and the whole to which it belongs changes in the development of a dysfunction or pathogenic processes, and the practitioner senses whether there are parts or regions that have lost their autonomy in relation to the surrounding tissue, or that are exerting excessive autonomy relative to their surroundings or the body as a whole (so as to appear relatively isolated or decoupled).

In both cases the availability of the tissue or function to the body as a whole is impaired. The practitioner uses palpation to approach this complex that is relatively either self-enclosed within too harshly defined boundaries or tending to merge with its surroundings. The aim in this first approach is to encourage its differentiation.

The emphasis is twofold: to resolve pathogenic influences and integrate those parts that have lost or exaggerated their relative autonomy. Both serve to support the establishment of higher-order balance within the body as a whole. The result is generally to increase its capacities and options for compensation, which in turn aids its ability to heal itself.

The history

In taking the history, practitioners will generally begin by collecting information and impressions that give an insight into the patient's capacities of perception, feelings and emotional life, cultural and social environment, and the disease course and the investigations carried out to date. This information remains in the background, however, during the palpation, and the practitioner's hands and sensory organs can focus on the history that the body and its tissues have to tell with as little prejudgment as possible.

The history usually begins with a description of the main complaint. The patient must be allowed time to explain freely, and is occasionally encouraged as necessary to give a fuller description. If anything is unclear, it should be clarified. Patients may well hold back with their description of feelings and emotions, thinking that these are irrelevant, so you should assure them that you are just as interested in these as in other facts.

Once the patient's free account is finished and you have made a chronological note of the disturbances involved in the course of the complaint, it is time to ask direct questions about anything that is still not clear. In the first instance you are looking for the causes of the symptoms; then for those factors that are maintaining them. This will not only include physical symptoms but the patient's self-perception and emotional life, family, cultural and biosocial environment. Try to develop a deep, rounded understanding of the patient as a whole. The nature of the symptoms – characteristics, type, intensity and progress – and how long they have been present and the time when they first began are of course extremely important. Are there any other symptoms, associated with those described? What eases the symptoms? What exacerbates them? What kinds of treatment have already been given? All the available information concerning the patient should be systematically noted.

It is usually necessary to make written notes so as to maintain an overview and to be able to assess the

---

[†]Dissociation is meant here as a partial or complete splitting off of psychological functions such as patients' memories of their own past, their own feelings (pain, fear, hunger, thirst, etc.), awareness of their own bodies and environment.

healing process in subsequent treatment sessions. The chronology of the problems and any accidents and trauma, including traumatic experiences, from birth to the present time, are especially significant.

The history should also give the practitioner an indication as to which major body systems are particularly affected in the imbalance that has disturbed the homeostasis of the body as a whole. This may, for example, be the musculo–fascio–skeletal system, the autonomic nervous system, the circulatory, visceral, or endocrine system. It may be external influences such as diet, environmental pollutants, or psychological stress. Are there interactions between these systems? These insights will provide a guideline to show which types of investigation are next indicated as helpful or essential. Even broad categories can give a basic hint as to treatment (males tend on the whole to be rationally inclined, autonomous, and goal-directed, while females might have a more emotional inclination, be more concerned with relationships, and take a more global approach). Recognition of the general personality category – more introverted or more extroverted – can also be helpful for the therapeutic interaction.

The most important points for the history

Hereditary influences:
Damage to the germ cells (e.g., through X-ray radiation, chemical substances)
Parental diet
Endocrine or metabolic disturbances in the parents.

Influences before and during pregnancy:
Maternal age
Maternal health (rubella, pre-eclampsia, etc.)
States of deficiency
Drug use, heavy metal, or pesticide pollution, etc.
X-ray radiation
Systemic disease
Endocrine disturbances
Stress suffered by the mother during pregnancy.

Number and course of previous pregnancies:
Miscarriages, stillbirths, or malformed births
Premature or late delivery.

The birth process:
Duration and strength of labor pains
Quantity of amniotic fluid
Presentation: face presentation (resulting in extreme extension), cephalic presentation of occiput (resulting in extreme rotation).

Duration of birth process:
Too long (e.g., hardening of the perineum, tense cervix, disproportionate difference in size of fetus and mother's pelvis, extreme lumbar lordosis of mother)
Too rapid (e.g., multiple births).

Conditions obtaining at the birth:
Poor hygiene
Excessive use of anesthetics
Excessive use of agents to stimulate contraction
Forceps delivery or vacuum extraction
Caesarean section.

Appearance and behavior of the newborn:
Asymmetric skull shape
Excessive bulges or depressions in the cranial bones
Overlapping of the cranial bones that does not resolve
Bluish discoloration of the skin (cyanosis).

Functional disturbances:
Abnormal crying or shedding of tears
Inability to suckle
Difficulties in suckling
Disturbances affecting the eyes (nystagmus, strabismus, etc.)
Opisthotonus
Spasticity or paralysis of limbs
Convulsions
Fever, tremor, and excessive drowsiness.

Development of the child:
(The most critical period is from the 6th month of gestation to the 2nd year of life.)
Incomplete closure of the fontanelles
Disturbances in the movement of the limbs and cranium

Asymmetries of the limbs and other body structures
Disturbances of the eyes
Accidents and falls
Abnormal behavior, e.g., banging of the head against walls or doors.

Serious diseases in childhood:
Scarlet fever, measles, whooping cough, otitis media, pneumonia, encephalitis, meningitis, etc.

Emotional status, family situation, psychological trauma in childhood:
For example: abuse, separation, death of family members, adoption, etc.

Serious disease in adulthood and trauma:
Time of occurrence
Childhood: accidents, falls
Adolescence: e.g., sports accidents
Adulthood: e.g., automobile accidents
Type, severity, region of body affected, and direction of force suffered
Dental procedures, e.g., extraction, bridge, brace
Operations
Accidents, whiplash injuries, concussion, fractures
Sunstroke, heatstroke, extreme cold
Psychoemotional: separation or death of a partner or close relative, loss of employment, abuse, etc.
Behavioral changes and symptoms following trauma.

Nature and location of pain or other symptom:
Description of pain/symptoms and location
General symptoms: reduction in performance, tiredness, loss of appetite, weight changes
Cardiovascular: palpitations, arrhythmias, chest pain, cyanosis, breathlessness
Respiratory organs: breathlessness, cough, expectoration, chest pain, hoarseness
Digestive tract: pain, feeling of pressure, nausea, vomiting, belching, bloating, colic, constipation, iarrhea, fatty, bloody or mucous stools, and stool color
Genitourinary system: color, smell, and quantity of urine; blood in urine; pain on urination; pain in the lumbar region; facial swelling; menstruation (length of cycle, quantity of blood, pain); menopause; libido

Blood: color of skin and mucosa, skin and nasal bleeding, tendency to hematoma
Nervous system: disturbances of sensation, pain along course of nerves, reflexes
Disturbances of the sympathetic nervous system with functional disturbances of internal organs
Abnormal sensations in the region of a suture
Locomotor system: pain localization; pain or tenderness to pressure; association with movement, stress, position, or time of day; pain on initiating movement, with stress, or at rest; movement restriction, etc.
Fascial Distortion Model: this offers ways to differentiate pain with direct treatment strategies of localized areas (see Chapter 20)
Pain with a distinct place: herniated trigger points (HTP), triggerband (TB), so called folding distortion (FD), and continuum distortion (CD)
Pain without a distinct place: so called cylinder distortion (CyD)
Pressure pain: in case of TB, HTP, CD
Pain in case of loading: TB, CD, HTP, uFD
Pain during lying: rFD.

Status praesens/patient's condition at the present time:
The patient's present condition should be established by inquiry at each session in order to assess the course of treatment.

Patient's activities:
Type of work
Sleeping position
Type and extent of sports exercise
Life circumstances.

Psychological status/social environment/family history:[5,6]
The patient's sociocultural environment and the dynamic interaction between individual and environment will also play their part in diagnosis and treatment. The manner in which the patient is able to balance inner physical need, energetic state, and psychological needs with the demands of the environment is significant for therapy and so should be elicited.

	Where	Patient's consciousness	Consolidating	Problematical	Transformational
Beige Archaic–instinctive	Newborn infants, people with learning difficulties, severely confused or traumatized individuals. Approx. 0.1%• of the adult population, 0% of the power	Prepersonal: level of simple survival; (actions are habit and instinct-driven); in newborn infants, dependent on development	Ensuring basic needs: food, warmth, physical protection. In the case of those suffering from Alzheimer's, caused by disease	Healing of psychological trauma, esp. relating to the non-fulfillment of basic needs and existential anxieties¶	Healing of psychological trauma, esp. relating to the non-fulfillment of basic needs and existential anxieties¶
Purple Magical–animistic	18 months until age 2 years, Developing World, gangs, sports teams, etc. 10% of popn., 1% of power	World is governed by magical powers (acc. to development until 2nd year). Problematical, e.g., "Someone is thinking bad thoughts about me and now I'm ill"	Use of positive "good" desires as magical power	Everything that removes the element of magic from this worldview: everything that creates objectivity, or reinforces the power of the self	Everything that removes the element of magic from this worldview: everything that creates objectivity, or reinforces the power of the self
Red Power gods	From 2 to 4 years of age. Toddlers' tantrums ("terrible twos"), rebellious youth, gang leaders, New Age narcissism, wild rock stars. 20% of popn., 5% of power	Egocentric, individuals doing what they want: "I can do anything as long as I want to" (up to age 4 years, depending on development)	Use of this (egocentric) wishful thinking for the purpose of therapy: trust in own strength and will. Consolidation of boundaries of self (what I do and do not want). Guided meditation as a hero's progress, in which hero conquers disease and is triumphant; strengthening of the self	Associated lack of insight. Treatment tip: to "sell" to patients what is right for them in such a way that they think of it as their own idea. Sometimes it can also help to suggest that the self will suffer more if the advice is not followed.	Anything that takes them beyond the boundaries of the self: all that creates an objective approach; also, any leads that can point to powers greater than the self (which in fact eases the way toward blue)

	Where	Patient's consciousness	Consolidating	Problematical	Transformational
Blue Mythic order, conformist rules	From age 4 years until age 7. Fundamentalism, patriotism, ethnocentricity, etc. 40% of popn., 30% of power	Sociocentric (follows the rules of the given group norm, religion, culture, or "ism." Individuals realize that they cannot direct the world according to their wishes, but do believe that there is a power that can (father, God, religion, sometimes even science). What are the norms that feed the life of this patient?	It is important to recognize what the "religion" of this patient is like; where it exerts its healing (consolidating and integrating) effects, and where (if appropriate) its effect is to make ill	An understanding of the norms that apply to the patient is essential: therapeutic intervention is possible by remaining within them; patients cooperate if the therapy accords with their norm, and tend not to if it doesn't (or must attempt to persuade)	Expose beliefs and convictions of which the patient is (still) unaware (food, sexuality, sickness/health, etc.), and (a) discuss sensitively with the patient where these stand in the way of health; (b) strengthen and confirm where they assist the healing process
Orange Scientific achievement	Approx. from age 7 years. Enlightenment, rising middle classes 30% of popn., 50% of power	Technical/ functional (guided mainly by measurable objective criteria, e.g., cost/ usefulness/ efficiency/ practicability, etc.)	Essential for patients to be given rational explanation of the facts as they are, to enable them to be open to the methods proposed••	Scientific objectivity sees mainly just external "hard" facts as proper justification; realms of inner experience tend to be devalued or excluded	Everything that leads patients into their inner realms of experience[¶¶]

Green The sensitive self	Postmodernism, humanistic psychology, Greenpeace, political correctness, diversity movements. 10% of popn., 15% of power	Pluralistic/ alternative (open to the diversity of possibilities) general preference for alternative/ unconventional methods over conventional ones	Relation to the greater whole; often, however, without sufficient differentiation ("all is one"). Gives full recognition to pluralism, inwardness and sensitivity, thus consolidating effect; has no difficulty with nearness, so practitioner should (also) take care to regulate distance	Pluralist viewpoint can go too far, resulting in patients rejecting distinctions based on assessment (which are also necessary in any treatment)	Support patient's capacity to make distinctions, so as to aid the emergence of "wholes" out of pluralistic "isolated entities"; concept of development should be stressed
Yellow Integrative	1% of popn., 5% of power	Holarchical, flexible (acts on the basis of knowledge and competence rather than power or status). Equal recognition and justification given to the self, nature, and culture, and all of these are equally experienced	Highly articulate patients. Attitude of full, independent responsibility for own lives; only slight therapeutic prompting is needed. They know about the significance of ALL levels of development and integrate them into their lives. Clarity in the experiencing of their own self, but without identifying with it. Full acknowledgment of cultural socialization, the surrounding world of family and friendship (incl. beneficial values and traditions). The scientific approach is utilized and integrated. Sensitivity, multiculturalism, and pluralism are put into practice, and they in particular are integrated into a living holarchy instead of being set out alongside or in opposition to one another		
Turquoise Holistic	0.1% of popn., 1% of power	Unites feeling with knowledge; sees the different levels of interaction and recognizes resonance and flow	Common, conscious flow of therapeutic interaction; independently able to integrate multiple impulses. In addition to the "yellow" qualities, a subtle (dream) state becomes increasingly prominent; consciousness extends into sleep; most noticeable in therapy is an increasing unity of body and spirit, experienced with immediacy		

TABLE 18.1: Levels of development according to Habecker/Liem, based on spiral dynamics[‡‡,§§]

‡‡All levels build one upon another in sequence, and should be approached working upward from below. (Thus, a hungry person (level 1) should first of all be given something to eat; a preconventional individual first needs to become conventional before progressing to the transconventional state.)

§§There is an increase in the extent of insight into the self, working down from top to bottom. Nevertheless, the basic functions of the "lower levels" are fully preserved, and can be reactivated at any time.

•Percentages are approximate only, and will not therefore total 100%.

†The need for healing of traumatic physical and psychological experiences can arise within any level; in relation to the main themes of the particular developmental stage(s) this applies especially at the time these experiences make their appearance physiologically (e.g., in "Red": the sudden extreme or persistent suppression of egocentric tendencies or of the individual's own strength).

••Patients at this level are not usually able to make the distinction between what is truly transrational and what is prerational magic. Since they confuse the two, they tend to reject both. It is therefore best to avoid saying anything that is not strictly logical, even if it derives from higher insights.

¶It could be explained to patients that these too (subjective and intersubjective) can be investigated scientifically.

Level of development

In order to establish contact satisfactorily with patients, it is essential to know their level of development, so as to meet them at the place where they actually are. If, for example, a patient's developmental state is at the orange level, and an explanation based on the consciousness of inner, shared conscious flow (turquoise) is offered as part of the therapeutic interaction, then that treatment would present problems for the patient.

A second point to be made is that patients' understanding of their health varies depending on the level they are at. It is also a general rule that no level can be bypassed. It is simply not possible for a patient on the red level to make the jump straight to the orange level. For such patients, the translative approach is first to support them in reinforcing the egocentric boundaries of the self. The transformative approach involves confronting them with powers that transcend the self, so as to accompany them to the blue level. For patients who are at the blue level it can help to offer a more reasoned interpretation of those aspects of their rigid viewpoint that are hindering their health. On the blue level, it makes sense to draw on scientific findings, such as a study on the success of osteopathic treatment in cases of sinusitis.

The degree of responsibility that patients are able to assume for their health on the basis of their development also varies considerably according to level.

Circumstances that perpetuate disease

These include conditioned reflexes, such as fear in anticipation in the case of asthma (e.g., anxiety about triggering an attack can cause autonomic nervous changes that actually provoke an attack), or exaggerated forms of treatment that lead to further damage.

Some examples of disease causing stress

- Life-changing stress (deeply distressing experiences such as the death of someone close to them, becoming unemployed, etc.)
- Biological stress (environmental causes → pollution, noise, electrosmog; modern lifestyles → "junk food" poor in nutritional value or laden with chemicals, harmful recreational substances, time pressures, too much or too little exercise, constant or unexpected changes in schedule)
- Emotional stress (frustrating demands → too much to do, too many telephone calls, etc. All

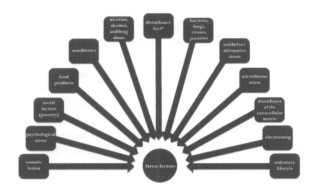

Figure 18.1.1
Overview of stress factors. Many of these factors interact and overlap - eg xenobiotics and oxidative/nitrosative stress, etc.)

those sources of unrelieved stimulation that activate the autonomic nervous system)
- Mental stress
- Spiritual stress (inadequate belief systems, unconscious fear of (or longing for) death)
- Social stress (big city life, crowds, social isolation).

Other aspects to be borne in mind are the level of psychospiritual development and how the individual deals with stress. Denial and suppression of problems have an adverse effect on health, as do attempts to avoid them or to attribute blame, or absence of emotion. Actively attempting to find a solution, on the other hand, and talking about the matter, are healthy.[7,8]

True as it is that the main route by which an osteopath makes a diagnosis is by means of the hands, verbal communication is also useful as the means of taking the case history; indeed, alongside the measurement of blood pressure and temperature, laboratory tests, and X-rays, the interview is an essential aid to arriving at a diagnosis. By taking the history, the practitioner hears about the disease from the patient's point of view. With practice, practitioners can recognize coded messages in what is said. Another benefit is that it brings them into contact with their patients' psychoemotional worlds. For beginners in osteopathy in particular, it is helpful to have a set routine to follow when taking the history.

Applying Stuart and Liebermann's BATHE technique

Stuart and Liebermann[9] investigated what it was that distinguished doctors who were successful in their dealings with patients from those who were less successful. Their study yielded the following technique for questioning patients, which enables more effective listening and therefore better patient contact. It consists of a quick succession of five questions:[10]

B: The first question enquires into the **B**ackground. It involves asking what is going on in the person's life. Questions might be, "What happened?" or "Tell me what happened to you." Stuart and Liebermann say that it is then important to listen without interruption for three minutes. If they continue to listen for longer than this, the patient tends to wander off into details and overlook the most important element – their feelings. The next question should therefore follow on immediately.

A stands for **A**ffect: "How did that make you feel?"

T asks about **T**rouble: "What troubles you the most?" This question is important because it looks at the heart of the matter. It helps untangle the confusion by directing attention to whatever it is that is causing most pain. The principle behind it is the need to find the point where the pain is profoundest, and then, using that as the starting point, to work back upward to the top.

H asks about **H**andling the problem: "How are you handling that?" A helpful question is: "What helps you most to deal with it?" This directs the patient's attention to the resources that their environment offers to help them overcome the disease/problem/challenge. The practitioner's confidence in a kind of self-healing and self-regulation is key here. Although the patient's need is for help, it is not a matter of presenting them with a solution, but of putting them into the position where they are able to find solutions themselves.

E is for **E**mpathy: "That must be very difficult"; "I am sorry to hear what has happened to you"; "I am very moved by what you say." Patients need to sense that you truly mean what you say. It is enormously helpful

for them to know that someone cares about what has happened, that another person feels genuine sympathy and so for that short time they are not alone with their suffering.

Inspection

The inspection involves the overall observation of the patient's posture and movement. Like the history, the inspection proceeds in a deductive way, from the general to the specific. The practitioner studies the patient from in front, from the side and from behind, noting any anomalies, such as variations in "gravity lines." Closer examination of individual structures may also be made, but without losing sight of the organization of the body as a whole. Is one ear, scapula, iliac crest, or posterior superior iliac spine higher than the other? Are the pelvic bones asymmetrical? What is the position of the feet and the knees? What curvatures of the spine are present? How is the head held? Is there any twitching of an eyelid or of the masseter muscle? Is there redness on a defined area of the body? Patients can be asked to perform a particular movement and a comparison is made of the amplitude so as to identify restrictions. Inconsistencies are another point to be noted: is there, for example, a mismatch between the patient's voice and appearance? Further reading offers more advice on the inspection.[11–15] Observation of patients' gestures[16] can also offer important insights for treatment strategies.

Palpation

The very first step to be taken at the start of palpatory examination concerns the practitioner's inner attitude: the practitioner must always begin each time by defocusing, by consciously avoiding all focus, so as to make contact with the whole patient and the tissue in an unprejudiced and intention-free way. This enables the practitioner to carry out the palpation of the tissue, as far as possible, without preconceived ideas.

The examination proceeds from the general to the specific, working from the global to the local and back again to the global. There is a process of focusing and defocusing, oscillating between the two in a rhythmic study of the local and global interaction, and in this way homes in on the individual organizational pattern of the patient, with greater precision. The practitioner is "listening" by means of palpation and seeking to discover the interaction between the workings of the innate life forces or homeostatic forces and the way in

Diagnostic methodology – possible approaches
History; inspection Barral's manual thermal evaluation Following supporting feelings of security and safety, in activating resources of the myelinated vagus and balancing the autonomic nervous system (see Chapter 20)

Global examination:

• Global detection of the disturbance according to McKone
• Posture: postural patterns (e.g., according to Hall); Barre's vertical alignment test; fascial patterns and organization according to Zink; gravity lines according to Littlejohn
• Identifying major character structures
• Examining the chakras
• Palpation of energy fields: ethereal (vital life force), astral (emotional), mental, and causal
• Barral's manual thermal evaluation
• Global palpation of developmental dynamics
• Barral's listening test, see "Palpation of fasciae"
• Global rhythmic examination by passive synchronization with inherent rhythms (pulmonary respiration, primary respiration, etc.)
• Global examination by active testing of mobility:
  – in synchrony with involuntary rhythms
  – independently of these rhythms
  – by exogenous rhythm or oscillation testing
• Palpation of fasciae – passive or active
• Palpation of fluid patterns – passive or active
• Screening of tissue elasticity
• Global palpation of tissue density
• Differentiation of level of dysfunction

Local examination:

• Local examination according to McKone
• Local palpation of developmental dynamics
• Local listening test (Barral), see "Palpation of fasciae"
• Surface qualities
• Palpation of form
• Local palpation of tissue elasticity
• Local palpation of tissue density
• Local tenderness to pressure
• Palpation of muscle tone
• Local rhythmic examination by passive synchronization with inherent rhythms (pulmonary respiration, primary respiration, etc.)
• Local examination by active testing of mobility:
  – in synchrony with involuntary rhythms
  – independently of rhythmic phenomena
  – by exogenous rhythmic or oscillatory testing

- Palpation of fasciae:
  - undirected palpation of fascial tensions, e.g., according to Barral
  - testing of fascial "pull"
- Palpation of fluid patterns:
- passive palpation of fluids
- fluid drive diagnosis

TABLE 18.2: Diagnosis

which they are conditioned and bound or fixed through such factors as the habits and circumstances of life, physical or psychological trauma, or the experience of past illnesses (biokinetic energy). For this examination it is helpful to begin by helping the patient to experience feelings of security and safety, in activating resources of the myelinated supradiaphragmatic vagus to down-regulate hypersympathetic arousal or deactivate vagal unmyelinated immobility reactions and balancing the autonomic nervous system (see Chapter 20).

According to Becker,[17] whenever contact is established between practitioner and patient, three different viewpoints come together:

1 Patients' views and expectations about the likely causes of their symptoms. They typically describe these in terms of their life history and general medical knowledge. The emotions and life events they mention will be those they consider relevant to their complaint. Patients are sensitive to the verbal and non-verbal link between them and the practitioner, and the openness of the practitioner's approach to them. The way in which patients see the problem is an important step toward healing; frequently, they almost unconsciously circle around the actual problem. Identifying this "blind spot" calls for sensitivity and experience on the part of the practitioner.

2 The practitioner's view of the causes and process underlying the symptoms. Training, experience, and knowledge of the anatomical, physiological, embryological, and psychological associations help practitioners to form a particular picture of the disturbances from which the patient is suffering. They can order X-rays or laboratory tests, and can carry out physical or bioelectric examinations. Their experience and knowledge of these matters may be greater than those of the patient, but practitioners can nevertheless only build up a mental concept of the organization of the disturbances and whole-body interconnections.

3 The knowledge that the anatomical and physiological whole, made up of the patient's body, person, and tissues, have of the problem from which the patient is suffering. The patient's body contains the entire spectrum of interconnections. It stores the tensions and patterns of the dysfunctions as a result of the constant interaction of function and structure. These interconnections can make their appearance in any of the organ systems of the body. Once practitioners have noted the patient's view of what is happening, made a diagnosis and formed their ideas, they should set these aside in order to be open to what the tissue has to tell them.

Palpation enables the practitioner to make direct contact with the information that is present in the tissue. It is from the tissue that the practitioner discovers when the disturbances began and how they will continue to develop. The tissue itself tells what happened, how, when, and where. This kind of information cannot be obtained from X-rays, CT scans, or laboratory analysis; the tissue, however, can reveal it, and it does so through palpation. The practitioner's hands mold to the patient's body through gentle, sensitive touch. Palpation seeks not so much what the touch of the practitioner's fingers can discover as what the patient's body communicates through that touch. The development of this awareness is one of the great arts of osteopathy.

It is comparatively simple to sense the tensions caused by the trauma and disturbances in the tissue. Within them, however, and focusing these tensions, is something termed the "potency."

There is a point of rest in every dysfunction of the body, and this point embodies the potency of the particular dysfunction. Every change in this point of rest also produces a change in the associations of form and function in the pattern of tensions.

Global examination

Palpatory diagnosis (modified, according to McKone)

1 First impressions count!
   a Observation is an active process that demands discipline. Each individual palpation should be performed for a few seconds only. If it is carried on for longer, there is a tendency to slip into a conditioned, reductionist mindset without realizing. With this change to analytical thinking, focused attention, and even confusion with preconceived ideas, there is a risk of distorting perception.
   b When palpating, it is important that you do not concentrate on the region between your eyes. (This alters the quality of the concentration, which then becomes too invasive.)

2 Sensory/physical perception: practitioners need to have an awareness of themselves in the process and the presence of the particular phenomenon they are sensing and palpating.

3 Gestures:
   a It is important to perceive the patient's body, person, and gestures as a whole.
   b Make use of your imagination.

4 Once you have gained some practice in the diagnostic steps described in the following text, begin to sense within yourself what you palpate in the patient.

I. Palpation of specific regions, e.g., the back of the neck

The order in which the following description is given is for training purposes. After a certain period of practice it will be possible to start at step 3. Steps 4 and 5 can be combined with any other palpatory approach used in diagnosis, e.g., together with palpation of surface qualities, form, density, tissue elasticity, muscle tone, involuntary rhythms, mobility testing, etc.

1 Palpate and examine the skin, muscles, ligaments or membranes, joints, bones, and fluids. Once you are able to distinguish these, release your hands.

2 Palpate the nape of the neck. As soon as you begin to sense something and receive the first impression, release your hands.

3 Think of your own feet (i.e., switch off all expectations): while palpating the nape, think about your own feet. As soon as you perceive the first impression, as before, you remove your hands. The effect of palpating in this way is to prevent your approach to the patient from being one of thought penetration and to set you free from conditioned expectations based on previous palpatory experiences. The attitude of expectation prevents you from making contact with what your hands are actually touching.

4a Build up your mental impression of the patient by working upwards. As your hands palpate, resting motionless on the patient's nape, think from the patient's feet upwards, working in the direction from the feet toward the practitioner, letting your thoughts move onwards into your hands and thinking of the patient as expanding and becoming bigger. This enables you to hold the idea of the patient as a whole in your mind.

4b Plus mobilizing diagnostic approach. As in 4a, you should think about the wholeness of the patient while performing the palpation of the nape of the neck. Thus, the direction in which you think of the patient is upward from the feet toward the practitioner. At the same time, your hands make a mobilizing examination of the nape region (including all the tissues). The situation that often confronts practitioners during this process is the sense of being in their own way, and the urge to lapse into an analytical, reductionist focus.

5a Think about the patient in an upward direction, toward the practitioner, and at the same time think about both patient and practitioner in an ascending direction. The procedure is twofold: as in 4a, think about the wholeness of the patient while performing the palpation of the nape of the neck. The direction of thought is upward from the feet toward the practitioner. In addition (at the same time) you should think, expansively and in an ascending direction, of both patient and practitioner.

5b Plus mobilizing diagnostic approach. While palpating the nape of the neck with your hands you can simultaneously make a mobilizing examination of the nape region (including all the tissues).

II. Global detection of the disturbance

1 Shift (in terms of either actual physical movement or direction of attention) from the whole to the individual parts.

2 Do not hold onto the impression that is experienced; otherwise, it is lost. Instead you should allow yourself to dwell on the dynamics of direct, immediate experience. Practice constancy of attention to this.

3 Instead of trying to penetrate down to what is inward, allow it to emerge outward, to develop. *Note*: here you should pay special attention to palpation of developmental dynamics (see p. 294) and regressive tissue palpation phenomena. Findings based on an understanding of the relationship between structure (tissues, energy) and function (objective: physiology; subjective: consciousness).

4 Observational judgment.

This palpation involves an additional new element: intuition. You do not so much seek as find the dysfunctional aspect in the patient's body. Once more, you should think of the patient expansively and in an ascending direction, towards yourself, the practitioner. This enables you to sense the dysfunctional aspect of the patient in your own body, and in this way to localize it. Here, the practitioner's imagination comes into effect, operating as a creative element in the diagnostic process. You need to imagine, or allow yourself to envisage, where the problem, disturbance, or dysfunction is located within yourself. The focus of attention now is the body and person of the practitioner as a whole. Once again, during the palpation you must avoid focusing on the region between your eyes. Note: as in II(c).

Posture

Hall analyzed various features of patient posture to describe particular types of postural pattern: (Table 18.3).[18] Littlejohn described certain lines of force or "gravity lines" to which the body is subjected (Figure. 18.2). Mayr described postural patterns that arise in reaction to visceral changes, in particular in the digestive system.[19]

Postural pattern	Ventral (anterior type)	Dorsal (posterior type)
Joint problems	Increased lordosis of cervical spine. Restriction of cervicothoracic transition. Increased tension of posterior back muscles and ligaments. Restriction and increased tension at T11 and T12 (T10–L1). Load at lumbosacral transition	Occiput in extension (and compression). Stress at cervicothoracic transition. Increased thoracic kyphosis and weaker lower thoracic spine. Compression of sternocostal joints. Increased lumbar lordosis. Load at sacroiliac joints
Respiratory/circulatory	Tensions in diaphragm (often on inhalation). Weak, overstretched abdominal muscles	Tensions in diaphragm (often on exhalation). Disturbances in relative pressure between abdominal and chest cavities. Increased tension of abdominal wall
Visceral	Tendency to prolapse or sinking down of organs. Relaxation of parietal peritoneum. Tendency to hernias and irritation in the lesser pelvis	Increased pressure on abdominal and pelvic organs. Tendency to circulatory disturbances. Tendency to respiratory problems. Tendency to constipation

TABLE 18.3: Postural patterns
According to Hall, Wernham, and Littlejohn.[18]

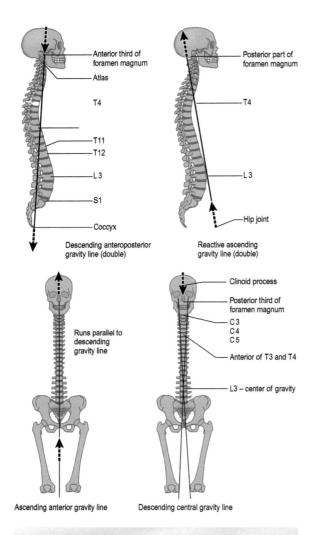

Figure 18.2
Gravity lines according to Littlejohn.

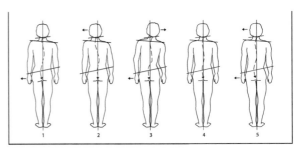

Figure 18.3
Barre's vertical alignment test.

Negative results: all reference points are found on the perpendicular. This should be held for at least four seconds.

Ascending chain may briefly be inhibited by standing on a Tempur cushion: neurovegetative dystonia: lateral shift.

Or four: shifted to the same side: completely decompensated (strong hypertension on one side (not clear why, maybe high toxic load, severe visceral problems) testing heart rate variability (NerveExpress testing)

1 Ascending dysfunction (pelvis displaced to one side): short leg, low back pain; dysfunction in the foot, knee, hip, or pelvis.

2 Descending dysfunction (head/neck displaced to one side): neck pain, dysfunction of the clavicle, shoulder, or mandible; previous (old) craniocervical trauma or disturbance of eyes or vision.

3 Ascending and descending dysfunction (head/neck displaced to one side; pelvis displaced to the opposite side).

4 Compensated state: where this state exists, any therapeutic intervention risks causing decompensation.

5 Monolateral hypertonus (head, upper body, and pelvis displaced to the same side): occurs in cases of central nervous or vestibular disturbance, perhaps also related to strong intoxication.

Barre's vertical alignment test (Figure. 18.3). Heels touching, forefeet diverging.

If possible the patient should not focus, which will put further demands on the proprioceptive system.

Build a perpendicular from bottom to top. Starting point is the contact point between the two calcanei.

Three reference points are examined: anal fold, processus spinosus C7 and vertex.

Fascial organization according to Zink (Figures 18.4, 18.5 and 18.5.1)

Zink described the interaction between fascial patterns and postural organization. He points to the transition zones – the craniocervical (AO joint), cervicothoracic, thoracolumbar, and lumbosacral regions) – as being of particular importance for diagnosis and therapy. In the ideal case, fascial organization would mean a body without any restrictions of fascial mobility, and in which rotation was equally possible in all directions. In reality, such a situation is impossible, since fascial organization reflects a number of factors: not only trauma but also asymmetries of gait, disturbances affecting the organs, and the general circumstances of life.

Compensated fascial organization The situation most commonly found in healthy individuals is compensated fascial organization. Here, the direction of fascial mobility changes so as to alternate from one zone to the next.

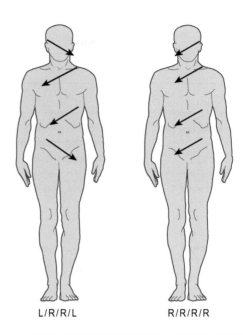

L/R/R/L   R/R/R/R

Figure 18.5
Decompensated fascial organization.

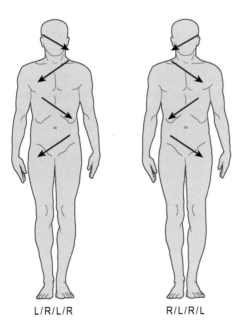

L/R/L/R   R/L/R/L

Figure 18.4
Compensated fascial organization.

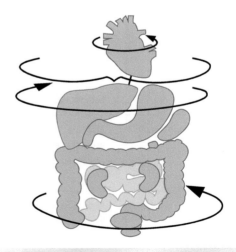

Figure 18.5.1
Physiological pattern of rotation according to de Bakker, modified from the handout of S. Kales OSD, 2016

	Schizoid	Oral	Psychopathic 1
Origin	Pre-/peri-/postnatal	1st year	Years 2–4
Mainly expressed as:	Reduced self-expression; withdrawn behavior and radiates apparent coldness	Needy; behaves childishly to gain attention	Superior; affects to have everything under control; hides weaknesses
Transformation	Desire to arrive in the world	There is support for me that I can rely on	I am loved, despite my needs and weaknesses
Body structure	Slight, constricted; tightly in-drawn, fragmented; movements "angular"	Slumped, body long and thin, long, skinny arms and legs, sunken chest (Compensated: strong body)	High center of gravity, top half of body dispro-portionately strongly developed, rigid; lower half of body slight
Body tension	Tense; chronic muscle tenseness at cranial base, diaphragm, shoulders, pelvis, hip joints, and feet	Low tonicity, muscula-ture underdeveloped, appearance of body as if collapsing	Diaphragm, waist, eye and occipital regions usually tense
Energy pattern	Dammed-up, lifeless at the core; energy held back from outer parts of body: face, hands, genitalia, and feet. Division in terms of energy at waist: upper and lower halves of body not well integrated	Lack of strength and energy (esp. in lower half of body), poor breathing, listless	Head has excessively high energy charge, resulting in hyperstimula-tion of mental system; pelvis has insufficient degree of charge
Contact with world around	Mask-like; lack of liveliness in the eyes and lack of eye contact; possibly squint	Wistful, contact-seeking, dependent. Eyes weak; possible myopia	Eyes especially alert/ highly charged or mis-trustful. Opportunistic
Psychological	Mistrust-ful, shy; oversensitive, lack of self-esteem, low degree of aggressiveness	Finds it hard to stand on own feet, wants support; sense of inner emptiness	Dominant, manipulative; an achiever; denies feel-ings, e.g., need for other people

Psychopathic 2	Masochistic	The rigid character types	
Years 2–4	From approx. 18 months	Years 5–6	Years 5–6
		Hysterical	Phallic
Conforms to the world around in order to control it	Suffering and enduring	Expressive and clinging; constantly seeks attention; avoids separation	Attention and recognition are hard earned
I am loved, despite my needs and weaknesses	I am allowed to be spontaneously happy and content with myself	I am loved on my own account	
Hyperflexibility, esp. of the back, very well proportioned	Compact, stocky; often abundant body hair; neck and waist short and thick; pelvis projected forward; buttocks flattened; low center of gravity	Back often tense and forcibly straight; upper body – especially heart region – tends rather to be small and contracted	High basic state of tension, especially of the extensor muscles of the back: gives the body the appearance of energy and readiness
Hyperflexibility	Thighs and buttocks heavy, pelvic floor drawn up, neck constricted	See above	
Excessively high charge, but not linked with core	Outer organs and parts of body have insufficient charge; waist slumped; energy flow choked off in neck and waist	Full of energy as regards external points of contact with environment; strong tendency to activity; especially in the hysterical type, this tendency can sometimes be extreme	
Seductive, charming, opportunistic, manipulative	Passive resistance	Seductive, good contact; creative and eloquent	
Seductive	Guilt, shame; overburdened; slow. Behavior: low degree of aggressiveness/self-assertion	Exaggeration of feelings and events; constant anxiety about not losing contact	Seeks refuge in activity; sees everything as a task to be fulfilled; very conscientious; rushes from task to task

TABLE 18.4: Main aspects of the different character structures

The most common compensated fascial organization (80% of cases) is expressed as ease of rotation in the direction sequence: craniocervical to the left, cervicothoracic to the right, thoracolumbar to the left, and lumbosacral to the right (= L/R/L/R). Compensated fascial organization in the opposite form, R/L/R/L, is found less frequently.

Decompensated fascial organization This is characterized by a situation in which the direction of fascial mobility does not change from one zone to the next. It can arise, for instance, as a result of trauma.

Diagnostic procedure The osteopath should test the zones described above with the patient standing and also supine. The first step is to determine the relevant compensated fascial organization. The next is to identify the levels that deviate from this compensated organization. Successful therapy is usually accompanied by a return to compensated fascial organization.

Identifying major character structures

Reich, Lowen, and Pierrakos, among other authors, described character structures associated with certain typical body–tissue–energy patterns. For example, the association between the schizoid type and a lanky body structure, uncoordinated body tension and "ring" tension, weak joints, cold hands and feet, hyperactivity and pronounced asymmetries (Table 18.4).

Examining the chakras

(See also Chapter 20, Treatment of the chakras)

Chakras can be perceived in the gross, subtle, and causal body (see also Chapter 25). Usually, however, it is their subtle expression that is sensed. Place your hands on the various locations of the chakras, about 10–90 cm away from the surface of the patient's body. The palm of your hand is directed toward the opening of the particular chakra.

Approach the physical body until you sense gentle resistance and/or a sense of presence or contact. Palpate the subtle expression of all the chakras, from caudal to cranial. The sensation by which palpation of an active chakra is identified is a powerful, large field and perhaps also a sense of warmth.

A weak chakra can be recognized by a weak field, as if your hand is falling into a hole, possibly also by a sense of coldness and a slow turning motion. In extreme cases a chakra, or parts of it, may hardly be detectable at all. Chakras can also appear distorted or displaced. If possible, the brightness, purity, and color of the chakra can be assessed.

Different procedures can be used:

1 The osteopath examines the chakras at the beginning of the treatment session; these can be re-examined at the end, to discover what changes have occurred. Specific treatment can then be given to the chakras.

2 The osteopath examines the chakras, and proceeds immediately to treat them.

Palpation of subtle and causal energy fields

(See Chapter 25 for further detail)

- Ethereal (vital) energy field (corresponds to vital energy and "potency," in terms of such matters as phenomenological significance of the bioenergetic field).

- Examination of the ethereal body is performed by holding the palm of the dominant hand (or palms of both hands) towards the patient's body. Gradually approach this hand towards the body until resistance is sensed. (This happens around 1–7 cm from the body.) Having sensed the resistance, move the hand over the entire body with a motion like a windshield wiper. Assess the strength and quality of resistance of the field, both in general and in terms of regional and local differences. Avoid remaining for any length of time in one spot.

- Another option is to place your hands on the patient's body, and quickly palpate the various regions of the body, working upward from the feet. At each place you should assess the vitality of the tissue, a kind of subtle oscillation inherent in all living tissue. For the procedure also see Chapter 20).

- The astral (emotional) energy field: this extends to around 40 cm above the surface of the body.

- Mental energy field: this is palpated up to around 90 cm above the surface of the body.

- Causal energy field: this is palpated up to around 90–110 cm above the surface of the body.

Chakra	Color	Location	Chakra opening
1. Muladhara	Red	Perineum	Caudad
2. Svadhisthana	Orange	Approx. 3 cm below navel	Anteriorly
3. Manipura	Yellow	Between navel and solar plexus	Anteriorly
4. Anahata	Emerald green	Heart/sternum area	Anteriorly
5. Vishuddha	Blue or turquoise	Neck	Anteriorly
6. Ajna	Purple or indigo	Centrally between the eyebrows	Anteriorly
7. Sahasrara	White	Highest point of head	Craniad

TABLE 18.5: Chakras

Examination of the individual fields

This tries to sense such features as the strength of that field, distortions, unevenness, depressions, contractions, bulges, dark patches, thickening or thinning, and tears or holes.

J.P. Barral's manual thermal evaluation[20]

Heat is one of the many ways in which energy is expressed (for example, in the electromagnetic spectrum in the form of radiation in the infrared or other wavelengths). Body heat is the end result of various metabolic processes. The sympathetic nervous system plays a significant role by regulating the muscle tone of blood vessels and so the circulation of the blood and distribution of heat throughout the body. This close connection is even reflected in the fact that in anthroposophy there are heat-producing processes of all kinds; both somatic (i.e., metabolic processes) and spiritual or emotional processes (fear, anger, envy, etc.) are grouped together in the concept "heat organism." The interaction and interrelationship between spiritual and physical heat-producing processes causes this to be regarded as the medium through which the human ego acts.[21] Changes in heat therefore have an effect on the ego.

Body heat is constantly given off through the skin as long as the ambient temperature is lower than that of the body. Although humans are warm blooded, and so maintain a fairly constant body temperature, there are nevertheless minor variations in skin temperature. These depend on which organ is below the skin, and on how that organ or tissue is functioning or malfunctioning. The temperature of the skin therefore reflects the inner state of the body. Skin regions associated with organs that are affected by acute disease processes, such as inflammation or irritation, appear warmer than the surrounding skin. Areas affected by degenerative changes appear very slightly colder than their surroundings. Degenerative changes also give rise to irritation of the surrounding tissue, so that this radiates increased heat. These temperature differences are held to appear before the emergence of clinical symptoms. They can be sensed, either by means of the temperature receptors, or by the mechanical receptors of the skin.

Method

1 Thermal evaluation is performed mainly using the palm of the dominant hand.

2 Palpation is usually done using the thenar eminence, less commonly the hypothenar eminence or the center

of the palm. The spot that is most sensitive to heat is the one that reacts most strongly to a slight mechanical stimulus. The way to find this spot is to stroke your palm gently with your finger. The place that is most sensitive to this is also the most thermally sensitive.

3 During thermal palpation, your hand should be relaxed, with hand and fingers slightly bent.

4 Position your hand about 10 cm (4 in) above the surface of the patient's skin. You can find the right

Characteristic	Diagnostic indicator of
Points of heat, sharply defined	Structural changes, e.g., tumors, calcifications
Linear, sharply defined	Sutures, blood vessels, visceral channels
Circular, large, sharply defined	Parts of an organ, e.g., lobe of brain or liver
Linear, large, sharply defined	Elongated structures: esophagus, small intestine, etc.
Circular large, ill-defined	Disturbances of visceral function or emotional causes

TABLE 18.6: Thermal evaluation: areas of heat

Distance from skin surface	Dysfunction
Approx. 10 cm (4 in.)	Somatic, visceral dysfunction*
20–30 cm (8–12 in.)	Emotional dysfunction**
100 cm (40 in.)	Hereditary disposition

TABLE 18.7: Thermal evaluation: distance from surface of body
*Usually directly above the affected structure.
**For example, above the frontal eminence.

Characteristic	Diagnostic indicator of
Excessive heat	Excessive blood accumulation, acute infection, or acute trauma. Acute infection/trauma usually accompanied by edema in neighboring tissue
Slightly raised temperature	Minor infection or dehydration of tissue
Excessive cold	Blood deficiency or chronic degenerative condition
Slightly reduced temperature	Blood deficiency caused by scar tissue or mild anemia

TABLE 18.8: Temperature abnormalities according to Pick

position by placing your hand almost on the skin in a thermal area; then gradually raising it until the radiation of heat feels greatest. From there, gradually lower your hand again until you reach a place where slight resistance is felt.

5 During thermal evaluation, your hand should always follow the contours of the body, so that the palm of your hand is constantly parallel to the surface of the skin.

6 To perform the diagnosis, move your hand gently from side to side, like a pendulum. It is very important not to let your hand remain in one place for too long, otherwise heat radiating from your own hand raises the temperature of the skin location being examined as compared with its surroundings.

Areas of heat

Significant thermal areas are most usually somatic/visceral. The second most common cause is emotional, and the least common hereditary.

The areas examined by Barral's method are always the areas of heat. The method developed by Pick, on the other hand, investigates both kinds of temperature abnormality: warmer and colder areas. According to Pick, such abnormalities usually indicate either an excess (heat) or a deficiency (cold) of blood.[22a]

Global palpation of developmental dynamics

Developmental dynamics are treated in detail in Chapters 7-11. The osteopath's hands should synchronize with the developmental dynamics of the structure being examined, and follow the morphodynamic developmental "movements." When doing so, the practitioner should sense whether any dysfunctional variations in tension appear. An alternative diagnostic approach is to position the tissue as it appears in its mature morphological form. Then, in this position, the practitioner traces whether any developmental dynamic tensions are present.

Two essential points need to be observed: the first is to synchronize with the relevant tissue fields and developmental dynamics. The second is to allow the establishment of understanding and resonance with the accompanying aspects of consciousness in the patient. See for example Table 18.9.

Synchronization with the developmental dynamic vectors of force is easier if gentle compression is used. This pressure constrains the surroundings and so intensifies the clarity of the vectors of force of the developmental dynamics and the relationship patterns of the tissue. Intensified in this way, the relationship between the tissues and the workings of the internal organization of the forces at work become easier to palpate and perceive. It becomes possible to see the underlying fulcrums and hidden conflicts. For example, the cranium would react to practitioner-induced compression with its original rotation pattern (i.e., the pattern that arose in the prenatal, perinatal, or postnatal period); according to Heede it would indicate a fulcrum or point of mechanical balance for this pattern.[23] This localized fulcrum contains within it the potential that can reorganize this pattern and transform blocked energies by restoring their flow.

This kind of compression is especially indicated when the dysfunctional forces and tension patterns are not clearly evident. This is particularly the case in dysfunction patterns that have been present for some time, when the "biokinetic" forces in the dysfunction have become organized in such a way that the relation between the structures involved has become "frozen."

Compression fields are also of central importance in the treatment of tension patterns related to developmental dynamics (see Chapter 20).

- Example: palpation of developmental, folding, and re-unfolding (elongation) dynamics in the embryo.

- Hand position: place your contact with the craniad hand on the patient's occiput and the caudad hand on the sacrum (see Chapters 6, 7, 8 and 10).
  - In the second week of gestation, elongation occurs due to external forces.
  - Folding or infolding takes place until approximately the fifth week. This process creates the formation of an internal space.
  - From about the fifth week, the dynamics change; the process merges into one of unfolding and elongation of the embryo. Development of the internal aspect produces polarization, the head and the nerve/sense pole becoming the upward direction and the tail end and metabolic pole the downward direction. An opening forms and the limbs begin to develop.
  - As head and pelvis uncurl, the neck is defined, and a little later, a waist. As the unfolding and

Stage	Positive emotion/regression	Negative emotion/regression
Development of oocytes		
Production of oocytes: Ancestral importance: inheritance from the maternal line, which can include psychological and biological influences deriving from the grandmother. Profound cellular experiences enter the psyche and are reflected in individuals and in cultures	Communal life. (Eggs exist in a benign communal situation, in mutual awareness of others' wellbeing, in the prophase state until FSH is released.)	Re-experience of apocalyptic situations; watching "sisters" in the act of leaving the community and that of dying
Ovulation	Experience of divinity, e.g., the fairy tale experience of attaining heroism on drinking a magic potion (FSH)	Having existed for many years in the company of its sisters, the oocyte changes in appearance; suddenly it is to begin a solo journey. Some competition among the sisters who all try to claim as much FSH as possible for themselves → jealousy, aggression. Survivor guilt (I am the oocyte that succeeded, and you are the remainder that will die)
Drift	During this stage the egg cell simply drifts (with no means of propulsion) → transition and trust on the cellular level. "Magic carpet." Enthusiasm and excitement; sense of being swept along, e.g., bungee jumping, surfing	Loneliness: on the cellular and psychological level. Depending on the quality of the relationship with the person's biological parents and their lifestyle, psychological disposition of mother → fear of being alone; possible sense of powerlessness and capitulating or giving up (trust or passivity)
Odyssey: Peristaltic movements carry the oocyte to the ampulla. It is now the largest cell in the body. (The oocyte should now be sensible of the mother and her emotions.) The oocyte has now arrived in a place of safety (sense of security and welcome). At the same time the oocyte is engaged in an expedition into new territory	Soul has fully adopted bodily form – deep sense of self worth and personality: a new living being has come into existence! Gives rise to lush feeling if the mother really wants the child and is emotionally healthy	If the mother does not want to become pregnant → fallopian tubes become "ice cold" and the journey through becomes quite uncomfortable → low self-esteem and sense of being unwanted. Toxic load (cigarettes, drugs, alcohol, poor diet). **Homesickness, divine longing:** separation from God is a huge loss. Although this feeling can be a very painful one, defiance of the divine separation makes the odyssey a restful time, and the journey down the fallopian tube, usually unaccompanied by negative feelings, a time of repose

Fertilization stage: When the sperm touches the zona pellucida, the oocyte stops moving, then begins once more (but in the other direction). The oocyte is no longer its own entity; new tasks have fallen upon it (from being queen to being full time mother)	Ecstasy, attachment	Terrible fear; the decision as to which sperm will enter is made in part by the oocyte → sense of being "used" by men, treated as an object, not given recognition, or sense of being manipulatively protected by mother or female friend; encounter of two lives and life goals → loss of control, loss of freedom; sperm dies → a kind of death experience
Development of sperm: Time of waiting in the epididymis (Fusion with the father on the psychological, spiritual and organic levels)	Rest and trust (in "brothers"/in "the team")	The sperm wait like soldiers en route to the place of battle; various emotions can be transmitted, esp. aggression
Ejaculation: Sudden, rapid movement of the sperm after the time of waiting (similar to that of an elevator, subway train, or rocket)	Excitement; epinephrine-induced excitement	Loss of protection, of the strength of the father; anxiety related to speed, free fall, flying, the new; desire for extreme sports, horror films, pornography, designer drugs
Entry of sperm into vagina: The sperm (soldiers) have landed (in vagina). Destructive chemical environment in vagina (unfriendly foreign territory). Attack, chemical destruction present despite parents' love	Shock as survival tactic, both on cellular and on organic level. Shock can either kill or save lives	Heat (greater warmth in vagina than in testes). Collective shock (around 25% of sperm die as a result of chemical reaction in vagina). Depression; possible regression on learning of loss, death, injuries
Entry into uterus and migration toward fallopian tubes	Strong, excited. Ecstasy, cooperation – sperm not battling against each other, but giving mutual support. Resurrection: if really the "chosen one," then following the phase of reduced mitochondrial activity the individual can begin another, new phase of activity – it can become indomitable! Soul had already adopted bodily form earlier on, but now comes recognition: "this is my cell, not my father's!" → courage and strength to continue; fertilization is near; sperm can now also recognize the strength of the oocyte. Recognition of field of influence (magnetic, electrical, chemical, etc.); recognition of its destiny; pursues course like a "shark that has scented blood"; direction and intuition	Confusion (where do we go next?); death, deformities, and destruction lurk behind every corner; speed increases as result of mitochondrial activity, but sense of death as activity dies away; exhausted and unable to continue as others rush past. On reaching oocyte: falling into a black hole – there's no return

Stage	Positive emotion/regression	Negative emotion/regression
Fertilization: Encounter with oocyte, which is 100 000 times larger. Acrosome tries to penetrate oocyte, which begins to rotate	Sense of being bathed in light of the full moon; strong attraction exerted by oocyte. Energizing of parietal region; contact and acceptance	Disorientation – falling into a swirling whirlpool; irresistible strength of attraction from oocyte. Experience is so powerful that it can produce experience of shock and soul departs again from the cell. Sensations of death, because for the oocyte the sperm means dying as an independent egg cell; for the sperm, the oocyte means death. Sensations of torture: all is being destroyed – head, tail; Who am I; where am I?
Pregnancy: Sense of being wanted; not wanted; rhythm, harmonization, difference.	Experiences of harmony and connectedness → feeling strengthened, invigorated, and sustained in eternal fullness and satisfaction.	Sense of being unwanted, threatened → feelings of worthlessness, of being superfluous, or of no account, or of threat and existential anxiety; retreat into protective postures or mood of irritation and disturbance; feelings of guilt and self-loathing.
Experience of space	Sense of floating, weightlessness; experiences of movement.	Prison, exposure → discontented and disturbed mood, irritability, sensitivity to stress and pessimism.
Nicotine → accelerates heart rate Hypoxia → compensation by decrease in movement and increase in blood supply to the placenta, esp. with relaxation of pelvis, abdomen and legs (femoral artery)		Recurrent depressive mood; child tends not to tense pelvis and legs and not to move about as much as other children.
Alcohol and other drugs: fetus tries to absorb as little alcohol-poisoned blood as possible: reduction in heart rate; legs drawn in and pelvis tensed to compress the points of origin of the umbilical arteries into the groin		Hypertonus, sleep disturbances, hyperactivity, not calmed by suckling, poor concentration; mistrustful of mother's milk, tense pelvis (iliopsoas muscle) and legs (internal rotation)

Birth		
First stage of birth process: Increasing intensity of labor, feet offer counter-support. Head presses against undilated or slightly dilated cervix	There is a way forward; the effort is worth it	Sense that there is no way out, of being crushed or imprisoned; uselessness and despair; anger → depression → giving up; problems of personal identity; claustrophobia, overreaction in situations where individual is made to wait (traffic jam)
Second stage of birth process: Rotation of head Turning (in a circle) Turning (to and fro)	Sense of being guided by wonderful forces, discovering how to turn the corner and find a way by actively twisting and turning	Inability to find direction, panic, activity but in the wrong direction, hopelessness, fear, anger, and sense of inability to find a solution, feeling that there is no solution. Sense of being torn to and fro, inability to make firm, reliable decisions, dogmatism, resistance to suggestions
Third stage of birth process: Movement to stretch head, feet offer counter-support Emerging, but head not yet visible Face against sacrum/coccyx (or pubic bone) Possible accompanying lack of oxygen Emerges, head becomes visible (→ flat occiput) Postnatal trauma Sense of abandonment, separation from mother too long	Last great effort with diminishing resources, absolute necessity of surmounting the next hurdle	No sign of light at the end of the tunnel, sense of no way out, wanting to give up, great weariness. Exhaustion, fear of failure, fear of death or elemental anger and despair. Difficulty in finishing projects Fear and panic when entering new territory. Endless pain and infinite longing; avoidance of nearness

TABLE 18.9: Hypothetical correlation between prenatal and perinatal developments and potential emotions
According to Ciranna-Raab and Liem, based on Terry, Janus, Dowling.[22b,c] (See also Chapter 11.)

elongation proceeds, the most marked polarizing axis becomes clearly evident: this is the craniocaudal axis. It is no longer external forces that drive this development, as in the second week, but the internal forces of the embryo.

- It is possible to sense the act of enfolding and concentration by palpation of the head (consisting of the rounding of the neurocranium and the forward orientation of the viscerocranium). The outward growth of the limbs, in contrast, is an act tending outwards to the periphery and opening up to the world.

- Example: upper and lower limbs (Figure. 18.6). The shape of the limbs (and indeed of all other structures) develops out of a growth movement, or as the final stage of a movement that has now come to rest. The manner in which the growth movement is carried out is an important determining factor for later function.

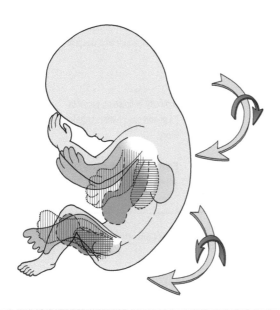

Figure 18.6
Developmental dynamics of the upper and lower limbs.

Palpation of developmental dynamics on the arm

- Flipper-like upper and lower limbs are polarized within the craniocaudal axis. Initially they appear to point towards each other. Further growth movements bring them towards the center, oriented in a way that converges around the middle (the navel) of the inbent body of the embryo.

- At the arm, there is a movement resembling an inward rolling or pronation. This is accompanied by a bending of the elbow, causing it to point downwards and outwards.

- Shoulder joint: abduction and anteversion (in a line of extension of the spine of the scapula) and slight external rotation of the arm.

- Elbow: 90° flexion at the elbow, slight external rotation of the forearm.

- Hand: slight dorsiflexion of the hand; abduction of the thumb; fingers slightly spread and forefinger more splayed than the others; palm towards the region of the heart. The hand position is recognizably one of grasping, with fingers bent and thumb against the palm, in immediate relation to the other fingers.

- Hands and arms point towards the heart, or rest on the heart region. Arrangement of heart and hands directed towards it express the notion of "here." This gesture appears one of release from gravity and from the bounden state that holds it to the periphery.

The practitioner should try to sense whether these developmental dynamics are able to have free expression, or whether there are contrary morphodynamic patterns of tension. Gentle pressure directed along the length of the arm can be exercised as an aid to this diagnosis. A possible alternative method is to place the arm in the position of the fully mature limb and to sense any developmental dynamic tensions.

Palpation of developmental dynamics on the leg

- The leg adopts a position resembling external rotation, creating a connection with the umbilical cord (the point of significance here is the polarity between the umbilical cord and the heart in the process of circulation).

- Knee: bends and points outward.

- Foot: supination and dorsiflexion. (Grows as it kicks against the abdominal wall.) The foot is flat, as the toes are not flexed.

- The arrangement of the feet, which point toward the umbilical cord, and the umbilical cord express the notion of "there." The legs and their closed chains of muscles exhibit a gravity-related architecture.

As before, the practitioner should try to sense whether these developmental dynamics are able to have free expression.

Global rhythmic examination by passive synchronization with inherent rhythms

When carrying out palpation of movement or mobility of bilateral structures, it is helpful for practitioners to coordinate their hands from a fulcrum. On the head, the hand position of choice is the cranial vault hold, with the tips of the thumbs touching. This helps the practitioner to sense any asymmetries. On the rest of the body, if possible, the fulcrum can be provided by resting on the elbows.

Homeodynamic activity and developmental dynamics are both expressed in the body by rhythmic fluctuations (or motion) in every body structure. Pulmonary respiration, for example, and the oscillations of inhalation and exhalation in the model of primary respiration, or other rhythmic phenomena, can be palpated (e.g., microvibration of 4–8 cycles per second). There are the cardiovascular and respiratory rhythms, blood pressure variations of 5–10 cycles/min and 0.6–5.4 cycles/min, the lymphatic flow of 6–10 cycles/min, the rhythm of 2–3 cycles/min reported by Jealous, the "long tide" or "large tide" of 6–10 cycles/10 min reported by Becker, the 1-minute ground rhythm of the smooth muscles, and the phasic pattern of motion of brain density of approximately 1 cycle/5 min (see also Chapter 10) (Table 18.10).

The rhythmic phenomena and various kinds of motion can occur either locally in a particular tissue or generally in the body as a whole. The osteopath can sense the phase of pulmonary or primary respiration, movement restrictions, or abnormal tensions in which restrictions or abnormal tensions occur.

The osteopath should synchronize with these involuntary inherent rhythmic motions and fluctuations, and register the findings. An assessment is made of the naturally occurring disengagement during each inhalation phase, and of the retraction or increase in nearness in each exhalation phase (for example, that of the interosseous and intraosseous structures). It is often helpful to assist the patient to down-regulate before the palpatory examination is started (see Chapter 20).

Method

- Practitioners should begin by requesting permission, in a non-verbal way, to sense the inherent forces in the patient.

- They should then seek awareness of their own inherent dynamics, and establish self-composure in active dynamic stillness, allowing their consciousness to rest in the present.

- They should then synchronize with the rhythm of the inherent involuntary dynamics and rhythms in the patient, all the time maintaining contact with their own inherent rhythms.

- They must observe, as far as possible, without exerting any influence or making any judgment.

- Practitioners should sense or, in other words, allow their attention to be drawn by the homeodynamic forces they are palpating to the regions of the patient's body in which these forces are most evidently active or "at work." A qualitative change in the rhythm can usually be felt in this region.

- At the same time, practitioners should focus their attention on or beyond the horizon (see pp. 348f., 353) and on the type of interaction that the homeodynamic forces are engaged with in the problem region of the patient's body.

Inhalation (inspiration)	Exhalation (expiration)
Expansion	Retraction,* collection
Natural disengagement Divergent motion	Drawing closer Convergent motion
Flexion, external rotation	Extension, internal rotation
Flow of life force from within to outside, toward periphery, centrifugal	Flow of life force from outside to inside, to the center, centripetal
Extroversion, moving out from the center, being beyond oneself, developing the self	Introversion, coming to the center, deepening toward the center, return to origin
Breadth, space, distance	Closeness
Redeveloping oneself anew	Regression
External world	Internal world
Expressive	Receptive
Interpersonal	Intrapsychological

TABLE 18.10: Oscillation in the inhalation and exhalation phases
*The intention here is to describe a natural, spontaneous movement directed toward the center, which draws the structures closer. The terms chosen do not mean "retraction" in the sense of reactive contraction, or delimitation, or state of calling a halt, which would hinder free flow and prevent an unconstrained body physiology. These are more characteristic of a dysfunction.

Symmetry

The symmetry of the rhythms is assessed by comparing the qualities of the rhythm for bilateral body structures. It can be used to locate all types of dysfunction in the body, e.g., scars, disturbances of the joints, adhesions, or bioenergetic differences. The asymmetry indicates the location but not the type of the dysfunction. Resolution of the asymmetry can be interpreted as an indication that the dysfunction causing it has also been resolved.

Frequency

The frequencies of the various phenomena (respiration, arterial pulse, lymph flow, craniosacral rhythm, 2–3 cycles/min "long tide," etc.) can also be examined.

Amplitude

Amplitude is the extent or fullness of motion of inhalation and exhalation (pulmonary or primary respiration), of systole, diastole, etc. The practitioner should note the neutral zone between the individual fluctuations/motions so as to judge whether that phase is occurring normally. Reduced amplitude usually indicates a reduction in vitality or a low energy level in the body. When found together with a strong, considerably accelerated rhythm, however, reduced amplitude can be an indication of hardening or restricted elasticity of the structure concerned, as for example following inflammatory processes. In such cases the inherent rhythms have to work against increased unphysiological resistance.

End feel

Does the movement come gently to a close at the end of the inhalation or exhalation phase, or does it arrive at its end point abruptly? A hard end feel usually indicates a restriction. What kind of hardness is felt: bony, rubbery, etc.? The quality of this end feel provides an indication of the type of tissue and forces involved in the restriction.

Natural disengagement

Can the structures be felt to disengage gently from each other? Can one structure disengage and slightly distance itself from the other (and vice versa)? For example, does the temporal bone disengage from the occipital bone, and the occipital from the temporal bone? Is the stomach released from its surrounding tissues (diaphragm, spleen, liver, colon, kidney, pancreas)? If this does not happen, who or what is preventing it? Or, where is the dysfunctional fulcrum? Where can the potential for change be found?

Natural compression/closeness

Do the structures approach each other, or permit the closeness created between them as they do? Can they experience the relaxation of tension as pleasant, or is there an increase in tension?

As the closeness or constriction increases, does a dysfunctional pattern emerge between structures, or is an existing dysfunctional pattern intensified? If so, where is the dysfunctional fulcrum; where is the potential for transformation?

If the patient either breathes more deeply or pauses in breathing at the end of inhalation, this can intensify perception of the patterns of activity present in the dysfunctional regions. Gentle pressure can also intensify dysfunctional patterns so that they appear more clearly (see Chapter 20).

Ease of movement

This gives an indication of the resistances that are present in the tissue that may be hindering or altering the free expression of the rhythms.

Strength

The strength of the rhythm (i.e., weak or strong?) provides an indication of the general vitality of the patient.

Fullness or emptiness

Is there more of a sense of fullness or emptiness in the tissue? The interpretation of these qualities is done in a similar way to the rhythmic fluctuations/motion. As a general rule, fullness corresponds to an excess of energy and emptiness to a lack of energy.

Asynchronous motion

Asynchronous motion features are an indication of dynamic dysfunctional patterns in the tissue.

Tensions

These indicate dysfunctional patterns of relationship in the fasciae.

Global examination by active testing of mobility

This can be used either to confirm the findings from passive palpation or as an independent method of examination. The practitioner should deliver a gentle impulse in the direction to be tested and follow the movement so induced with passive attention through to its end point. Apart from the initial impulse, the practitioner should give no further guidance as to the direction of movement, but simply accompany the movement. This testing is carried out in respect of the biomechanical state of the tissue or its developmental dynamics, among other considerations.

The practitioner should seek to detect whether the movement is permitted or restricted, to sense the quality of the movement and discover the direction and manner in which the structure reacts to the subtle movement impulse. The start and end feel of the mobility should also be noted.[‡,24]

This examination can be carried out in the following ways:

- In synchrony with involuntary rhythms, e.g., that of primary or pulmonary respiration. Testing can be

---

[‡]Note with regard to cranial osteopathy: since there is no further physiological articular movement (mobility), in the narrower sense, at the cranial sutures from a certain age onward, Guillaume takes the following approach regarding mobility testing at the sutures. He prefers the concept of compliance, by which he means the capacity of adaptation or elasticity in relation to a particular force.

done at the beginning of the inhalation or exhalation phase. For example, at the beginning of the inhalation phase, an impulse can be delivered to the particular tissue, to encourage movement in line with the same parameters as the inhalation.

- Independently of these rhythms. It is preferable, whenever possible, to carry out testing in synchrony, i.e., to deliver an impulse to movement in accordance with the parameters of inhalation, at the beginning of the inhalation phase. The examination of joint misalignment, somatic dysfunctions (restrictions of joint mobility, etc.) can be done using a great variety of methodologies. To describe them all in detail would greatly exceed the bounds of this book.

- By exogenous rhythm or oscillation testing (e.g., body adjustment, general osteopathic treatment, harmonic techniques, etc.). Testing can sometimes also be oriented in relation to the body's own inherent rhythms.

All articular and tissue connections, the glide of all the body's fascial structures, and the symmetry of their capacity to glide can be tested by this method.

Oscillation tests

Example with patient standing:

- The practitioner should sit behind the patient, who is standing.

- Place your hands bilaterally on the patient's ilia or regions of the spinal column.

- Your knees should be placed next to and in contact with the patient's legs.

- Administer oscillatory impulses to the patient's body with your knees, using gentle lateral impulses.

- Assess the extent to which the oscillation is freely transmitted to various regions of the body and spinal column, or is hindered.

Palpation of fasciae**

Passive/undirected palpation of fascial tensions

A dysfunction or fascial restriction exerts a centripetal "pull" on the surrounding tissue structures, as a result of the changes described above. The practitioner can use this effect to localize dysfunctions. The process is one of deduction, working from the general to the particular.

The practitioner should begin with a global examination such as Barral's listening test, standing and sitting, to identify the points of greatest tension. One hand is placed on the cranial vault, and the other, aligned lengthways, on the patient's lower back or sacrum.

Active palpation of fascial tensions, e.g., testing of fascial "pull"

Dysfunctions are usually accompanied by chemical changes and polymerization, an increase in collagen fibers and distortion of elastic fibrous structures. As a result, when there are adhesions, fibroses, inflammation, or other dysfunctional processes, there is usually a reduction in the slight capacity of the fasciae to glide.

Fascial glide is tested by applying gentle traction. Normally, the fascia yields slightly and glides along with the traction. If there is a movement restriction, gentle traction can pinpoint exactly where the restriction is located. The practitioner senses just how far the traction has been transmitted, up to the restriction. The nearer to the disturbance, the greater the restriction is found to be.

**The Fascial Distortion Model offers ways to differentiate movement restrictions in localized areas but generally is more focused on patient gestures and does not depend on palpation skills. A global active and passive restriction in an area points towards an inability of fascial surfaces to glide, the so-called tectonic fixation (TF). Restriction of movement in one or more axes of one joint hints towards a distorted fascial band, so called triggerband (TB). Restriction of movement in one or more related joints refers to an abnormal protrusion of tissue through the fascial plane, the herniated triggerpoint (HTP). Restriction of movement only in one joint and one axis indicates an alteration of the transition zone between ligament, tendon, or other fascia and bone (continuum distortion (CD)).

Testing of fascial tension can be carried out on any part of the body. The testing of the dural and myofascial structures of the spinal column by means of caudal traction at the sacrum, and by cranial traction at the head, are both of proven value. When testing the limbs, gentle caudally directed traction can be applied on the heel, lower leg, or thigh, or on the hand, forearm, or upper arm. The symmetry of the mobility should be compared, and the practitioner should sense where fascial mobility appears to be restricted.

In order to distinguish between primary and secondary dysfunctions, traction can be maintained for a while at the site of the restriction. If the restriction then disappears, it is probably a secondary dysfunction or compensation. If it remains, a primary dysfunction can be assumed to be present at this site.

Palpation of global fluid patterns

Fluid patterns (extracellular fluid, cerebrospinal fluid) can also be palpated. These can change and exhibit abnormal patterning as a result of trauma. For example, functional disturbances in the flow detected from the point of view of developmental dynamics, can be precursors of disturbances of the supportive function provided by the vessels. (See Chapter 23).

Passive palpation of fluids

Following the same principle as in the undirected palpation of inherent fascial tensions, the practitioner's attention should now be directed to the fluid components of the patient's body, looking for asymmetrical movements.

This palpation is able to sense, for example, directions of force that have acted on the body and been imposed within. To do this, the practitioner's hands should be placed very gently on the patient's body. It helps to visualize the body as a collection of fluids, and to rest your hand on the patient's body as if on the surface of a body of water. With practice, it becomes possible to sense a subtle flow, or a direction in which your hand is being drawn. The direction, in which your hand is drawn, is determined by the direction from which the force of the trauma impacted on the body. It can be sensed even when there have been no processes of reconstructive alteration in the fasciae.

Active palpation of fluids

If fluid patterns have been detected in the passive fluid palpation, these can be confirmed by active testing. To do this, a gentle impulse is delivered through the fluids in the direction of the restriction.

Screening of tissue elasticity

Tissue elasticity provides a means of examining osseous, muscular, fascial, visceral, and vascular structures.

Place your hands on the various parts of the patient's body, working rapidly upward from the feet. As you do so, exert brief, gentle pressure on each part of the body, releasing it suddenly, as in gentle recoil. Assess the response of the tissue (resistance) to this pressure: note the ease and extent of deformation, and the way the tissue reacts to the release of the pressure (resilience). The screening is performed first over the entire body, then focusing on the regions, and finally locally. Testing in this body screening is done with the palm of the hand, symmetrically and bilaterally at each particular body region.

Palpation of tissue density[25]

The examination of tissue density and hardness can provide an indication of the severity of the dysfunction, and can also be used to assess the course of therapy. Hardening can be due to such causes as chronic scarring or previous posttraumatic injuries.

- Slight finger pressure is used to assess the density/hardness of the tissue being examined. The expression of softness or hardness is found in the interaction of force between pressure and counter-pressure. Hardness produces increased resistance to palpation.

- The examination is carried out first globally (over a large expanse of tissue) and then locally.

Differentiation of the characteristics found by this examination does require a degree of practice, e.g., in order to arrive at a precise description of a sense of firmness. Is it, for example, cement-like, more like a rubber band, or like chewing gum? Should this firmness be described as like wood or stone, hollow or full, tense or relaxed? Auxiliary aids to diagnosis can be used in addition to palpation, such as X-ray, ultrasound, etc.[26]

Differentiation of the level of the dysfunction

The practitioner has to decide the level at which the dysfunction is present: osseous, fascial/membranous, visceral, or fluid.

Practitioners have two options: the conscious decision to make contact with one of these levels, by establishing resonance between their hands and the level in question; or to allow themselves be led to the level where the dysfunction is located (e.g., by means of a listening test).

Ethereal (vital energy), astral (emotional), mental, and causal energy fields (see earlier in this chapter), and electrodynamic fields and complex wave forms can be differentiated.

It is important for the treatment process to understand the relationship and interaction between the patient's symptoms, tissue findings, body physiology, energy body, and subjective inner experience of the patient.

Local examination

Local palpation of developmental dynamics (see also p. 297 and Chapter 20)

Example: palpation of developmental dynamics in the stomach

The practitioner should take up a position on the patient's right side, and palpate the stomach with the right hand. This hand should be placed on the patient's stomach with fingers pointing craniad, thumb bent and resting on the pylorus. The fingers should be cupped around the stomach so that it lies in the palm of the practitioner's hand and the lower border of the stomach is held in the base of the practitioner's hand and wrist.

The following parameters of developmental dynamics can be palpated:

Symmetry
Frequency
Amplitude
End feel of the particular phase
Natural disengagement at the end of the inhalation phase
Natural compression/closeness at the end of the exhalation phase
Ease of movement
Strength/force of movement
Fullness/emptiness in the tissue
Additional asynchronous chaotic motions during the (sub-) phase(s)
Tensions

TABLE 18.11: Qualities to look for in the assessment of the homeodynamic forces sensed by palpation

- Downward migration of the stomach.

- Clockwise rotation of the stomach (by about 90°) around its longitudinal (and dorsoventral) axis, so that the ventral wall moves to the right and the dorsal wall to the left, growing more quickly to produce the greater curvature.

- Clockwise rotation of the stomach by 30° around its sagittal axis, so that the cardia shifts to the left and sinks slightly, and the pylorus to the right, ascending slightly.

- A marked polarity exists between the upper and lower portions of the stomach. In the upper portion there is a morphological developmental dynamic tending posteriorly, laterally, and to the left; in the lower portion the dynamic tends inferiorly, anteriorly, and to the right.

The practitioner should sense whether these developmental dynamics can be freely expressed or whether there are anomalous morphodynamic tension patterns present. Diagnosis can be assisted by gentle pressure on the stomach and examination continues as for global palpation of developmental dynamics.

Surface qualities

The surface qualities of the different dermatomes can provide an indication as to the condition of the underlying segment of the spinal cord: relaxed or tense areas of skin, displaceable or immobile skin zones, pigmentation, raised areas of skin, swellings or other noticeable features should be noted. Dampness of the skin is another feature to observe, since damp areas can be a sign of the dysfunction of segments of the sympathetic nervous system; reflex responses along nerve pathways can cause increased or reduced activity of the sweat glands in the zone concerned.

Palpation of form (of bones, tissues, and organs)

The shape of the tissue can also give an indication of altered function, e.g., scoliosis, a raised posterior superior iliac spine, gastroptosis, fishhook-shaped stomach, or protruding frontal eminence.

Local testing of tissue elasticity

This is carried out in the same way as global testing. Depending on the structure being examined, in local testing it is possible to use just the fingers to perform the examination.

Local palpation of tissue density[27]

This is carried out in the same way as for global testing.

Local tenderness to pressure

Local tenderness to pressure, e.g., a trigger point, can be an extremely valuable sign in diagnosis.[28] On the head, local tenderness to pressure at the sutures can indicate a suture dysfunction.

Palpation of muscle tone

The examination of muscle imbalance and muscle chains has been extensively described in the osteopathic literature, for example, by Struyf-Denys, Busquet, etc.[29–32]

Local rhythmic examination by passive synchronization with inherent rhythms

This is carried out in the same way as for global testing.

Local examination by active testing of mobility

This is carried out in the same way as for global testing.

Local palpation of fasciae

Passive/undirected palpation of fascial tensions

To perform local testing, the practitioner's right hand should be placed on the region to be examined, e.g., the abdomen. Exert very slight pressure with this hand, and follow with your attention the first impulse that is detected, through to its origin. In effect, you allow your hand to be guided by the tensions present in the direction of the greatest restriction. It is very important to perform this diagnostic technique completely without any prejudgment and without projecting your attention in any particular direction toward particular tissues. Instead, wait with passive attentiveness to discover where your hand will be led by the tension. Only then should you translate your perception into anatomical, physiological connections. A similar procedure can be followed at the sphenobasilar synchondrosis/synostosis (SBS); for that, contact is taken up with the hands at the greater wings of the sphenoid and at the occiput. The background to this lies in the fact that the fascial system is in a sense suspended from the SBS, so that dysfunctions in other tissues are reflected via the fascial system at the cranial base. From that contact at the SBS, the practitioner can follow the fascial tensions to their place of origin, the location that is responsible for the restriction at the SBS. In this way, extensive regions of the body can be examined for abnormal tensions, tensile forces and to identify the original dysfunctions behind movement restrictions of certain particular structures such as the SBS or an organ (e.g., liver). Another possible approach is for practitioners to examine each individual tissue for abnormal tensions; to do this they should direct their attention to the layer concerned. In the abdominal region, for example, these would be: skin, subcutaneous tissue, fascia, muscle, peritoneum, the tissue surrounding the organs and adnexa, the organ itself, and so on. Using this method to palpate the head, you would direct your passive, non-invasive attention to the scalp, epicranial aponeurosis, cranial bones and cranial sutures, the intracranial dural membrane system, the cerebrospinal fluid, and cerebral tissue.

Active palpation of fascial tensions

Every fascial connection between structures is capable of being specifically examined. If necessary, this examination can be done by exerting a slight pull in the direction in which the fascia or ligament runs. Assess the resistance to this traction.

Palpation of local fluid patterns

Passive palpation of fluids

Local fluid fields (e.g., of a bone) can be palpated using the same approach as for global fluid palpation.

Active palpation of fluids/fluid drive diagnosis

1 In fluid drive diagnosis, a gentle impulse is delivered through the fluids (extracellular fluid, CSF, etc.) toward the location to be tested. The practitioner should then sense and assess the reaction of the fluid wave at this location.

2 Another option is to deliver a fluid impulse directly to the bone to sense how the fluid wave propagates within the bone. This enables the practitioner to assess the elasticity and dynamics of intraosseous structures (e.g., of the ulna or radius). For example, the practitioner can touch the two ends of the ulna, and send an impulse down the bone from one end to the other. The hand at the other side senses whether and how the wave arrives.

Additional investigations

Differentiation of acute and chronic dysfunction

Palpation of the tissue can also reveal evidence to indicate whether a dysfunction is acute or chronic (Table 18.12).

Criterion/structure	Acute dysfunction	Chronic dysfunction
Temperature	Raised	Lowered
Skin	Tense and immobile	Tense, with marked immobility
Muscle	Increased tonus	Markedly firmer and more fibrous
Deeper-lying tissues	Edematous swelling	Usually no swelling

TABLE 18.12: Tissue characteristics in acute and chronic dysfunctions

Sensing of spatial organization

- How is the structure organized, e.g., the stomach, its tissue elasticity, wall tonus, and motility?

- How is the structure organized in relation to its local surroundings, e.g., the gliding surfaces of the stomach relative to the surrounding organs or structures (diaphragm, pericardium, and left pleura, duodenum, large intestine, liver, pancreas, spleen, left kidney, adrenal glands, and blood vessels)?

- How is the structure organized within its regional surroundings, e.g., the stomach in relation to the abdominal cavity (e.g., through the linkage of the ligaments and fascial connections, gastrophrenic ligament, gastrocolic ligament, lesser omentum, gastrosplenic ligament, and esophagus)?

- How is the structure organized in relation to the rest of the body as a whole, e.g., the stomach relative to the rest of the body?

In addition, the organization of various parts, or of the body as a whole in relation to gravity, can be palpated. This can be done, for example, by differentiating the findings from palpation with the patient standing, sitting, and supine. Another possibility is to assess the organ in relation to the chakra system or the layers of the aura.

Palpatory differential diagnosis

The section dealing with the palpation of inherent fascial tensions (see p. 308) suggested a possible method for identifying connections between dysfunctions and their reciprocal effects. A further method is described below, which makes it possible to distinguish whether a movement restriction affecting one structure (e.g., SBS) is caused by another body structure (e.g., liver).

Begin by supporting one of the two structures (e.g., liver), and establish a point of balance in this structure, or resolve the restriction there by another method. Investigate whether the inherent motion or mobility of the other structure (e.g., SBS) has changed. Normalization would be indicated in this example by an increase in amplitude and symmetry of the inherent motion at the SBS and of its mobility. If this occurs, this indicates that the liver was affecting the SBS. If it becomes worse, this indicates that the SBS was using the liver either as support or to achieve compensation.

Fields of non-physical energy

Fields of non-physical energy cannot be palpated with the hands. Practitioners can establish contact with them by directing their inner perception toward the structure to be examined, and note the pictures or content or forms or whatever it may be that takes shape in their consciousness.

Palpation of emotional tissue loading

Emotional and mental or spiritual levels have a corresponding part of the tissue to which they relate. In principle, gentler emotions tend to be localized on the anterior and aggressive ones on the posterior side of the body. Feelings belonging to the heart tend to be found in the upper abdomen, while the lower abdomen holds feelings of sexuality. In the neck and chest, it is often feelings of tenderness that circulate, and the shoulders tend to express anger. For example, constriction affecting the thoracic cage is usually associated with suppressed feelings of the heart and exhausted center of sexuality. Stiff neck can be associated with a basic attitude of non-acceptance and a lack of flexibility, usually occurring together with a tense facial expression and weak chest region. "Diaphragm block" is often the expression of states of shock and disturbances connected with the ability to give and receive. A schema of typical body–tissue–energy patterns can also be found in the character structures set out in an earlier section of this chapter (Table 18.4).

Diffuse tension, the precise bounds of which are difficult to define and which often takes the form of vibration in the tissue, is often an indication of emotional involvement; indeed, some therapists also sense particular emotions rising up within themselves. A sudden, spontaneous halt in the rhythmic tissue dynamics can be a further sign of emotional involvement. Where there is emotional tissue loading, a change often occurs in the homeodynamics of the body as a whole on taking up contact with the affected region. This usually takes the form of autonomic nervous system signs, and might typically involve: respiration (e.g., deeper or shallower, slower or faster), sighing, vascular pulse (slowed or accelerated), skin (pale, moist; temperature), and other involuntary rhythms (primary respiration, etc.), twitching that extends through the entire body, change in the bioenergetic field, or a change in the patient's consciousness.

In the author's experience, however, any attempt to categorize different kinds of emotional load too inflexibly is unhelpful. True as it is that certain findings tend to appear together, it is always necessary in the individual case to explore what kind of emotional load exists in which significant regions. Patients should be invited to exercise an awareness of their inner experience during the treatment and to permit the release of emotional load. They can also be asked, if appropriate, to say what emotional, mental, or spiritual changes occur.[§,33–35] It is also possible to find associations between mental or spiritual experience and certain somatic dysfunctions (see Chapter 20).

Which points should the practitioner note?

The following questions help the practitioner take up contact with the tissue and with the patient:

- Where is the health in the patient, or place of originality in the patient, located?

- Where is the balance of the imbalance located? (This can be either inside or outside the body.)

- What is the patient's body trying to tell me?

- What is the patient's deepest need?

- What happened?

- Where does the tissue want to move, and where does it not want to move?

- When did this motion restriction or tension pattern first come about?

- Is the motion restriction or the tissue tension primary?

- Is it the result of another motion restriction or tension?

- If so, where does this tension or motion restriction come from? Which other body structures are associated with this strain pattern (fasciae, muscles, sutures, CSF, ligaments, membranes)?

- In what way are the other dimensions in the patient associated with the tension pattern (e.g., perception of self, family, and cultural environment, biosocial environment)?

- How did the body function in the past, and what influences led to its present way of functioning?

- What happened in this person when this tension pattern or this motion restriction came about?

- What has changed since that time?

- How does the energy field of the dysfunction and that of the body feel?

- What forms of coordination and organization maintain the body's present homeostasis?

- How have the body and the person as a whole adapted to the new situation?

- How has this changed their perception of the world?

- How will this body, with its present organization, function in the future?

- What would change in the patient if these strain patterns were not there?

- Where is the potential that maintains this dysfunction?

- Whereabouts in the patient is the potential that would allow the dysfunction to be resolved and become integrated?

- What is the direction in which the imbalance tends: toward what potential balance? What is the potential challenge?

- Why does the patient want to become well?

- Is the structure that has been treated happy?

The osteopath's ability to establish a non-invasive contact with the characteristics of the tissue, without prejudgment, is important. This will not only bring an

§Despite several attempts to do so, the author has not so far been able to establish reliable correlations between palpatory findings and states of psychological development (e.g., according to Piaget or spiral dynamics). Certain patterns found in the body and characteristics indicative of psychological constitution have been described by authors such as Keleman, Kurtz, and Latey.

increase in the differentiation of the findings as to the state of the tissue; the greater and the more differentiated the contact that is established, non-invasively and without prejudgment, the greater will be the resonance of the hand contact. Here is a list of the kind of characteristics that may be noted:

- Fullness/emptiness

- Immobile, stiff/mobile

- Warm/cool

- Hot/cold

- Dry/moist

- Smooth/rough

- Firm/soft

- Stiff/pliable

- Protruding/retracted

- Permeable/impermeable

- Contracted/extended

- Drawn in a given direction/repelled

- Wooden/stony

- Muddy/watery

- Angular/round

- Elastic/firm

- Mushy/stony

- Knotty/soft

- Sunken/taut

- Massive/ethereal

- Tense as a violin string/saggy as a worn waistband

- Happy/unhappy

- Cheerful/sad

- Angry/fearful

- Light/dark

- Excitable–prone to react/unexcitable–unreactive

- Willing/unwilling

- Solid–undeformable/fluid–deformable

- Inflexible/pliant

- Resistant–strong/fragile–weak

- High density/low density

- Compressed/expanded

- Stolid, inertial/light, airy

- Tense/relaxed

- Bloated/atrophied

- Vitally alive/dead and lifeless

- Twisted–torsioned/straight

- Up/down

- Left/right

- Lateral/medial

- Forward/backward

- Drawing apart/pulling together

- Expansive/retractive

- In the same direction/in opposite directions

- Vibrating/still

- Trembling/at rest

- Uneasy/calm

- Mobile/stiff

- Agile/sluggish

- Great, expansive movements/imperceptibly small movements

- Rolling/sliding

- Flowing/pounding
- Quick/slow
- Pulling/pushing
- Sucking, drawing in/gushing out
- Subsiding/repelling
- Timid/wild
- Rearing up/settling down
- Loud/quiet
- Hesitant/abrupt
- Controlled/impulsive
- Twisting and turning 1200 angles/monotonic
- Flowing/rigid
- Swirling/directed
- Aggressive/gentle
- Seething/stagnating
- Seeking protection/challenging
- Large amplitude/slight amplitude
- Soft end feel/hard, abrupt end feel
- Powerful/weak
- Light/ponderous
- Chaotic/ordered
- Multidimensional/one-dimensional
- Taking/giving
- Glutinous/free-flowing
- Involved/detached
- Goal-oriented/aimless
- Grounded/insufficiently grounded
- Symmetrical/asymmetrical.

Further reading

Arbuckle BE: Effects of the uterine forceps upon the fetus. JAOA. 1954;53:499–508.

Armitage P: Diagnostic touch: its principles and applications. Society of Osteopaths, Cranial Group. Newsletter. 1981;11:7–12.

Bates B: A guide to physical examination and history taking. 4th ed. Harper; 1987.

Besser-Siegmund C und H: Kursunterlagen NLP; 1993.

Chapman JD: Perinatal factors causing brain injuries. Osteopath. J. of Ob. and Gyn. 1962;X(1).

Dobbing J, Sands J: Vulnerability of developing brain. IX. The effect of nutritional growth retardation on the timing of the brain growth-spurt. Biol. Neonate. 1971;19:363–378.

Donovan JB: Nutrition and cranial problems. J. Osteopath. Cranial Assoc, Cranial Academy, Meridian, Idaho; 1958:57–80.

Dovesmith E: Growing skull and injured child. AAO Yearbook. 1967:34–40.

Drew EG: Diagnosis of acute brain injuries. JAOA. 1937;36:517–518.

Frymann VM: The trauma of birth. Osteopath. Ann. 1976;4:8–14.

Gelb HL, Arnold GE: Syndromes of the head and neck of dental origin. AMA Archives Otolaryngol. 1959;70:681–689.

Gillespie B: Dental considerations of craniosacral mechanism. J. Craniomand. Pract. 1985;3:381–384.

Goodheart GJ. Jr.: The cranial sacral and nutritional reflexes and their relationship to muscle balancing. Detroit: Privately published; 1968.

Gross J, Schmitt FO: The structure of the human skin collagen as studied with the electron microscope. J. Exper. Med. 1948;88:555–568.

Kimberly PE: Osteopathic cranial lesions. JAOA. 1948;47:261–262.

Lay E (ed.): An outline of osteopathy in the cranial field. Department of Osteopathic Theory and Methods. Kirksville: KCOM; 1981.

Magoun HI: Idiopathic adolescent spinal scoliosis: A reasonable etiology. D.O. Magazine. 1973;13(6): 151–160.

McCatty RR: Essentials of craniosacral osteopathy. Bath: Ashgrove; 1988.

Page E: Diagnosis of intracranial lesions. JAOA. 1926;26:55–56.

Page EL: Osteopathic fundamentals. London: Tamor Pierston;1981.

Peters JE, Romine JS, Dykman RA: A Special neurological examination of children with learning disabilities. Dev. Med. Child Neurol. 1975;15:63–78.

Schooley TL: Correlated mechanics of the secondary respiratory mechanisms. J. Osteopath. Cranial Asoc. 1953;1:48–53.

Sutherland WG: The cranial bowl. Mankato, Minnesota: Free Press Company;1939.

References

[1a]Chila AG: AAO Convocation, Birmingham, Alabama, USA; 2006.

[1]Wales AL: Cranial diagnosis; 1948. In: Swan K (ed.): J. Osteopath. Cranial Assoc. Meridian, Idaho: The Cranial Academy; 1988:19.

[2]Esteves JE, Spence C: Developing competence in diagnostic palpation: Perspectives from neuroscience and education. International Journal of Osteopathic Medicine 2013;16(1):52–60.

[3]Aubin A, Gagnon K, Morin C: The seven-step palpation method: A proposal to improve palpation skills. International Journal of Osteopathic Medicine 2013;17(1):66–72.

[4]Liem T: Pitfalls and challenges involved in the process of perception and interpretation of palpatory findings. Accepted for publication in International Journal of Osteopathic Medicine.

[5]Baum A, Posluszny DM: Health psychology: mapping biobehavioral contributions to health and illness. Annu. Rev. Psychol. 1999;50:137–163. Review.

[6]Salovey P, Rothman AJ, Detweiler JB, Steward WT: Emotional states and physical health. Am. Psychol. 2000;55(1):110–121.

[7]Goleman D: Die heilende Kraft der Gefühle. Gespräche mit dem Dalai Lama. Munich: dtv; 2004:120ff.

[8]George LE: Integral Medicine. AQAL: Journal of integral theory and practice. 2006;1(2):1–22.

[9]Stuart MR, Lieberman JA: The Fifteen Minute Hour. Practical Therapeutic Interventions in Primary Care. Philadelphia: W.B. Saunders Company; 2002.

[10]Servan-Schreiber D: Die neue Medizin der Emotionen. Munich: Verlag Antje Kunstmann; 2004:237–242.

[11]Bates B, Berger M, Mülhauser I: Klinische Untersuchung des Patienten, 2nd ed. Stuttgart: Schattauer; 1993.

[12]Digiovanna E.: An Osteopathic Approach to Diagnosis and Treatment, 2nd ed. Lippincott-Raven; 1997.

[13]Liem T, Dobler T: Leitfaden Osteopathie. Munich: Urban und Fischer; 2002.

[14]Liem T, Dobler T, Puylaert M: Leitfaden viszerale Osteopathie. Munich: Urban und Fischer; 2005.

[15]Ward RC (ed.): Foundations for Osteopathic Medicine. Philadelphia: Lippincott Williams & Wilkins; 2003.

[16]Typaldos, Stephen. FDM: Clinical and Theoretical Application of the Fascial Distortion Model Within the Practice of Medicine and Surgery. Orthopathic Global Health Publications, 2002.

[17]Becker RE: Diagnostic touch: Its principles and application, Part I, AAO Yearbook. 1963:33–34.

[18] Fossum C: Allgemeine Diagnostik. In: Liem T, Dobler T (eds.): Leitfaden Osteopathie. Munich: Urban und Fischer; 2002.

[19]Liem T, Dobler T, Puylaert M: Leitfaden Viszerale Osteopathie. Munich: Elsevier; 2005.

[20]Barral JP: Manuelle Thermodiagnose. Munich: Urban und Fischer; 2004.

[21]Steiner R: Über Gesundheit und Krankheit. Grundlagen einer Geisteswissenschaftlichen Sinneslehre. 3rd ed. Dornach, 1983.

[22a]Pick G: Cranial Sutures. Seattle: Eastland Press; 1999:3–8.

[22b]Dowling T: Pränatale Einflüsse auf die frühe Mutter-Kind Beziehung: Auswirkungen auf die Beckenspannung. Manuskript für Liem T, Altmeyer P, Kleemann E, Zweedijk R: Osteopathie in der Pädiatrie. Stuttgart: Hippokrates; 2006.

[22c]Terry K: The sperm journey. The Egg Journey. Santa Maria la Ribera: Editorial Colibri; 2005.

[23]Heede van den P: Der natürliche Geburtsvorgang. Osteopath. Med. 2001;4:10–12.

[24]Guillaume JP: Entwicklungen und Perspektiven der kraniofaszialen Osteopathie. Osteopath. Med. 2002; 2:9–12.

[25]Guillaume JP: Entwicklungen und Perspektiven der kraniofaszialen Osteopathie. Osteopath. Med. 2002; 2:9–12.

[26]Guillaume JP: Entwicklungen und Perspektiven der kraniofaszialen Osteopathie. Osteopath. Med. 2002; 2:9–12.

[27]Guillaume JP: Entwicklungen und Perspektiven der kraniofaszialen Osteopathie. Osteopath. Med. 2002; 2:9–12.

[28]Travell JG, Simons DG: Myofascial Pain and Dysfunction: the Trigger Point Manual; vols 1 and 2. Baltimore: Williams and Wilkins; 1999.

[29]Struyf-Denys G: Les Chaînes Musculaires et Articulaires. 4th ed. Brussels: ICTGDS; 1987.

[30]Busquet L: Les Chaînes Musculaires. Vol. III. La Pubalgie. 2nd ed. Paris: Éditions Frison-Roche; 1993.

[31]Busquet L: Les Chaînes Musculaires. Vol. IV. Membres Inférieurs. Paris: Éditions Frison-Roche; 1995.

[32]Myers TW: Anatomy Trains. Myofascial Meridians for Manual and Movement Therapists. London: Churchill Livingston; 2001.

[33]Latey P: Feelings, muscles and movement. J. Bodywork and Movement Therapies. 1996;1(1):44–52.

[34]Keleman: Verkörperte Gefühle. Munich: Kösel; 1992.

[35]Kurtz R, Prestera H: Botschaften des Körpers. Munich: Kösel; 1979.

19

The practitioner and the therapeutic interaction

Torsten Liem and Michael Habecker

Compassion means a feeling of sympathy toward oneself or others who are experiencing some type of difficulty. A softness, a tender heart that is sympathetic and willing to open to all of life, but at the same time, possessing a strength that is not weighed down by difficulties and sorrows. That is, one can identify with the difficulty but maintain a degree of Equanimity and Strength to deal with the situation calmly and wisely in order to find the best solution.

R. and S. Weissmann[1]

Introduction

Although body, soul, and spirit are linked one with another and interact, each part has its own set rules of functioning, so that the practitioner must pay due regard to these when providing therapy. This means that osteopaths need to bring patients' thoughts, feelings, and beliefs into the treatment just as surely as the physical findings. If this input is missing, they will be evaluating only one dimension of a multidimensional person.[2]

This means of course that professional education and training in osteopathy must teach practical competence in these areas. A good practitioner will not use the placebo effect to deceive the patient, but with the purpose of developing expectancy, meaning, and consciousness. According to McGovern and McGovern, patient contact is based on the attitude:

I want to treat your body, mind and spirit; I want to help you gain meaning, and use your unity, structures, mechanisms, and responses. I want to allow you to access your healer within![3]

The Dalai Lama quotes a proverb that tells us that the effectiveness of treatment depends not so much on the skill of the doctor as on his selflessness and empathy.[4] If we trace the words back to their origins, we even find a link between the root of the word "medicine" and that of "meditation," pointing to a connection between them. Meditation, interpreted in the widest sense, can be understood as a way of life, as the capacity to expand the attitude of care and concern and turn it into an integral quality of the individual's own life. This is not a matter of manipulating attentiveness at particular times, e.g., during treatment, but rather of nurturing an attitude of attentiveness so that one's whole life becomes an expression of the practice of meditation.[5] What is required is more than just knowledge and the mastery of principles and manual skills; it is also the ability to overcome the hierarchical patient–practitioner relationship that is the general norm.[6] It is not "either-or," but rather an integration of approaches, quantitative and qualitative, descriptive and inductive.

In an integral treatment approach, which osteopathy aims to be, the responsibility for the success of treatment does not only lie with the osteopath, but also with the patient. The task for patients is that of assuming responsibility for their lives and for their healing process. The role of the osteopath is to make patients sensitive to their task. There are good methods of achieving this, and others that are less good.

The key to reaching patients is for them to feel directly touched in their hearts – not simply in their intellect or tissue. What the patient does is not at all the same as taking a car to the garage to be repaired, just handing over their bodies for treatment as they might to a skilled mechanic. All parties involved – patient, osteopath and the treatment method: osteopathy – have a share in the success of the healing process.

This chapter falls roughly into three parts. The first discusses the role of the practitioner, viewing it from a perspective that is usually referred to as the placebo effect. This section discusses those qualities that hinder and those that help. The second concentrates primarily on the therapeutic interaction.

The third presents the many different perspectives and dimensions involved in taking up contact with the tissue. These include the phenomenological, hermeneutical, structural, objective, and interobjective dimensions. Differentiation of such aspects enables the osteopath to take a more conscious and integral approach to the tissue in palpation.

The practitioner

The requirements on the part of the osteopath, from the morphodynamic point of view, extend beyond the familiar ones (knowledge of the interactions of form and function in the body and person as a whole, their application in giving treatment, conscious performance of palpation, etc.). They also include the ability to synchronize with the dynamic stillness in and around the person's body as a whole, and above all to take due account of the evolutionary dynamics in the patient. The sense of separation from all else and from others is a narcissistic illusion. Progressive release from this sense brings the benefit not only of a widening of sympathy, but also an increase in therapeutic healing potential.

The osteopath assists the patient's body and person to use the available resources for that individual's own particular pattern of health.[7] The practitioner, or the interpersonal relationship between practitioner and patient, acts as a catalyst in releasing existing bound forces and bringing about a new, higher-order integration; it assists the body's efforts to focus its forces to resolve the problems present within the patient. Even the earliest stages, the observation and examination, have an effect on this process.

It is not merely the hand contact itself which acts as a catalyst to the spontaneous reactions of healing and harmonization; even the presence and spatial proximity of practitioner and patient in the same room, the personal interaction, and the intention on the part of the practitioner have an effect, through the electromagnetic and other field resonances. The dynamic interaction, based on authenticity, and the open state of resonance between patient and practitioner are primary treatment factors.

Qualities of a good osteopath

- For Brody, active "listening" is an essential part of treatment.[8] Patients are given the opportunity to tell their story, and as they do so they receive attention and feel that they are being taken seriously.

All this strengthens their confidence in the practitioner and the method being used. Listening strengthens the conditioning toward a healing reaction, along with the expectation that it will be achieved, and with the advent of greater meaning it brings a reduction in disease. Meaning, in the sense of patients' better understanding of the symptoms and of the suffering in their lives, is achieved through explanation of the symptoms and the prospect of better control over the disorder, and the congruence of method and practitioner.[9] Hawkins, writing about ways of optimizing non-specific effects in therapy, mentions a number of studies relevant to the present subject.[10]

- A study by Thomas looking at patient consultations with medical practitioners produced the result that simply being more positive during the consultation led to a 25% improvement in clinical outcome.[11]

- The following qualities were listed by patients in answer to the question as to what makes a good practitioner.[12] These were: friendliness, the desire to listen, sympathy, patience, tolerance, and understanding. Such qualities not only satisfy the patient's wishes, but also produce a better therapeutic outcome.

- Montgomery found the following aspects to be significant for the patient–practitioner interaction: paying attention to our own health, working on our own emotional blocks, better time management, longer consultation times, better continuity of patient care, caregiving, training in communication, regular feedback from patients, and the quality of closeness in the therapeutic context.[13]

- Also of importance are studies indicating that empathy, warmheartedness and respect can also in practice have a direct effect on the practitioner,[14] and can directly improve the coherence of heart rate variability.[15]

- In a study observing 255 medical graduates over a period of 25 years, the death rate in the group whose hostility score was above average, consisting of 119 participants, was six times the average for the study population as a whole.[16]

In considering all these study results, one point that must be borne in mind is that a person's own genuine growth and development, sympathy and serenity can never be forced but only promoted. Empathy, for example, is not some invariable commodity but undergoes marked changes in quality in each phase of development. Only very few people have in fact developed completely unconditioned empathy for all living beings. Calmness and circumspection, humility, and an authenticity that recognizes one's own level of development are all helpful qualities to maintain so as not to descend into pathological and dissociated extremes.

Possible hindrances to treatment

- Distance: often confused with respect for boundaries, and often seen as therapeutically necessary. However, the life force is in fact able to unfold more freely and with less hindrance in the patient if we allow the practitioner's own vulnerability, honesty, openness, presence, and consciousness, and realization of our deep connectedness to be brought into the treatment. If practitioners try to shield themselves from patients' feelings and to hide their own feelings from their patients, this creates separation.

- Excessive focus on technique and on facts: acquiring more knowledge and techniques does not automatically make us better osteopaths. There can be no doubt that technical skills and abilities are indispensable for the practice of osteopathy. Nevertheless, we must avoid limiting healing potential by too exclusive a focus on technical performance and intellectual knowledge.

- Over-identification with the role of the osteopath: osteopaths quite often hide behind their technical ability and professional role. These, however, are the expression of what we do and should not take over the practitioner's whole identity. Inflexible identification with a professional role or with role structures in general shackles the very powers needed to expand our experience and to be responsive and open. The therapeutic work carried out in patient contact is limited in various ways according to those aspects of personality – or conditioned, compensating personality patterns – that actually occupy the secret positions of power. Whereas the search for compensation by means of

technical, intellectual, spiritual, or other elitist therapeutic models is something that can never be completely avoided, practitioners can make themselves sensitive to such things and develop an awareness that they are happening. If, for example, the practitioner's own compensated low sense of self-worth produces an over-identification with theoretical knowledge or excessively rigid patterns of patient–practitioner relationship, it helps to face the underlying feelings and open up to them. Every time a practitioner makes therapeutic contact with a patient, it is as a general principle an opportunity to mature.

- Projection: patient contact repeatedly has the effect of facing practitioners with elements in their own consciousness that are bound up with anxiety. If the practitioner does not acknowledge these feelings and open up to them, it often causes patients too to suppress their own perceptions. This can make the course of healing and of the achievement of awareness much more difficult on certain levels.

  Such situations offer practitioners an opportunity to integrate an experience full of anxiety (for example), instead of shutting themselves off from certain elements within the patient. It is helpful for practitioners to permit these unpleasant elements of consciousness, without however identifying with them (in practice this would mean increasing awareness). This frees the bond tying them to the many anxiety-avoidance strategies that people tend to adopt; it releases them from the resulting compensatory patterns of over-stimulation, or indulgence in moments of artificially stimulated euphoria conjured up in order to feel temporarily more alive or experience more intensively. This is not a process that can ever be forced, any more than it is possible to force the healing process in the patient.

- Reductionism: this involves the reduction of the levels of subjective experience (e.g., emotional; mental elements) in patients to the simple level of tissue findings in a way that is inappropriate to treatment. It may cause us to interpret them through the lens of an exclusively one-dimensional, mechanical viewpoint. This does insufficient justice to the multiple and varied, interacting evolutionary developmental dynamics in the patient.

Trusting your own body

Andrew Taylor Still said that osteopathy begins with trust in the body. This trust is something that osteopaths must first develop in respect of their own bodies, before they can attempt to bring about any changes in the patient's body. Osteopaths experience, in themselves, how every expression of disease also carries the potential for change, and this should not be squandered by precipitately banishing the symptoms by suppressing them. Practitioners need to restrain themselves from inducing changes in the patient when they have not first accomplished them in themselves.

The osteopath's consciousness

- Davis states that the information we receive from our patients, and also the information we transmit to them, is determined by our own state of consciousness, i.e., by what we are in ourselves.[17] There is a direct connection between the process of the practitioner's own consciousness and the available therapeutic options, if the aim of these is indeed to treat the wholeness of the body and person. Practitioners' own personal maturity and inner balance, their centeredness in the present, in stillness and in "being," their ability to open themselves up to life (instead of trying to control and manipulate it), and to give wholeheartedly of themselves, to access their own vulnerability and consciousness of self, all have a direct effect on the patient. It is through these things that contact can be made with homeodynamic forces, something that is not possible by the simple application of a technique.

- The kind of consciousness needed is not simply one that is limited to therapeutic practice. Rather, it is the outworking of a consciousness that is lived in every part and every moment of life, the effect of which extends into the therapeutic contact and therefore makes it easier for patients to experience the wholeness. That in turn helps patients to experience deeper insight into their relationship to life as a whole. The presence of the practitioner has a healing effect in its own right; it brings about a higher state of energy in patients, inspiring them to take this path themselves. Time brings the development of an increasing consciousness in the practitioner for the interactions

of the forces and events in a wider sphere of connectedness of reality. A continuity of consciousness comes into being, tending toward vitality and emptiness and aiding the practitioner to engage with the patient.

Emptying oneself

- It is essential to become empty when giving treatment. The more fully developed this emptiness is in us, the better we are able to experience everything that happens as an expression of the divine, and to treat everything that the patient tells us with judgment-free empathy. "I love my fellow man because I see God in his face and in his form" (Still).[18] There is nothing dull and wan or lukewarm in this state of emptiness; every moment vibrates with vital strength and intensity, since we are able to experience originality in every sensation, down to its very roots. The veil has been lifted, the mist of hazy perception that surrounds our ego has cleared, and what lies behind is revealed.

- Emptiness cannot be reduced simply to a kind of treatment technique or concept, or indeed any other kind of concept. It exists beyond concepts as an immediate perception of boundlessness, the most original and pure form of awareness and knowing. This formless, space and timeless consciousness is, as it were, the ultimate ground of all that exists, with all its forms, spaces, and times. It is emptiness as the purest form of "letting be" – without imposing any order, without manipulating or reacting to it in any way. This does not mean denying or ignoring the world of appearance – this too would be no more than a reaction to its appearing – but instead includes it, comprehending the body, emotions, mental processes, etc. without attaching itself to them. Although emptiness on the part of the practitioner improves the therapeutic interaction, this emptiness is not something that can be forced, in practitioner or patient. We can however decide to open ourselves up increasingly to emptiness, whether by realization of our originality or by deconditioning or release. Realization of emptiness occurs in a stepwise process of dialectical, increasing consciousness. Another way in which this can be explained is as an increasing convergence of consciousness by which the consistency of emptiness makes its appearance.

- It is in this emptiness, in this space, that the essence and the aspects of the patient can best be expressed and understood. When we permit this emptiness, this space, we enable the deeper aspects and dynamics in the patient to become evident, together with the patient's true needs and the inherent transformational forces in the patient.

Openness, synchronization

In every case, openness and the flow of energy make demands on the personality of the practitioner; they call for a corresponding capacity of collectedness and stability within the personality.

The practitioner must not ignore or downplay the fact that an attitude of greater awareness toward life does not only involve those experiences that we might regard as desirable, but also undesirable ones. In fact, as we begin to open up, the aspects of consciousness that are intensified are precisely those that we do not wish to find.

As practitioners we begin by freeing ourselves as best we can from any rigid views as to what ought to constitute health for the individual. Instead we allow ourselves to enter a state of un-knowing and absence of prejudgment. This state forms the starting point from which to allow the wholeness of the patient and the circumstances that surround that patient's life to work upon us.

We should also direct our attention to the fullness of life in the patient, which is a priori our fulcrum. We give this fullness our entire and unlimited devotion.

The final step is to give ourselves the space and time to tune in to the patient and to synchronize with the Breath of Life and the inherent motions and rhythms and oscillations within the patient, both as a whole and in each part.

Belief systems

Belief systems are not simply the kind of system that can be altered at will. Their significance for the individual is a part of that person's identity, and for whatever time it applies it represents a "home" for the person's self. The belief system is a kind of contraction; narrowed confines into which something infinite is compressed and presenting to the world a pattern of limited and selective perception. In principle, absolutely anything is capable of serving as a belief system; most particularly, it would seem, those things that represent high ideals, ethical or religious models (and in the field of therapy these would be, for example, the "holistic" models).

This continues to be the case until the self feels too constrained within those confines, and consciously or unconsciously there is an opening-up into expansion and transcendence of the belief system takes place. This opening-up cannot be forced, but only facilitated, and invited when the moment is ripe. Quite apart from this, we find a natural tendency toward overcoming restrictive viewpoints and selective perceptions, and a dialectical process. The tendency is toward a fundamental attitude that is increasingly open.

Symptoms arise when a threshold is crossed and the person is no longer able to achieve the imperceptible integration or compensation of certain elements (matter, body, psyche, mind, etc.) in the same way as before: by suppression and dissociation in the narrow confines of the belief systems, by depriving these elements of their relative autonomy, or by exaggerating it. In these threshold periods, the egocentric defense of the particular personal belief systems can reach an unexpected intensity. Those finding themselves in this situation want to retain their sure, familiar, narrow bounds at all costs, and at the same time trying to make themselves and all the world believe that these narrow bounds deserve to be acknowledged as a broad vista and represent the highest of goals, to be striven for and admired. The inner contradictions of this process usually cause it to develop in the direction of a labile and chaotic state that can be a period of transition to the establishment of higher-order integration. This phase can be associated with many disease symptoms. The symptoms tend to have symbolic character, and are the expression of divergent forces. This might for example be the effort to maintain the best possible balance on the present level and with the present belief system, set against a striving for another level of balance that is of a higher order. (One reason for this would be that the potential for integration that exists on this level is no longer adequate to resolve the challenges before it.)

In a certain sense the self can be regarded as the original or oldest dysfunction from which the rest springs, or, perhaps better, as the main challenge facing the person. However, this self is not a monolith but a pattern of organization that is structured in itself and phylogenetically, ontogenetically, socially, biosocially, and culturally conditioned. It is a kind of fulcrum or virtual center of gravity of the personality, around which the powers possessed by that person are distributed and the core that conditions the person's perception. This self takes on various quite specific characteristics of resistance, contraction, narrowness, selective world view, and expression in the tissue, depending on its conditioning. However, these patterns of organization in the body tissue should be seen rather as a symbol of this conflict between the self and the highest achievable consciousness. The treatment will lie somewhere between the state of tension of what might be called the original dysfunction and what we might call the original state of health – in the sense of an undivided consciousness. The more consciously the practitioner is able to perceive this state of tension, the closer the treatment will come to being an integral approach and the better it will be able to comprehend the patient in entirety or in part. This consciousness therefore has a decisive effect on the therapeutic interaction. The more "unconscious" and one-sided the disposition of the practitioner, the more the treatment comes to resemble an equation with two or more variables. Practitioners themselves are one of these variables to the extent that (depending on their own conditioning) they are able to recognize only a certain view of causality and potential or evolutionary finality (understood, for example, as a telos, see Ch. 1, p. 22) in the patient and take account of it. This is neither good nor bad in principle, but if we – as practitioners – are able to recognize this dilemma it gives us greater ease of access and empathy as we recognize our own steps in development. The point at which these two subjective "variables" (practitioner and patient) meet is helpful, seen from a higher viewpoint, even though consciousness is hazy on both sides, if only because of the coherence, that is, the inherent forces at work that have led to this meeting of practitioner and patient.

A great number of levels become apparent in this meeting of practitioner and patient. The ones described in this chapter represent only a small sample.

Therapeutic interaction

In osteopathy we do not treat disease symptoms but try to recognize and understand the patterns of relationship operating in the patient's body as a whole at that particular time, primarily through the medium of the tissue.

The therapeutic context has as its starting point the perception and acceptance of the symptoms and the patterns of dysfunction, which we approach as far as possible in a judgment-free way and accept even if we find them to be contrary to our expectations. By acceptance of the symptoms and patterns of dysfunction and letting go of any attempt to control, we open ourselves to the information they contain within them and to the way they relate to the whole.

Wright and Sayre-Adams[19] see the observation that we are energy patterns in resonance with other energy patterns as giving rise to clear consequences for the therapeutic interaction with patients. The reason is that, from this point of view, there is no real distinction between practitioner and patient, and no relationship of the kind that proceeds from one party alone to the other can exist between practitioner and patient. Long-term health processes seem highly dependent on the extent to which patients are helped to a conscious perception of their relationship to life, emotional attitudes, the external world in space and time, and to rhythmic regulators, etc.

The risks of excessive focus on technical performance

According to Still, osteopathy is not a collection of hopefully healing techniques. If osteopathy is reduced to the mere manipulation of tissues, and therapeutic contact to nothing more than technique, this creates an artificial separation between osteopath and patient and reduces the vital flow between them. Such an approach seldom provides any real insights into life processes for practitioner or patient.

This approach is based on a mechanistic worldview. True as it is that it is possible to achieve certain effects by means of certain techniques, and in certain ways influence the body as a whole, the key to the heart of a problem or to profound changes is not simply a matter of technique; it is not even anything we can affect directly.

The situation is in fact quite the opposite: the more we develop our capacity to release control and allow our authenticity, openness, and vulnerability to engage in interaction with the patient, the greater the accessibility we develop in ourselves for the wholeness and healing resources in the patient and for the immediate experience of vitality in the patient and in ourselves. It is impossible to overstress the fact that this process cannot be forced.

The patient's intention to be healed

It is important to sense the patient's motivation to be healed, or indeed which elements in the patient desire healing. It is entirely possible to find that the part that wants to be healed of the symptoms is the very part that lies behind the emergence of these symptoms. The practitioner is then confronted with a situation in which the patient has come with the desire to have the existing avoidance strategies confirmed and the symptoms eased away; yet these same strategies have a problematic dual role: they are designed to avoid certain elements in the patient's life, and at the same time are the cause behind the symptoms. Such patients want everything to stay the same in their lives, including their lifestyle, their narrow attitude to life, and limited perception of it, just without the symptoms. This hunt for the magic cure – medication, manual technique or all-surpassing meditation or psychological method – is in fact often an attempt to avoid the challenges of life instead of facing them. There is a risk here: if we unconsciously identify with the main, egocentric wish that brings these patients to us and perform the manipulation to enable them to continue to function as they did, we participate in reinforcing a restrictive pattern. In this situation, an approach involving greater consciousness would be to make clear to such patients the choice they have available to them, either to take the opportunity to change (since the symptoms can in fact contain within them the chance to open oneself) or to remain within the old system of experiencing. This is by no means simply a decision between true and false, and it is not our place to judge it; only to act in accordance with it.

Seen from another point of view, however, or from another level of consciousness, certain symptoms can be interpreted in other than the traditional way. Appearing in a different connection they are no longer phenomena to be resisted but can be viewed, for example, as part of a process of growth and change or healing. A disease or collection of symptoms can then indicate the relationship between an open system – in this case, the patient's self, energy state, or state of consciousness – and an external force. The disturbances or symptoms that call the external force into effect in the body as a whole could also be part of a process that raises the currently existing balance to a new balance. It often seems that each experience and each illness bears within itself, almost inherently, the potential for transmutation, if the patient can only open up sufficiently to allow the forces of disharmony and unpleasant experiences or symptoms and surrender completely to them.

Processes of development

- Human beings as biological entities are continually active giving rise to entropy that forms part of a constant exchange of energy with their surroundings. As in all dissipative, self-organizing systems, development occurs through the destruction of order in the neighborhood of states of balance, while, far away from the state of balance, order is able to be maintained or new order created, passing through states of instability.[20] In the course of biological, emotional, intellectual, and spiritual developmental dynamics, we pass from a state of order to a phase of disorder, then spontaneously back to a state of order on a higher level. We see a tendency for there to be order and stability with phases of disorder – which can also find expression in the form of disease symptoms – that are necessary for the development of a new state of order.

  The patient goes through a phase of instability so that old patterns of order which are no longer adequate can disintegrate and a new, higher-order structure or integration can develop. A necessary state of disorder is the precursor of the new order. Superficially, this process can sometimes seem like disintegration on the part of the patient, but practitioners should not make the mistake of remaining on that superficial level or aiding patients to reorganize and stabilize their old or dysfunctional patterns of order. Instead, they should take up contact with the motions and homeodynamic forces occurring inwardly and accompany the spontaneous processes of reorganization. An improvement in general wellbeing (despite the appearance of temporary symptoms such as withdrawal symptoms, the reappearance of old, suppressed symptoms and the reversion of chronic conditions to an acute stage) is usually a sign that a process is occurring in the direction of health, as is also a developmental tendency bringing greater enlightenment, sense of meaning, and security.

- We fail to do justice to the dynamics of the process of life if we look at the present state of the patient – state of health and dysfunctions – in a purely static way. For deeper understanding and a broader view we also need to include the growth processes and developmental dynamics in which the patient is involved. This approach will also encompass a cognitive, palpatory, empathetic and intuitive perception of the patient's physical, mental, emotional, and spiritual development on both the subjective and objective levels. These developmental processes are not concluded on reaching adulthood; on the contrary, being human involves lifelong growth processes. If we understand them in this context, the symptoms or dysfunctions that arise assume a quite different significance from the one they have when they are viewed in a purely static way. This view enables practitioners to arrive at a deeper meaning and significance for the symptoms and dysfunctions and to provide treatments that are more integral and adequate to the case. Much of the present book concerns itself with the morphodynamic development that takes place during the time in utero. It would be wrong to mistake the consideration given to morphodynamic development for a romantic, transfigurational idea of deliverance into health found in the embryonic or childhood state. Health is not to be sought in the embryo or in early childhood, even though we may need to turn to that early stage of development when working to bind forces, so as to ease or enable further development and integration of a higher order in the patient.

Suppression of symptoms

- If our efforts in providing treatment are exclusively aimed at the short-term relief of symptoms and the maintenance of the status quo, we hinder the potential for integral healing that is inherently present in the disease symptoms. Although manual therapy that is given palliatively to suppress symptoms can indeed banish them for a while and mask conflicts in the body of the patient as a whole, it happens at the cost of a more fulfilled sense of being, in unmediated contact with life itself and more richly energized. For practitioner and patient alike, the more we reduce the intensity of the moment – whatever the interaction that brings this about – the more we hinder the natural flow of healing forces.

- Further disease can even occur during this course, the expression once again of underlying unconscious conflicts or suppressed symptoms. The suppression of particular undesired physical, emotional, or spiritual phenomena can sometimes have the long-term effect of intensifying the suppressed forces or displacing them to another level. An example would be the suppression of certain experiences, the result of which tends on the whole to intensify that aspect of consciousness on another (or deeper) level.

'Opening up'

According to Still, the way to achieve an increase in health is not by the focus on disease or dysfunctions, but by focus on and unconditional surrender to the immediacy of vitality.

The aim of therapy is not necessarily to manipulate the external world, the dysfunction, or the patient in whatever way we or they believe to be appropriate, but to encourage a state of openness, perhaps better a dynamic of openness and non-control, during which healing forces are released to such extent that the result is very often the establishment of health.

If we resist the urge to do something at all costs and to exert control with the desire to get rid of the problem, and if instead we are open to the deep patterns of energy underlying the dysfunctions and to the meaning that the painful symptoms may have for the patient, this can bring us to a deeper understanding of dysfunctional pattern. The osteopath opens up to an understanding of the underlying, invisible patterns of order in the organization of the body and in the dynamics of the body, including the dysfunctions, which are space–time dependent and can acquire a quite different significance or interpretation when seen from the viewpoint of the immediate experience of wholeness.

- If we are open, we are vulnerable. Chronic, systematic avoidance of this makes it impossible to establish authentic, empathetic contact. The protection and control that we have built up in our consciousness and in our bodies (in the form of dysfunctions) in response to past unpleasant experiences and trauma is usually what shuts us off from life in the present. Protective mechanisms are essential, but those that we have unconsciously absorbed can reduce vital energy if they have become too inflexible to respond adequately and appropriately to the particular situation.

- The practitioner uses palpation to help patients to "let go" of everything that hardens them against immediacy of experience.

- "Opening up" is usually the first step in the healing process. In the course of the treatment the patient opens up increasingly to immediate experience and so also to energies that are often uncomfortable at first. Consciously or not, patients have often avoided or even suppressed the experience of these unpleasant energies. As they come to understand these energies better, they also become better able to let go; for example to let go of defense strategies that are no longer helpful. The change occurs with this increasing awareness and as this "letting go" increasingly comes to replace egocentric, conditioned control. The act of giving up the conditioned, forced control and replacing it with awareness, plunging into the unknown and into experience, forms a significant part of the therapeutic interaction. The length of time needed to adapt in this way varies according to the dysfunction.

- The process of opening up and complete surrender to the deep interconnectedness and inseparable wholeness of all life processes offers direct access to vitality and healing for both practitioner and patient. The transmutation of a dysfunction (which is the release and transformation of bound conditioned forces and elements within the consciousness) occurs when these are experienced to the very depths along with all their somatic, visceral, emotional, mental, spiritual, social, cultural, and other components.

- To conclude, it is essential for patients to learn to permit themselves to open up in different life situations, and to experience the permeability of the body, the flow of bodily energies and this surrender in everyday life, consciously and without the aid of the practitioner, to allow the relative balance between protection and openness to be reset and to set about their lives in the strength of their newfound energy with creativity and an awareness of responsibility.

- It cannot be too much stressed how important it is to maintain the connection between the therapeutic interaction (and indeed one's own personal development) and love, sympathy, trust, surrender, and consciousness. These balance the other aspects – the reduction of dysfunctional patterns (or exercise of control) – during the process of opening up into an enlarged perception of reality.

'Tuning in'; resonance

- Osteopathic treatment always consists of different elements, functional and structural, "listening" receptively and "speaking," "being with the patient" and actively "doing." Resonance, "listening" and "being with the patient" create a dynamic environment in which the patterns that tend toward wholeness in the patient can come to the fore. This process calls for patience and attentive waiting. It is in these conditions that the right approach to "doing" becomes clear to the practitioner: the technique that is helpful, that takes account of the whole or parts and is in harmony with the homeodynamic forces. However, if the aspect of "doing" comes to dominate over the "listening" in the therapy, this tends to promote control, dependence, and displacement of symptoms rather than the experience of greater order and awareness.

- There is a clear difference between the way a practitioner would behave in an endeavor to bring about a change, and tuning in to establish resonance with the patient, so as to allow changes to take place. Becker points to this distinction in his account of the three viewpoints that come together in palpation (see p. Ch 18, p. 283). This is an essential distinction, since living organisms – as opposed to inanimate objects – do not interact in precise and predictable ways. The quality of personal flexibility in the practitioner is an essential element in the therapeutic interaction.

- A dysfunction is not simply a matter of local tissue mobility and tissue tension, any more than cigarette smoking is just to do with the lips and mouth. It is always an interactive process, interconnected to varying degrees with other issues. So, just as the cigarette produces certain hormonal and autonomic reaction patterns and effects on underlying mood (sense of safety and security, feelings related to oral regression such as suckling at the mother's breast, etc.), making it all the more difficult to give up smoking, in the same way there can be hormonal, neurological, and psychoemotional patterns associated with a somatic dysfunction of the tissue. Therefore, it is fundamentally important to be aware of the possible interactions there may be between tissue restrictions or changes and the patient as a whole if we are to provide healing that is "holistic." The ability of the osteopath to achieve resonance with these patterns of dysfunction by palpation is the key skill that marks out the difference between a maneuver performed in a purely mechanical way and the conscious application of touch in relation to the person as a whole.

- Osteopathic treatment enables the patient to make contact with the deeper, greater levels of existence that form part of a person's life. Resonance with the patient or "tuning in" by the practitioner in therapy relates not only to the tissue dynamics, but also to the emotional, mental, and spiritual patterns. The practitioner allows the emergence of resonance with stillness, the stillness that exists between words and sentences, the stillness of a dysfunction and the stillness that represents the point or state of balance of the patterns of relationship in the body. The osteopath can also tune in to the patient's potential state of being, that is, the potential of a freer, more creative and transforming manner of experience in the body.

- The authenticity, empathy, and love on which therapeutic contact is based determine to a great extent the level on which resonance can be established with the source of vital force in the patient and with certain patterns of dysfunction. This also seems to increase the effectiveness of whichever technical approach is used. Therefore, the outcome of the therapeutic interaction also depends on the quality of surrender and genuineness with which patients open up to their own experience, the extent to which they confront their fears and anxieties (and are prepared to let them go) on their vitality and their preparedness to be seized by life as a whole. If, during therapy, they have consciously experienced a state of opening of the heart or permitting the flow, this experience will serve as a fulcrum in daily life, and enable them to develop increasing confidence and the right kind of surrender when facing the challenges of life.

- The body is a resonance structure for processes of balance between individual and collective forces. The solidity of anatomical structures should not deceive us into ignoring the fact that the body is a highly dynamic and resonant milieu that is responsive to experience. Practitioners hone and develop their receptivity to perceive how deeply and in what way the dysfunctional patterns are rooted in the individual person, and how they can attempt to integrate given elements in the person's consciousness which may underlie certain disorders.

Consciousness and the therapeutic interaction

The structuring of the personality develops in response to various influences: it is determined, for example, by genetic and epigenetic, cultural and sociobiological influences and the biography of the individual, etc. It finds expression in the form of certain conditioned views and reflects the way that our consciousness relates to the continuum of forces. It represents a kind of filter in the perception of the external (and internal) world, one element of which involves preselected perception by the senses as the stimulus is received by the sensory organs, transmitted, processed, and interpreted. The tissue likewise reflects these influences, just as elements of consciousness that have been suppressed or energies within the body are expressed in it.

We are consciousness, in consciousness we live and consciousness surrounds us (Wright, Sayre-Adams 2001).[21] Healing takes place when all those involved consciously participate in the healing process. It is founded on the direct healing intention and the consciousness of all who are participating in this process. It is a relationship that involves not only practitioner and patient, but all and everything around. The interaction that takes place between the consciousness of practioners, patients, their family, and social environment and against the background of the sociocultural collective qualities of consciousness is a factor in the healing process that must not be overlooked. Perception of this multi-layered, multidimensional interconnectedness reveals what healing can mean in the individual case and how it can be achieved. Mind, body, soul, and emotions are not separate entities, but intimately interwoven parts of the person, who in turn is embedded in the entirety of existence. The aim is to promote the patient's own consciousness.

Consciousness, according to Jantsch, is the extent of autonomy of a system in its dynamic relationship with the external world. It therefore determines the level or complexity of the interactions of a system with the external world. According to Newman (1986),[22] health is a state of continual expansion of consciousness, while diseases represent the effort to achieve a higher level of consciousness. Similarly, for Mishel (1990)[23] the uncertainty that arises during an illness offers the possibility for individuals to alter their viewpoint in life and raise it to a new, more complex order. Focusing on health means not so much the dissolution of disease symptoms as arriving at a consciousness of the integration of the current process of symptoms and dysfunctions into a larger, wider scope of connection and order. Once health is understood in these terms, a patient in the latter stages of serious illness can nevertheless be completely "healthy" in the sense of achieving broadened consciousness.

Profound change or the transmutation of patterns of organization that maintain the dysfunction can be achieved by expanding the consciousness to include an awareness of the many-layered interconnections and the meaning to be found in the functional significance of the dysfunction. It has been demonstrated many times that the function of the body is influenced by the consciousness. All this should be borne in mind during our dealings with patients.

The entire pattern of tensions and associated psychological, neurological, hormonal and immunological conditioning are experienced together with the patient, in the utmost possible degree of consciousness. It seems to be part of the innermost nature of all things – in a way the essence of the magic that brings about change – that this kind of focus, in tune with its own rhythm, leads on to release and unwinding. The moment of unwinding is unpredictable; it can take seconds, minutes, hours, months, or even years.

The establishment of meaningful therapeutic interaction

It is important to understand that the specific patterns of conditioned habits, fears, desires, yearnings, aspects of the personality, or areas of ignorance, that are dis-

liked or rejected, and the conflicts and worries which arise from that, all serve to form the basis of the person's experience of self and of the world. The interweaving of all these things with the person reaches down into the deepest depths of the personality; the individual identifies with them. They therefore make up the person's identity and perception of the world at a very deep level. This is why we are not immediately aware of them; they are not instantly accessible, and in fact the contrary is true.

Even if patients are intellectually convinced of the necessity for change in these areas, both practitioner and patient face the problem that this is not believed deep down in the patient's unconscious.

The important task of the practitioner is to establish contact, not only with the intellect but also with the heart of the patient, including the depths of the unconscious. This opens up the possibility of sensing the meaningfulness in the patient's and the practitioner's striving for health, even on these levels. A purely rational explanation is of only slight help to the patient. It is necessary to perceive and understand the powerful forces that arise from the depths of the person's physis (natural life and growth), bios (physical life), psyche, soul, and spirit.

What we are concerned with here is not a matter of delivering general words of wisdom or performing a few technical maneuvers. It is a matter of establishing contact with patients by attuning to their experience with all the personal baggage that has accrued from events lived through, physical conditioning, emotions, belief systems, and thoughts. Patients will be unaware on a deeper level that, for example, certain desires lie at the root of the disorder. Following on with such an example, if patients are simply urged to give up smoking, without making any more fundamental connections, the benefit to them is no more than one of translation, affecting superficial features. The point is rather to seek out the forces at work behind the problem, so as to realize that identification with certain desires is the cause of the disorder and suffering.

When patients experience on this level and discover how a desire can be an obstacle to happiness, it enables them to let go of it and integrate it.

At this deep level, patients have no sense of differentiation and cannot distance themselves from the desire. On the contrary, the inmost part of the self is firmly and fully convinced of actually being that desire or that fear.

It is perfectly, intimately bound up with the personality of the individual as a whole, to such an extent that the person's entire life's experience seems to have been lived out in the attitudes concerned. Only after arriving at differentiation do patients gradually begin to find a kind of process of release in which they see that the fears, desires, or selfishness are not identical with their own selves. This recognition has transforming potential. It is inherent in the process of life, and it is the dialectical momentum of this kind of recognition that confronts the osteopath in the healing process.

Osteopaths are tasked with the role of applying touch, speaking to, communicating with, and interacting with patients in such a way as to bring them into relationship with their life.

If they do not achieve this, they will not be able to support patients in their process of achieving consciousness. This is then not available to appeal to in arriving at an understanding of personal responsibility regarding the situation and context of their lives. In this sense, each treatment situation is an extremely personal and intimate matter.

How, then, can an osteopath establish contact with the patient?

- First of all the osteopath should try to take into account the patient's entire context, developmental dynamics, degree of consciousness, and inner experience, in both diagnosis and treatment.

- Secondly, the practitioner should tune in completely to the patient. This means that practitioners do not try to take up contact from their own perspective, but from that of their patient. This is necessary in order to achieve the maximum possible resonance with the whole being of the patient. It is their whole being, body, gestures, touch, their emotional, intellectual, and spiritual self and consciousness that embody patients' greatest needs at that given moment, in that particular place, and in those particular circumstances. This is imprinted on their every touch, word, gesture, and tone of voice. Consequently, osteopathic treatment is not only directed at treating the tissue; it should touch the tissue, heart, and spirit of the patient in equal measure.

- This being so, osteopaths will not give their patients revealing statements about their lives, universally applicable insights about life in general, exercises, tips, or nutritional advice; nor carry out techniques, any of which may perhaps be significant for their own lives, but inappropriate in the context of the therapeutic interaction because they do not relate to the patient's experience. The patient would not be able to appreciate their deeper significance at that time, or put them into practice.

- Osteopaths should recognize the patient's situation and deep needs in life, the point of contact where the conditioned and restricting aspects encounter and conflict with the unconditioned aspects in the patient. In the therapeutic interaction they will then establish a link to this point of contact. They should then lead their patients to the place where they can perceive the forces that are at work within them and standing in the way of healing and higher-order integration. All depends on the precision with which the practitioner chooses the moment to allow an appropriate, attuned, and coherent therapeutic encounter to take place.

- In all this, of course, we inevitably encounter boundaries, and these cannot just be wished away. These boundaries are ultimately based on the practitioner's own level of consciousness and quality of osteopathic touch. This therapeutic capacity is dependent on the practitioner's own level of development, which determines the perspective from which practitioners are able to experience the internal and external world, and determines the aspects in the patient to which they are able to construct a relationship. The ideal practitioner is one who can make contact with each patient from the perspective that enables greatest coherence between practitioner and patient.

The meaning of empathetic contact

- Therapeutic touch as understood in osteopathy also includes the aspect of touch as an expression of unconditioned empathy and love. Because the therapeutic interaction is subjective, it requires the empathetic participation of the practitioner, drawing on the experience of both practitioner and patient. Intimacy, not of course in a sexual or childish sense, is essential. The greater the clarity with which practitioners are able to sense the presence of wholeness in their own experience, the easier they will find it to let this happen in the therapeutic interaction. Our patients are part of our heart, and helping them to heal themselves heals our own hearts at the same time.

Patients learn to trust their own experience

- We invite patients to trust their own immediate experience, to open up completely and unreservedly to it, and to enter into deep connectedness with all of life.

- The body can be experienced as a medium by which we harmonize our emotions and consciousness and open up to them.

- The experience that patients have during an osteopathic treatment session of the dynamics of the body and the energy processes taking place in it help them to achieve greater consciousness in their lives.

The focus is on health

- Still teaches, as a fundamental principle, that the aim and direction in therapy is health. All that we do in therapy is directed by the search for health, vitality, and support of the direct experience of wholeness. Its basis is not problem-oriented, i.e., not the search for primary or secondary dysfunctions. A problem-oriented procedure defines us in terms of our restrictions, dysfunctions, and disease symptoms, and our attention is then focused on problem areas. We are then so occupied by the problem areas that almost everything we do happens within those limits and the system of rules that govern them. This approach can still produce release, but it uses only a fraction of the potential vital forces and the possibilities potentially available to us. If by using it we unconsciously deny wider associations in terms of meaning, and identify our role as one of looking for the dysfunction, we even risk intensifying the reality of the problem areas and confirming them. Only when we as practitioners focus unreservedly and devotedly on the immediacy of the moment can we help our patients find a

route in this direction. (What is meant here by focus on the immediacy of the moment is not an absolute status quo, but a process of development in which both practitioner and patient draw benefit from each other.) As we strengthen our focus in this direction, working with the greatest possible devotion in this process we find ourselves able at the given moment to see the hindrances, conditioning, and fairly rigid somatoemotional and mental patterns or dysfunctions that need to be considered in order to enable still deeper opening or "letting go." This helps us on our way to unconditioned, conscious experience and deeper acceptance of the fullness of life. In a sense, this process can be seen as like that of dying. It sees the dissolution of an old, physical–spiritual perception of self (a certain tissue–energy–consciousness complex), a particular attitude to life, or a dysfunctional pattern, so that a new, more comprehensive one can come into being. These former patterns are not wrong in themselves. As protective mechanisms they are the expression of particular states of consciousness, aimed at defining the individual relative to former horizons of experience.

- The osteopath's task is to arrive at conscious awareness of the health in the patient, the health that never sickens, and to support it.

- According to Van Den Heede, healing is able to take place in a state of unknowing. Healing begins when the practitioner accompanies the patient into the state of unknowing.[24]

- Every therapeutic intervention is based on the ability to perceive normal function, normal patterns of tension and their associated normal range of movement or elasticity. This involves the differentiated perception of bones, membranes and ligaments, fluids, soft tissues, electromagnetism, potency, etc. and of dynamic, active stillness in the patient. It enables the osteopath to distinguish health from disease, that is, to recognize the difference between healthy and unhealthy tissue, and normal and abnormal tension patterns. The ability to sense the expression of body rhythms in a differentiated way makes it possible to localize and identify the findings, and in addition assists in treatment by supporting the body as a whole in achieving a state of balance in the way that the body itself intends.

- The prime aim is not to free the person from symptoms, but consists in the experience given by the challenges of life, which enables us to participate more profoundly in the fullness of existence and to live in a state of conscious being.

The process of release

- The amount of time needed for release of the dysfunction, in which binding forces are resolved and emerging forces integrated, depends firstly on the depth and strength with which the somatoemotional, neurohormonal tissue pattern is anchored in the personality structure. It also depends on the ability and the trust of both practitioner and patient, which enable them to observe the process of release without suppressing it, whilst maintaining contact with vitality. The inherent dynamics of this process may take minutes, hours, months, or even years, depending on the dysfunction. The signs that signal release are, in addition to an increase in energy, a feeling of fulfillment, vitality, and presence. It cannot be restated too often that these processes can only ever be offered and encouraged, never forced.

- The release of dysfunctions, in a sense, also calls for a loss of control of old patterns of identification that find their reflection in the body. Softening of body patterns combined with opening of self-perception allows a new order to come about in the body as a whole, so that the person can retain contact with the new energies that the process makes available.

- Once the boundaries have been opened up they need time to stabilize so that the more refined sensitivity, freer flow of energy and increased energy state can become integrated into everyday life. Osteopathic treatment can also follow patients in this stage; conscious palpation helps them by strengthening the patterns of body energies in their perception. Patients learn to use their bodies as a feedback system for spiritual processes.

- A number of different stages may become evident, especially when treating chronic conditions. Old patterns may become strengthened, and hidden body patterns or suppressed symptoms may appear. Both practitioner and patient learn to observe these processes without suppressing or manipulating them. A change occurs from a certain point in the process onward: a transmutation in the pattern of dysfunction. It can be compared to Becker's "something happens," (see pp. Ch 15, p. 243).

- There is a period of re-organization and stabilization, in which the individual learns to integrate the newly available energies and to make creative use of them.

Perspectives on therapeutic interactions in osteopathy

An interaction takes place between osteopaths, with all the various perspectives, lines, and levels of development that characterize them as sentient beings, and their patients with theirs (see Ch. 1, p. 23ff). The perspectives are those of subjectivity (I), intersubjectivity (you/we), objectivity (it), and interobjectivity (they, systemic). The levels that are important are not only the physical, biological, emotional, mental, and spiritual levels of the patient but also those of the practitioner.

The osteopath's contact with the tissue, in terms of Wilber's quadrants model

(a) Subjective dimension

The subjective components of tissue elasticity are an example. The subjective dimension comprises all the inner perceptions, thoughts, feelings, and associations on the part of the osteopath that arise during the palpation of tissue elasticity, i.e., when examining for external findings. Influences that color, condition, or otherwise affect the practitioner's perception include:

- Previous experiences (prenatal, perinatal, postnatal, childhood, physical, and psychological trauma, etc.).

- Experiences in professional practice.

- Understanding (intellectual, empathetic, and manual) of the interactions of structure and function and osteopathic issues.

- The osteopath's own state of consciousness, state of mind and mood at the particular time, suppressed, repressed, or projected matter, etc. (and much of this quite unconsciously).

- Cultural (intersubjective) and social (interobjective) influences (see below).

The facts as found in the tissue (objective) and interpretations of these findings (subjective) are inseparably, though distinguishably, linked. The realities of the tissue and the patient are always present within the osteopath's perspective when exercising perception. Consequently there is an element of interpretation in all perception. This does not however mean that we are free to interpret perceptions freely at will (i.e., postmodern absolutism).

The internal, individual, or subjective conduct of palpation can be further analyzed into the following aspects:

- Phenomenological: what feelings and associations, etc. arise for me as the practitioner during palpation? The phenomenological flow of my own subjective experience.

- Structural: what patterns can I identify during the conduct of my palpation (recurrent feelings, associations, etc.)? These things objectivize what lies within. They present me, as the osteopath, with charts setting out my own inner workings. In this way, osteopaths may discover connections between certain processes happening in the tissue and their own inner associations, or certain perceptions of tissue qualities and psychological phenomena.*

---

*On the intersubjective level, this can create a broad, solid basis for observation. It can also acquire objective character (see below). One method of applying this would be for practitioners to keep a diary of their own phenomenological impressions during treatment, and to evaluate it at a certain distance in time. This would reveal the patterns and rules governing their own perception (i.e., structural approach). This would give them an awareness of their own inner subjective structures such as recurrent patterns of feeling, and patterns and associations of thoughts and emotions during palpation. (Structuralism = phenomenology+time/distance.)

(b) Intersubjective dimension

In the intersubjective dimension, osteopaths acquire their approach to understanding as individual members who are part of a professional group. These approaches to understanding are formed by the cultural history of development of osteopathy, the common background of method, similar courses of osteopathic training (similar principles of diagnosis and treatment taught in the curriculum), and the similarity in the cultural background of osteopathic medicine. The conscious and unconscious influence from the background of the individual's own cultural history is often underestimated because it is not directly visible. The group settings that influence the individual osteopath include not only the professional context, but also any number of other relationships, professional and private, past and present, and each exerting its own particular influence.

The internal, intersubjective approach to understanding can be further analyzed into the following aspects:

- Hermeneutic approach: our palpation experience as osteopaths, as a professional group. For example, the intersubjective components of tissue elasticity, i.e., the collected knowledge of osteopathy with respect to: "What associations and interpretations arise when palpating tissue elasticity?" The individual experience of the "culture" of osteopathy can be expressed as: "We osteopaths are..."

- Structural approach: for example: "What common, recurrent patterns can be found by palpation in particular types of tissue elasticity (i.e., interpretative charts relating to tissue elasticity)?"† Structuralism can enable us to investigate patterns of recurrent interpretations in the diagnoses of osteopaths, as formulated or postulated in standard works of osteopathy. Other practitioners, such as homeopaths or practitioners of Chinese medicine, will have different patterns of interpretation in their diagnoses.

---

†These charts are inner ones when dealing with psychological interpretation, and external when dealing with anatomical interpretation. The question "what does it mean?" would render it subjective. The question, "what is it?" renders it objective.

There is another "we" present in the treatment situation, and that is the one that exists between practitioner and patient. There is a common "cultural" background and imprint, forming the basis for reciprocal understanding. The practitioner–patient relationship has a beginning, and it develops. As it does so, a common "history" with its own dynamic comes into being. In the treatment situation, this "we" is a matter of direct experience. If, for example, after three sessions with the patient, the osteopath reflects on what has been experienced, then (dynamic) structures and patterns that have formed in the context of this intersubjectivity may become evident. Possible examples of such patterns are:

- Recurrent touching of particular parts of the body associated with particular emotions or bodily sensations.

- Certain sequences of moods and feelings in the course of treatment.

- Features characterizing the nature of the atmosphere.

- Patterns of (inner) nearness or distance, etc.

(c) Objective dimension

The elements that make up the objective dimension are the timeframe within which the treatment takes place, and the external facts or objective parameters that apply during palpation, e.g., tension, inherent motions/rhythms/mobility, density, elasticity, amplitude, etc. The objective components of tissue elasticity are findings of the type that would be made by an instrument of measurement, or as an objectively observable change in the tissue in response to objective examination by the osteopath, using pressure or traction. External features of the physical world can be evaluated using objective methods of examination. The advantage of such methods is that they place limits on subjectivity. The evidence can be presented to others, asking the question, "Look; this is what I observed. What do you see?" This can then lead on to an assessment that is as objective as possible (i.e., as free as possible from subjective, individual interpretation): the triumph of objective science. It applies to those things that are external. When we are dealing with those that are internal (feelings, belief systems, values, ethics, art, etc.), subjectivity and intersubjectivity have a fundamental role to play. Objective observation alone will never be able to explain the meaning of a book, the hand of an osteopath applying touch, or the reason for a patient's tears: the great flaw of objective science.

This approach does not stand in isolation, of course; it still involves all four quadrants, meaning that everything can be seen from at least four viewpoints:

- The osteopath applies pressure. Intentionality on the part of the osteopath lies behind this, with several subjective, "I" backgrounds (rational, emotional, conscious, unconscious, suppresses, etc.).

- There are also many intersubjective, "we" backgrounds to this intentionality (conscious and unconscious, etc.), and deriving from the osteopath's professional and personal relationships, cultural environment, the present "we" relationship existing with the patient, etc.

- At the same time, there are also external and collective aspects to the situation: the treatment room, e.g., its architecture, furniture, equipment, and lighting; and the infrastructure, e.g., the structure of the health system, and official regulations (which kinds of therapeutic intervention are permitted, and which are not?).

- Objectively measurable qualities, e.g., pressure in terms of force/area.

(d) Interobjective dimension

With regard to this dimension, the views present in the individual osteopath are generated by the social course of development of osteopathy and the social systems within which the osteopath has grown up and now lives. The influence of this social determination is often underestimated; for example, the invention of the internet, originally for a quite different purpose, has had the widespread effect of influencing people's behavior and even consciousness. The (partial) truth expressed by Marx is relevant here, that "(material/systemic) existence determines consciousness." An important example of an influence that affects osteopathic practice is the health system and its structures, regulations and provisions, etc.

Reactions by the patient to the therapeutic interaction

Patients enter therapy bringing with them their entire history (all quadrants, lines, levels, states, and types).

The therapeutic process operates in more than one dimension, affecting on the one hand the interactions of tissue and physiology and patient behavior (the objective dimension) and on the other, the individual's ego-space and consciousness (the subjective dimension). Examples of this would be the impressions that patients have of the role of the osteopath (e.g., status) and of the therapeutic intervention (satisfaction, frustration, anxieties on account of the symptoms).

All these changes can be studied in various ways: phenomenological or structuralist, or by the use of physiological parameters and instruments of measurement.

The therapeutic interaction can extend to include the patient's cultural environment. This is done by involving the patient's family in the healing process, through the exchange that takes place in self-help groups, through better patterns of relationship between patients and those around them (relatives, friends, and work colleagues), and through new attitudes or re-orientation in the field of work, etc. Patients' belief in the osteopath's authority in the healing process, or enquiry into the role that the osteopath performs will depend on their particular cultural background. Their approach will in turn have a considerable effect on the extent to which patients enter into the treatment and engage actively in the healing process.

The social environment can also be integrated through the treatment. Examples of this are the reduction of environmental toxins and fields of disturbance in the home, participation in social projects, beautification of the home and workplace, further improvement of conditions at work, and commitment to finding financial support, etc. The influence will extend to other dimensions depending on the setting (private practice, hospital/clinic) and social structures, e.g., in the health system (reimbursement through health insurance).

These changes can be studied in various ways: phenomenological, hermeneutical, or structuralist, or using objective means of measurement, either in the individual patient or in a group (intersubjective). This may open up ways of investigating such things as connections between certain osteopathic treatment methodologies and a change in the patient's condition. It is

also possible to investigate cultural influences such as the place accorded to osteopathy in that society. This and other kinds of sociological information can provide individual osteopaths with useful insights to help in their work, e.g., the extent to which the method is known or accepted in society.

Summary and conclusion

All these aspects come together in the treatment situation. Osteopaths' perceptions are conditioned by the ways in which they themselves have been formed. This influences their perception of the subjective and objective dimensions of their patients and their capacity to influence patients' inner lives (e.g., level of development, personality, states of consciousness, conditioning and incidences of trauma, cultural and family influences, social status of the patient, etc.). The resources available to osteopaths include the knowledge and experience of their own (and other) traditions, e.g., anatomy and physiology, psychology, cultural and sociological knowledge relating to medical issues (e.g., the effect of social systems on health). At the same time, knowledge of their own ego-space also has an important role. This is explored, for example, through meditation. The more individual osteopaths look at this aspect and set it in order, the less of it will be projected onto the patients.

In all these dimensions there is an evolutionary dynamic. Starting on the basis of past influences and their formative effects on the practitioner and the patient, a new element is added by the creativity of the moment. This then becomes a formative influence in its own right, for the next moment, and operates as a morphogenetic field or as karma.

References

[1]Weissmann R, Weissmann S: With compassionate understanding. St Paul, Minnesota: Paragon House; 1999:201.

[2]McGovern J, McGovern R: Your healer within. Tucson, Arizona: Fenestra Books; 2003:145.

[3]McGovern J, McGovern R: Your healer within. Tucson, Arizona: Fenestra Books; 2003:145.

[4]Goleman D: Die heilende Kraft der Gefühle. Gespräche mit dem Dalai Lama. Munich: dtv; 2004:296.

[5]Goleman D: Die heilende Kraft der Gefühle. Gespräche mit dem Dalai Lama. Munich: dtv; 2004:155.

[6]Still AT: Der Natur bis ans Ende vertrauen. Pähl: Jolandos; 2003:1415.

[7]Becker RE: In: Brooks RE (ed.): The stillness of life. Portland: Stillness Press; 2000:2.

[8]Brody H: The Placebo Response. How you can release the body's inner pharmacy for better health. New York: Harper-Collins Publishers; 2002:88.

[9]Brody H: The Placebo Response. How you can release the body's inner pharmacy for better health. New York: Harper-Collins Publishers; 2002:84,100.

[10]Hawkins J: How can we optimize non-specific effects. In: Peters D (ed.): Understanding the placebo effect in complementary medicine. Edinburgh: Churchill Livingstone; 2001:72, 83f.

[11]Thomas KB: General practice consultations: is there any point in being positive? Brit. Med. J. 1987;294:1200–1202.

[12]Sachs H: Can patients influence health decisions? J. Royal College of Gen. Practit. 1982;32:691–694.

[13]Montgomery CL: The care-giving relationship: paradoxical and transcendent aspects. Altern. Therap. 1996;2(2):52–57.

[14]Rein G, Atkinson M, McCraty R: The physiological and psychological effects of compassion and anger. J. Advancem. Med. 1995;8(2):87–105.

[15]McCraty R, Atkinson M, Tiller WA et al.: Effects of emotions on short-term power spectrum analysis of heart rate variability. Am. J. Cardiol. 1995;76(14):1089–1093.

[16]Barefoot JC, Dahlstrom WG: Williams R.B. Hostility CHD incidence and total mortality: a 25-year follow-up study of 255 physicians. Psychosom. Med. 1983;45:59–63.

[17]Davis W: Energetics and Therapeutic Touch. In: Heller M (ed.): The flesh of the soul: the body we work with: Selected papers of the 7th Congress of the European Association of Body Psychotherapy, 2–6. September 2001, 59.

[18]Webster GV: Concerning osteopathy. Norwood, Mass, USA: The Plimpton Press 1910; 2.

[19]Wright SG, Sayre-Adams J: Healing and therapeutic touch: is it all in the mind? In: Peters D (ed.). Understanding the placebo effect in complementary medicine. Edinburgh: Churchill Livingstone; 2001:172.

[20]Jantsch E: Die Selbstorganisation des Universums. Vom Urknall zum menschlichen Geist. Munich: Hanser; 1992:61–63.

[21]Wright SG, Sayre-Adams J: Healing and therapeutic touch: is it all in the mind? In: Peters D (ed.). Understanding the placebo effect in complementary medicine. Edinburgh: Churchill Livingstone; 2001:172.

[22]Newman MA: Health as expanding consciousness. St Louis: C.V. Mosby; 1986;43:20.

[23]Mishel MH: Reconceptualization of the uncertainty in illness theory. Image J. Nurs. Sch. 1990; 22(4):256–62.

[24]Course notes: P. Van Den Heede: Pädiatrische Osteopathie. OSD Hamburg; 2003.

20

Treatment principles

Torsten Liem

L'ostéopathe est d'abord une présence

C. Bochurberg[1]

Introduction

It is the fundamental principles of osteopathy that unite the great variety of treatment approaches within this field. The following account of treatment principles is by no means exhaustive, and it is not the purpose of this book to present or list all those that exist. This does not however mean that these cannot be applied just as effectively in an "integral" osteopathic treatment. Each of the methods described here can be adapted or modified; it is also possible to integrate parts of these into other osteopathic methods.

The following provides treatment guidelines specific to osteopathy as well as further essential guidelines for treating patients, from a holistic osteopathic point of view. Are they based on the principles of A.T. Still? Most certainly! The physical material (the tissue correlate), the external element, is present throughout, to the highest level of the internal aspect (i.e., the highest consciousness) (see also Chapter 1). Consequently, there is an inseparable link between, for example, regressive palpation (in essence, the palpation of developmental dynamics in the tissue) and certain inner dynamics of consciousness (see also Chapter 37). Therefore, tissue dysfunctions in particular stages of development of the tissue can often be associated with certain conditioned dysfunctional patterns of consciousness in the patient. It is not enough to treat only the tissue correlate if we wish to provide adequate treatment for the wholeness of the patient. It is equally important to be able to take account of the inner components of consciousness that appear. The practitioner needs to distinguish the osteopathic principles/viewpoints that are appropriate in terms of method, and similarly in terms of the interaction between structure and function. Practical approaches need to be worked out that will take account of the elements of inner consciousness in the patient and integrate these in the treatment of tissue dysfunction complexes.

It is essential in this respect to recognize the dynamics and interactions of objective and subjective factors of the patient's internal and external world, and also those of the practitioner, as integral, inseparable components in the healing process, and to include them. The tissue energy status or physiological parameters, and the physical, emotional, mental, and spiritual levels of consciousness all form part of the internal world, while the sociocultural context and environmental conditions form the external.

In the models of healing current until recently, the patient has tended more to be the passive recipient of what is done. If the method assumed the existence of homeostatic forces that were responsible for the actual process of healing, this seldom required the active participation of the patient. Authority and responsibility lay with the practitioner and the treatment method employed. In the postmodern paradigm, however, healing is an active process and always an internal one. It is necessary to examine the effect on health of all the attitudes, convictions, emotions, and patterns of perception of all levels of the patient. The challenge to the patient, and the task that the patient must fulfill, is to let go of negative and restrictive patterns. The success of healing vitally depends on the prime fact of patients' cooperation in the task. Without this, an essential element in the healing process is missing. This consists in the expansion of the patients' consciousness to be able to perceive the link between the symptoms occurring in their lives, and their personal share in what is happening, and then their active application of this gain in insight. Recovery and relief of symptoms can of course occur without this work, but the profound transcendence of the meaning of the disease, the profound resolution of the disease pattern and its conscious translation into healthier patterns of order will all be lacking. If this does not occur, then sooner or later the unconscious, conditioned patterns will often find renewed expression in similar or transposed symptoms.

Patients usually consult an osteopath to cure or ease their symptoms. They seldom realize that their attitudes, models of belief, and conditioning and their level of development are also involved. It then becomes the practitioner's duty to make them aware of how they are connected. It is likewise their duty to exercise insight regarding their patients' individual developmental process, to exercise respect, and indeed to recognize their decision not to deal with these connections at the time of the consultation and nevertheless to provide them with the best possible treatment. Osteopaths are therefore mainly concerned with translative work in their day-to-day practice (i.e., healing within the patient's level of development). They should nevertheless be receptive and open to the possibility of transformative processes at any time during treatment, i.e., the possibility of transformation to arrive at higher-order states of balance in the body, as a whole, and higher stages of development and consciousness in the patient.

Extensive knowledge of the body is fundamental to osteopathic treatment. A.T. Still, for example, was so familiar with every bone in the body that he could assemble a human skeleton with his eyes closed. Our bodies also consist of ligaments, muscles, soft tissues, nerves, blood vessels, organs, etc. and of various associated energies and fields. The qualities of these are an expression of our life histories, of morphogenetic and genetic factors, of our experience and our consciousness and also our family, cultural, and biosocial environment.

Osteopathic treatment demands many abilities of the practitioner. It is essential to be able to perceive, differentiate, and interpret tissue qualities and morphological dynamics in the body as a whole, to place these findings in the total context of the life history and environment of the patient, and have a command of the osteopathic influences on every kind of tissue–energy–consciousness complex. Another important element is the ability to synchronize with inherent homeodynamic processes in the body.

To translate findings that are human or interpersonal exclusively in terms of anatomical and physiological processes carries the risk of reducing the person. Whereas we can justifiably see dynamics of form and function as a condition of such human findings, they are not the entire cause. Perhaps the most universal oscillation, or the most profound, is that of unconditioned love, which finds its purest and most direct expression in the causal state. Synchronization with this is not a technique in the conventional sense but sympathy made manifest and deconditioned consciousness beyond the traditional practitioner–patient duality.

If we understand treatment, or healing, as the quickest and most efficient way to dispose of symptoms, then technical considerations will be paramount.*

However, technical approaches are of necessity based on a minimum of directly experienced findings. In other words, the findings are reduced to those elements or facts that are necessary to the particular technique. Apart from the (entirely justified) "technocratic" osteopathic approach that seeks to relieve disease symptoms as quickly as possible by tissue manipulation, osteopathic treatment can also serve the purpose of supporting dynamic processes directed at higher-order integration in the patient. If we approach it from this point of view we should avoid excessive focus on technical performance that might limit the healing potential.

One way of applying this is to regard treatment in the context of a holistic or integral concept of osteopathy. This will include setting out a hierarchy of levels of dysfunction and compensation. Some of the concepts (and "philosophies") involved in this are presented and discussed in the present book.

Another way of applying this is contained in the therapeutic intention of "being" with the patient instead of the aim of "doing"; this enables patients to contact the quality of being. This may or may not be accompanied by a relief of symptoms.

While tuning into this quality of being, there may be a change in the potency. This is the effect that Becker described as "something happens" in relation to the therapeutic interaction on the tissue level. The experience of being finds expression in a special quality in which transformation can take place without any need for the practitioner to focus on the transformation. From the point of view of therapy, the experience of being is important not only in respect of contact with the tissue; it naturally also includes contact with the patient as a whole person.

---

*Osteopathy must also be compared with other methods in this respect, e.g., traditional allopathic medicine. It is also necessary to examine such issues as whether osteopathy does indeed, as often maintained, help to achieve more enduring relief of symptoms than for example traditional allopathic medicine, and whether osteopathy produces fewer side effects.

It would be naive to think that a purely intellectual grasp of what is said here might be enough to develop the quality. This cannot be done by reading these lines, listening to exhortations by lecturers (who may not necessarily have achieved the quality in their own lives), or by attending a few courses. (In a Tibetan monastery, it takes some 30 or 40 years to learn composure, awareness, and sympathy.) The best support that osteopaths can find in developing the necessary qualities is provided by actively nurturing their own emotional, mental, and spiritual awareness, and by various kinds of regular practice.

True synchronization with the deeper levels of being in another person calls for an authentic awareness of simple being on one's own account. This awareness encompasses all aspects of the aspiring practitioner's life and opens up a constant consciousness, stage by stage. This is experienced not only in the waking state but also in the dreaming state and in deep, dreamless sleep. The potency of this present awareness has the power to inspire patients to the depths of their being. Patients too must take this path for themselves. At the far end of this process (which usually proceeds in stages) lies transcendence of the practitioner–patient role, of every other kind of seeing in terms of subject and object, and of every kind of conceptualization.

It must be stressed that this is not an attempt to "polarize" these three different therapeutic approaches. Rather, the aim is to integrate the quality of being in the therapeutic contact with the essential, fundamental principles specific to osteopathy, which relate to the dynamics of form and function and the body conceived as a whole entity. This emphasis will become apparent in the following description of treatment principles.

The world that presents itself to us, including the body tissue that we touch in our work as osteopaths, is not solid, but a temporary phenomenon. It is the expression of circumstances and evolutionary forces interacting with each other. All depends on a vast number of other dependent facts and factors. We need to distinguish these factors. Perception of the patient and of the interplay of the tissue and physiological elements needs to be set in relation to the patient's current state of development, and the dynamics and interactions of objective and subjective factors in the inner world of the patient.

(This involves both the organization of the interwoven anatomical and physiological elements, and the physical, emotional, mental, and spiritual levels of the patient's consciousness.) Secondly, the external world of the patient must be brought into the picture. (This involves the cultural setting and the patient's worldview and biosocial environment, including the economic conditions, which make up the context of the patient's life.)[†]

Another aspect to be considered in the therapeutic intervention is the patient's level of development (e.g., the individual's physical, emotional, mental, and spiritual level). So we form an integral picture of the patient, and the more comprehensive that integral concept of the patient, the more appropriate the course of the therapeutic interaction will be, because the resonance we can establish will be stronger and more significant. It involves more than just an intellectual understanding to create this state of relationship; it involves an empathetic and intuitive perception of this dynamic interweaving of existence. Therefore, if we are to achieve holistic treatment, the patient's subjective experience must be integrated, and, in palpation, resonance must be established both with the tissue dynamics and with the subjective world of experience in its various aspects (see Chapter 11). Even when all these aspects have been taken into account, practitioners can still not be certain what role they are in fact playing in their interaction with the patient in this "cosmic" realm of "karma."

Healing is not a one-way process from practitioner to patient. Another extremely important element appears to be the conscious participation of all concerned in the healing process, together with empathetic insight into how symptoms are related, as well as the connectedness, the interrelationship, and the evolutionary or "involutionary" dynamic of all that lives.

[†]The subjective inner and external world of the patient is expressed in such things as the experience of "the potential of the space-time nature of existence, physicality, coexistence in a shared world, the determined nature of existence, the general openness of existence and the development of these fundamental potentialities toward freedom of existence" (Medard Boss).[1a]

Treatment aims

- Experience of simple being, of things being as they are.

- Support the maintenance of the integrity of self in order to prevent, overcome, and heal damage from system pertubations inflicted by the internal and external milieus.[2]

- Support that encourages higher-order levels of integration in the patient.

- Support for the evolutionary dynamics in the patient and for the capacity to sense, interpret, and act on data available from parts of the whole and the environment, and learn from those experiences.[2]

- Support for the experience of meaning in the phenomena and areas of life and experience that affects the patient.

- Differentiation and resolution of trauma (physical, biological, emotional, mental, or spiritual) and support for the integration of body–energy–consciousness complexes.

- Support for immanent regulatory tendencies such as those of self-preservation, self-adaptation, immanence, and transcendence, increasing autonomy, differentiation, integration, and increasing complexity. On the biological level, for example, this would involve support of the energetical management to maintain self-organization, enable self-transcendence, and to support the energetic requirements of essential functions of a living system,[2] including the body's own healing forces and defenses and homeostatic forces, so that the processes of fluid, neural and energetic exchange can fulfill their function. These effects are:
  - normalizing the function of the nervous system
  - resolving congestion and barriers and normalizing the movement of various fluids (flow of blood and lymph, the dynamics of intercellular and intracellular fluids and CSF)
  - achieving a dynamic physiological balance of fascial tensions in the body (including that of membranes and ligaments)

- releasing of restrictions of movement and pain
- improving the reaction of body tissues to stress
- improving the statics and dynamics of the body
- improving the energy level of the patient.

Still[3] called the human body "God's drugstore," containing every sort of remedy the individual needs to maintain and restore health. We simply need to let these remedies redevelop and flow freely, and ensure that they function harmoniously together in the body. In osteopathy, symptoms are not "banished" and the sick person is not "cured." The process is rather one of dialog with the tissues of the body and with our knowledge of the physiological relations in the body as a whole, by which we create the structural preconditions to enable the individual as a whole person to become "healthy". For example, osteopathy supports the resolution and integration of structural and emotional barriers, so that the biological circulatory processes can function in the best possible way.

Many of the diseases and disorders suffered in the Western world are chronic conditions brought about by our lifestyle and habits. If we wish to treat these, it is not sufficient to restore some element of mobility like a watchmaker setting a couple of cogwheels back in motion in the mechanism of a clock.

The demand that this makes of patients is to learn to adapt their behavior, lifestyle, and diet to the needs of their body as a whole, enabling that inner "drugstore" to perform its task. This kind of healing takes time. It is not achieved in a 15-minute session, but requires constant effort on the part of the practitioner to form an idea of the organization of the patient, which is in constant motion. It also requires the dynamic interaction between patient and practitioner, hand and tissue, understanding and the individual's own assumption of responsibility, between tissue and energy, consciousness and environment.

Not all causative factors are capable of being resolved. Genetic influences are an example. Irreversible changes and malformations cannot be reversed. In such cases, treatment needs to aim at achieving the best possible adaptation by the body to these circumstances, so as to give the patient as trouble-free a life as possible.

Not every predisposition necessarily results in a disorder. A predisposition to an allergy is an example. Patients can heed those factors that promote their health and avoid those that encourage the predisposition to develop into the disorder. Manual osteopathic treatment can meanwhile promote and support the homeostatic forces in the body as a whole. This addresses a further important field in which osteopathy can be applied: prevention.

This point also explains Still's constant stress on the idea that, in osteopathy, everything begins and ends with the anatomy and physiology of the living human being.

Osteopathic treatment is always an individual matter, since no patient is exactly like another, and even the same patient changes from one day to the next in all sorts of ways: in the state of tissue tension, in energy potential, and in emotional, mental, and spiritual state.

Translation and transformation

Translation and transformation belong in the context of the evolutionary development of human beings, and in osteopathic treatment, and it is also here that they derive their meaning. Every therapeutic intervention involves sensing two different but very important functions in relation to the levels of development of the patient. The first of these is a horizontal/translative function, the other a vertical/transformative one.

The first has to do with recognition of the level of development attained, perceiving how it is structured, becoming acquainted with it, and assuming ownership of it. It involves acquiring competence, consolidation, and healing. The second seeks to transform, to leave behind, and release (and integrate) what has been in the past, up to that point. A natural tension exists between the two. The first brings comfort and security, a sense of safety and calm. The second creates disquiet, insecurity, a mood of change and uncertainty. Both are important, since one without the other enmires the individual in a state in which change is blocked, or produces dissociation and disintegration (development in which the lower levels are not carried forward).[4] Day-to-day osteopathic practice tends to bring significantly more dealings with translative work, although the possibility of encountering transformation is always there.

Translation involves reinterpreting or shifting dysfunctional patterns (for example, to another tissue or body system, shifting "from the lungs to the skin" or to another physiological state, or from soma to the emotional field, etc.). This shift may ease the patient's symptoms or pain to some degree for a while – short, medium, or long term. The osteopathic manipulation in effect offers the patient a fresh interpretation of the conditioning that lies behind the dysfunctional pattern, by shifting or relocating the dysfunctional pattern. There is no enquiry into the conditioning and forces behind the dysfunctional pattern, nor does this address the fact that the conditioning (i.e., the level of development) is part of what makes up the person of the patient. Instead, support is given to patients as they are stabilized in their present level of development, and their manner of perceiving the world and themselves. This is an essential and important part of the process of growth.

Transformation looks at the patient in person. The dysfunction complex is not simply a part that imposes restriction on the patient; the complex is something that has significance within the patient. Release (or overcoming of the dysfunction complex) is encouraged when we recognize the patient as part of the state of limitation. The type of treatment that is aimed at translation hardly touches the deep, fundamental pattern of the particular patient. Therapeutic interaction aimed at transformation, in contrast, recognizes the involvement of the integral, interwoven elements – material, biological, and mental – in the patient in the particular dysfunction pattern, and incorporates this aspect. The therapeutic interaction makes it easier for patients to see and understand the dysfunctional patterns in themselves that are restricting them, giving them a better understanding of the way these patterns find expression in the symptoms and automatic conditioned reactions. Osteopaths need to sense these things (in themselves), or enter into resonance with them (in the patient), in order for this to happen. They also need to support patients in establishing contact with their own potential and resources, giving them the means to free themselves, if possible, from the restricting patterns. Doing so creates the conditions for transcendence and transformation. This "transcendence" is not of course meant in an absolute sense; it should be understood as a stepwise, evolutionary process of transformation, which therapy can encourage but never force to come about. Each transcending step within the process brings integration, and each time with a higher order. In translative procedures, one of the prime aims is often to relieve the symptoms as quickly as possible (bringing the risk of displacement of symptoms). The prime

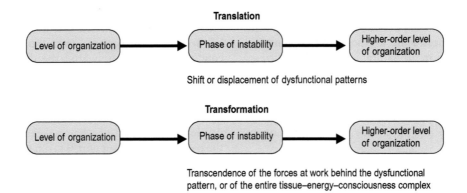

Figure 20.1
Translation and transformation.

endeavor in transformative processes is to understand and arrive at a consciousness of the deep association between the somatic dysfunction and the symptoms with which it is interwoven in the associations of meaning within the patient, and to allow this realization to mature. This understanding and this realization form the foundation that can support transformative processes in both practitioner and patient.

Factors to heed in treatment

The following points are very important to the healing process. The practitioner can both accompany the process and provide the impulse. For patients, the task is to reassume responsibility for their own well-being and assume an active role.

1 Regulation of eating habits: food, alcohol consumption, and smoking. Osteopathy has always regarded the diet as one of the factors affecting health and disease. These matters should therefore be explored and careful consideration given to the positive and negative importance and effects of alcohol and smoking etc. on the individual as a whole.

2 Elimination of sources of disturbance. In cases involving such problems as arthritis, neuritis, and other complaints, it will be necessary to identify the focus of any recurrent infection and eliminate this. Sources include: root-treated teeth, chronic inflammation of tonsils, sinuses, appendix, gall bladder, etc. The actual focus of infection is often found to be producing no symptoms at all. Chronic heavy metal poisoning, and other such problems, should also be considered.

3 Attention to chronic local or generalized infection; treatment to eliminate the infection. Osteopathic treatments often have a positive healing effect on these infections. However, due consideration must be given to the possible need for specialist medical treatment in addition.

4 Elimination of toxic substances. Heavy metal pollution, hydrochlorofluorocarbon, indoor toxins (funguses, toxic colours, wood coatings, toxic carpet adhesives, solvents), and environmental pollutants (insecticides, pesticides).

5 Regulation of the work/rest balance and wake/sleep rhythm. A balance of activity and rest and the rhythm of wakefulness and sleep that is suited to the individual are important in providing the right amount of stimulation on the one hand, and time for regeneration and recovery on the other. Relaxation exercises are particularly helpful for those affected by the stress levels of Western society. The method of relaxation developed by Harvey is an example of this, with practices to help relax the muscular, autonomic, emotional, mental, and spiritual levels.[5] On the muscular level, relaxation is based on the idea of progressive relaxation of the muscles; on the autonomous level, it is achieved through slow, calm breathing or mindful observation of breathing. Emotional relaxation comes about by bringing to mind and resolving negative images of the self and negative belief models, supported by breathing and movement exercises and by talking about the matter. Mental relaxation can be achieved by sensory focus, concentration, and meditation. Spiritual relaxation is brought on by strengthening trust and belief through contemplation of nature, prayer, singing, reading sacred scriptures, and meditation.

6 Resolution of emotional patterns that play a part in structural and functional disturbances. Structural changes can lead to altered emotional perceptions. Similarly, past or present experiences, memories, and belief systems, whether personal or professional, short-term, traumatic, or sustained, can play a part in the development of abnormal tissue tensions and in functional impairment of body physiology. These experiences can affect the body as a whole. For example, thoughts can lead to the production of specific neurotransmitters and hormones. These in turn cause the body and tissues to react in a certain way.

The reactions by the tissues – the particular activity, physiology, and energy – in a sense reflect the experiences. In this way, experiences can bring about or sustain disease symptoms and dysfunctions.

Healing becomes possible as patients become aware of the emotional attitudes underlying the problem, and learn to perceive and integrate their various, often contradictory, personality aspects and needs in a more differentiated way. Patients have to learn to trust and respect their own perceptions and inner impressions. The approaches developed by Harvey (see point 5), visualization, affirmation, and psychotherapeutic support can all be helpful.

7 Body consciousness and regular, appropriate physical activity, preferably in the fresh air and in an unspoilt natural environment. Physical activity has many benefits. It promotes the flow of body fluids, exercises the cardiovascular system, drains and vitalizes body tissues. It also has a balancing, positive effect on the psyche, for example by producing endorphins. Activities that are helpful here include running, cycling, swimming, yoga, aikido, etc. Intensification of body consciousness can be achieved by the following methods: patients are asked, for example, to lie supine, without moving, and successively sense the various parts of their bodies, developing an inner awareness of each part. Another possible approach is progressive muscle relaxation using the method proposed by Jacobsen as well as HRV - biofeedback - or neurofeedback practice.

8 Involvement in local cultural groups. Self-help groups, community groups, meditation groups, play groups, walking groups, social conversational groups, cultural associations, etc.

9 Involvement in social projects. Help for the homeless, human rights groups, famine relief groups, groups for the protection of animals, nature, etc.

10 Finding meaning in one's life. Individuals can find a sense of direction if they have a spiritual fulcrum to guide them, if they find meaning in their life, and if they perceive the link between them and the rest of the cosmos. In this context growth represents an increase in the immediate awareness of this link with existence as such, other people and the rest of nature, and the integration of the various aspects of the personality. Viewed in this way, disease symptoms can be a sign that the person's lifestyle may not be in accord with the person's psychological and physical nature. This can give the patient the opportunity to change and grow as a whole being. Helpful approaches to achieving this are: exercises in consciousness, sitting in meditation, reading spiritual texts and

sacred scriptures, and contemplation of inner knowledge and perception; also unselfish activities such as work in the social field, dedication, and exercises to develop spiritual control.

11 Achieving awareness of compensatory patterns of behavior. For example, compulsive eating, smoking addiction, excessive alcohol consumption, TV, power, money, sex, work, etc., and underlying (often suppressed) traumas and unpleasant experiences.

Palpation: general treatment principles

"Allowing oneself to be grasped" and actively "grasping"

In osteopathy, palpation was applied from the outset in a manner that combined the functional and the structural, in other words, combining the "listening" and "speaking" forms of palpation. On the one hand, in palpation osteopaths allow themselves to be "grasped" by the organization of the tissue and by the tissue fields; on the other, they also "grasp" the initiative through their hands, to assist the establishment of higher order in the body as a whole. "Listening" and "speaking," functional and structural, receptive and active, allowing themselves to be grasped and actively grasping are all essential elements of each therapeutic intervention.

The capacity to allow oneself to be grasped, to allow something to happen, to permit and to forget the self is extremely important. It is so fundamental that it is the first requirement when starting to perform any technique. It is the prerequisite for the active part of therapy, which consists in "grasping" and carrying out the technique.

A distinguishing characteristic of the art of osteopathy is the continuous dialog between the osteopath's hand and the patient who is to be treated, the person and the tissue.

A predominantly "listening" technique such as balanced tension still involves an active element, and, similarly, a predominantly "speaking" technique such as HVLA (high velocity, low amplitude) or ART (articular technique) requires a degree of gentle listening and tuning in to the tissue.

Allowing oneself to be grasped: working receptively, the practitioner senses all the involuntary rhythmic and chaotic motions and changes in tension and density that appear in the tissue. To do so requires an inner receptive and neutral attitude on the part of the practitioner.

Grasping: actively, the practitioner leads the tissue out of the areas of tension, and strengthens, reduces, or modifies inherent tissue dynamics, confronts or does not confront various motion and tension barriers, etc. Attention is also directed at perceiving the reaction of the tissue to this approach. (Figure 20.2)

"Letting oneself be grasped" and actively "grasping": the practitioner synchronizes with rhythms in the tissue such as pulmonary breathing or or other involuntary rhythms while:

1 Gently supporting one phase, for example the inhalation phase, without causing any change in the amplitude of movement in this phase

2 Gently accompanying, (focusing attention on) chaotic, aberrant motions (i.e., additional dysfunctional movement) in a particular phase

3 Fractionally reinforcing the amplitude of chaotic, aberrant motions in a particular phase

4 Gently reinforcing the amplitude of a particular phase, etc.

The secret of successful treatment essentially lies in the ability to establish resonance between the hand of the osteopath and the different levels of tissue and inner experience of the patient.

Listening palpation

Much has already been written in the osteopathic literature about the very great variety of treatment approaches – the specific osteopathic activity – including the use of palpation to listen in the particular way required by that method; also about listening techniques used in diagnosis (such as that developed by Barral). This section seeks to deal in more detail with the significance of listening palpation, to probe further into its essence and explore its inherent characteristics and therapeutic effects.

Listening palpation is a way of making contact with the patient and tissue and establishing a link. It means learning a fundamentally open, accepting attitude and respect toward the patient as a complete being, both in general and in the palpation of the tissue in particular. Its essence is not that of resting with the tissues

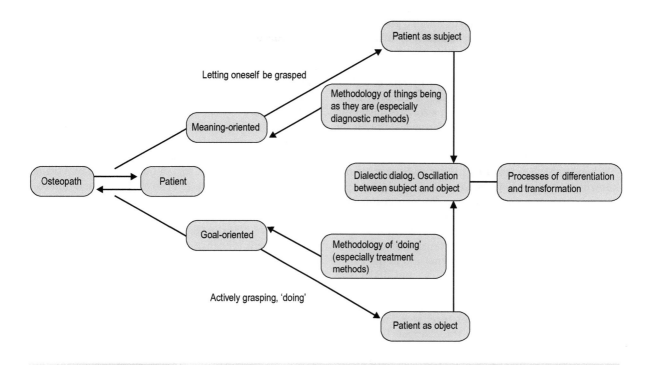

Figure 20.2

"Letting oneself be grasped" and actively "grasping" in the therapeutic interaction.

in a particular way, fixing or concentrating attention on them. The osteopath palpates with an attitude of attentiveness, to sense or perceive, but not change, strengthen, or diminish the dynamics of the tissue or force them in any given direction. We are generally taught to act upon nature, other people, and ourselves in a manipulative way, and this is what we are accustomed to doing. We are constantly seeking the ultimate magic bullet or trick, some simple technique that will solve all the patient's problems (and of course our own). However, this is not how healing and growth work.

Our fundamental attitude is the key to its simplicity: we let go of expectations and preconceptions as to how health in the patient will present itself. Instead, we make contact with the patient and tissues from a state of not knowing, and leave open the question as to where change will appear and what kind of change it will be.

We consciously restrain the conditioned urge that makes us want to change processes, tissue patterns, tissue tensions, movement restrictions, somatic dysfunctions, psychological patterns, and energy fields, etc. in the patient. (The urge to do so often springs from our technocratic scientific knowledge, our culture, our personality structure, and not infrequently from our osteopathic training.) This may well sound quite counter to osteopathic aims, as we ask ourselves what, then, is the purpose of the treatment? Can we really know what the tissue, or the patient, needs? Certainly we have some inkling; our past experience, the principles we have been taught, studies we have read or performed and the culture that surrounds us have all given us certain ideas and conditioned expectations as to how matters should be or how they should change. Yet, when we listen honestly and intently deep inside ourselves, we find that behind every answer lies a further question, and behind every cause that we label as primary there is a further cause: a context within a context. Listening honestly and intently, we reach the conclusion that we do not in fact know what the patient needs, and cannot really know how things should develop.

When we have reached this point of insight, of not knowing, then as osteopaths we can decide simply to permit the process to happen. We can decide this because we sense that something new can happen, beyond our own conditioned expectations, and because inwardly we sense and trust that change is the natural state of all living systems and of the entire cosmos. All life is in flux, a cyclical and dialectical process of change. Surely, this is what we find: that we come closest to the potential for change when we keep our personalities out of the picture, along with their incessant attempt to control the change? The extent of our ability to keep our own personalities out of the picture does of course depend on the osteopath's state of consciousness. It cannot be forced without becoming dogmatic, restrictive, and imposed; it needs to be gently encouraged.

The desire to change another person, or to be changed, is not the same thing as change; in fact, the opposite is the case: it hinders the natural flow of change. This is because the desire to do so bears the stamp of past conditioned ideas about what should change and how. It therefore tries to force through these ideas and to manipulate reality in line with them. The momentum contained in the desire to change tries to direct matters and so does not permit change to simply "be." Our therapeutic preconception of how things should be, what should be changed, and what that change must look like hinders our engagement in the here and now in the therapeutic interaction. In effect, the desire for change stands in the way of change, because we deny change: the inner process that is taking place in all life. We replace it with a conditioned idea of change, and it is this that we pursue. It escapes our attention; we remain, for the most part, quite unaware of how invasive and manipulative our intervention in natural processes is. We do not see the violence we are doing to the flow of change by our attempt to force it into the mold of our narrow horizons of experience, directing it instead of allowing ourselves to be drawn along by the flow of change to new horizons of experience. It is this act of direction that embodies the momentum not to permit change. It turns the therapeutic action into hindrance and resistance.

The situation then becomes one in which patients have not only their own, natural process of change, which they are resisting through their own concepts of change, but additional ideas of change being imposed by the practitioner. What sort of outcome will that bring? All that remains is a faint echo of the original inherent force of change, vitality, meaning, and freedom.

If we try to induce change in the tissue or in the patient, we place obstacles in the way of the natural development of change. Change will still happen, but as a reaction to our influence.

This influence achieves its greatest potency when operating in complete harmony with the developmental force inherent in the cosmos. Its greatest coherence (in consonance or together in concert) is found allowing what happens to unfold: the attitude of "Thy will be done."

The act of synchronization of the self, entering into this change, produces a revelation, a realization, of the highest form of freedom. This coherence or synchronization is again something that cannot be forced, and pretence is no use. This only emphasizes the disharmony. We can however try to feel our way into our patterns of consciousness, molded as they are by contraction of the self and the dualism of subject–object, seek to penetrate our feelings and emotions, thoughts and intuitions, our unstoppable urge to manipulate, our impatience, mistrust of self-regulation, our inadequacy – we can try to allow what is there to happen and respond with awareness to the act of "allowing to happen." It is above all through that attentive, patient act of feeling one's way to understanding, of sensing and awareness of this inexpressible performance that sympathy comes into being, at whatever time and place, at first perhaps almost imperceptibly, later perhaps clearly felt: a sympathy for our own selves. This sympathy has the capacity to expand to embrace others. This sympathy teamed with awareness is able to induce transformation. As long as we do not try to fight or shake off this further self-contraction of our awareness, a further development occurs: when we exercise pure perception and feel our way single-mindedly to understanding, then the perception and feeling itself becomes quite free of all self-contraction and conditioning, and becomes instead a fulcrum of the greatest freedom. It becomes ever stronger, as the fulcrum of an awareness that has always been and aware of itself as transforming, loving consciousness.

In the tissue, the development is similar: if we allow processes to take place and allow to happen, what will; if we avoid being invasive, avoid wanting to manipulate and change things, and instead use our hands and our entire attention to see, hear and feel in a loving and empathetic way, observing what is happening in the patient and the tissue at that moment, it enables the tissues and associated objective and subjective patterns of relationship to "clear" in their own time. We have to give the tissue space, along with all the structural, physiological patterns of relationships, and the subjective patterns of consciousness involved (as well as the cultural and biosocial patterns affecting both), to allow it to attune itself with the course of the tissue dynamics, to simply be, allowed to be present and to express its dissociations. Then comes what we might call clarity.

Our hands synchronize with the forces and patterns at work in the body and with the conditioning of the patient that tends to self-contraction. We do not hinder or reinforce them, or change them in any other way. So doing, we meet the inherent forces halfway, and achieve the clarity in the patterns of relationships in the tissue itself and in the related subjective elements (feeling and sensation, thinking and intuition) and understanding can come into being in the patient. Non-invasive empathy and synchronization dissolve resistance and allow change to unfold, change that is impossible to ignore.

The secret of such therapeutic change and change in ourselves lies in the selflessness of action, allowing what happens to come about, not obstructing it but "getting out of its way," as Becker explains.[6]

Listening palpation is intimately linked with stillness. In the state of stillness, palpation can develop without any preconceived idea. For Becker, stillness is essential not only to understand the teaching of Sutherland, but also as the factor that is in fact responsible for producing change in the patient,[7] since it is in stillness that the art of palpation without preconception is able to develop.

The above is not meant to be interpreted dogmatically. The situation may vary, both qualitatively and quantitatively, according to the individual case. If there is a splinter in the patient's foot, the obvious thing to do is to remove it, and similarly if the patient has a broken leg, it would be stupid and irresponsible to allow events to unfold instead of treating it. Osteopathy by its nature expects us to weigh carefully the balance of listening and doing. What distinguishes it from the more "technocratically" inclined methods of treatment is the greater weight given to listening in treatment, as against "doing" and the practicable. It is this that produces the greater emphasis on meaning, and gives the "doing" more of the quality of meaning and being, with respect for circulatory systems and self-organization.

Examples of this emphasis can be found, for instance, in the fact that even when performing HVLA techniques, the osteopath listens to the inherent tissue dynamics before delivering the directional thrust. This is not to say that we leave determination of the site where the thrust is delivered to its own devices; the treatment is quite specific and we are performing a manipulation to bring about change in a targeted way. Nevertheless, as we perform the manipulation, we listen; listening is an integral part. The more we listen, attune, and synchronize with the whole, the greater the meaning that the thrust at the joint has for the body and patient as a whole. Each osteopathic treatment method has its own particular kind of listening.

Listening palpation is also found at the point of balanced membranous/ligamentous tension. We establish a point of balance in the tissue as a voluntary act in which the osteopath decides where to work, and decides to create a point of balance. Once it has been established, however, we allow the tissue to carry out the correction.

This treatment principle is fundamental to most of the approaches presented in this book. In disengagement, for example, the tissue is given space, but no direction is imposed on the dynamics that occur within that space; nothing is forced; it is allowed. The osteopath listens to the processes unfolding in the patient.

The practitioner's receptive capacity to take in a state of stillness is essential, and the higher the level of consciousness in practitioners themselves, the greater the depth of this capacity. This is something that can be developed. The ability to experience a state of stillness cannot be forced, but is an expression of the practitioner's own particular development. Conditioned attitudes and views cannot be changed overnight by a deliberate act of will. They do nevertheless determine the extent and quality of the stillness the practitioner can access.

The use of listening palpation as a type of treatment technique represents only a small part of its potential. If we include the entire development of the practitioner's awareness, then its dimension is far greater. Different aspects, shades of differentiation and levels of development exist, and, as a type of technique, listening palpation has a direct effect on the patient at the physical, biological level. Consciously, to varying degrees depending on the practitioner's development of awareness and intention, this technique also has an effect on all the other levels within the patient that are involved.

In this sense, listening palpation is able to exert an effect on the emotional, mental, and spiritual levels and even in the non-dual realm, if the practitioner can consciously establish resonance with the patient from these levels and realms. The more comprehensive levels of listening palpation do not exclude previous approaches; rather, it integrates them, and they can still be used as necessary.

One final point to consider arises from the fact that, in osteopathy, the main means of approach to the patient is by palpation of anatomical structures. This brings certain advantages, but also limitations, because it so clearly and naturally directs the therapeutic focus toward the somatic element in the patient. This is not to deny the influence on the psychological and spiritual level through interactions of structure and function. However, the psychological and spiritual levels are primarily internal and subjective dimensions of experience and consciousness in the patient, so exclusively external, objective knowledge on the physiological and anatomical level is simply not adequate to treat them. The coherence between practitioner and patient on these levels is improved by recognizing the significance of a person's own development of consciousness in the context of treatment; coherence is also improved by integrating mental and psychological levels in the methods of diagnosis and treatment, putting these into practice and taking up contact in a suitable way. There is a correspondence between inner levels and external forms, and this provides a way to influence the inner levels. There is a danger, however, in attempting to influence the inner state and inner experience through the external alone, because it risks reducing the subjective to the objective level, and reducing the spiritual and psychological to the physical and biological level. A further danger is that of reading spiritual and psychological significance into the physical and biological level

when it is not there. It is not uncommon for indications of spiritual or mental levels of being to be read into the biological, when no such access between the two yet exists.

The fulcrum

A fulcrum is a kind of point of rest, a movable fixed point that enables a weight to be moved. The power inherent in it acts as an organizational factor to direct patterns of movement and patterns of organization. To give an example from nature, a fulcrum might be seen in the eye of a storm.

In the human body there are many fulcrums. The pivot points of the cranial sutures are one kind. (These are the particular point along the border of the articulating bones at which the inward-facing beveled edge meets the outward-facing bevel.) They act as fulcrums for the movement of the cranial bones.

The sternal end of the clavicle acts as a bony fulcrum for the function of the whole arm. There is also a bony fulcrum at the SBS (sphenobasilar synchondrosis), a membranous one at the straight sinus, and a nerve fulcrum at the lamina terminalis. Sutherland also detected a fulcrum in the fluctuations of the CSF.[8] There are also believed to be fluid fulcrums in the body, for all kinds of fluid functions. Sutherland and Becker also described spiritual fulcrums.[9,10]

Meditation, when practiced regularly, a particular religion, principle in life, or guiding principle such as "love your neighbor as yourself" are all examples of these. We are able to realize the potential power of the principle as we allow it to direct our lives. Just as regular meditation provides a point of rest and reflection, like a ship on the vast ocean of life, so a fulcrum can be a regular chance to take stock, to become empty and open, as Chila points out, both before and during treatment: open to the wholeness of the patient.

All the inherent motions, patterns of movement, tensions, and physiological processes taking place in the body are organized by fulcrums, as are dysfunctions and abnormal patterns of tension and movement.

A fulcrum acts as an organizing factor for movements, and possesses potency, rather like the eye of a hurricane.[11] A fulcrum can be seen as a concentration of potency. Cells and tissues organize themselves in relation to the potency and the fulcrums.

All natural fulcrums act as automatic shifting suspension fulcrums. This means that their position changes in synchrony with the respiratory cycles. Dysfunctional fulcrums, in contrast, the organizational factors within a dysfunction, present an obstacle to motion, a movement restriction, a place where energy or matter becomes denser and inertia increases.

The eye of the hurricane or point of rest bears within it the potency and the pattern of that storm. In the same way, there is a point of rest within the dysfunction, which embodies the potency of the dysfunction. The abnormal forces and tensions in a dysfunction are centered here, in this potency in the fulcrums. It acts as a kind of additional fixed point or point of orientation in the body, around which it is organized.

This "eye" of the dysfunction, or region of rest in the patterns of tension in the tissue, is the place that represents the specific potency of that dysfunction; we can see it as the spirit of the dysfunction, the energy, the movement manifesting itself, which maintain the pattern of tension. Every change that happens at this place produces a change in the pattern of tension and affects its structural and functional relations. The osteopath can learn to palpate and identify locations.

The fulcrum: the "automatic shifting suspension fulcrum"

This concept, also termed the "suspended automatically shifting fulcrum," refers to a point of rest, or point of orientation, which is suspended in such a way that it can move or "shift" automatically.

The eye of a storm or hurricane is a striking natural example of this, and gives an indication of the potential power of a fulcrum. Becker describes it as the point of rest and potential source of power for the whirlwind's strength. It is at the same time a suspended automatically shifting fulcrum as it moves across land and sea. The axle of a wheel is another example, with the fulcrum as the point of rest around which the wheel turns. At the same time it is a suspended automatically shifting fulcrum in that it moves along, together with the bicycle, while still retaining its function as a point of rest for the movement of the wheel.

All natural fulcrums in the body act as automatically shifting suspension fulcrums, which enables then to act dynamically in response to external and internal events and continuous rhythmic impulses.[12]

They are responsible for organizing the equalization of reciprocal tension in the body. Sutherland chose this expression to describe a functional region on the course of the straight sinus, at the union of the falx cerebri, falx cerebelli, and tentorium cerebelli, also known as the Sutherland fulcrum. It represents a movable point of rest for the reciprocal tension membrane in the cranium and spinal canal. The membranes need to operate out from a fulcrum or point of rest in order to maintain an equal balance of membrane motion and tension in all directions. This point of rest needs to be suspended if it is to be able to move or shift automatically. This shifting ensures the equal distribution of tension in the dural membranes when subjected to pressure or tension.

Sutherland wrote that the change in position of the automatic shifting suspension fulcrum could be palpated at the beginning of respiration. This occurs along with a sense of warmth, brought about by the circulation of the cerebrospinal fluid.[12,13]

The fulcrum: dysfunctional fulcrums

This is the name given to fulcrums that operate as an organizing factor for dysfunctions, i.e., for abnormal tissue tensions and movement restrictions. In contrast to natural fulcrums, these can react to only a limited degree, if at all, to rhythms such as pulmonary breathing or the Breath of Life, or to physiological demands in response to internal and external stimuli, or shift, or move.

Rather, they can be viewed as disturbance factors that make demands on the body for special compensation and react to the natural fulcrums, so that the best achievable balance of tension can be maintained. As a result, these dysfunctional fulcrums do not only exert a local effect but also affect the entire body, depending on the degree of the disturbance. There are various models that help explain the effects of the fulcrums; such as the tensegrity model, electromagnetic fields, biophoton fields, the fluid crystal properties of organisms, and morphogenetic fields as proposed by Sheldrake. Other, neurophysiological and endocrine effects may also be at work.

The dysfunctional fulcrums result in acquired states associated with resistance to or restriction of movement, or restrictions in the tissue and fluids, which involve particular patterns of movement and tension, changes in elasticity, local intensification of energy or matter, or increases in inertia; these vary in quality and extent from one individual to another.

These effects can be seen as representing the history of the individual as it is imprinted on the tissue. They are the result of events whose intensity or duration was too great to be completely resolved by the homeostatic forces alone. These include such causes as physical trauma or birth trauma, illness or psychological trauma. Becker calls these forces "biokinetic energy." According to Becker, biokinetic and biodynamic forces are at work at the heart of every dysfunction. The biokinetic forces are centered by the "potency." This describes a homeostatic process that endeavors to resolve the biokinetic forces, either to release them to the environment or, if this does not succeed, to compensate as well as possible.

The practitioner will try, by means of palpation, to "listen" to the interaction between the activity of the immediate life forces/homeostatic forces and the conditioned clustering, restriction, and fixation of these forces brought about by the circumstances or habits of a person's life, physical or psychological trauma, or diseases that the person has suffered, etc. (biokinetic energy). A certain pattern emerges at the moment when what is suffered so impairs the system that the body cannot remember how to heal itself.[15]

The center of the dysfunction

The center of a dysfunction is, according to Becker,[16] rather like the center or eye of a hurricane. This center contains within it the potency and force of the dysfunction. Becker describes it as a kind of energy field, which can be detected by consciously performed palpation.

Note, during the course of treatment, it may become necessary to direct part of your attention to the center of the dysfunction. This should not detract from the first essential that the treatment needs to be deeply rooted in the health of the patient; that is, the resources available to the patient. Even while synchronizing with centers of the dysfunction, constant contact must be maintained with these resources.

Palpation of the fulcrum

The osteopath can learn to palpate and localize the fulcrums, both in health and in a dysfunction. Place your hand on the patient's body. Your elbow should be placed on the treatment table to provide a further fulcrum. Allow the dysfunction to lead your hand to the point of rest of the dysfunction. With relaxed attentiveness, you should now sense where in the dysfunction this point of rest is located. This is the indirect technique, and therefore serves at the same time both as a

means of diagnosis and of therapy. When your hand finds the position in the tissue where the tensions of the joints or tissues involved in the dysfunction are restored to a state of balance (the fulcrum), that is the moment when the change to normal physiology can take place. This is not an act of "doing" on the part of the practitioner; rather, it is the inherent potency, the power of the patient that performs the work.

The stages of treatment

Some important tissue fulcrums have been described, and since these exercise a certain organizing function, they receive special attention in diagnosis and treatment. In the cranial field, a bony fulcrum has been described at the SBS, a membranous fulcrum at the straight sinus, and a nerve fulcrum at the lamina terminalis. Sutherland also identified a fulcrum in the fluctuations of the CSF.[17] A therapeutic approach goes far beyond these observations, however. There is considerable variation in important fulcrums, in development, and in treatment, and this must be taken into account. There are fulcrums for every organ, every tissue, and every moment in its development. In this respect, to establish contact with the correct fulcrum in the patient is to arrive at treatment that is significant for the patient.

Three stages of treatment

- The first step in treatment is to make contact with the inherent stillness in the patient, and with the homeodynamic forces in the body of the patient as a whole.

- Secondly, find the abnormal tension patterns and more subtle patterns of energy, and the fulcrums around which they organize themselves, or are organized. This will involve exploring the relationships between the tissue tensions and the dynamics and interactions of objective and subjective factors in the patient's inner world (physical, emotional, mental, and spiritual levels of consciousness) and external world (sociocultural surroundings, environmental influences, etc.).

- Thirdly, establish a kind of therapeutic fulcrum, around which the motion/energy can organize itself so as to bring about a higher-order integration as the abnormal patterns of tension and energy are resolved.

What happens, in effect, is that the abnormal tension and energy pattern is exactly copied and a new, therapeutic state of balance established, one that copies the suspended automatic shifting fulcrum of a healthy system. The newly established fulcrum enables the inherent homeodynamic forces to change the abnormal tension/energy state, transforming it into a higher-order state of balance (i.e., greater freedom). This sets free the forces that had been bound by the abnormal tension/energy patterns, and they are now able to integrate into the physiological activity of the body as a whole.

Creation of an adequate therapeutic fulcrum calls for an understanding of the patient from the point of view of the evolutionary or "involutionary" dynamics of the person; this understanding is the only basis to achieve it. The new fulcrum is therefore more than an expression of the local release of underlying tensions. It is at the same time related to all the forces that are at work in the body of the patient as a whole to maintain local and global homeodynamic processes.

The establishment of a new fulcrum is most certainly not a return to a former "ideal" state of balance that existed in the past. A kind of manual regression therapy may well be helpful and even necessary, to integrate old, past abnormal conditioning. The issue here is not to bring back past ontogenetic stages of development, along with their quite specific patterns of health or personality, and establish those. What we try to do is rather to resolve or integrate misdirected conditioning that stands in the way of further development in the present. The aim is to support the homeodynamic forces that are at work in this process, from an understanding of the person's individual process of growth. This goes far beyond a materialistic view of health that simply seeks to resolve symptoms, and beyond a romantic view that looks to the embryo in an almost magical doctrine of restored health.

A "point of balance" in the fluids or reciprocal tension in the potency (reciprocal tension potency; RTP) can be established using a similar method to the one described later in this chapter to establish a fulcrum or "point of balanced membranous tension."

Another possible approach is to encourage a still point in the fluctuations of the CSF, so establishing a point of rest/fulcrum to set healing processes in motion and provide the body with an opportunity for reorientation. At the moment when the still point occurs, a point of rest emerges that enables the body to establish a new

relationship with its own wholeness; a point at which transformation can take place.

Sutherland also spoke of being able to sense the fulcrum or still point in the fluctuations of the CSF and the reciprocal tension membrane, and of maintaining the fluctuation of the CSF at the "balance point."[17]

Sutherland not only describes the potency in the CSF as fundamental to the functioning of the primary respiratory mechanism (PRM);[18] he also says that the potency in the fluctuation of the CSF can be used in diagnosis and treatment.[19] The CSF is even said by Sutherland/Magoun to have an intelligence of its own.[20]

It is even thought that the fulcrums of development relating to developmental dynamics (the axes of the developmental dynamic growth processes) can be sensed in the tissues of the patient, and that it is possible in this way to forge a link for the patient with the homeodynamic potential at work in these processes. To an extent, the tissue is the expression of its past developmental dynamics. However, the experiences that have overtaxed the homeodynamic forces in the tissue, in particular, condition the tissue dynamics in a manner that can restrict a person's overall potential. Some osteopaths in fact believe that it is possible to sense, at the cranial base and the diaphragm, the result of the forces that led to the development of the septum transversum (which later developed in the downward direction to form the central tendon), as well as minor functional deviations of this developmental process. In the ideal state, the developmental dynamic motion of the structures ought to occur in a balanced state of tension, and deviations from this can be palpated in the case of disturbances.

Synchronization with these embryonic forces is thought to support the present homeodynamic forces and the correction of minute functional deviations. Osteopaths can also use the assessment of these inherent motions of the tissue as a guide when deciding when to end a technique, since this can be done when balanced physiological "developmental dynamic" movement can once again be sensed in the tissue. The osteopath can also sense the points of rest/fulcrums of the wholeness in the patient, or the potential for wholeness, independently of space and time. By doing so the osteopath can communicate an immediate experience of the wholeness of body, mind, and spirit to the body and person as a whole. This is a sensation that may have been obscured by stress and disease, though the fulcrum or orientation it provides for the patient, tissue, and function of that tissue makes it enormously important for the ongoing healing process. The experience of wholeness can be a very special experience and a relief, especially for those who are seriously ill, and it is unaffected by the extent of illness suffered by the person's body in the present.

Note, the ideas presented above are hypothetical in nature and refer to highly subjective perceptions of the tissue dynamics.

Focus of attention

Osteopaths' ability to direct their attention and intention consciously during the course of the therapeutic interaction is a decisive factor in the healing process taking place in the patient. They should begin by directing attention inward, centering the self. This process can be assisted by orientation in relation to a particular fulcrum (e.g., the solar plexus, the region of the heart, the third ventricle, emptiness, a mantra, inner images, etc.).

The therapeutic focus can be on wider relationships and forces of order, or on the life forces present in the depths of a dysfunction. In both cases, our attention is centered in the homeodynamic forces at work, and as we do so the relative status of the dysfunctional patterns becomes evident. Our aim is to see the whole. The fact that the practitioner is making contact with the health and the homeodynamic forces in the patient gives special significance to the therapeutic contact.

It is helpful if the first touch is made with unfocused attention, as far as possible with a deliberate lack of focus. This keeps our perception open to as much as possible of all that is to be learnt from the body. In the second step, it may then become necessary to focus our attention on particular regions and then, finally, specific locations.

The best way to describe the process of gentle palpation with relaxed attention is to say that, instead of our hands invading the structure we are treating, we allow the tissue to come into our hands. This way of proceeding could be called "local focusing." Practitioners learn to focus their palpatory attention very precisely on the structure to be treated and the tissue qualities of the structure, without in any way becoming invasive.

Practitioners also learn to become aware of the regional surroundings of the structure to be treated, the dynamic balance of tension of the whole body and the field around the body, as well as allowing their attention to rest in the wide expanse of nature. This is done by allowing attention to relax and expand to the horizon, out into the wide expanse, as we do when we let our relaxed, unfocused gaze reach out into the far distance. It eventually becomes possible to arrive at a perception beyond the horizon.

With a little practice, practitioners can develop their ability to focus beyond conscious focus to conscious choice of the degree and quality of focus. They become increasingly able to allow their attention either to rest simultaneously on the regional surroundings of the structure to be treated, the entire body, the field around the body, the broad expanse of nature and beyond, or to oscillate continually between them, and to do so while carrying out techniques involving precisely directed local focus. This oscillating manner of focusing the attention is like the continual oscillation that happens in the accommodation of the eye, in which there is constant adjustment between focusing and defocusing.

Training in palpatory perception is the most fundamental requirement for the successful application of all the techniques below. The more conscious the perception during palpation, the greater the resonance that develops between the practitioner's hand and the tissue. The more the humanity of the patient finds an echo in us, and the more direct our acceptance of this field of experience, the more we find emerging a reciprocal field of contact that carries within it the potency of healing touch.

Shifting of attention

In the course of synchronizing with the homeodynamic forces of the body and being of the patient as a whole, it may happen, at a particular moment in the treatment, that the practitioner's consciousness changes or shifts. It is also an indication that a clearer perception of the wholeness of the patient is entering into the palpation.

The importance of stillness in treatment

Stillness, according to Becker, is the key to understanding Sutherland's teachings. According to Becker, the ability to perceive stillness as a conscious act is essential to treatment, and is indeed the true factor that brings about change during treatment.[21] He says that stillness is the source of all energy and centers the whole body and every molecule of which it is made up. Physiology is the external expression of this stillness. There is a

Box 20.1

Focus of attention

Local, on the structure to be treated

Regional, on the area surrounding the structure to be treated

Global, on the entire body

On the field surrounding the body

On the horizon, expanding out into the distance

Beyond the horizon/beyond space and time

balanced rhythmic and dynamic process of exchange taking place between the physiology and the stillness, that is, between health and the stillness: a process that relates to the entire system. In health, this exchange flows freely. However, even disease and dysfunctional patterns are organized by stillness.[22] Energy flows out of the stillness into the physiology of the body, and from the physiology of the body into the stillness, like the movement of the tides. Becker states that it is possible to sense the interchange taking place in both directions in every healthy tissue. Even in sickness or dysfunction, it is possible to sense the interchange of the stillness with the pathogenic forces in the tissue.[23]

Method

1 First, direct your attention to the unity of the stillness in the body as a whole. The stillness itself cannot be palpated with your hands; what can be done is to cultivate an awareness for the stillness in the patient and for the interchange between the stillness and the physiology of the body.[24]

2 In healthy tissue, it is possible to sense the free interchange with stillness. This palpation involves sensing the way that stillness represents, to a degree, the ultimate foundation and fulcrum for the physiology in the tissue, and how the potency of this stillness finds expression in the dynamics of the tissue.

3 As soon as you become aware of the stillness that organizes the dysfunction patterns, your hands begin to palpate a change in the dysfunction pattern.[24]

4 Palpation enables you to sense the changes in the tissue, whose motive power again lies in the stillness. It is possible to sense interactions between the homeodynamic forces and the problem (or the dysfunction) in the patient. These interactions are aimed at resolving the biokinetic forces, or releasing them to the outside world.[25] It is the specific way in which the body physiology is organized, in interaction with the stillness and stimulated by the stillness, that brings about a change in a dysfunction pattern.[26]

Note, a still point can represent a means of access that enables you to make contact with the stillness.

Intentional approach according to McKone

See also Chapter 18.

This approach is based, not on the principle of cause and effect, but on the paradigm that the whole is reflected in its parts. Therefore it is not a polyreductional approach, but an organic one. The fulcrum of the treatment is in the realm of the mind, because the aspect of the patient that we are approaching is to do with thought. Intention is an essential element of the procedure. This is a qualitative method, whose basis is experience. This kind of technique is a formless idea.

If we focus only on a tissue, this yields an approach more in line with Newtonian or Cartesian thought. If we look at the patient as a whole, it is uninterrupted and the outcome is continuous transformation.

Seen from the viewpoint of Goethean thought, the relationship between practitioner and patient can be described as a reciprocal one, constantly in motion, between the two participants.

The same morphology is reflected in both embryo and adult. Specializing in embryology risks placing these connections out of context. The context of morphology can be maintained, seeing the adult as a grown-up embryo and the embryo as a not-yet-grown adult. There is a polarity between the surrounding material and the content, so that, for example, the brain is soft and vulnerable, but surrounded by hard bone.

The most important region in mammals is, in Goethean terms, the middle one, because it mediates between the upper and lower regions and has to perform an integrating function. Similarly, according to McConnell the middle region is of particular importance as the connection between the celestial and the terrestrial, and is an important fulcrum in sickness and health. McConnell states that lesions of the ribs are particularly liable to impair the autonomic vasomotor system, through their effects on the ganglia of the sympathetic trunk; a disturbance in this region has a particularly significant weakening effect on homeostasis. A disturbance here also tends to impair function in the head and abdominal regions.

In line with the approach indicated by the threefold concept we would seek, for example, to build up the relationship between the three spheres: head, thorax, and abdomen. We need to keep this system at the back of our minds while palpating (see Table 20.1).

Preparation

- Palpate and examine the patient's skin, muscles, ligaments/membranes, joints, bones, and fluids. Release your hands again once you have managed to differentiate these.

- Palpate the region, immediately releasing your hands as soon as you receive the first sensation or perceive the first impression.

- Think about your own feet (i.e., free yourself from preconceived expectations). As soon as you start to perceive the first impression, release your hands again. This kind of palpation keeps the practitioner's mind under control, preventing it from making leaps or penetrating by thought into the patient, and causing it to let go of conditioned, preconceived expectations based on previous palpatory experience. Expectation hinders you from making contact with what your hands are in fact touching.

Treatment

After some practice you will be able to omit the preparation stage (i.e., step 1 in the following list) and begin straight away with steps 2 and 3. These can be combined with any other treatment approach: for example, with balanced tension, exaggeration, disengagement, compression, etc.

1 Think of the patient in an upward direction: palpate the region again with motionless hands, thinking upward from the patient's feet, i.e., from there toward yourself and into your hands, so that the patient is expanding and becoming larger, extending outward into openness. Keep in your mind the concept of the patient as a whole entity. At the same time, perform an appropriate therapeutic interaction, for example, balanced tension.

2 Think of the patient in an upward direction, toward yourself; in addition, think jointly of the patient and yourself, in an upward direction: As in step 1, you think upward, expanding, from the patient's feet toward yourself; at the same time you should also think of yourself and the patient in a shared upward movement, a common expansion.

Note, you need to learn to regulate the balance between drawing upward toward you and maintaining the distance between you and the patient. At the same time, perform an appropriate therapeutic interaction, for example, balanced tension.

a Change in temperature/perfusion: your intention affects temperature and perfusion in response to changes in warmth and circulation in your own hand.

b Increase in temperature: think outward (i.e., think of something pleasant, perhaps a pleasant experience or event), expansively, thinking of outward movement, enlargement, and space. The region you are touching becomes warmer.

c Reduction in temperature: if there is inflammation, think inward, into the structure or downward, in order to reduce the temperature and the perfusion of the affected part of the body.

Note, you should not maintain this for more than one minute, as it is extremely exhausting.

Intention, breathing, technique

The conscious linking and integration of intention, breathing, and movement/palpation increases the potency of the therapeutic interaction, increases resonance and entrainment, improves the establishment of vectors of force and energy, reduces negative reactions to treatment, and reduces the risk of exhaustion or depleting the reserves of the practitioner.

Closed (completely surrounded by bone)	Ectoderm/emphasized in the "ectomorph" C	Cranial sphere	Vibration
Half open (partly surrounded by bone)	Mesoderm/emphasized in the "mesomorph" C	Thoracic sphere	Rhythm
Open (surrounded by bone to a minor extent only)	Endoderm/emphasized in the "endomorph" C	Abdominal sphere	Motion

TABLE 20.1: The threefold concept, after Goethe

C, constitutional type.

- Intention: the intention of the practitioner is a very important factor in every therapeutic approach, and can permeate to all levels. Practitioners should have a sure consciousness of their intention whenever they take up contact or perform palpation, whatever the type. Intention occupies first place: practitioners must make the conscious decision to take the initiatory in-breath, and to perform a particular therapeutic interaction/technique/taking up of contact with the tissue.

- Breathing: the practitioner's breathing sets in train the therapeutic intention. Conscious breathing on the part of the practitioner precedes and accompanies the taking up of contact with the tissue.

- Performance of the movement/tissue contact and tissue interaction: the final step is the movement performed by the practitioner or the establishment of the therapeutic fulcrum and breathing. For example, when establishing balanced tension in the spinal column, hand contact is made on the in-breath. On the out-breath the practitioner follows the inherent tissue dynamics; then, with the next in-breath a point of balance (for example) is established. The practitioner's breathing (and indeed that of the patient) can be used to intensify the therapeutic tissue dynamics (see pp. 356 and 371).

Special treatment principles in palpation

It is the underlying basic principles of osteopathy that provide the link between the great variety of methods of osteopathic treatment. For example there are techniques to stimulate the flow of body fluids. There are other methods whose aim is to resolve hindrances to the free flow of body fluids. Yet others are based on reflex mechanisms.

The treatment principles presented below are by no means an exhaustive list. It is not the aim of this book to provide a comprehensive account of all osteopathic treatment methods. This should not be thought to imply that other osteopathic approaches can not be used just as effectively or indeed more so, in the context of integral osteopathic treatment. Any of the methods described in the following text can also be adapted or modified, or parts of them incorporated into other osteopathic methods.

Note, every therapeutic intervention described, in this and subsequent chapters, should be understood as part of a dialog with the tissue/energy, and represents a kind of invitation to the tissue. The decision as to whether to accept the invitation is made by the tissue itself and the body of the person as a whole. It is therapeutically highly important for the practitioner to respect that decision. The uncontrolled, imposed application of force is not the way to approach treatment; it is the consciously conducted dialog with the tissue that opens up access to an understanding of the organizing forces and activates the body's healing potential.

Letting oneself be grasped and actively grasping, listening palpation, fulcrum palpation, focus of attention, stillness, and intention according to McKone can be applied and integrated into all the following treatment principles.

In order to achieve the necessary quality of meaningful palpatory contact and a therapeutic fulcrum it is

Box 20.2

Treatment principles

- General: can be integrated into all approaches to a greater or lesser degree: letting oneself be grasped and grasping; listening palpation, fulcrum palpation, focus of attention; stillness; intention according to McKone; intention/breathing/movement

- Balancing the autonomic nervous system

- Synchronization with the patient's space

- Treatment of developmental dynamic tension patterns

- Sensing the vitality in the patient

- Treatment through rhythmic impulses

Balanced tension

- Point of balanced membranous/ligamentous/(fascial) tension (PBMT/PBLT)

- Establishment of a local, regional, and global point of balanced tension (PBT):

Possible assistance of balanced tension by the following methods

- Exaggeration

- Direct technique

- Disengagement

- Compression/decompression

- Opposite physiological movement

- Molding

- Recoil techniques

- Multiple-hand technique

Assistance of self healing through the following

- Fluid impulses

- Breathing

- Myofascial system

- Sensorimotor integration

essential to know the biomechanical relations, vectors of developmental dynamics, and morphogenetic fields of the tissues and to be able to build up meaningful touch that can access these and the wholeness of the patient, which will include the person's subjective experience.

Balancing the autonomic nervous system

A balanced autonomic nervous system reduces the stresses of adjustments brought about by everyday life. It starts and supports the process of shifting into a more coherent state. The reciprocal tensions in the body, and the aspects of body, mind, and spirit work in a more consistent connection.

Healing and transformation of dysfunctional patterns becomes easier and accessible in the best possible way. Negative consequences are reduced to a minimum and the endpoint of a treatment is felt more easily. Patients are better able to sense changes in their bodies and minds.

Many approaches are possible, e.g. supporting an empathic relationship with the patient, stabilisation exercises, butterfly hug (see Chapter 37), 'patient's neutral' according to J. Jealous (see also T. Liem, Cranial Osteopathy: A Practical Textbook. Eastland Press; 2009) 'the Osteopathic Felt Sense' or Osteopathic Heart-Focused Breathing.

In the 'Osteopathic Felt Sense', the osteopath palpates regions of greatest rhythmic flow and vitality in the patient (see also p. 358). These can also be regions which the patient recognizes as being strong and flowing. At the same time, the patient focuses on visual, auditory, kinesthetic, olfactory, and gustatory sensations related to the palpated regions. The osteopath observes whether the sensations strengthen the well being of the patient, and recalibrates the awareness of the senses with palpated regions of strengh and flow.

Osteopathic Heart-Focused Breathing

This is an adapted exercise based on the Heartmath Program (http://www.heartmath.com/), aiming to increase cardiac coherence, which can take between two to five minutes.The osteopath palpates the field around the heart and slowly, by lowering the resistance, the hands approach the tissue level and palpate the heart region, following the tissue dynamics.

At the same time, patients softly direct their attention into the heart region in the center of the chest whilst

> **Box 20.3**
> Zones, according to Jealous (modified)
>
> From the midline to the local and global soma
>
> From the midline to the field around the body
>
> From the midline to the horizon, expanding far outward
>
> From the midline to beyond the horizon/ beyond space and time

breathing in and out, imagining a red balloon in that area while breathing. A slower and deeper breathing than usual will arise. The breathing could be - if necessary - consciously regulated at a 10-second rhythm, 5 seconds breathing in and 5 seconds breathing out.

Synchronization with the patient's space

1 Synchronize with the particular zones, and sense the function and qualities in the zone in question (Box 20.3).

2 Examine to find the zone in which the presence of the patient is most clearly evident:
   a In which zones is the expression of health most evident?
   b In which zone is the identity of the patient most strongly centered? Or in which is the focus of consciousness of the patient?

3 Synchronize with that zone, so as to strengthen its presence.

The treatment of developmental dynamic tension patterns

From the morphogenetic point of view, the development of position influences that of form, and that in turn influences the development of structure. Metabolic movements, organized in metabolic fields or fields of tension, are the components of these processes. These always take place against resistance from their environment (see Chapter 7).

Mechanical stresses play a major regulatory role in many cellular and morphogenetic processes. Examples of this are: the generation of pressure in cavities and vacuoles, contractile activity by cells, and directional forces brought about by the active elongation of microtubules (also, to a lesser degree, by microfilaments). Mechanical stress is also believed to be one of the components in the signaling pathways that keep cells from apoptosis.

Developmental dynamics are founded on precise inductive interactions of tissues and self-regulatory elements, e.g., between patterns that produce active mechanical stress and passive stress such as stretching or compression. Mechanical stimuli affect cells by producing chemokinetic activation or inhibition of production, cleavage, and diffusion. The model of hyperrestoration developed by Beloussev and Mittenthal describes an active mechanical response to mechanical stress, which, aimed at restoring initial stress values, regularly overshoots in the opposite direction. As a result, stretching leads to active compression stress, and compression to active, directional stretching.

Resistance, fields of compression and stretch, i.e., compression and tensile stress (as well as shear stress) are important components in the formation of tissue. Residual tensile and compression stress can thus be found in many tissues.

From the descriptive point of view, Blechschmidt has described models of mechanical stresses in the developmental dynamics of human embryos, where specific compression forces are at work, for example, in corrosion, densation, contusion, and distusion fields. Specific tensile forces operate for example in the suction or dilatation fields, and shear forces in detraction fields (e.g., in regions of formation of bones of the cranial vault).

Physiological loci of compression that appear during development and growth act as points of balance for the body. Not to be confused with compression dysfunctions caused by pathological excessive force, these are part of the expression of homeostatic mechanical organization, with the capacity to absorb misdirected energy and serve as sites for the exchange of energy between different tissues. Osteopaths therefore take especial account of these sites of compression in diagnosis and treatment, and ensure that they are able to fulfill their homeostatic function.

Compression and tensile fields are important components in the treatment of dysfunctional developmental dynamic tension patterns. Gentle compression (or stretching, e.g., in the form of disengagement) of patterns of relationship, either of tissues or of developmental dynamics, makes the force vectors more clearly evident. However, the main purpose of their use is synchronization with physiological mechanical stresses related to developmental dynamics, and with dysfunctional tension patterns in the patient, with the intention of supporting the release process to resolve dysfunctional force vectors and patterns of relationship.

It should be noted that many of the following treatment models are simply attempts to take account of certain tissue–energy–consciousness complexes. Many other methods are possible, and may be as appropriate, indeed even more suitable, for the support of healing in the patient.

- The most important aspect of this treatment principle is the synchronization with morphological developmental dynamics; also the ability of the osteopath to achieve resonance and understanding of the accompanying inner aspects of consciousness in the patient (see Chapter 18).

- The osteopath performs a gentle, differentiated form of compression (or traction) on the dysfunctional developmental dynamic pattern. Example: when treating cervical structures, creation of a compression field by gently pressing in a caudal direction from the head and in a cranial direction from the heart.

- It is essential to apply the compression or traction components of treatment in a differentiated way that depends on the particular tissue to be treated.

- While applying the gentle compression or traction field, the practitioner should register all the dynamics in the tissue, without intervening in them.

- The formation of a fulcrum will be sensed within the compression (or traction) field.

- The practitioner should maintain the gentle compression (or traction), following the process of release that comes about in the compression (or traction) field. This emerges in the form of a spontaneous disengagement (or greater closeness) between the tissues concerned.

- It is important to do no more than maintain the gentle compression (traction) field, simply following the disengagement or greater closeness. The practitioner must avoid influencing the direction of the developmental dynamic tension patterns, or exerting any influence at all on these.

- During the palpation of a tissue, the osteopath should allow whatever elements may appear of psychological, mental, and spiritual significance, that might be associated with that region, to emerge and evolve (see p. 371 and Chapter 37). By avoiding the invasive imposition of a change of pattern on the tissue dynamics, and instead pursuing dialog that gently supports release, the osteopath provides space. This space enables all these significant elements to reveal themselves in the course of the release process and become integrated.

- Balanced tension is established.

- It may sometimes also be possible to induce the release of tension without creating a compression (traction) field, by simple synchronization with the inherent tissue dynamics.

The establishment of balanced tension is described in detail on p. 360 ff.

Developmental dynamic treatment can be assisted by focus on the vitality in the patient, and by fluid impulses, pulmonary breathing, sensorimotor or myofascial systems, or emotional, mental, and spiritual integration (see below).

Sensing the vitality in the patient

The vitality, the energy or life force that distinguishes the inert from the living, and the non-biological domain of the physiosphere from the biosphere, is fundamentally significant for the treatment of living organisms. Different ages and cultures have given it different names, such as chi, ki, orgone, etheric energy, mana, etc.

In the system of yoga, vital energy is called prana. It is renewed as we breathe, but is more than simply breathing; the meaning of the word prana is far greater than that. All the forces of the body and all the functions of the senses are an expression of the force of prana. At the same time, it corresponds to the quantum potential of fundamental physics. At the beginning of creation, matter is believed to have appeared in the world as a kind of crystallization and condensation of prana.

Control of the breath can exert a specific and deliberate effect on vital energy (pranayama: prana = vital energy; yama = control). Breathing begins immediately after birth with a baby's first breath, marking the end of life in the womb. A person's breathing is a direct reflection, not only of their physical state, but also of their spiritual and emotional state, and it integrates them in a functional unit. It does far more than to provide the body with oxygen; in Indian yoga it is through breathing that prana or the life force enters. It is the activity of breathing that marks the point where the constant, inner realm of the body meets the circumstances of the constantly changing external world.

A possible way of making contact with the biofield and intensifying the vital force is to direct the focus onto breathing.

Attunement by the practitioner

All the following techniques need to be learned slowly and gradually, ideally working with a teacher. They should be stopped immediately if starting to feel unwell or if any dizziness is experienced.

Caution, before using any of the techniques, with the exception of 1–3, it is important to be taught them in person by a competent teacher. These breathing techniques are practiced at your own risk and should not be performed without approval of your medical doctor. No advanced breathing techniques are presented here, since these would be dangerous (above all for the practitioner, but also potentially for the patient) without sustained previous practice and purification of the body.

It is helpful in all the techniques to adopt an upright, relaxed posture, since this encourages natural, unforced alertness and attention on the part of the practitioner.

1 Awareness of inhalation and exhalation: on inhalation, the osteopath silently says the words "breathe in" and on exhalation, "breathe out." The osteopath can then begin breathing techniques specifically aimed at intensifying the life force.

2 Combined abdominal and chest breathing: the osteopath should perform three complete breaths. Inhalation should begin with the abdomen, next drawing the breath into the sides and chest, and finally up to the clavicles. During exhalation, first the clavicles fall, then the chest and sides, and finally the abdomen. The practitioner should begin by observing a 4:4 rhythm of breathing; that is, breathing in on a count of four, and

out again on a count of four. With practice, this can be extended to an 8:8 breathing rhythm. On inhalation, the practitioner should sense the energy rising from the feet and legs, then medially through the trunk to the top of the head. On exhalation the practitioner senses the energy flowing into arms and hands.

3   1:4 Rhythm: the further raising of intensity of the practitioner's own bioenergy (or prana) can now begin: the practitioner does this by selecting a 1:4 rhythm, inhaling on a count of one and counting up to four during exhalation. Once again (as described for the previous breathing technique), the prana can be directed into the practitioner's own hands.

4   Chest breathing with guttural sound: this type of breathing is performed together with gentle tensing of the pelvic, diaphragm, and throat bandhas, and intensifies the vital force. In yoga, it is also called ujjai breathing. It involves deep, regular breathing, in and out, through the nose into the chest, observing a 4:4 rhythm or slower rhythm. It is important to hold the bandhas that retain energy at the pelvic floor (by gently raising the perineum), diaphragm (drawing in the abdomen and pressing the diaphragm upward), and throat (inclining the chin down toward the breastbone). Each breath produces a guttural sound like the distant sound of the sea. This sound is caused by narrowing of the epiglottis that enables control of the flow of breath.

5   Breath of fire (similar to the yoga technique of kapalabhathi): this involves fast breathing using the abdomen and diaphragm. In this technique, exhalation is focused, and inhalation takes place gently and naturally, of itself, lasting a little longer than exhalation. Exhalation is performed quickly and strongly, by drawing the abdominal muscles sharply backward to force the air out of the lungs. As soon as this happens, the abdominal muscles relax again, the diaphragm is lowered and air flows into the lungs. Breaths are taken in quick succession. To begin with, while learning the technique, up to 15 breaths are taken in each phase (beginning at first with around 3 phases per patient). This can be increased each week by about 10 breaths per phase. Once again (as described above), the prana can be directed into the practitioner's own hands. This breathing technique provides very strong stimulation of energy.

6   Bellows breathing: this provides the strongest possible build-up of prana or vital energy. Unlike the breath of fire technique, it makes full use of the entire respiratory system, and not simply of the diaphragm. Inhalation and exhalation are of the same length. Do this short and powerful breathing around 20 - 30 times. It is best to breathe through the nose, but for this form of breathing (exceptionally) it is possible to breathe through the mouth. Exhale completely and then take a deep last breath to your maximum but without forcing the body, and hold your breath as long as you can. Then take a full breath and hold it for 5 - 20 seconds. At the same time, bend your chin towards the sternum and place your tongue against the palate. Patients can also perform bellows breathing during treatment to support the release of tensions in the body. During breathing, energy or warmth is sent to the restricted areas, and during apnea patients may become aware that the circulating sensation of energy releases restrictions.

Tingling sensations and light-headedness can occur during this breathing exercise. If you experience pain or dizziness, this technique should be stopped immediately.

By way of preparation and in order to "charge" the hands to a high level of excitation energy, you may wish to begin by holding your hands, palms facing each other and a few centimeters apart, in front of your lower abdomen. Meanwhile, you direct vital energy into your hands with each exhalation, producing a gradual increase in the energy field between your hands. This creates a feeling of increased resistance between your hands.

It is important to maintain your breathing in a conscious way during the treatment. Breathing provides a vehicle through which to influence the flow or intensity of vital force in yourself and in your hands during treatment, and to apply it in a precisely directed way. It is essential to maintain the coordination or synchronization of your breathing with the performance of the technique. During exhalation, vital force is directed into your hands, and you allow the energy to flow. If you sense weak energy, halting, or holding back ujjai breathing, breath of fire or bellows breathing can be used to strengthen the energy or restore its flow. Whether or not you use a particular type of breathing, you should in any case follow the flow of energy in the patient and in the patient's tissues with your attention.

It is also essential to hold "body locks": the pelvic, diaphragm, and throat bandhas.

- The pelvic floor should be drawn gently upward.

- The abdomen should be drawn in, toward the back, and the diaphragm raised in the cranial direction.

- The throat bandha should be activated: by drawing the chin toward the chest.

Maintenance of contact with your own flow or source of vitality is fundamental to the performance of the following method. Only once you have sensed this flow in yourself, this sense of being "in the flow," do you begin to direct your loving, non-invasive attention toward the patient, without losing contact with the flow in yourself.

Therapeutic approach to the patient

Examination Let your hands glide over the patient's body. Direct your attention toward those parts of the body that are especially vital; for this, do not use your hands only, but all your senses. Where is there motion? Where is there vitality? Where is there pulsation?

During this initial stage, do not attend to anything that is stiff, lifeless, immobile, tense, dysfunctional, restricted, or stagnated, but concentrate instead on what is soft/elastic, alive, mobile, relaxed, functioning, free, and flowing. The characteristic sensations on palpation of tissue vitality are tingling, vibrating, or hammering. Heat can also be an expression of intense vital force. Another may simply be that you sense a kind of hard-to-describe vital energy. The stronger the sensations, the stronger the vital force in the areas concerned.

Alternative method An alternative approach for the osteopath to use is region by region. To do this, you first place your right hand on the patient's right foot and your left hand on the patient's lower leg, and sense the strength and ease of the flow of energy between your hands. You then place your right hand on the patient's right lower leg and your left on the patient's thigh, and so on, examining the whole of the patient's body and applying treatment straight away as necessary (see below).

According to Gordon, five main patterns can be palpated in the course of energy. The present author has, to a great extent, been able to confirm this in palpation (Table 20.2).[28]

- Making contact with regions of good vitality: once you have found or been led to the region with good vitality, the next step is to make contact with the patient in this region. Place your hands on the region in question and direct attention and empathy to it. Simply by doing this you can strengthen the vitality and the flow in the patient. Permit whatever this region of greatest health expresses – whether through the tissue or by a means beyond it. Allow the vitality and originality of the patient to "touch" you, and give expression to that touch by means of your hands. Taking up contact in this way takes very little time. It would make no sense to remain in this region of greatest rhythmic flow and greatest vitality, because free flow is already present here; on the other hand, moving on immediately to the place of greatest restriction (i.e., trying to bring about a change at the place where immobility is most pronounced) may very well be too invasive. This would mean that you were "doing" something rather than allowing the patient's body (in its fullest sense) to act.

- Taking up contact with the intermediate zone: your next step is to sense the region of the body where the free flow encounters resistances, restrictions, and contractions. It is important to detect this location accurately. At this stage it is not the place of greatest immobility that you are trying to contact, but the place where a relatively large amount of flow, rhythm, and pulsation is present; the dividing line between softness and rigidity. The rigidity or immobility has not yet developed fully at this location; it is here that you support the inherent rhythm and flow, because it is here that health can spread relatively easily, ease the reduced mobility and soften the resistances.

Motion restrictions and blockages are released by the natural tendency of the vitality in the body to spread. Patients acquire greater consciousness, and so also responsibility as to how they treat their lives or their bodies so as to assist rather than block the flow. It is not the practitioner who acts.

It is important, in order to achieve this, to be able to sense in yourself what is happening in the body of the other person. The sensing of health is not to be understood simply as a kind of technique or manipulation in the traditional sense. It is just as essential for you, as the practitioner, to be in contact with your own flow and originality, to develop a consciousness

Course	Diagram	Sensation palpated	Occurrence
Normal course	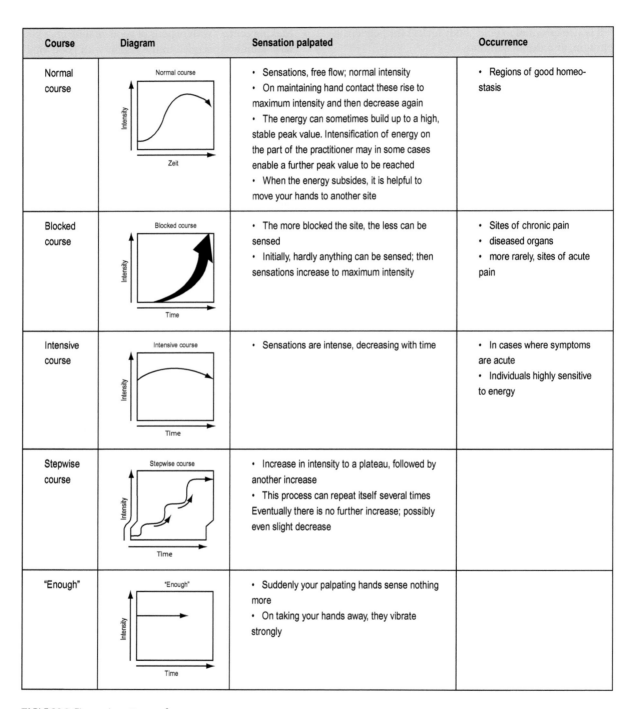	• Sensations, free flow; normal intensity • On maintaining hand contact these rise to maximum intensity and then decrease again • The energy can sometimes build up to a high, stable peak value. Intensification of energy on the part of the practitioner may in some cases enable a further peak value to be reached • When the energy subsides, it is helpful to move your hands to another site	• Regions of good homeo-stasis
Blocked course		• The more blocked the site, the less can be sensed • Initially, hardly anything can be sensed; then sensations increase to maximum intensity	• Sites of chronic pain • diseased organs • more rarely, sites of acute pain
Intensive course		• Sensations are intense, decreasing with time	• In cases where symptoms are acute • Individuals highly sensitive to energy
Stepwise course		• Increase in intensity to a plateau, followed by another increase • This process can repeat itself several times Eventually there is no further increase; possibly even slight decrease	
"Enough"		• Suddenly your palpating hands sense nothing more • On taking your hands away, they vibrate strongly	

TABLE 20.2: Five main patterns of energy

According to Gordon (modified).[28]

of your own immediate sensation, with the capacity to allow a sense of intimacy and closeness, and to permit processes to occur without needing to intervene. The extent to which you are in contact with this originality and with your own flow determines the extent to which you will be able to establish this same contact with the patient.

Once the practitioner has established this contact with the patient and located, welcomed, and respected the flow in the patient, it becomes possible to assist the patient's body, in the way that suits the nature of that individual, to release dysfunctions and restrictions that obstruct the free flow and the homeostasis of the body. It is in this way, direct contact can be made with locations of restriction.

- Taking up contact with the restricted region: the more restricted the region, the less that can be sensed; however, if the practitioner's hands are allowed to rest for a while on the region, then usually a rise in energy can increasingly be detected. If the location is severely restricted this may take some time. What is generally found is that, over whatever period of time it may take, the intensity of the vital force arrives at a maximum. Sometimes, however, the energy remains at this level for some time before rising to a higher plateau of intensity.

- The therapeutic interaction in the intermediate zone and in the restricted region. Method: follow the motions in the tissue. These are the expression of the vital potential in the patient, the visible tips of the patient's health that can be seen on the surface, and you follow them – through the layers of adaptation that have occurred in response to internal and external influences – to their place of origin. Your hands should always follow the tissue motions/dynamics in the direction of free movement. The tissue motions and dynamics can be sensed even in severely restricted tissue. Do not let the motion restrictions in the restricted region or in the intermediate zone detain you; when you sense restriction of any kind, direct your relaxed attention back toward the motion that you can sense. As you do so, you can use any of the breathing techniques described above, in order to strengthen tissue vitality. However, it is very important not to engage in actively "doing" anything, and not to

try to direct motion or rush ahead in anticipation of it. Instead, remain restfully in receptive, open, relaxed perception and follow the flow of health in the patient with your hands, through the tissue structures to its origin, the mesenchymal primal ocean, the potential, and meaning. When you have followed the tissue motions through to the end, to their origin and the vital potential of the patient, there is a qualitative change in the tissue palpation, felt as free flow. Motion ceases to be expressed in a particular direction, but is instead sensed as a rhythmic expansion and retraction. Here, the body in its fullest sense can reorient itself in direct, immediate experience and make the transition from the fulcrum of disease to the fulcrum of health.

Treatment by means of rhythmic impulses

The use of different methods of applying rhythmic impulses, or synchronization with rhythmic dynamics, can address different facets, levels, and states of consciousness, and assist various processes of integration.

- Synchronization with microvibration (4–8 cycles/sec) can influence the autonomic nervous state and vitality.

- Synchronization with homeodynamic rhythms such as heartbeat, circulatory, blood pressure variations, and respiratory rhythms lends support to their activity. See, for example, "dynamic balanced tension."

- Experiment whether synchronization with different types and frequencies of rhythms support possible access to emotional, mental, causal energy fields and states of consciousness and non-dual states. Avoid rigid models.

- Synchronization with the 1-minute fundamental rhythm of the smooth muscles aims to influence the perfusion of the skin, mucous membranes, and muscles and of the hollow organs.

- Synchronization with rhythms of lymphatic flow, e.g., rhythm of approximately 10 cycles/min.[29]

Contraindications: acute infections, serious disorders of blood vessels (e.g., thromboses), serious cardiac disorders (e.g., acute myocardial infarction or acute angina pectoris), hemorrhage, acute anuresis, and malignant disease (not operated on or under medical control). Relative contraindications are lymphedema, menstruation, and (where there is a change in metabolism) certain medicines.

An express warning needs to be given here against misapplication of this aspect. The simple perception of rhythms, or the synchronization with rhythms, should not be treated as a kind of magical technique for treating disturbances of inner worlds of experience, and physiological or dysfunctional states of all kinds.

Another possibility that osteopaths might employ appears to be synchronization with, and consideration of, other rhythmic phenomena (see Chapter 4).

Balanced tension

The "balanced tension" approach has a key place in the treatment of patterns of tension linked to developmental dynamics. There are many different ways of applying balanced tension. One example is the point of balanced membranous tension; this is a defined place, in space and time, in the range of motion of a joint or of a specific state. The fascial structures involved are in a state of balanced tension at this point, which is located between normal tension and dysfunctional factors or increased tension. The concept of balanced tension can also be applied to fluid structures and electromagnetic fields.

Balanced tension techniques can be used to bring dysfunctional patterns of tension into resonance with homeodynamic forces, so integrating and releasing them. Establishment of a state of balanced tension leads to the release of the bound forces in patterns of tension due to developmental dynamics, by enabling the tissues to resolve the relationships between them. Inherent homeodynamic forces come into effect in the dysfunction, enabling a dynamic state of balance to be reestablished. This, in contact with the dysfunctional fulcrums, can set healing reactions in motion.

The balanced tension of a pattern of tension due to developmental dynamics has to balance or offset all the forces related to this dysfunction and all the associated worlds of experience. These had previously led their own life, separate from the whole, incompletely integrated and unconsidered or in some other way suppressed or repressed. Balanced tension becomes all the more effective, the more it is able to relate to the morphodynamic "movements" of development, orient itself to the whole, and make contact with a host of individual and collective forces, both in the tissue and in various levels of consciousness. This kind of balance of tension cannot be forced. Its potential is also dependent on the aspects of the patient that practitioners are able to perceive and permit, which will depend on their own views and patterns of experience, conditioned and limited as they are. It would be inadequate to reduce this kind of balanced tension to the mere performance of a mechanical technique. During the therapeutic interaction, the practitioner's perception should do more than concentrate on the state of balance and the interaction of the forces of restriction and release; it should also rest in the best possible state of unconditional attention.

Several factors are important for the outcome of treatment: exactness and empathy, attentiveness and relaxation, physical and psychological stability, or groundedness and flexibility; but it is the inherent forces in the patient[30] – the forces acting from within – that carry out the correction:

- The disengagement at the end of each inhalation phase

- The retraction/drawing closer at the end of each exhalation phase

- The synchronization (see also entrainment model)[31]

- Transmutation, etc.

All the forces and tissues in the body that are involved in any way in the dysfunction pattern can express themselves during this process (for example, in the form of tensions, aberrant motions, heat, trembling, memories, emotions or thoughts arising in the patient, or other kinds of expression) and bring about a new relationship to the affected tissue and to the area around those forces or tissues. When palpating the

---

‡It should nevertheless be noted that no satisfactory explanation has yet been arrived at as to the ontogenetic substance of these rhythms. These remarks are therefore hypothetical. See also T. Liem. *Cranial Osteopathy: a Practical Textbook*, Eastland Press, 2009, p. 34ff.)

morphological developmental dynamics, the osteopath should be open to all the biological reactions in the tissue, and also to all elements of meaning of the psychological, mental, and spiritual kind. By gently assisting release in dialog, and avoiding any invasive imposition of a change of pattern on the tissue dynamics, the osteopath allows space for all these elements of meaning to emerge and become integrated in the course of the release process.

When a region's dysfunctional pattern changes, there is also a change in the relationship of the whole, or of certain body regions and functional spheres, to that region. That will then lead to further changes in the body as a whole. This process begins during the therapeutic interaction, but for the most part continues to take place after the consultation, in the interval between treatments. Balanced tension finally leads to the resolution or reduction of dysfunctional fulcrums; the tissue and inherent forces are able to realign themselves in the direction of the natural fulcrums, and bound energies or experience become once more accessible as a resource for the dynamics of the homeostatic forces operating in the body and person as a whole. A new, higher-order state of balance can be established in the body.

Note, whereas, in the biomechanical approach, motion barriers are tested and addressed in therapy, vitalist approaches avoid testing and confrontation of motion barriers, both in diagnosis or testing and in the therapeutic interaction. Of course, you can use both models for testing, but try to do only one at a time. In vitalist approaches, a shifting of attention in the practitioner serves as a kind of indicator for the presence of primary respiration, which is held to act as the active, directing force in the therapeutic interaction.

Point of balanced membranous/ligamentous/fascial tension (PBMT/PBLT/PBFT)

Biomechanical approach

The osteopath tries to find the point of balance of the dysfunctional articular structures. This is the position in which the ligaments, membranes, or fasciae involved in the dysfunction are in the best possible state of balance relative to one another. This position lies between the normal range of motion in one direction and the restricted range of motion in the other direction. The

point of balance of the membranous, ligamentous, and fascial structures is then harmonized with the fluid point of balance and developmental dynamic patterns. This is the result of the inherent homeodynamic forces taking over the therapeutic work.

Once the PBMT has been reached, the practitioner experiences a sense of lightness in the tissue, like a state of floating. This is accompanied by the onset of an inherent chaotic tissue dynamic in the membranous/ligamentous structures. Anne Wales described this as "the ligaments/membranes go shopping." The practitioner now needs to hold the articular structures so as to enable this inherent play to continue. Holding the articular structures at the point of balance enables the inherent power in the tension of the dural membrane, the ligaments, or the fascia in general and the potential power in the fluids of the body to work as effectively as possible to restore better mobility.

Frequently there comes a moment of stillness or a functional still point, when all motions seem to come to rest and a change occurs. The expression Becker used to describe this was "something happens." Afterwards, motion can be palpated again and the dysfunctional pattern is found to have changed toward normalization and health. A more physiological balance of tension has now become established, and release of the restriction and normalization of fascial tension (and that of membranes and ligaments, etc.) can be sensed.

Vitalist approaches

Vitalist approaches, in contrast to the biomechanical approach, do not confront motion barriers, and establishment of a point of balance is done without any testing of the tissue barriers.

Practitioners also direct their awareness to the "automatic shifting" that takes place at the moment change occurs.

Establishment of a local, regional, and global point of balanced tension (BT), e.g., at the stomach

1 Establish a local BT, e.g., in the tissue elasticity, tonus of the stomach wall, or motility of the stomach.

2 The next step is for the osteopath to allow a local BT to become established between the stomach and its surrounding organs/structures (diaphragm,

pericardium, left pleura), duodenum, large intestine, liver, pancreas, spleen, left kidney, and adrenal gland (and vessels).

3 In the third step, a regional BT becomes established between the stomach and the whole abdominal cavity.

4 Finally a global BT develops between the stomach and the entire body.

Dynamic balanced tension (DBT)

The osteopath synchronizes with the morphodynamic "movements" of development and senses the way in which the forces at work in the tissue are acting.

According to Jealous, during the inhalation phase (especially the 2–3 cycles/min rhythm) the self-correcting forces produce a state of balanced membranous tension, so that hydraulic forces can bring the tissues and fluids back to their normal relation to the embryonic fulcrum and its organizational fulcrums during the exhalation phase.[32] It is usually sufficient to support this homeodynamic process gently during the inhalation phase, and then, during the exhalation phase, to stay with the change with passive attentiveness. (This method for the most part corresponds to Jealous's preferred procedure for the establishment of balanced membranous tension.)

Method

- Synchronize your hands with the morphodynamic developmental "movements" during the patient's involuntary rhythms.

- The biggest part of the practitioner's attention remains with the homeodynamic rhythms of the body, and the rest follows the dysfunctional or asymmetrical, aberrant tissue dynamics.[32]

- Do not confront any tissue restrictions or tissue barriers in the dysfunction.

- From a certain moment on in the therapeutic interaction, a shift occurs in the practitioner's consciousness.

- During the inhalation phase, you should bring about a very slight intensification of the dysfunctional or asymmetrical, aberrant motion/tension present in the tissue, but without altering the speed of these motions.

- To amplify the perceptions of palpation dynamics, they can be expressed in the body of the therapist. In this way the therapist uses his own body proprioceptors to intensify the impressions of palpation.

- During the exhalation phase, simply follow the tissue tensions passively.

- Repeat this process until, at the end of an inhalation phase, there is a clearly perceptible disengagement that is quite spontaneous and not elicited by you. (This disengagement is more pronounced and greater than the one that occurs at the end of every inhalation phase.)

- This is usually accompanied by automatic shifting.

- Forces that were not induced by the practitioner begin to operate. During the next exhalation phase, these forces lead the affected tissue out of the dysfunction. What happens is in effect a self-correction.

- You may sense a lateral fluctuation at the level of the affected tissue.

- There may also be a transition to a still point.

Balanced fluid tension (BFT)

Every organism passes through a fluid stage in its embryonic development, and this is marked by fluid dynamics. The complex interactions of fluid motions and chemokinetic, biophysical, morphogenetic dynamics lead finally to the emergence of the visible shape of the body's solid material form. Even the adult human body still consists of about 70% of fluids. The BFT technique is designed to act on the fluid aspect of the body and synchronize with fluid developmental dynamics.

Method

- Synchronize your hands with the qualities of the fluids (motion, speed, density, expansion/retraction phase, etc.).

- If a directional fluid pattern is palpated, follow this pattern to its natural end point. Very often a switch or an inherently, spontaneously appearing disengagement, can be perceived.

Box 20.4

Establishment of a PBMT: summary

Structural approach

- Testing parameters of movement and consequences in the direction of ease/greater mobility; this may be assisted as necessary by slight compression of the tissue (or the developmental dynamics) patterns of relationship

- Permit inherent motions/tensions that occur: "membranes/ligaments go shopping"

- A kind of functional still point comes about, in which all motions appear to come to rest and a change occurs ("something happens")

- Movement can be palpated again: release of tissue tension, new balance of tension.

Vitalist approaches

- Establish PBMT by following passively (without preceding this with motion testing); this may be assisted as necessary by slight compression of the tissue (or the developmental dynamic) patterns of relationship

- Permit inherent motions/tensions that occur: "membranes/ligaments go shopping"

- Sense shifting of attention during the therapeutic interaction

- A kind of functional still point comes about, in which all motions appear to come to rest and a change occurs ("something happens")

- Sense "automatic shifting"

- Movement can be palpated again: release of tissue tension, new balance of tension

- A balance of the fluids is established.

- There is an interaction between the local fluid pattern and the whole fluid body.

- Also other procedures of balanced fluid tension exist and can be applied. Another method would be to synchronise with the motion of the fluids, the speed of their motion, and the inherent, spontaneously appearing disengagement.

Balanced electrodynamic tension (BET)

Initial position

Position your hand above the skin, at the level of the structure to be treated. Slowly lower your hand until you reach a point where you sense a resistance. Another possible approach is to set the hand down and establish contact with the origin of the electromagnetic field of the particular tissue.

Method

For example in treatment of the origin of the electromagnetic field of the occipital bone, sphenoid, and ethmoid bones after Heede (modified):

- Gently place the pads of your index finger, middle and ring fingers bilaterally on the patient's head, level with the bones to be treated.

- Place your thumbs, touching each other, bilaterally on top of the patient's head to provide a fulcrum.

- Your fingers should synchronize with the electromagnetic fields of these bones.

- Permit all the various motions of these fields, until they come to rest or until you sense symmetrical motion.

- From a certain moment on in the therapeutic interaction, a shift in your consciousness occurs.

- An automatic shifting takes place.

Other methods of achieving balanced tension

Additional methods that may be needed to arrive at a state of balanced tension are presented below. The method depends on the age and condition of the patient, on the acuteness and type of dysfunction(s). The practitioner tunes in to the fluid fluctuations and the tissue that offers the most suitable means of achieving balanced tension. The osteopath can use the following maneuvers as a means of diagnosis, to sense the reaction of the tissue to these "invitations," and also as a means of treatment to achieve a new dynamic balance of tension.

Two main basic tendencies may be found in the dysfunction complex:

- An entity that is relatively isolated or decoupled from the body as a whole.

- A loss of relative autonomy in the dysfunction, relative to its surroundings, in the sense of a weakening of its natural boundaries.

In both cases, the tissue or its function in the body as a whole is no longer available to the optimum extent. The practitioner should use palpation to approach this complex, which is either relatively self-contained or, more usually, relatively merged with its surroundings, and should begin by encouraging its differentiation.

Parts that are isolated and self-contained can be invited to relate to their surroundings and to the body as a whole, by gently compressing the tissue parts or inducing nearness between them. Merged parts can be invited to distance themselves from their surroundings or the related parts with which they are involved, by gently bringing about space between the tissues concerned.

In this nearness or space, the existing patterns of relationship may become more pronounced; they may differentiate; the forces of balanced tension may develop, and the self-isolation or merging may finally be overcome.

Finally, there is a process of integration in which the relatively decoupled entity is brought back into dynamic relationship with the body as a whole and its resources once more become available to the body; or, the relatively merged parts regain the relative autonomy regarding their surroundings which is needed for their optimal function.

These processes must not be forced, since this would hinder or prevent the differentiation and integration of the subjective, intersubjective, and objective factors (physical, biological, emotional, mental and/or spiritual) related to the dysfunction complex. In other words, all the parts associated with the dysfunction complex must be given sufficient space and time to show and differentiate themselves.

Exaggeration

Several methods are also possible for the exaggeration technique.

Biomechanical approach

In the exaggeration technique, an impulse is delivered to the tissue, organ, bone, or fascia in the opposite direction to the restriction; in other words, in the direction of greater mobility or ease.

This time, however, you do not simply accompany the tissue in the direction of ease to the stage where a point of balance is established. The practitioner takes the tissue a little further beyond the point of balance, in the opposite direction to the restriction.

In structural approaches, the tissue is led to (or at least near to) its physiological limit. The practitioner should wait for the tissue to relax, resulting in greater mobility, and then lead the tissue to its new physiological limit. This procedure is repeated until no further relaxations of tension are sensed.

Contraindications In some cases of acute trauma, when there is a risk that exaggeration might exacerbate the symptoms.

Vitalist approach

In this approach, unlike structural approaches, the tissue is led gently out of its field or state of tension in the opposite direction to the restriction without confronting any tissue barriers or motion barriers. The practitioner senses the tissue dynamics during involuntary rhythms without intervening. Finally, a new balance of tension becomes established.

Method

- Synchronize with involuntary rhythms.

- Establish resonance with the developmental dynamic dysfunction pattern.

- Gently lead the tissue out of the state of tension in the opposite direction to the restriction.

- Do not confront any tissue barriers.

- Passively sense the tissue dynamics that become established.

- A shift in consciousness may be sensed during the therapeutic interaction.

- Automatic shifting may be sensed.

- A new balance of tension becomes established.

Direct technique

In the direct technique, pressure, or traction is applied in the direction of the restriction. The tissue or structure is led gently in the direction of reduced mobility. The amount of force applied is slight, and constantly remains below the threshold where the tissues involved exert counter-contraction. The force used in this should not hinder the inherent rhythmic homeodynamics.

Indications

In acute dysfunctions arising from trauma, since there is a risk that exaggeration might exacerbate the symptoms.

It can also be helpful to combine direct and indirect techniques, and in such cases, the practitioner always begins with the indirect technique.

Vitalist approach

In this approach, developmental dynamic tension patterns are simply eased gently in the direction of the restriction without confronting tissue barriers or motion barriers.

Method

- Synchronize with involuntary rhythms.

- Establish resonance with the developmental dynamic dysfunction pattern.

- Gently lead the tissue out of the state of tension in the direction of the restriction.

- As you do so, do not confront any tissue barriers.

- Passively sense the tissue dynamics that become established.

- A shift in consciousness may be sensed during the therapeutic interaction.

- Automatic shifting may be sensed.

- A new balance of tension becomes established.

Disengagement and traction field

This treatment method can be applied for various purposes:

- Disengagement as an invitation to the tissues to allow space to be created between them. Used biomechanically, this technique involved easing the articular surfaces concerned gently away from each other and separating them so that they are able to allow the creation of balanced tension. Used to release tension at sutures, limb joints, traumatized and severe chronic restrictions, and fascial fibroses.

- This treatment approach is also indicated when the forces present in a dysfunction produce excessive closeness on account of the underlying trauma. Either the compressive forces are too great, or the bound forces in the dysfunction are too densely compressed for balanced tension (BT) to be able to release the forces in this tissue from their bound state, making them accessible once more to the dynamics of physiological forces. Another possibility, though more difficult, is to make contact with the underlying dysfunctional fulcrums by means of balanced tension; however, this contact is insufficient to counter the compressive forces.

  If we translate this into terms of personal relations, the first stage in resolving conflict between two closely associated individuals can be to create space between the conflicting parties. In other words, the two are sufficiently separated from each other for them to be able to listen to each other again. The partners in the conflict are each in turn able to air their view of the conflict, while the other is instructed not to interrupt, but simply to listen. In just the same way it is possible to give a "hearing" to the relations between tissues. We are not trying to drag apart the structures and forces concerned by force, but rather, firstly, to direct our attention to the space that is still available in the dysfunction and so set an expansion under way. Secondly, by gently easing them apart in resonance with the forces that are present, the tissues and fluids involved are invited to create space. The manner in which this is done can differ according to the situation, i.e., in one case it may mean applying a kind of movement, in another, the mere intention of disengagement. It is important to realize that this easing apart is not done in order to eliminate the forces that are operating, but so that you can sense or palpate the way they are operating and their inner order, to reveal the underlying fulcrums and allow these forces to act in balanced tension. Once this has been achieved, it creates its own dynamic, in the course of which further spontaneous disengagement usually occurs, followed by integration of the bound forces.

- Disengagement can be also used to unfold tissue around joints after a folding injury, e.g., a shoulder, which was drawn out forcefully. The palpatory finding in this case would be, the tissue does not like to be compressed and the patient disrelishes compressive forces at this joint but favors pulling forces. Patients often embrace the joint with their hands and describe a deep pain inside the joint as well as a feeling of joint instability.

- This treatment principle also serves the further purpose of synchronization with developmental dynamics expressed in the tissue as active pressure stress. Differentiated traction fields are involved in the formation of such tissues as thin "limiting tissue" and "inner tissue," or that of glands (suction fields) or muscles (dilatation fields). The practitioner induces a traction field, within which it is possible for developmental dynamics to be re-experienced in a kind of tissue regression. This enables the differentiation, integration, and release of dysfunctional tension patterns.

Note, the osteopath should not induce movement in any particular direction or release, apart from the invitation to disengagement, but should simply allow inherent motions or tensions to find expression. No change should be made to the speed of these expressions of tension, which should take place at their own pace.

1 Structural approach (Box 20.5):
 a Synchronize with involuntary rhythms.
 b Listen and establish resonance.
 c Establish a BT; however, the compressive forces present will be too strong for any spontaneous release of tension to occur.
 d Disengagement as an invitation to the tissue, e.g., gently disengage two neighboring joint components from each other.
 e Establish balanced tension.

f Your attention should be directed toward the activity of the inherent homeodynamic forces.
g Alternative method: holding one component of the joint, gently disengage the other: BT. Then hold the other component of the joint and gently disengage the first.

2 Vitalist approaches (Box 20.5):
 a Synchronize with involuntary rhythms.
 b Listen and establish resonance.
 c Establish BT (do not confront any tissue barriers). Any spontaneous release of tension is prevented by the compressive forces present, which are too strong to allow release.
 d Disengagement as an invitation to the tissue, e.g., gently disengage two neighboring joint components from each other.
 e Establish balanced tension (do not confront any tissue barriers as you do so).

Box 20.5
Questions to pose to the tissue (or) direction of therapeutic attention

- Did the tissue develop in a traction or compression field?
- Does the tissue require a traction or compression field?
- How much space is available?
- What is the quality of this space?
- How much nearness is available?
- What is the quality of this nearness?
- How much space do the forces involved allow? (Or, how do the forces involved react to the invitation to disengagement?)
- Where is the fulcrum of this dysfunction?
- How do the forces react in the BT?

See also questions about the PBT.

f Your attention should be directed toward the activity of the inherent homeodynamic forces.

g You may sense a shifting of attention during the therapeutic interaction, at the moment when a change occurs.

h You may sense automatic shifting.

3 2 (a) Developmental dynamic approach (Box 20.5):
a Synchronize with involuntary rhythms.
b Listen and establish resonance with developmental dynamic tension patterns.
c Establish balanced tension (do not confront any tissue barriers). Any spontaneous release of tension is prevented by the compressive forces present, which are too strong to allow release.
d Induce a traction field (e.g., at the oculomotor nerve, achieved by the application of gentle traction at the eyeball, see Chapter 33).
e Register the tissue dynamics, without intervening.
f Create a fulcrum.
g Maintain the traction field, following the release process that emerges. This usually makes its appearance as a kind of increasing nearness (as if the muscles of the eye were drawing the oculomotor nerve nearer).
h Simply follow the process of release (if appropriate, it can be gently intensified); you must not however guide it in any particular direction or influence it in any way.
i A state of balanced tension becomes established.
j You may sense a shifting of attention during the therapeutic interaction, at the moment when a change occurs.
k You may sense automatic shifting.

4 2 (b) Spontaneous disengagement:
a Here, according to Jealous, the disengagement occurs spontaneously, during the process of balanced tension. It is not induced by the practitioner, but is the expression of inherent forces that express and form part of the body's own self-correction.

Method

1 Direct your attention toward the wholeness of the patient's body and being and surrounding field.

2 Neutral state.

3 The tissue as part of the field of tension of the body as a whole.

4 Sense the inherent dysfunctional tensions and fulcrums.

5 Establish balanced tension.

6 Your attention should be directed toward the horizon.

7 A shifting of attention is sensed during the therapeutic interaction.

8 Long tide: the potency of the Breath of Life comes into the midline from outside and operates through the dysfunctional fulcrums.

9 Spontaneous disengagement occurs in the tissue.

Compression/field of compression

This treatment principle can also be applied for various purposes:

• Combined application of compression and decompression. This is indicated particularly for all severely restricted joints, e.g., at the SBS (sphenobasilar synchondrosis/synostosis), sutures, membranes, fasciae, etc. First the tissue is compressed and eased into the lesion; then decompressed in the opposite direction. It therefore, in a certain sense, combines the indirect and the direct technique. The best way to understand this is to imagine releasing a jammed drawer. If we begin by pushing the drawer in, this can release the blockage and we can then pull the drawer out quite easily, with no need to use force. In other words, we start by moving it away from the blockage in order to release it. Compression does not actually alter the dysfunction pattern initially, but it does produce relaxation. We apply it until we sense the tissue giving a kind of sigh. Then we make a fluid transition to decompression. Gentle decompression brings about an unwinding of the tissue, like untangling a telephone cord by letting the weight of the dangling receiver do the work.

- Compression can be used to create a situation in which the relationship between tissues is intensified; within this situation, hidden conflicts become visible, or more easily palpated. This is indicated, for example, in the case of dysfunction patterns that have been present for a long time, when the biokinetic forces in the dysfunction have become organized in such a way that the relationship between the structures involved has become "frozen." This is not a case of forcefully compressing the structures and forces concerned, but rather of using gentle compression to bring the structures and fluids involved into resonance with the forces that are present and to allow a dynamic to arise. Once this has happened, BT can be established, and activity by homeodynamic forces can come into play in balanced tension. In the course of this, spontaneous disengagement usually occurs and there is integration of the bound forces. Apart from the invitation to nearness there should be no attempt to move the tissue in any particular direction; instead, the inherent motions or tensions should be allowed to find expression. You should not alter the speed of these expressions of tension, but allow things to happen at their own pace.

- Another use of this treatment principle is to achieve synchronization with developmental dynamics that were expressed in the tissue, for example as active, directed stretching by the tissue itself. Differentiated compression fields are involved in the formation of such tissues as thick limiting tissue, the mouth region (corrosion fields), the bones of the arms (densation fields), joint cartilage (contusion fields), or the sphenobasilar synchondrosis (distusion fields). The practitioner induces a field of compression in which developmental dynamics can be re-experienced by a kind of tissue regression. This enables the differentiation, integration, and release of dysfunctional tension patterns.

- Compression can also be used to refold tissue around joints after a folding injury, e.g., falling onto a shoulder. The palpatory finding in this case would be that the tissue does not like to be decompressed and patients disrelish decompressive forces at this joint. They often embrace the joint with their hands, rubbing across it and describing a deep pain as well as a feeling of instability in the joint.

Method

1 Structural approach (Box 20.6):
   a Synchronize with involuntary rhythms.
   b Listen and establish resonance.
   c Establish BT but spontaneous release of tension is prevented by rigid biokinetic forces and unclear dysfunction patterns.
   d Compression as an invitation to the tissue, e.g., gently easing two neighboring components of a joint closer to each other.
   e Establishment of balanced tension.
   f Your attention should be directed toward the activity of the inherent homeodynamic forces.
   g Alternative method: hold one component of the joint and gently ease the other closer: PBT. Then hold the other and gently ease the first closer.

2 Vitalist approaches (Box 20.6):
   a Synchronize with involuntary rhythms.
   b Listen and establish resonance.
   c Establish BT (do not confront any tissue barriers) but spontaneous release of tension is prevented by rigid biokinetic forces and unclear dysfunction pattern.
   d Compression as an invitation to the tissue, e.g., gently easing two neighboring components of a joint closer to each other.
   e Establishment of balanced tension (without confronting any tissue barriers).
   f Your attention should be directed toward the activity of the inherent homeodynamic forces. You may sense a shifting of attention during the therapeutic interaction.
   g You may sense automatic shifting.

3 Developmental dynamic approach:
   a Synchronize with involuntary rhythms.
   b Listen and establish resonance with developmental dynamic tension patterns.
   c Establish BT (do not confront any tissue barriers). Any spontaneous release of tension is prevented by the compressive forces present, which are too strong to allow release.
   d Induce a compression field (e.g., at the neck, by gentle caudad pressure from the head and gentle craniad pressure from the region of the heart, see Chapter 29).

Box 20.6

Questions to pose to the tissue (or) direction of therapeutic attention

- Did the tissue develop in a traction or compression field?

- Does the tissue require a traction or compression field?

- How much space is available?

- What is the quality of this space?

- What is the nature of the dynamics of the forces involved?

- How clearly can the dysfunctional pattern be perceived?

- How do the forces involved react to the invitation to compression?

- Where is the fulcrum of this dysfunction?

- How do the forces behave in the BT?

- See questions relating to PBT

e Register the tissue dynamics, without intervening.
f Create a fulcrum.
g Maintain the field of compression, following the emerging release process. This generally starts to appear in the form of a kind of distancing (disengagement) between head and heart.
h Simply follow the process of release (if appropriate, it can be gently intensified); you must not, however, guide it in any particular direction or influence it in any way.
i A state of balanced tension becomes established.
j You may sense a shifting of attention during the therapeutic interaction, at the moment when a change occurs.
k You may sense automatic shifting.

Molding

This treatment method is one of the direct techniques. In molding, the practitioner tries to change the shape or pliancy of the bones by the application of external pressure or traction. This technique is mainly used for intraosseous dysfunctions.

Understandably, molding is more frequently used in childhood, since the bones are much more pliable at that stage of life than in adulthood, and the growth of the bones is more open to influence in childhood. However, even in adulthood, impulses can be delivered to influence the organization of osseous structures.

Recoil (modified variant based on the method of Chauffour and Prat)[33]

In this method, too, the osteopath begins by synchronizing with the developmental dynamic vectors of force, e.g., at the elbow (90° flexion and slight external rotation of the forearm). Here, too, a gentle field of compression can be applied in addition. The dysfunctional vectors of motion are determined. There are two possible methods:

1 Direct:
    a Step 1: precisely determine all the components of tension/motion (vertical, horizontal, rotational, torsional, side-bending, tension vectors running in the direction either with or opposite to the rest), working in the direction of the restriction.
    b Step 2: explore further to discover the moment during deep inhalation or exhalation when the tissue tension in the dysfunction is at its greatest. Recoil is performed in the breathing phase at which tension in the dysfunction increases. You can in addition ask the patient to stop breathing momentarily at the stage during breathing that is associated with the greatest tissue tension. The recoil is carried out at that moment of apnea.
    c The procedure can be performed in essentially the same way, but incorporating synchronization with involuntary rhythms.
    d Step 3: deliver a very gentle, brief, and very rapid impulse toward the barrier. This has the effect of creating a vibration, and this aspect of the technique is believed to be able to release not only the local developmental dynamic tension patterns, but also the dysfunction chain, assuming that the dysfunction treated is a key, primary one.
    e Emotional integration: a further possibility is for the patient to imagine an emotional problem. As the patient does so, the osteopath assesses the

tissue tension. If this increases when they imagine the emotional problem or situation, you should ask them to retain the thought. Perform the recoil at the moment when tissue resistance is strongest.

2 Indirect:

Determine all components as above, but perform this in the direction of greater mobility or freedom.

Other treatment principles

Some treatment principles emphasize the treatment of local symptomatic areas (e.g., pain), such as trigger point therapy, strain/counterstrain, and fascial distortion model (associated with the gesture of patients). These treatment principles can be integrated into an osteopathic treatment session, e.g., in order to treat local areas of pain or restriction of movement.

Burning or pulling pain along fascial structures can be treated by deep strokes along the area of pain. Patients who often push a tender area with their fingers will be treated with strong pressure likely to push an abnormal protrusion of the tissue back through the fascial plane. Or, pain in non-jointed areas (and to a lesser extent in jointed areas) which cannot be reproduced or magnified by palpation and which often is associated with paresthesia, numbness, weakness, or spasm, can be treated with massage-like techniques. Achy joint pain, with patients usually cupping the affected joint with their hand, can be manipulated with compression or decompression forces. In stiff joints, high velocity manipulation and mobilisation (also self mobilisation) can be used.

Many other treatment principles are described in the osteopathic literature and therefore do not need to be described in detail here; however, some will be characterized later on in the book by means of a description of specific techniques.

Assistance to self-healing

The therapeutic factors presented below can assist the treatment of developmental dynamic tension patterns and the establishment of balanced tension, and can be used with all the techniques described earlier. They have the effect of directing the self-regulating forces toward the processes of integration and differentiation, thus reinforcing the self-correction of the body as a whole. Attention can also be paid in the treatment to additional levels of being that may be involved in the dysfunction complex.

Assistance by means of fluid impulses

Fluid impulse techniques (e.g., fluctuations of the CSF) are used to send gentle impulses via the body fluids toward the site that is being treated, or to direct fluctuations toward that place in the body. A fluid impulse can be sent from the point opposite the location of the dysfunction.

A fluid impulse can also be delivered from the sacrum or from the foot of the contralateral side of the patient's body. Release of the restriction can also be assisted by dorsiflexion of the foot on the opposite side to the dysfunction, or dorsiflexion of both feet. When fluid impulses occur spontaneously in the body – as part of homeodynamic processes – these can also be utilized therapeutically to assist healing activity and regulatory processes.

Assistance by pulmonary breathing

Thoraco-abdominal breathing can be used to assist the release of restrictions. This technique arose as a result of experience, since it was found that the release of tissue restrictions often occurred at the end of the particular breathing phase, when coughing, or (in small children) when crying/screaming.

In a restriction of tissue mobility in inhalation (i.e., exhalation dysfunction), or an extension/internal rotation dysfunction, patients should be asked also to hold their breath for as long as possible at the end of exhalation. In a restriction of the mobility of an organ in exhalation (i.e., inhalation dysfunction), or a flexion/external rotation dysfunction patients should be asked also to hold their breath for as long as possible at the end of inhalation. The correction takes place at the end of the period of apnea, when the transition to spontaneous inhalation or exhalation occurs.

Note, breathing can sometimes, in the right circumstances, be used in such a way that a force is generated in the direction of the motion restriction (direct technique). To do this, in an exhalation dysfunction of a tissue, patients should be asked to hold their breath at the end of inhalation.

Assistance by the myofascial system

In extension/internal rotation dysfunctions, patients can be asked additionally to stretch their hands and feet (plantar flexion) during the exhalation phase of pulmonary breathing or independently of it. In flexion/external rotation dysfunctions, they can be asked additionally to bend their feet (dorsiflexion) during the inhalation phase of pulmonary breathing or independently of it.

The position of the patient is normally arranged so as to intensify the dysfunction of the tissue concerned (indirect): by means of rotation/sidebending of the head, or the positioning of the legs and trunk (sidebending, etc.).

Sometimes, the body can be positioned so as to induce a force in the direction of restricted mobility (direct technique).

Assistance by sensorimotor integration

Therapeutic interaction

Tuning in by the practitioner

- Sense your own bones, as elements involved in compression, and your soft tissues, as elements involved in tension.

- Stand with both feet firmly planted on the floor; if sitting, also position your seat bones firmly on the chair.

- Through your contact with the ground you will be aware of a force, which you feel rising up through your bones with an uplifting effect.

- You can strengthen this sensation by exerting a downward push with your muscles and feeling the reaction of pressure in your bones.

- This entire process lasts just around 10 seconds.

- You can direct your attention back to your own sensorimotor system from time to time during the treatment, whenever you need to, for example when carrying out manipulation of a joint of palpating the tensions in the body as a whole. Patients can be asked to move their fingers, feet, tongue, and eyes simultaneously to and fro while holding their breath.

Additional therapeutic methods There are many osteopathic techniques that are ideally suited to influencing the body's sensorimotor system; these include, among many others: body adjustment, general osteopathic treatment, harmonic technique. These are fully described in the osteopathic literature and do not therefore need to be detailed here.

Assistance by means of emotional, mental, and spiritual integration

In the state of balanced tension, integration of emotional, mental, and spiritual matters within the patient can take place. During palpation of developmental dynamic tension patterns or of other dysfunctions, or during balanced tension, certain retrograde/retroregressive recalls (e.g., pictures, words, sounds, kinesthetic sensations, etc.) or emotions (close body-related feelings such as anxiety, fear, anger, irritation, hate, desires, etc.) can occur. Similarly, on the mental level, symbolic and inner images can arise, as well as transrational higher archetypes or visions on the spiritual level. Usually the dysfunctional tissue qualities that can be palpated will be intensified.

If the inner resources of the patient are active and the patient is stable enough, the treatment can go on:

- The patient could be asked to remain present within the inner process, e.g., emotional, mental, or spiritual matter and/or to intensify the perception of whatever tissue sensations, emotions, images, etc., arise.

- Often bilateral stimulation, e.g., visual, kinesthetic or auditive is very helpful in this process.

- Alternatively or in addition, the osteopath is assisting the patient to complete his retrospections (kinesthetic, visual, auditive, smell, and gustative aspects of the event).

- Practitioner and patient can work together to put the matter into words to render it concrete and differentiate it. The patient will sense tissue dynamics as this is being done.

During this process the practitioner is present and in resonance to the tissue dynamics (and/or performs balanced tension), energetic compotents, and the patient as a whole. Spontaneously occurring disengagement at this stage is usually an indication that integration and transformation of the matter is taking place.

A differentiated method of emotional, mental, and spiritual integration is presented in the following text.

Emotional integration**

Psychological tension and stress lead to shallow, rapid breathing. If anxieties or suppressed aggression persist, this will then lead to a chronic change in respiratory motion.

Not all tissue dysfunctions are emotionally charged. A straightforward tissue dysfunction with no associated emotional element will be easier to resolve than one that is maintained or constantly renewed by a particular emotional charge or thought pattern. Patients can use their health problems as an opportunity to gain insight into their lives and see the connections between the circumstances of their lives, and their behavior, and the physical and psychological reactions.

During the approach to the tissue (see earlier), or palpation of a particular tissue, the osteopath palpates (for instance) increased resistance or a marked increase in tension. This tension may be linked with an emotion, e.g., anger or a deep sense of injustice.

Sometimes, during palpation, bodily sensations, memories, images, or situations linked to these emotions may arise in the patient (and/or in the osteopath). If the osteopath is unfamiliar with this feeling, or unable to integrate and accept it, this may lead to transference, i.e., the practitioner experiences a feeling of anger and may perhaps direct this toward the patient. It is also possible that practitioners will direct this anger at themselves.

According to Levin, there are four components to the experience of trauma: an exceptionally strong sense of agitation, psychophysical contraction, dissociation, and stiffening combined with a sense of helplessness.

Requirements for the integration of those parts within the patient that have become dissociated

1 A situation affording security to the patient, both within and outside of therapy. Providing this will sometimes require inner and external resources to be established, i.e., it will be necessary to stabilize the patient, provide familiar surroundings, integrate everyday life, etc.

2 Good, empathetic contact between practitioner and patient.

3 Patients need to be anchored in their resources and in their homeodynamic forces. If necessary, their inner and external resources may need to be expanded. Their defense strategies form part of their resources, so no attempt should be made to eliminate these. (This may also include identifying and acknowledging those parts within the patient that have no interest in working with suppressed unpleasant experiences.) Anchoring in this sense can be done in a number of different ways. One might be to ask patients to imagine a pleasant experience that makes them relaxed; it can be something that really happened, or an entirely imaginary experience. Another possible method is to direct patients' attention, just briefly, to various regions of the body, e.g., their breathing, heart rate, foot, abdomen, chest, or shoulders. It is important for this tour of the patients' attention to be a brief, fleeting one, since the contemplation can otherwise have the opposite effect and cause patients to plunge deeper into their traumatic experience.

4 There needs to be some capacity to halt the therapeutic process, for example by activating an anchor or by dual awareness; in this, patients learn to accept the inner reality of regressive emotions and at the same time anchor their consciousness in reality. This they can do by imagining a slightly stressful experience and registering their reaction in terms of bodily sensations and physiological aspects (heart, breathing, etc.). They are then asked to direct their attention toward present perceptions by their senses in the treatment room (items of furniture, colors, smells, temperature) and register that here there is nothing really to fear. Patients ultimately remain simultaneously conscious both of their immediate surroundings and regressive emotions and bodily sensations. Finally it is important to become anchored once more in the immediate present.

**see also Chapter 38

5 The effect of traumatic experiences is rather like a pressure cooker, which means that, when dealing with regressive traumatic experiences, the pressure should, as a rule, be reduced, not increased.

Therapeutic approach to the patient

(a) Practitioner The osteopath tries to hold the tissue tension in a kind of limbo with this feeling: to permit it. Success depends on the extent to which practitioners find themselves confronted by unmastered matters in their own consciousness. If this happens, it presents an additional challenge as well as an opportunity to allow integration to come about. If, at that moment, it is more than the osteopath can deal with or the emotion more than can be held in this suspended state of limbo, it is advisable to seek a different approach to the patient. Practitioners in this situation might alternatively choose to separate themselves emotionally from that tissue dysfunction. In this case, they should seek a neutral place from which they can work without being forced to react emotionally when confronted with these feelings.

(b) Patient According to Levine, every complete memory of an experience consists of the elements set out in the SIBAM model (Fig. 20.3): **S**ensation, **I**mage, **B**ehavior, **A**ffect (emotion), and **M**eaning. In traumatic situations, however, at least one element is separated-off, so that the experience can no longer be completely recalled to mind. The SIBAM model helps to resolve dissociation in patients in post-traumatic states, because it makes it possible to discover which elements of an experience have become dissociated, so that they can, if necessary, be re-integrated into the patient's consciousness.[36]

Healing occurs when all the elements of the experience become accessible once more, and inner experience and external facts about the experience are brought together. The somatic dysfunction should be brought into relation with SIBAM.

If there is an associated sensation such as anger during the approach to the tissue (see earlier in this chapter) or during palpation of somatic/visceral dysfunctions, the following steps can be applied:

1 Assess the autonomic state of the patient by:
   a Asking the patient to rate the following on a scale of -5–10: depressive/empty/impassive (-5) to quite calm (0) to maximum emotional agitation (10).

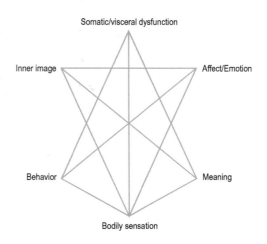

Figure 20.3
Somatic dysfunction and SIBAM.

   b Observation: the practitioner maintains observation throughout the therapy session.

In addition and if necessary, patients can also be asked about their state:

   c Strong arousal (Table 20.4) at the very latest is the moment when the therapeutic process must be halted (positive anchor; dual awareness, see earlier in this chapter). This can become necessary at any moment in the therapeutic interaction; otherwise there is a risk of retraumatizing the patient!
   d In the motionless or "frozen" state (Table 20.4), on the other hand, it is necessary to encourage the patient gently and carefully to participate again in the therapeutic process and become "alive" again; this can be done by gently stimulating the perception that patients have of sensation, and supporting them in the process. The following questions and statements can be helpful for this purpose:[37] I am here with you; can you feel that? Tell me how you feel. You don't need to hide. You are safe here; can you feel that you are? We won't continue until you're ready to let me. Remain in your heart. Everything's all right; it's OK.

Emotion	Sensation	Physical expression	Behavior	Expressed as
Sadness	Tears in the eyes Lump in the throat	Tears; eyes red	Weeping	Dissolving in tears
Anger	Tension, especially in jaw and shoulder	Tense lower jaw, reddened neck	Fighting, shouting	Becoming very red
Disgust	Nausea	Turning up nose, curling lip	Turning away	"I feel sick"
Happiness	Deep breathing, sighing	Eyes wide, eyebrows raised, trembling; pale	Laughing	Bursting with pleasure
Fear	Pounding heart, trembling	Cringing, rigid (with fear)	Running away, trembling	Butterflies in stomach
Shame	Feeling hot, especially in the face	Blushing, looking away	Hiding	Unable to look you in the eyes

TABLE 20.3: Emotion and body

After Rothschild.[35]

2 When asking the patient to recount the situation being recalled, this can be done in stages, which should follow in the order below. Patients experience an increasing degree of arousal as the account becomes more detailed.

a i. The patient is asked to name the situation being recalled, or the experience/trauma that accompanied it.

b ii. The patient enumerates the main events/occurrences

c iii. The patient recounts each in detail.

3 Step 2 can be omitted. In that case, the patient will begin directly to recount the experience. If all the requirements for proceeding safely are present, and if the patient's level of arousal is only slight, the osteopath can encourage the patient to say what feeling or emotion arises, to permit that feeling/emotion and, if appropriate, intensify it, along with the accompanying bodily sensations (e.g., tense, constricting feeling in the chest or region of the heart), inner images (sometimes also sounds, smells, or even a particular taste), behaviors (e.g., changes in depth of breathing, urinary urgency, swallowing, tensing of the jaw, neck, or upper abdomen, etc.) and the meaning or significance, that is, to arrive at an understanding of the circumstances of a particular experience. It is usually only when the meaning of a suppressed experience is seen and understood that integration becomes possible. The act of remaining with the accompanying, changing bodily sensations can help the patient to approach the suppressed situation.

4 The osteopath must hold the tissue tension in a kind of limbo, and take up contact with it without seeking to eliminate it. The contact, and the act of maintaining the state of the tissue in limbo, assists the achievement of awareness and the integration of the associated psychosomatic pattern. Healing occurs with the conscious linking together of all the aspects of the SIBAM tissue dysfunction complex, producing a kind of unwinding. The key to achieving this is to maintain this complex in that state of limbo without suppressing it.

	Autonomic state	Respiration, heart, skin, pupils, etc.	Patient
I. Relaxed state	Moderate activation of PSN	Breathing deep and easy, heart rate low, skin tonus normal	Calm and relaxed
II. (a) Slight arousal	SNS tone slightly to moderately raised	Respiratory/heart rate accelerated with normal skin color. Skin pale and slightly moist with normal respiratory/heart rate, pupils possibly slightly dilated	Joy or manageable unease
II. (b) Moderate hyperarousal	SNS tone markedly raised	Respiratory/heart rate accelerated with skin pallor, pupils slightly dilated	Difficulty in integrating therapeutic process or appearance of considerable fear
III. (c) Strong hyperarousal	Further rise in SNS tone	Respiratory/heart rate accelerated with skin pallor, pupils, cold sweat, etc., pupils dilated	No longer able to integrate
III. (d) Dangerous hyperarousal	SNS + PNS both markedly raised	Skin pale, with very low heart rate. Mydriasis with marked reddening of skin; very low heart rate with accelerated breathing; very slow breathing with markedly elevated heart rate	Strongly traumatized state
IV. Motionless state (frozen)	Strong activation of PNS	Patient motionless, immobile. Breathing slow and imperceptible, heart rate low, skin cool	Lack of participation, withdrawal from therapeutic process and own body, depressive, weary, withdrawn, dissociated

TABLE 20.4: Autonomic nervous system and condition of patient[35]

PNS, parasympathetic nervous system; SNS, sympathetic nervous system. See also polyvagal theory according to Porges, Chapter 37. After Rothschild.[35]

If certain parts of the experience are not accessible to them, patients should be supported in re-experiencing and integrating these dissociated parts; however, in doing so the practitioner should ensure that these patients are not retraumatized.

This may not yet be entirely possible at that particular time. If this is the case, the tissue will react to the practitioner's contact with increased tension, and may "freeze" or appear more lifeless. The osteopath should on no account respond to this by applying increased pressure. The correct response should be to sense the tension and hold this reaction by the body in a kind of limbo (see also step 1). In a similar way, it may be too much for the patient to hold an emotion, such as anger, for example, in such a suspended state of limbo, and they may then sense suppression of anger. The osteopath must in no way try to forcefully hasten the process. Consciousness has its own rhythms of operating, acting like a light that illuminates and dissolves the shadow. Unwinding is a natural process. The symptoms and tissue tensions are the expression of a pattern, a combination of SIBAM and specific physiological reactions.

The practitioner needs to sense the way in which they are combined to form that pattern, to recognize it, and not to force the release of the tension and restriction. Instead, what the practitioner must do is to comprehend the pattern and discover the mechanisms that maintain it. This is an organic process, to bring together apparently unconnected phenomena. It is all too easy, under the pressure of patients' desire to be rid of these unpleasant symptoms, to feel we must respond and simply do just that: relieve the symptoms. This, however, would be more like an allopathic treatment method using manual techniques in place of an analgesic for the same end result. The desire to bring about health should not lead us to compel health by force, but to discover the patterns that maintain the disease, so as to make room for health. The situation is the same when dealing with a complex of somatoemotional tension. Meaningful touch is touch that forges a link; that enables insight to arise through touch. There is no particular recipe for achieving this; no purposeful tuning in to certain deeper rhythms. Rather, the procedure and the course of tension release are determined by the capacity of practitioner and patient to achieve integration. This is a process that develops; an organic, intuitive recognition of associations on a non-intellectual level; and an evolving awareness/perception that increasingly acquires the confidence to look at what is there. This always happens in interaction with the patient. It does however also call for specific memories, i.e., facts, to relate what was experienced to the patient's past in a meaningful way to see where it belongs.

Mental integration

Tuning in by the practitioner

A first step toward calmness and equanimity of mind can be achieved by way of the biological level through regular, conscious breathing. This does not usually resolve deep-seated mental or spiritual dysfunctional patterns of mental conditioning, however. The converse, a shift of consciousness into the noosphere, does often exert effects not only on the subtle energies of the noosphere (i.e., the spiritual level), but also on the vital energies of the biosphere, and on such matters as the rhythms of breathing.

Energy follows thought, whether such thoughts are unconscious, half-conscious, or conscious. Disciplined concentration can be a means of consciously directing vital energy in the therapeutic interaction. Through concentration, the practitioner can directly enter the noosphere and enable resonance to come about. In concentration, the mind is focused on an external object or inner idea, and all other thoughts excluded. A number of methods may be used, but it takes the practitioner many years to gradually achieve a degree of competence, because clear and increasing concentration requires deconditioning from restrictive dysfunctional beliefs, emotional patterns, self-images, etc. Exclusively applying techniques of concentration brings the risk of fading out or suppressing unwanted, unpleasant issues present in the mind, or forcing them down into deeper levels of consciousness instead of experiencing and accepting them, differentiating and integrating them.

The consciousness exercise presented below provides one method of differentiating, integrating, and transcending mental hindrances and opens up a gentle, conscious means of access to the noosphere.

We are all, to a greater or lesser degree, faced with experiences and elements in our consciousness that are unpleasant and tend to produce anxiety. Osteopaths find themselves in just the same situation as their patients in this respect. Our own inner growth is closely connected with our understanding and acceptance, ability to deal with, integrate, and achieve mastery over experiences and elements of consciousness of this kind. We can decide to confront these challenges consciously and deliberately, or to run away from them and compensate, perhaps with food, alcohol, smoking, excessive consumption, sex or television watching, or exaggerated endeavors to be needed or to be acknowledged, achieve power or money. Running away and compensating both have the effect, not only of maintaining the inner discord and separation from our deeper selves, but of placing a burden on the body and person as a whole, the people around us and our environment. On the other hand compensating is also an important ability in life. Everyone wants to be healthy and whole and at one with themselves, or at least to become so. (If we trace the words "healing" and "wholeness" back to their origins, we find that they embrace all these meanings.) Osteopaths who seek to integrate the forces of the mind for the purposes of healing have the challenge – on this as on other levels – to perceive and integrate their own dissonances. It is in this labor of consciousness that the potential lies which will enable us to master the forces of the mind, and these forces will become available to the extent that the osteopath makes it a reality. As they become increasingly available, so it becomes more possible to integrate parts of the emotional, mental/psychological, and higher mental/psychological fields into treatment. Without this labor of consciousness, a certain dissonance will always still be apparent and will be evident in the practitioner's therapeutic work; inevitably, the motive force behind it will be a technocratic, manipulative one instead of inner awareness and insight. (This is quite irrespective of whether the practitioners describe their therapeutic work as "holistic" or "spiritual" or any such term.)

The following consciousness exercise assists the process of "becoming whole" and the integration of all parts; even those parts of the self that are unconscious or as yet unaccepted. (Patients can also be taught to perform the exercise.)

- Sit on a chair, with both feet in full contact with the floor and both seat bones in good contact with the chair.

- Your spine should be erect and relaxed. Your chin should be slightly retracted and your cervical spine gently extended.

- If you have very good mobility in your legs, you can adopt a lotus or half-lotus position on the floor instead, placing a firm cushion under your seat so that both knees are flat against the floor. This sitting position ensures stability and a relaxed, upright spine.

- Gently direct your attention toward the breathing motion of your chest and abdomen, or of your nostrils, as you inhale and exhale. You should decide to concentrate on one or the other, either chest and abdomen, or nostrils, but switch your attention to and fro between them.

- Whenever you sense your attention wandering away, take mental note of the fact and exercise mindfulness as you carefully direct your attention back to your breathing. Try to acknowledge the thoughts, simply recognizing their existence and then letting go of them and returning to your breathing.

- It is quite normal to find your thoughts wandering, influenced by past experiences, and conditioning. It is not something that you can or should prevent. Each time you notice your thoughts drifting away and bring them back to your breathing, you are in a moment of mindfulness. This process is at the same time a gentle means of deconditioning.

Obstacles may tend to make their appearance during this mindfulness exercise as:

1 Dissociation, rejection, aversion, and hatred (of self or others)

2 Desire of all kinds (including expectations as to what feelings this mindfulness exercise should evoke)

3 Fear, anxiety, and unease

4 Sluggishness and weariness

5 Doubt.

When your attention wanders, use the opportunity to identify and acknowledge these energies, and then redirect your attention back to your breathing. The usual reaction to these is to allow our minds to become befuddled by them, either becoming preoccupied with them and losing ourselves in them, or reacting in rejection. In this exercise, however, we learn to recognize the basic pattern of certain states of mind at a very early stage, just as they are taking shape, to perceive their effect on mind and body, observe the energy that accompanies them, and discover that they are transient. If our response is neither to suppress them nor to lose ourselves in them, we gain in attentiveness and gradually come to comprehend their true nature. This gives us increasing sympathy for the suffering produced by the limits of these states, and the ability to accept them, to let go of them, integrate and transform them. This process enables you, in your role as practitioner, to recognize similar states of mind and emotional patterns in the patient in a value-free way, and to make contact with them in an adequate manner. At first it is only possible to register theses obstacles once we have been caught up in them for a while. Practice, however, develops the presence of mind to spot and counter them at an even earlier stage, exercising mindfulness.

If possible, this mindfulness exercise should be performed for 10–60 minutes, once or twice a day. It is best to perform it at the same time each day. You should either finish or begin the exercise by imagining yourself and the people closest to you, your friends and enemies, and say aloud or silently to yourself the following sentences:

May I/... learn, practice, and develop techniques, the tools and methods of mental/spiritual development, to enable me/..., to understand, accept, and overcome the difficulties and challenges of life. May I/... find inner peace.

Therapeutic approach to the patient

If symbolic images, inner images, or belief models on the intellectual level arise in the patient's consciousness, the osteopath can integrate these using a method such as that given below.

Spiritual (causal) integration

Tuning in by the practitioner

Practitioners can establish resonance with the causal consciousness and energy of patients by attuning to a causal fulcrum or to their own spirituality, e.g., the potential emptiness, the effective principle of love in the cosmos, the Christian Trinity of Father, Son and Holy Spirit, their own true self (Atman), etc.

Therapeutic interaction

The practitioner creates a realm for the causal: a region of experience encompassing the associated body, the huge background against which all problems are "relative" in the truest sense of the word, or dwindle to non-existence, and the individual's experience of existence extends into infinity.

The route to this, in the waking state, is that of radical testimony. If practitioners are to be able to assist their patients to consciously experience this realm, they first need to have had some degree of experience in the causal state. Synchronization with the "long/large tide" may perhaps offer some possibility of a technical version of this means of access.

Additional treatment approaches

Complex waveforms according to Abehsera

Modern physics was confronted by the paradox that matter, at its most elementary level, can take the apparent form of particles or of a field of energy waves. According to Abehsera, if this insight is transferred to the human body, each region can be seen as a collection of minute particles, or as complex waveforms, e.g., a wave-like liver.

These complex waveforms cannot be palpated directly using the hands, so the position of the hands is not critical. To establish contact with these, the osteopath creates a holographic image of the structure concerned (joint, ligament, muscle, organ, blood vessel, nerve, or suture) of the patient and projects this image, created as it were of pure thought-waves, so that it is held in the osteopath's hands. Via this image the osteopath can sense rhythms, abnormal dysfunctional patterns of the structure concerned, and can correct them according to the therapeutic principles already described (PBT, direct and indirect techniques, etc.), applying them to the holographic image. Abehsera found the results to be more effective, when the creation of the hologram was more precise. Sensing at this level makes it easier to register and influence the interaction of the organ with other parts of the body as a whole. The great advantage of this approach is that the flow of information between organs can be influenced directly.

Treatment of the chakras**

Tuning in by the practitioner As a means of tuning in to prepare for treatment, osteopaths can direct their attention to their own chakras, intensifying their presence for the individual centers of energy and consciousness. This should always be done beginning with the first chakra and ending with the seventh; for each, you should sense the direction of rotation and qualities of that spiral of energy and its gross, subtle, and causal aspects. You can assist the process by breathing into the individual chakras. It is also helpful to visualize the color of the particular chakra. After examining the patient's chakras, you can begin the treatment.

Physical alignment of the chakras

It is not uncommon to find lateral or vertical positioning of the chakras. Physical alignment can be a useful first step, especially to help harmonize the association between subtle and gross expression. Of course, this does not suddenly bring about a leap from one of the seven levels of development to the next without any actual consciousness work.

Chakra alignment can be achieved by gently bringing the spine upright. Meanwhile, the person's feet should

---

**see also Chapters 25 and 26

press downward onto the floor, and, in the sitting position, the seat bones should also be pressed down onto the chair. The practitioner can induce this alignment by means of gentle craniad traction with the patient in the supine or sitting position.

Cleansing, harmonizing, and strengthening the chakras

Place your hands on the various locations of the chakras, 10–90 cm away from the patient's body surface (or even directly on the surface of the body).

Hand contact Direct the palm of your hand toward the opening of the particular chakra. Hold it 10–90 cm away from the patient's body surface or place it directly on the surface of the body (you should if possible avoid doing this at the level of the perineum). The contact can be made using any of several possible options:

- Version 1: place the palm of your right hand on the chakra to be treated, from in front. For the first chakra, the palm of your hand should be 10–90 cm caudal to the perineum, palm facing the craniad. For the seventh chakra the palm of your hand should be 10–90 cm cranial to the top of the patient's head or resting on it, facing caudad.

- Version 2: place the palms of your right and left hand side-by-side, index fingers in contact, and thumbs crossed. The palms of both hands should face toward the chakra, from in front. (For the first and seventh chakras, positioned as for version 1.)

- Version 3: place the palm of your right hand on the chakra to be treated, from in front, and the palm of your left hand on the chakra from behind. In this version, energy is directed from the palm of the right hand dorsally from in front to the left hand. (For the first and seventh chakras, positioned as for version 1.)

Method

- Approach the physical body of the person until you encounter slight resistance or a sense of presence and contact. What is felt at each chakra is a kind of sphere of energy or rotating swirl of energy.

- With your hand, or with both hands, follow the direction, rotation, or movement that you sense in the chakra. You may be able to gently intensify the movement you sense. (If, at the beginning of treatment, the chakra is rotating anti-clockwise, you may well find that the direction of rotation changes at a particular moment in the treatment, and it begins to spin clockwise.

- At the same time, the presence of weak chakras can be supported and strengthened by flow of energy. Breathing techniques are another form of assistance (see p. 355).

- When dealing with a blocked chakra, you can direct energy into it. You should inhale and visualize the color of the chakra. Energy and color flow from the palm of your hand into the chakra as you breathe out.

- Dammed-up energy can be drawn out.

Balancing the chakras

Hand contact Place the palm of your right hand on the chakra with too much energy, and the left on the chakra with reduced energy.

Method The balance of energy between the chakra with excess energy and the chakra with reduced energy is brought back into equilibrium.

Note, the chakra system is a concept based on tradition and experience. In this concept we can assume that the chakras are already present and able to function in the child from birth, although still in immature form. Development normally occurs over the whole course of life, and even in advanced age it is exceptional for them to be complete in the causal and subtle planes. The idea that developmental processes, in the sense of the shift of the person's main focus of perception and consciousness or worldview from one chakra to the next, takes place over a period of many years, becomes easy to comprehend when we view the chakras as a model of developmental stages. As a result, this process, which embraces all areas of the patient's life, goes far beyond the methods presented for the treatment of the chakras. The primary purpose of treatment of the chakras is to assist their basic function. The treatment described

Chakra	Color	Location	Chakra opening
Muladhara	Red	Perineum	Caudad
Svadhisthana	Orange	Approx.. 3 cm below navel	Anteriorly
Manipura	Yellow	Between navel and solar plexus	Anteriorly
Anahata	Emerald green	Heart/sternum area	Anteriorly
Vishuddha	Blue or turquoise	Neck	Anteriorly
Ajna	Purple or indigo	Centrally between eyebrows	Anteriorly
Sahasrara	White	Highest point of head	Craniad

TABLE 20.5: Differentiation of chakras

Energy field	Distance of outer edge from body surface
Subtle	
Etheric (vital)	Approximately 1–7 cm
Astral (emotional)	Approximately 40 cm
Mental	Approximately 90 cm
Causal	90–110 cm

TABLE 20.6: Differentiation of energy fields

above cannot replace the development of consciousness in the patient, but can support and encourage that development.

Strengthening and cleansing the fields of energy

Delivering energy from the feet

Preliminary exercise for the osteopath You may allow your arm to hang loosely. As you do so, direct your attention toward the physical sensation, as though water is flowing down your arm. Eventually you begin to feel increasing pressure in your hand. You experience a similar sensation when transmitting energy through your hands. When you sense this, you are ready to allow energy to flow via your hands.

Position of the practitioner Place your feet securely on the floor, because you take in energy from the earth through your feet. You can aid this by imagining roots reaching down from the soles of your feet (and from your coccyx) to the center of the earth. If you are carrying out the treatment from a sitting position, your seat bones should be in firm contact with the seat and your spine should be upright. Your chin should be drawn slightly toward your chest, and you should feel as if a cord is attached to the top of your head and pulling it gently upward.

Method

- Allow energy to flow into your body and flow through you. Your role is simply to be a channel for the energy. You also need to establish a link between you and the universal field of energy.

- Breathing assistance can help to raise vital energy to the necessary level. As you breathe in, sense the way energy rises from the earth through your feet, on upward through your legs, pelvis, and the center of your body to your head; then, as you breathe out, feel it flowing down the sides of your head and into your shoulders, arms, and hands.

- Let energy flow through your hands into the patient's feet and onward into the whole of the patient's body.

- The energy will automatically spread to those places where it is needed, through the body's natural channels.

- Sense the cleansing, clearing, and strengthening of the patient's field. Often, what you sense will be, for example, that increased energy begins to flow on one side of the patient's body, and then evens out.

- If the energy declines again, that is, if the flow of energy in your hands becomes less, it is best to release your hands.

Harmonization of the energy fields (Table 20.6)

- Direct your attention and your presence toward the energy fields concerned.

- With your hands, palpate the outer boundary and shape of the energy field you are addressing.

- Correct any distortions, instances of unevenness, hollows, constrictions, bulges, dark patches, areas of thickening or of thinning, tears, or holes. This correction is performed using your hands, by direct technique at the location concerned. For example, you would smooth down a bulge, or draw out a hollow place.

- You then comb through the entire aura with your fingers, perpendicularly to the surface of the patient's body, working outward from a point close to the skin to the periphery of the aura. The palms of your hands should face outward as you do this. Begin at the patient's feet and work upward to finish at the top of the patient's head.

- Finally you can strengthen the outer skin of the aura by focusing on the patient's crown chakra, cradling the outer skin in your hand, and letting white light flow into the aura. Continue until the person's entire body is bathed in an ovoid field of white light.

- At the end of the harmonization it is important to re-separate your own energy field from that of your patient. This is done as follows: as the patient inhales, you should move your hands and yourself outward, out of the patient's field, and give a quick shake with your hands. It is all the more important to do this if your energy field and that of the patient have merged at all during the treatment.

Note: the description of energy fields is only a working model - as are most of the treatment principles in this chapter. If you sense differently from the description, please experiment with it and adapt it.

Treatment of fields of nonphysical energy: morphogenetic, intention and consciousness, synchronicity

Hand position The hand position is not critical. One possibility is for you to place your hand on the structure to be treated, to make it easier to sense that structure. However, it is also possible to work without hand contact.

Method

- Direct gentle attentiveness toward the structure concerned. It is very important that the practitioner should not be tense or apply excessively invasive intention when working. The approach needed is more one of opening up to the structure to be treated, tuning in to it and harmonizing with it. Do not perform the technique if no image of the structure appears or if the procedure involves a great deal of effort.

- When the structure concerned appears in your consciousness, note as many details about it as possible.

- Silently ask questions of this structure: Do you agree to let me make contact with you? If the reaction you sense is a rejection, do not perform the technique at this time.

- If the reaction you sense is one of consent, silently ask the structure to be treated to let go completely and express what is preventing it from achieving a better state of balance.

- While you maintain contact with this structure, permit all the images, words, and other phenomena that appear in your consciousness. Do not try to retain these or to assess or interpret them.

- At this point you may enter into direct dialog with the patient. Invite the patient to express openly to you all the emotions, sensations, or images, and all the tastes, scents, and sounds that they perceive inwardly.

- Continue to permit all this to happen until the images and phenomena come to rest, or until they reflect balance and harmony.

- At the end, direct a nonverbal question to the structure, asking it whether it needs anything else to make it healthy and happy.

- If effort becomes evident during the process, or if tension arises, you should bring the technique to an end. Similarly, you should bring the technique to an end if you sense a force rejecting or pushing you away.

- Sometimes you will find that you can continue the technique in subsequent sessions.

- If certain stress-laden phenomena occur, you can enter into direct dialog with them. Begin by asking their permission to make contact with them. If this is accepted, you can begin to ask questions about how they originated, their motives and, how they are related to the affected structure or to the patient.

Advice relating to treatment, end points of treatment, and reactions to treatment

Advice relating to treatment

At every moment of the treatment, the practitioner should give particular attention to the needs and reactions of the patient. The following sensations are indications that you should end the treatment currently being given:

- A qualitative hardening of the patient's tissues, like the putting on of armor and a sense of being rejected or pushed away.

- A sensation of losing contact with the patient as a whole. In this situation, it is helpful to listen, concentrating down into your own stillness, and silently (or in actual words) ask yourself what is happening at that moment and what the patient needs just then.

If you suddenly begin to sense rapid pulsations moving laterally to and fro, this usually indicates that you are palpating too invasively. You should reduce the physical pressure you are applying, and relax your intention and concentration. It also helps to change the palpation site.

Following a treatment session, the patient should be given the chance to rest for a moment on the treatment table, and should also be advised to take things as easy as possible even after leaving, and to avoid stressful situations. The body and person as a whole are more sensitive and vulnerable following a treatment session. It is all too easy to hinder, reduce, or disturb the integration of changes that have occurred during the treatment, or the continuing processes still taking place afterwards and their positive effects. Some time is evidently needed for these new experiences to become integrated and established in the body and person as a whole, both physically and psychologically.

The natural end point of a treatment session

In order to sense when the end of a session is reached, the requirement is a fundamental attitude that is non-invasive and does not seek to force the body and person as a whole in a particular direction. Instead, the attitude should be one of synchronization with the homeodynamic forces in the body as a whole.

The following points can help to sense the end point of a treatment session:

- The support of downregulation of the patient in the beginning of the treatment process.

- A consciousness that rests in the present[38] and awareness for the needs of the patient.

- Synchronization with homeodynamic forces in the patient.v

- The ability to sense whether the patient is "rebalanced" at the end of treatment.

- The appearance of balanced, good, and even amplitude and frequency rhythmic dynamics for at least three cycles is an indication of the end point of a treatment session.

- Reharmonization techniques can be carried out at the end of the treatment session so as to avoid the emergence of side effects. Reharmonization is especially helpful when motion barriers have been confronted during the treatment, or when there has been over-treatment, e.g., CV-4 (or EV-4), gentle disengagement at various central regions especially the cranial base, at C0/C1, L5/S1, without confronting any motion barriers,[38] midline techniques, and Robert Fulford's technique for treating the solar plexus.

Reactions to treatment

Changes during the period following treatment are very informative for the osteopath. Interpreting these changes is important for the ongoing course of treatment and for prognosis.

The healing reactions begin during the therapeutic interaction, but continue afterwards, over a period that can vary from a few hours to several days or even months. The course of the disorder may revert from chronic to acute. There can be further differentiation in changes that have occurred during treatment, and/or these changes may become integrated into the body and person as a whole and into patients' everyday lives. There may be further changes. Unwinding of dysfunctional bound energies occurs, and there is change in the relationship between various parts on a variety of different levels of structure and function (endocrine, vascular, autonomic, fascial, postural, etc.). These developments can also be accompanied by new patterns of perception and consciousness in the patient and can perhaps bring changes and new insights in daily life and in family and work environments.

Reaction to treatment	Interpretation
Symptom-free interval (or of reduction in the symptoms), which increases with each treatment	• Positive healing course, esp. with increase in patient's general state of well being, sense of meaning and consciousness
Temporary deterioration without improvement	• Condition reverts to previous state → primary dysfunction complex was not resolved • May have been brought about by contact and intention that was too forceful, forced, invasive, or otherwise inadequate, by wrongly directed application of traction, wrong hand position, or failure to treat associated patterns of tension in other regions
Temporary deterioration and signs of regression with improvement	• Part of the healing process • Patient should be informed of this possibility. Patient should if possible avoid taking any medicines without discussing this first • Previous, suppressed conditions (disturbances, pain, or emotions) (e.g., by medication or manual therapy) can reappear, existing ones exacerbate slightly, or new symptoms appear briefly • Signs of detoxification

	• Chronic clinical picture can revert to acute • Symptoms can also form part of the necessary period of instability that enables old, now inadequate patterns of order to disintegrate and a new structure or order to develop • Improvement after a few days: indicates treatment of a primary dysfunction complex
Distant reaction	• Symptoms at a distant site may indicate site of a primary dysfunction
Immediate freedom from symptoms, lasting at least 1 day	• It is helpful to repeat treatment at the same site. This should have the effect of lengthening the symptom-free period • If symptom-fee period lasts longer, this probably indicates that a primary dysfunction complex was treated
Immediate freedom from symptoms, lasting a few hours, followed by immediate return of symptoms	• Treatment of symptoms, e.g., ◊ temporary release of secondary dysfunction ◊ temporary transference phenomenon brought about by practitioner ◊ reaction-resistance on the part of the patient, caused by other factors (nutrition, psyche, life circumstances, etc.)
Delayed reaction (Improvement 1 day to 3 weeks later)	• If this lasts for at least several days, this indicates that a primary dysfunction was treated
Signs of a process tending toward health	• Improvement in general state of health, subjective well-being and general mood (despite appearance of possible temporary symptoms) • Improvement in general psychoemotional/spiritual well-being • Improvement in energy (calmer and more relaxed, greater energy and élan, happier, etc.) • Improvement/lessening of limitation of everyday life caused by symptoms, or more positive subjective interpretation of that limitation • Improvement in clinical symptoms in everyday life

TABLE 20.7: Reactions to treatment

Box 20.8

Possible causes of treatment complications

- Contact and intention that was too forceful, forced, invasive or otherwise inadequate

- Wrongly directed application of traction, compression etc.

- Practitioner's use of wrong hand position

- Failure to treat associated patterns of tension in other regions

- Excessive demands placed on capacity of patient's body and person as a whole for integration, e.g., by failing to respect natural end point of treatment, by resolving dysfunctions without establishing resonance with body and person as a whole, or by over-treatment

- Destabilization by removal of compensatory functional areas

- Desynchronization of patient

- Tissues led too much toward the limit of motion, or manipulations performed in the direction of the motion barrier[38]

References

[1]Bochurberg C: Une approche ostéopathique de l'angoisse. Paris: Maloine; 1988:66.

[1a]Boss M: Grundriss der Medizin und Psychologie. 3. Aufl., Bern: Hans Huber; 1999.

[2]Forrest CB: A living systems perspective on health. Medical Hypotheses; 2014: 82: 209–214.

[3]Still AT: Autobiography of A. T. Still. Indianapolis: American Academy of Osteopathy; 1981:182.

[4]Habecker M: Personal correspondence. 5/2005.

[5]Harvey J: Total relaxation. Healing practices for body, mind and spirit. New York: Kodansha America; 1998.

[6]Becker RE: In: Brooks RE (ed.): The stillness of life. Portland: Stillness Press; 2000:15, 16.

[7]Becker RE: In: Brooks RE (ed.): The stillness of life. Portland: Stillness Press; 2000:66, 67.

[8]Sutherland WG: Contributions of Thought. Sutherland Cranial Teaching Foundation. 1967:153, 208, 244f.

[9]Sutherland WG: Teachings in the Science of Osteopathy. Sutherland Cranial Teaching Foundation; 1991:14, 46.

[10]Sutherland WG: Contributions of thought. 2nd edn. Sutherland Cranial Teaching Foundation; 1998:238.

[11]Becker RE: Be still and know. A Dedication to William G. Sutherland D.O. Cranial Academy Newsletter. 1965;12:6.

[12]Sutherland WG: Teachings in the Science of Osteopathy. Sutherland Cranial Teaching Foundation; 1991:285.

[13]Sutherland WG: Contributions of thought. Sutherland Cranial Teaching Foundation; 1967:215.

[14]Becker RE: In: Brooks RE (ed.): The stillness of life. Portland: Stillness Press; 2000:8.

[15]Becker RE: Diagnostic touch: Its principles and application, Part I. AAO Yearbook; 1963:35.

[16]Sutherland WG: Contributions of thought. Sutherland Cranial Teaching Foundation; 1967:244f.

[17]Sutherland WG: Contributions of thought. Sutherland Cranial Teaching Foundation; 1967:166.

[18]Sutherland WG: Contributions of thought. Sutherland Cranial Teaching Foundation; 1967:153, 208.

[19]Magoun HI: Osteopathy in the cranial field. Kirksville: Journal Printing Company; 1951:59.

[20]Becker RE: In: Brooks RE (ed.): The stillness of life. Portland: Stillness Press; 2000: 66, 67, 69.

[21]Becker RE: In: Brooks RE (ed.): The stillness of life. Portland: Stillness Press; 2000: 68, 70.

[22]Becker RE: In: Brooks RE (ed.): The stillness of life. Portland: Stillness Press; 2000: 71.

[23]Becker RE: In: Brooks RE (ed.): The stillness of life. Portland: Stillness Press; 2000: 68, 70, 72.

[24]Becker RE: In: Brooks RE (ed.): The stillness of life. Portland: Stillness Press; 2000: 69.

[25]Becker RE: In: Brooks RE (ed.): The stillness of life. Portland: Stillness Press; 2000: 70, 71, 72.

[26]Jealous J: The Patient's Neutral No. 1. (audio CD series) 2001. Marnee Jealous Long, 6501 Blackfin Way, Apollo Beach, FL 33572, mjlong@tampabay.rr.com.

[27]Gordon R: Quantum Touch. Berkeley, CA, USA: North Atlantic Books; 2006. München: Goldmann; 2005: 74f.

[28]Chikly B: Theory and practice of lymph drainage therapy. An osteopathic lymphatic technique. 2nd edn. I.H.H. Publishing, 2004.

[29]Miller A: Pandura and Endura: The core-link twins. Oakland, California.

[30]Liem T: Cranial Osteopathy: A practical textbook. Seattle: Eastland Press; 2009:404ff.

[31]Jealous J: Automatic shifting. 2/1989.

[32]Chauffour P, Prat E: Mechanical Link, Florida: North Atlantic Books; 2002:46–52.

[33]Rothschild B: The body remembers. New York: Norton Professional Books; 2000.

Der Körper erinnert sich. Essen: Synthesis; 2002: 91f, 163f.

[34]Levine PA: The body as healer: transforming trauma and anxiety. Lyons, CO.

[35]Chikly B: Brain tissue, nuclei, fluid and autonomic nervous system. Hamburg: Course notes, Osteopathie Schule Deutschland; 2005.

[36]Jealous J: The Biodynamics of Osteopathy. Rebalancing. Nos 1,2 (audio CD series), 2001. Marnee Jealous Long, 6501 Blackfin Way, Apollo Beach, FL 33572, mjlong@tampabay.rr.com.

21

Total rhythmic balanced interchange according to Becker

Torsten Liem

I have but one law for all my opposed pairs of creating things: and that law needs but one word to spell it out, so hear me when I say that the one word of My one law is balance

And if man needs two words to aid him in his knowing of the workings of that law, let those two words be balanced interchange

If man still needs more words to aid his knowing of My one law, give to him another one, and let those three words be rhythmic balanced interchange

W. Russell1 (quoted by R.E. Becker)

Introduction

Becker's approach is not limited to treating the cranial structures, but represents one of the principles of osteopathic treatment.

Fulcrum point technique[2]

The special characteristic of this technique is that hardly any pressure is exerted on the tissue of the patient. The amount of pressure exerted by the hands placed on the patient remains the same, irrespective of whether they are palpating and treating superficial structures or deep structures of the tissue.

In order to establish resonance with the forces in the tissue, the osteopath uses a fulcrum or fixed point, established using another part of the practitioner's arm on the treatment table, to alter the pressure exerted. This pressure on the fulcrum enables the practitioner to perceive and treat structures deep inside the body or induce inherent activity in the tissue without increasing the pressure of the hands on the patient's body.

Method

- Place your hand on the tissues to be treated. The elbow or lower arm of the same hand should rest either on the treatment table or on your knee or thigh.

- This creates the fulcrum or fixed point. The exact position is whichever feels most relaxed.

- Increase the pressure by means of this point, to whatever extent is needed to direct your hand to the tissue depth required. If you want to project it to superficial tissue, the pressure at the fulcrum will remain light. If it is to reach farther down into the tissue, increase the pressure of your fulcrum (hand or elbow) on the treatment table. The pressure of your hand on the patient remains unchanged, but your hand follows the inherent motions or tensions of the tissue.

- Palpate the gentle give and take in the tissue. The therapeutic fulcrum position is directed towards the surrounding energy and towards the osteopathic dysfunction.

- Once you have established the fulcrum position, you can exert gentle compression.

As you maintain the fulcrum position, a 3-phase (or 4-phase) process usually occurs. The osteopath's attention is especially important for the success of the treatment (see also below):

- First, use your hands to establish resonance with the state of tension and energy in the tissue. In effect, your hands assume a support function for the ligaments/membranes/fasciae/fluids and also the energies and fulcrums.

- The energy fields and the tissues involved move and act according to their specific pattern towards the point of balance of that pattern. With respect to the ligaments, this corresponds to the situation memorably described by Anne Wales as "the ligaments go shopping."

- A kind of functional still point comes into being. In it, all movements appear to come to rest. At that moment, when the potency enters the focus, a change takes place: "something happens."

- There may then be a kind of unwinding process.

- Motion can be palpated once more, and the dysfunctional pattern has changed in the direction of normalization and health. The tissues that had previously been dysfunctional now orient themselves again to natural fulcrums and to the midline. Palpation detects a clear increase in the ability to vibrate in syntony* with rhythmic oscillations. The previously dysfunctional fulcrums are resolved.

Modified rhythmic balanced interchange techniques (RBIT) according to Becker[3]

These RBI techniques utilize the energy and resources of the physiology of the patient's body for the purposes of diagnosis and treatment. This comprises all the soft and hard tissues and body fluids.

The practitioner evaluates the rhythmic motions in relation to space and time. This provides a means of exploring the state of health of the body's physiology. These techniques enable the body to initiate healing processes to resolve the sequelae of trauma or other pathogenic states.

Indication

RBI techniques are used for the purpose of making contact with the physiological and anatomical needs of the tissue in health, in disease, or following trauma, and to set off healing reactions.

Localization of the region to be treated

See under diagnosis (Chapter 18).

---

*'Syntony' means resonance or a state of being responsive to and in harmony with the environment.

Hand position

Place your hands on and/or under the place to be treated.

Method

- Establishment of the fulcrum and of resonance: use your hands to establish resonance with the state of tension and energy in the tissue. Create a fulcrum on the basis of the patient's body physiology. The place at which the fulcrum is established is the location of the potency and the stillness (this is characteristic of all fulcrums) that the patient's body physiology can utilize. Exert moderate, controlled compression on the tissues to be treated.

- Support function: your hands take over the function of support to the ligaments/membranes/fasciae/fluids and also the energies and fulcrums.

- Increase in inherent motions: the energy fields and tissues concerned move or act according to their specific pattern toward the point of balance of that pattern. With respect to the ligaments, this corresponds to the situation memorably described by Anne Wales as "the ligaments go shopping."

- Adapt your hands to the dynamic changes in the tissues or to the tension/energy patterns.

- The conscious palpatory contact does two things: it senses the increasing RBI activity in the affected tissue, and is also part of the process. In a certain sense the practitioner's hands come to resemble these processes. The resonance engendered produces a similar effect to that in homeopathy, when the effects of the remedy coincide with the patient's symptoms.

- Functional still point: the inherent motions appear to cease. As the practitioner, you eventually sense the RBI activity bringing about a shifting of the potency.

- At that moment, when the potency enters the focus, a change takes place: "something happens." This is accompanied by a change in the pattern of the RBI activity of the affected tissue. A better state of balance is established for the particular tension/energy pattern.

- The fulcrum that you have established with your treating hand, which is associated with relative stillness and potency, is like the relative stillness that appears in the best possible state of balance of the tension/energy pattern of the tissue.

- Maintain the contact until the shift of the potency is complete and the RBI activity of the affected tissue indicates a change in that tissue tending toward healthier functioning and interaction in body physiology and improved dynamic balance.

- Motion can again be sensed: the dysfunctional pattern has changed in the direction of normalization and health. The previously dysfunctional tissues have re-ordered themselves to relate again to natural fulcrums and to the midline. Palpation detects a clear increase in the ability to vibrate in concert with rhythmic oscillations. The previously dysfunctional fulcrum is resolved.

- The time needed for this change to occur depends on the qualities and potency of the tissue concerned and of the body as a whole.

- You can now release hand contact, and if necessary move on to treat another dysfunctional region.

- Your attention should be directed towards the interrelationships between the structures and functions. Palpate whether there is a connection between the tissue that was initially treated and the tissue to be treated next, and assess the nature of that connection. You should also sense the relationship of both to the body as a whole.

Summary

- Establishment of fulcrum, resonance, support function: induce activity in the tissue

- Accompany into new state of balance

- Stillness: something happens

- Rhythm returns: observe healthier functioning and interaction in body physiology.

Ongoing procedure

- The change in potency and RBI activity in the first tissue acts as an initiator leading to further changes in the body as a whole. In the ensuing therapy, an increasing rise in potency is generally found in the tissues to be treated, along with greater responsiveness and faster change during treatment.

- The osteopath integrates the corrections that have been achieved in various tissues and allows the effects to interact and merge. To various extents this establishes a new order on the pattern of synchronous, dynamic rhythmic activity and the patterns of tension and energy in the body as a whole.

- The treatment concludes when the osteopath senses that the response from the physiology of the body is

---

Box 21.1

Questions to ask in diagnosis (see also pp. 310 ff.)

- What does health mean for the patient and the patient's tissue?

- What is the state of health of the patient and his tissue?

- What is the quality and tone of the tissue?

- Is this an acute or chronic process?

- When did the dysfunctional process begin?

- In which phase of the particular rhythm and at what stage of it does the dysfunction appear?

- Is the flow of vitality restricted in the inward or outward direction?

- Are other tissues or processes involved?

- What factors led to the original appearance of the dysfunction?

- Where is the fulcrum of this dysfunction?

Box 21.2

Questions to ask in therapy

- What is the nature of the tissue's receptivity to the RBIT?

- How long does the reaction to the RBIT in the tissue last?

- What processes occur in the tissue during the RBIT?

- How is a change in potency and RBI activity expressed?

- Do still points occur?

- How is the healthier functioning and improved interaction in the physiology of the body expressed, as sensed by palpation?

the maximum that the body as a whole is capable of producing (or willing to produce) at that time.

- Note: further treatment will also enable the inherent rhythmic system to perform its work with increasingly less assistance provided by the contact through hand compression via the fulcrum.

References

[1] Russell WA: New concept of the universe. 1989: 146 (revised edition; originally published 1953). Quoted from his previous book The Divine Iliad. Also quoted by: Becker RE: In: Brooks RE (ed.): The stillness of life. Portland: Stillness Press; 2000:92.

[2] Becker RE: Diagnostic Touch: Its Principles and Application, Part III, AAO Yearbook (162) 162, Part IV. AAO Yearbook. 1965:165.

[3] Becker RE: In: Brooks RE (ed.): The stillness of life. Portland: Stillness Press; 2000:74–92, 117.

22

Midline: development and introduction

Torsten Liem

Touch is *the interval and the heterogeneity of touch. Touch is proximate distance. It makes one sense what makes one sense (what it* is *to sense): the proximity of the distant, the approximation of the intimate.*

J-L. Nancy[1]

Importance of the site of sperm entry into the ovum

In the absence of information from the outside, unfertilized frogs' eggs do not have the capacity to develop bilateral symmetry. This information is imparted by the site of sperm entry into the ovum. Only then does differentiation occur between meridians or lines of longitude, i.e. one meridian becomes differentiated from all others. Without this information being imparted from the outside, the ovum cannot know which of the existing lines of longitude will be the future symmetry-determining line of longitude, epigenesis cannot begin, and no embryo will develop. In general, the sperm enters the ovum a little below the level of the equator. The meridian joining the two poles and the entry site becomes the median plane of the ovum. The first cell division follows this meridian and the side on which the sperm enters becomes the ventral aspect of the frog.

The ovum would divide and continue to develop into a fully-grown frog, the sole difference being that it would possess only half the normal complement of chromosomes and would not be able to reproduce.

However, frogs' eggs should not be regarded as exemplifying the development of symmetry in higher animals and in humans. The amphibian ovum is already organized prior to fertilization. The cytoplasm recognizes gradients that are located in the ovum in organized form. In contrast, this type of intracellular cytoplasmic organization in the as yet unfertilized ovum is thought to be virtually absent in higher animals and totally absent in humans.

Nevertheless, in the human ovum too, the site of sperm entry is of some importance because the two centrioles originating in the sperm spread out from this site

and organize the spindles of the first cell division. These align themselves with the poles at opposite ends and the first cell division plane arises in the 'equator' thus formed. However, as already known, this is thought to be unconnected with the later development of the symmetry plane of the body. In humans, this plane is not laid down until the emergence of the primitive streak and the primitive node.[2]

Cleavage planes

The first cleavage plane determines the right-left dimension, the second cleavage plane is perpendicular to the first, and the third is perpendicular to the first two, thus separating the animal pole from the vegetative pole.

The first three cleavage planes thus result in organization in the three dimensions of space. At this stage of the morula, however, the dimensions are not yet determined in the embryo, but surround it like a sphere.[3]

Gradient between center and periphery

Even at the 8- or 12-cell stage of the morula, no cellular or intracellular gradients are yet present, and thus no symmetry plane can be identified. The first gradient to appear in human ontogenesis is the gradient between the center (later to form the embryoblast or inner cell mass) and the periphery (later to form the trophoblast or outer cell mass). This first appears as a dynamic phenomenon, i.e. differentiation occurs as a result of metabolic relationships: the metabolic conditions confronting the cells at the periphery are different from those confronting the centrally located cells. Later, this difference also becomes established in genetic-morphological terms and structurally different trophoblasts and embryoblasts are formed.[2]

Dorsal and ventral aspects

The future dorsal and ventral aspects of the embryo are already morphologically identifiable at the start of the second week by the formation of the embryonic disk between the amniotic cavity and the yolk sac.[4]

The axis between the ventral aspect (endoderm: metabolic pole) and the dorsal aspect (neurosensory pole) has also been described by van der Wal as the axis of the will and of motion.[5]

The craniocaudal axis

For Rohen, the craniocaudal dimension already has its beginning with the emergence of the primitive node and the primitive groove. According to van der Wal, it is the attachment of the connecting stalk in the region of the future rump during the second week that determines the craniocaudal axis of the embryonic disk. While a cranial and a pelvic region have already started to differentiate, a thoracic and an abdominal region have not yet developed. The site of attachment of the connecting stalk determines the position of the rump and of the head at the opposite end. The craniocaudal axis simultaneously represents the axis of polar opposition (of the information and metabolic system) and of its rhythmic balance in the middle.

Blechschmidt and Gasser have noted that the cranial and caudal ends, the dorsal and ventral sides, and the left and right borders of the entocyst disc become established once the axial process has become distinct.[6] This principal body axis is also the principal axis for molecular orientation in the organism as a whole.

For osteopaths, the formation of the longitudinal axis expresses itself as a potency, which assumes a type of fulcrum function not only for the embryonic development of further structures, but also throughout the whole of life.

Polarity between the connecting stalk and heart

The embryonic disk, the 'earthbound central body', is linked via the connecting stalk at its pelvic pole to the 'skyward-oriented peripheral body'.

Blood vessel formation and hematopoiesis have their beginnings in the periphery. Hemodynamics come into being through osmotic forces and blood starts to flow in the capillaries of the chorionic mesoderm and collects in the connecting stalk. Finally, driven by metabolic forces, it flows from the connecting stalk via the yolk sac, the amniotic cavity, and the flanks to the head region, the cranial end of the embryonic disk. It is there that the primordium of the heart is ultimately formed, due to congestion of the blood. The blood 'comes to rest' at the cranial pole and then finally returns along other capillaries toward the periphery. For van der Wal, this is the moment when a 'presence' is formed in the embryo, a center that stands in opposition to the periphery. Now the embryonic disk becomes the center of attention, and developmental forces orientate themselves in the embryonic disk.[7]

To some extent, the connecting stalk and the heart represent polarities:

- The connecting stalk (later to become the sacral region) symbolizes an opening from the periphery.

- The heart (located cranially) symbolizes a 'coming to rest'.

Embryologically, this polarity is also expressed in the growth dynamics of the arms and legs: the growth direction of the arms is oriented toward the center, and that of the legs toward the periphery.

Further craniosacral polarity exists between the unconscious and the conscious: the more caudal the regions of the body, the more unconscious they are, and the more cranial the regions of the body, the more conscious they are.[7]

Development of left-right symmetry

At the cranial pole, which is closely associated with the heart, there is space for expansion, which is not present in the rump region due to the attachment of the connecting stalk. In the coccygeal region, therefore, the growth dynamic is directed inward and the impulse is created for the development of a new tissue layer, which is inserted between the ectoderm and the endoderm. This impulse ascends from below[8] and the result is the mesoderm. Starting at the cranial end, a thin strand (the chorda dorsalis or notochord) develops, and this ultimately establishes the median body axis, the axis between left and right. However, the future longitudinal axis of the body is already preformed with the development of the primitive streak.[9]

Cell movements to the right and left of the primitive streak characterize the beginning of bilateral symmetry in the embryo.[10] Differentiation in the sense of left-right symmetry appears at the start of the third week due to a polarity in the direction of movement of the cilia of the primitive node cells. These cilia beat synchronously to the left, causing fluid to flow over the dorsal aspect of the embryo. By this fluid motion, factors inducing left-right determination flow to the left side of the embryonic disk, causing flow-sensitive calcium receptors to be triggered only on the left side. The result is a left-right axis in the embryo in relation to its primordial organs. Blockade of ciliary movement (either experimentally or due to a genetic defect) leads to partial or total lateral transposition.*

The direction of the flow of intercellular fluid determines the cells in which a specific cascade of chemicogenetic reactions will unfold, which in turn will activate specific genes etc.[11] The same rule applies in this context: specific metabolic conditions and specific positional relationships come into being first, to be followed later by genetic 'determination'.

Whereas the ectoderm and mesoderm show a tendency to form symmetrical structures, endodermal structures tend to exhibit asymmetry. Thus, asymmetrical structures appear at a very early stage. As early as day 13 to 14, the later asymmetry of the organs, especially of the cardiac primordium, is identifiable by a slight divergence of the principal axes of the anterior and posterior endoblast chambers.[13, 14]

The development of three-dimensional structure

Despite this trilaminar form, the embryo still appears flat. It is only with the formation of somatic segments and the resultant onset of mesenchymal development that the body begins to take shape as a three-dimensional structure and the anterior-posterior dimension – already adumbrated in the axis between endoderm and ectoderm – becomes clearly apparent.

Electrical fields

Research with embryos from a wide range of animal species consistently confirms that in all body tissues the anterior-posterior axis is the axis with the greatest polarizing potential. From the axis with the highest voltage gradient in the electrical field of a frog's egg, Burr was able to detect the future direction of growth of the frog's nervous system.[15]

The fluid membrane matrix of the embryo is thought to be oriented within this median electrical voltage gradient. However, these investigations are limited to work in frogs' eggs.

Liquid crystalline properties of tissue

According to Ho, anterior-posterior or dorso-ventral polarization is based on the liquid crystalline structure of living organisms. In temporal terms, the antero-posterior axis is established before the dorso-ventral or proximal-distal axis. Ho regards the living organism in effect as one uniaxial liquid crystal.[16]

Depending on their expression, liquid-crystalline mesophases may range from more liquid structures with only one-dimensional orientation through to very solid structures with three-dimensional orientation. In embryology, large tissue components undergo development from a more liquid to a more solid liquid-crystalline structure. The properties of the liquid-crystalline structures act as a shaping force for the development of a uniform organism because they shape the parts into a unified whole. This therefore constitutes an important morphogenetic organization field. This has been substantiated by research demonstrating that non-linear vector fields were responsible for supernumerary or incorrect limb-bud growth.[17]

Middle (formerly ventral), dorsal, anterior and central midline according to van den Heede

The midlines arise from anatomical interrelationships; however, they represent functional qualities rather than being anatomical structures.

All organisms orient themselves around midline functions. Midlines represent orientational points and fulcrums in embryonic development. In phenomenological palpatory impressions, vital and dynamic potencies seem to spread in a fluctuating manner from the midlines toward the periphery and to be involved in the organization of structure.

---

*In contrast, Bateson believes that the information necessary to determine asymmetry must already be present in the frog's egg before fertilization, and he suspects the presence of a spiral of non-quantitative relationships, with the result that each meridian (regardless of where it is drawn) must be asymmetrical.[12] However, his data were obtained from experiments in frogs' eggs and, as has been noted already, this situation cannot be transposed automatically to that in humans.

Synchronously occurring tissue growth processes, expansions, differentiations and polarizations also stand in relationship to the functional midlines.

According to van den Heede[18], it is possible to distinguish a middle (formerly ventral) midline, a dorsal midline, an anterior midline and a central midline. The description here follows the chronological sequence of midline development.

Middle (formerly ventral) midline: (Figure 22.1)

The middle (formerly ventral) midline is seated in the area of the former notochord and continues as far as the sphenoid bone and the ethmoid air cells. After the development of the anterior midline, this midline will be the middle midline.

The balance point of the fluid middle (formerly ventral) midline is the heart. The nasion is the reference point for the development of the middle midline; the sacrum is also a reference point. It appears to be represented by the development of the notochord.

The middle midline acts as a support for the body[18] and organizes the biomechanical centerline of the body. It seems to have a cyclical expression and to have a stabilizing function in the densification of matter.

Dorsal midline: (Figure 22.2)

The dorsal midline seems to be seated in the area of the neural tube.

The balance point of the dorsal midline is Sutherland's fulcrum (in the area of the straight sinus).

It seems to represent a bioelectrical function of the nervous system. Exchange and memorization occur in the dorsal midline. This midline is dynamized by fluidic expansion of the ependymal canal and the ventricles.

The formation of the dorsal midline is related to the formation of the neural tube.

Anterior midline: (Figures 22.3 A,B)

The anterior midline travels from the nose through the hyoid bone, sternum, xiphoid process and linea alba to the symphysis pubis. The balance point of the anterior midline (to the dorsal midline) is the hyoid bone.

The potential body presents itself in the anterior midline. Its function seems to be to adapt and potentialize the vitality of the body. Convergence of the forces from

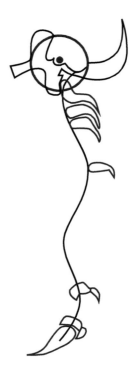

Figure 22.1
Middle (formerly ventral) midline.

the periphery and the integration of these forces take place in the anterior midline.

The formation of a third (anterior) midline – anterior to the formerly ventral midline – is triggered by the first two midlines. It develops through laterality or infolding and flexion of the embryo and the lateral encompassing of space and the anterior meeting of the two sides. The anterior midline is involved in the migration of neural crest cells – posterolaterally as melanocytes and ventrally as visceral plexuses.

Central midline

Known as the electrical midline, it is located directly anterior to the spinal column. The prevertebral plexuses belong to it.

The central electrical midline is thought to arise as a result of the interaction of fluidic and bioelectrical

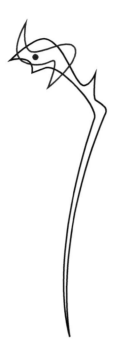

Figure 22.2
Dorsal midline.

components of the nervous system. Via the migration of neural crest cells the dorsal midline induces the formation of the anterior and central midlines and their potentialization. Cells from the neural crest have migrated there and form the prevertebral plexuses.

According to van den Heede, expansion occurs through the lateralization of the midline. However, the development of expansion requires the concentric force of the midline as polarity.

Treatment of the midlines according to van den Heede, modified

- Therapist: take up a position to one side of the supine patient, on a level with the navel.

- Hand position for middle and dorsal midline (Figure 22.5):

- Place one hand at the back of the patient's head.
- Rest your other hand at the sacrum.

The central midline can be palpated with this handhold; alternatively, the area of the prevertebral plexuses can be contacted with your hands at the body's anterior midline.

- Hand position for anterior midline (Figure 22.6):
  - Place your hands along the anterior midline by spreading your fingers along the line from the nose to the symphysis pubis.

- Alternative hand position for anterior midline (Figure 22.7a-d)
  Place each hand on one side of the pelvic area with your thumbs meeting above the symphysis pubis and along the linea alba.
  - Next place each hand on one side of the lower chest area with your thumbs meeting along the sternum.
  - Then place each hand over the shoulder area on one side with your thumbs meeting in the vicinity of the suprasternal notch.
  - Finally place your hands over the patient's face, with your thumbs meeting over the nasal area, index fingers at the intermaxillary suture and middle fingers at the point of the chin.

- Method:
  - First synchronize with the qualities of health and with the homeodynamic forces in the patient. This can be done by synchronizing with kinesthetic sensations during palpation, or by focusing on inner visual pictures, colors or other sensory impressions during palpation that are related to health and homeostasis in the patient.
  - During the technique maintain contact with the sensed qualities of health.

- Middle (former ventral) midline:
  - Begin by palpating the functional unit of the middle (former ventral) midline qualities in the area of the former notochord from the sacrum as far as the sphenoid bone and the ethmoid air cells.
  - Sense the quality of support for the body of the middle midline and the balance point in the area of the heart.

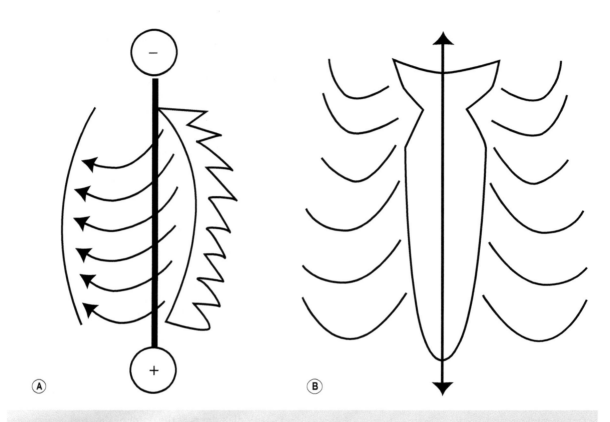

Figure 22.3
Anterior midline.

- It may be necessary to exert a compressive force to support the inherent forces and bring them into action.
- If you sense any dysfunctional patterns, amplify them slightly during the inhalation phase while simultaneously remaining in contact with the qualities of health.

- Dorsal midline:
  - Focus on the functional unit of the dorsal midline, and palpate the area of the neural tube.
  - Establish contact with the fluidic, bioelectrical qualities of the nervous system and the balance point in the area of the straight sinus.
  - Here too, if dysfunctional patterns are sensed, amplify these slightly during the inhalation phase while simultaneously remaining in contact with the qualities of health.
  - Then sense the interaction between middle midline and dorsal midline function.

- Anterior midline:
  - Now palpate the functional unit of the anterior midline along a line from the nose through the hyoid bone, sternum, xiphoid process and linea alba to the symphysis pubis.
  - Establish contact with the balance point in the area of the hyoid bone.
  - Acknowledge the formation of this functional unit: the laterality or infolding and flexion of the embryo triggered by the first two midlines.

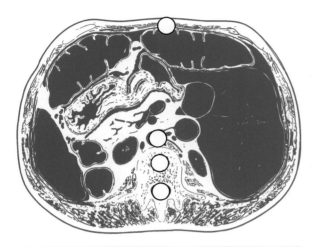

Figure 22.4
Notional positions of the midlines after van den Heede.

- If you sense any dysfunctional patterns, amplify them slightly during the inhalation phase while simultaneously remaining in contact with the qualities of health.
- Use the alternative hand position for the anterior midline to appreciate the forming quality of lateral encompassing of space and anterior meeting of the two sides.

- Central midline:
  - Focus on the functional unit of the central midline in the area of the prevertebral plexuses and on their qualities during palpation. Acknowledge the formation of this functional unit: the migration of neural crest cells between the myotome and sclerotome ventrally.

- Integration of all midline functional units:
  - Place one hand again on the back of the patient's head, with your other hand at the sacrum.
  - Finally connect the midlines to each other, sense also the space around these midlines while

Midline	Area	Balance point	Function	Formation
Middle midline	Former notochord; as far as the sphenoid bone and the ethmoid air cells	Heart	Support for the body	Represented by the formation of the notochord
Dorsal midline	Neural tube	Sutherland's fulcrum (area of straight sinus)	Fluidic, bioelectrical function of the nervous systems; exchange and memorization	Represented by the formation of the neural tube
Anterior midline	From the nose through the hyoid bone, sternum, xiphoid process and linea alba to the symphysis pubis	Hyoid bone	To adapt and potentialize the vitality of the body	Triggered by the first two midlines; laterality or infolding and flexion of the embryo. Lateral encompassing of space and anterior meeting of the two sides. Migration of neural crest cells: posterolaterally as melanocytes and ventrally as visceral plexuses
Central midline	Prevertebral plexuses		Electrical midline	Interaction of fluidic and bioelectrical components of the nervous system; migration of neural crest cells between the myotome and sclerotome ventrally, for example to form the prevertebral plexuses

TABLE 22.1: Overview of the midlines

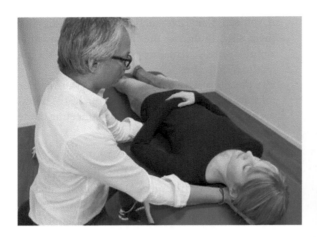

Figure 22.5
Hand position for middle and dorsal midline.

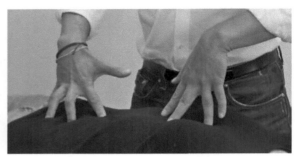

Figure 22.6
Hand position for anterior midline.

simultaneously focusing on the qualities of health and the homeodynamic forces.

- Allow the dynamics between the functional units of the different midlines to unfold and observe the formation of a new balance between the midlines.
- Synchronize with the rhythmic qualities and release your hands during the inhalation phase.

Further details

Orientation to the midline is re-established spontaneously when dysfunctional tension is released following osteopathic treatment.[20]

Each part of the body has its own midline, around which it is organized and around which it develops; according to Blechschmidt, for example, the vessels represent a type of organizational structure for the development of the limbs. (In this context, a space-time unit exists for each development.) Simultaneously, each structure also orientates itself around a specific primary midline or matrix of fluid potency, for example, around the primitive streak as a fluctuating midline or around one situated in the chorda dorsalis. Spiraled development movements organize themselves eccentrically and concentrically in relation to the midline.

However, the body is not absolutely symmetrical. Even the brain and the vertebral column are not symmetrical. There are midline structures, however, which represent an integration point for asymmetries and which exert a symmetry-stabilizing function.[19]

The term midline may also denote the mean or mesor of rhythmic phenomena. The emotions too are oriented around a specific midline. One important midline in diagnostic and therapeutic terms relates to the dynamics of energy uptake and release, and this also includes sensory stimuli. One of the first and most important diagnostic questions may be to consider whether patients consume more energy than they release or release more energy than they consume, and which tension patterns and etiologies sustain this imbalance in the patient.

Traumatic and other factors may disturb the relationship of median and peripheral structures to the primary midline. This is also of major diagnostic importance.

The midline of stillness

Create the conditions for stillness to come (see Chapter 19) and give the stillness space to become full.

Allow a dynamic stillness to become established between yourself and the patient.

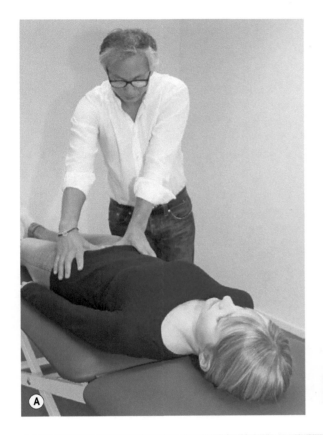

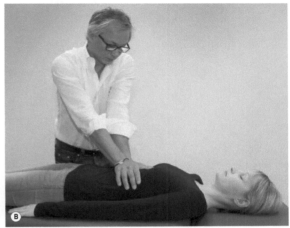

Figure 22.7A-B

Alternative hand position for anterior midline

This stillness may be regarded as a type of midline that is always retained during the techniques described below.

Midline from the vertex to the tip of the coccyx (Figure 22.8)

- Patient: Supine.

  Therapist: Take up a position to one side of the patient.

- Hand position: Place the index and middle fingers of your caudal hand on either side of the coccyx.

- Method:
  - First sense the midline, the space around this midline, and the potency in the midline.
  - Then sense the relationship between the vertex and the tip of the coccyx.
  - Establish a point of balance between the two.
  - If there is a lack of potency in the midline, direct attention to the tip of the coccyx.
  - Ascending from the coccyx, sense the flow of potency and the inherent tissue motions that accompany this flow of potency.

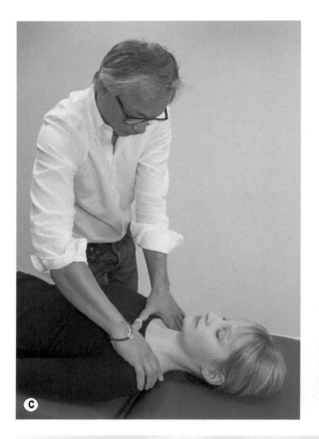

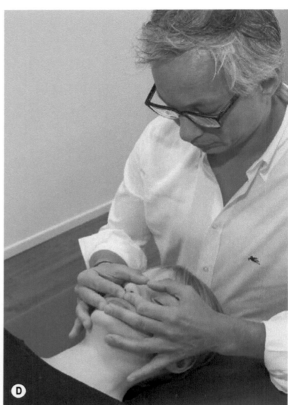

Figure 22.7C-D

Alternative hand position for anterior midline

- You may also gently amplify motion in the direction of ease (indirect technique).
- You will sense an influx of potency between the coccyx and vertex. Direct attention to the rising flow of potency from the coccyx tip in the midline around the region of the former chorda dorsalis as far as the third ventricle of the CNS. Finally, sense the spread of this potency throughout the entire body.
- Re-orientate the vertex and coccyx to the primary midline.

Sacrococcygeal-lumbosacral and thoracolumbar midline (Figure 22.9)

- Therapist: Take up a position to one side of the patient on a level with the pelvis.
- Hand position:
  - Position the index and middle fingers of one hand on either side of the coccyx.
  - Place your other hand on or span the spinous processes at the level of the lumbosacral or thoracolumbar junction.

chronous expression of primary respiration in these structures.

- While continuing to focus your sensing on the expression of primary respiration, additionally start to go with the tissue tensions and amplify motion in the direction of ease (indirect technique).
- Establish a dynamic tension balance.
- Establish a fulcrum between the structures involved in order to balance the tensions between the two structures.
- Through resonance with the forces contained in the fulcrum, release the bound potency and make it accessible again.
- Potency will flow into the structures involved.
- You will sense an increase in synchronicity.

The chorda dorsalis technique according to Jealous, modified (Figure 22.10)

- Indication: For example, to correct vertebral dysfunction.

- Therapist: Take up a position to one side of the patient on a level with the vertebrae affected.

- Hand position:
  - Take hold of the two vertebrae involved in the dysfunction.
  - Place your cranial hand on the upper vertebra.
  - Place your caudal hand on the lower vertebra.

- Method:
  - In line with the embryonic development of the vertebra, gently compress together the lower half of the upper vertebra and the upper half of the lower vertebra.
  - Then establish a point of balance between the two vertebrae.

A sacrosternal midline, and a midline of the two cerebral hemispheres or of the frontal lobes only may also develop, in addition. CV-3 may also be performed.[20]

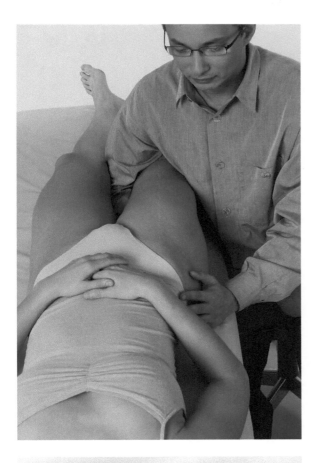

Figure 22.8

Midline from the vertex to the tip of the coccyx

- Method:
  - First sense the midline, the space around this midline, and the potency in the midline.
  - Sense the relationship of the structures involved to the primary midline.
  - Next assess the sacrococcygeal and lumbosacral or thoracolumbar structures in relation to each other. Focus your sensing on the expression of the primary respiration of the membranous-fluid aspects of the structures involved. Assess the syn-

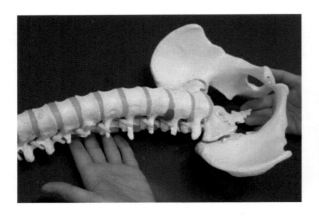

Figure 22.9

Sacrococcygeal-lumbosacral and thoracolumbar midline

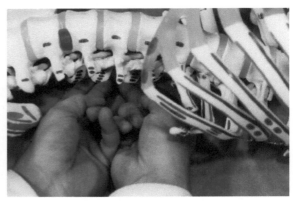

Figure 22.10

The chorda dorsalis technique of James Jealous

Sacrococcygeal-sternal midline (Figure 22.11)

- Hand position:
  - Place your cranial hand on the sternum.
  - Place the index and middle fingers of your caudal hand on either side of the coccyx.

- Method: Follow the steps described above.

Inion-SBS midline (Figure 22.12)

- Therapist: Take up a position at the head of the patient.

- Hand position:
  - Place your thumbs on the greater wings of the sphenoid on both sides.
  - Position the tips of your middle and ring fingers on the inion.

- Method: Follow the steps described above.

Nasion-inion (Figure 22.13)

- Therapist: Take up a position at the head of the patient.

- Hand position:
  - Place the tips of your index and middle fingers of one hand on the nasion.
  - Place the tips of the index and middle fingers of your other hand on the inion.

- Method: Follow the steps described above.

Bregma (Figure 22.14)

- Therapist: Take up a position at the head of the patient.

- Hand position: Place your thumbs on the bregma, with the tips of your other fingers on the squamous margin of the parietal bone on either side.

- Method: Follow the steps described above.

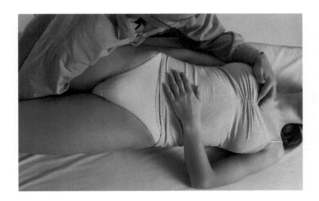

Figure 22.11

Sacrococcygeal-sternal midline

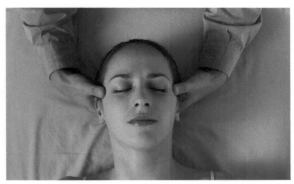

Figure 22.12

Inion-SBS midline

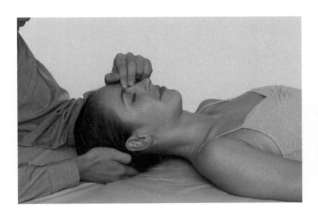

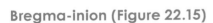

Figure 22.13

Nasion-inion

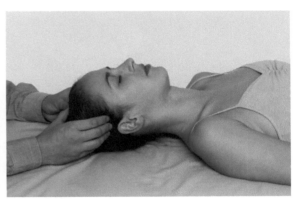

Figure 22.14

Bregma

Bregma-inion (Figure 22.15)

- Therapist: Take up a position at the head of the patient.

- Hand position:
  - Place the tips of your middle and ring fingers of one hand on the bregma.
  - Place the fingertips of your other hand on the inion.

- Method: Follow the steps described above.

Midline from the vertex to C1 (Figure 22.16)

- Therapist: Take up a position at the head of the patient.

- Hand position:

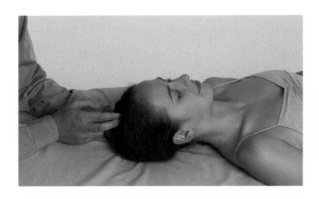

Figure 22.15

Bregma-inion

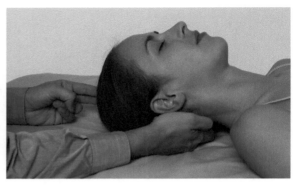

Figure 22.16

Midline from the vertex to C1

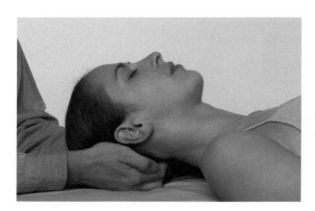

Figure 22.17

Atlanto-occipital midline

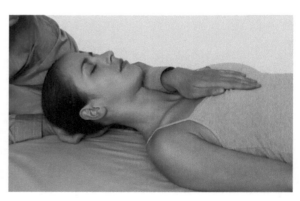

Figure 22.18

Occipito-sternal midline

- Place your cranial hand on the vertex.
- The fingers of your caudal hand should be in contact with the posterior tubercle of C1.

- Method: Follow the steps described above.

Atlanto-occipital midline (Figure 22.17)

- Therapist: Take up a position at the head of the patient.

- Hand position:
  - Cradle the occipital bone in your hands. Your middle, ring and little fingers should touch at the median line of the occipital squama, inferior to the inion.
  - Your index fingers should touch at the posterior tubercle of C1.

- Method: Follow the steps described above.

Occipito-sternal midline (Figure 22.18)

- Therapist: Take up a position at the head of the patient.

- Hand position:
  - Place your cranial hand beneath the occipital bone. Position your middle finger on the midline of the occipital bone, with your index and ring fingers next to it.
  - Place your caudal hand on the sternum.

- Method: Follow the steps described above.

Navel-occiput (vertex) midline (Figure 22.19)

- Indication: Important technique for use in birth trauma and emotional trauma.

- Therapist: Take up a position to one side of the supine patient, on a level with the navel.

- Hand position:
  - Place one hand on the navel.
  - Rest your other hand on the occiput or the vertex.

- Method:
  - First palpate the tension at the level of the navel and produce a resonance.
  - Next sense the midline and the space around this midline.
  - Then connect the navel and the midline to each other.
  - In individual cases it may be necessary to exert a compressive force to support the inherent forces and bring them into action.
  - Establish a point of balance between the midline and navel.

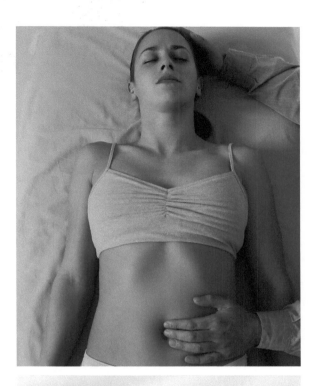

Figure 22.19

Navel-occiput (vertex) midline

References

[1]Nancy J-L. *The Muses*, trans. Peggy Kamuf. Stanford: Stanford University Press; 1996:17.

[2]Correspondence with Jaap van der Wal: 2003.

[3]Rohen JW. *Functional Morphology. The Dynamic Wholeness of the Human Organism.* Hillsdale/NY: Adonis Press; 2007:46.

[4]Hinrichsen KV. *Humanembryologie: Lehrbuch und Atlas der vorgeburtlichen Entwicklung des Menschen.* Berlin: Springer; 1990:112.

[5]Van der Wal J, Glöckler M. *Dynamische Morphologie und Entwicklung der menschlichen Gestalt.* Dornach: Freie Hochschule für Geisteswissenschaft am Goetheanum; 1999:82.

[6]Blechschmidt E, Gasser RF. *Biokinetics and Biodynamics of Human Differentiation.* Springfield, Illinois: Charles C. Thomas; 1978:34.

[7]Van der Wal J. Course transcript. Hamburg: German Osteopathy College; 9/2003.

[8]Van der Wal J, Glöckler M. *Dynamische Morphologie und Entwicklung der menschlichen Gestalt.* Dornach: Freie Hochschule für Geisteswissenschaft am Goetheanum; 1999:83.

[9]Hinrichsen KV. *Humanembryologie: Lehrbuch und Atlas der vorgeburtlichen Entwicklung des Menschen*. Berlin: Springer; 1990:113.

[10]Rohen JW. *Functional Morphology. The Dynamic Wholeness of the Human Organism*. Hillsdale/NY: Adonis Press; 2007:54.

[11]Poelmann RE. Er bestaat een gen voor links of rechts. Bionieuws 2003;10:3.

[12]Bateson G. *Mind and Nature. A Necessary Unity*. New York: E. P. Dutton; 1979:164.

[13]Blechschmidt E. *Die pränatalen Organsysteme des Menschen. Stuttgart:* Hippokrates; 1973:128.

[14]Blechschmidt E. *Humanembryologie-Prinzipien und Grundbegriffe. Stuttgart:* Hippokrates; 1974:21ff.

[15]Burr HS. *Blueprint for Immortality. 5th edn. Saffron* Walden: CW Daniel; 1991:33.

[16]Ho MW. *The Rainbow and the Worm*. 2nd edn. Singapore: World Scientific Publishing Co.; 1998:178.

[17]Ho MW. *The Rainbow and the Worm*. 2nd edn. Singapore: World Scientific Publishing Co.; 1998:180.

[18]Van den Heede P. Course transcript. Hamburg: German Osteopathy College; 3/2002.

[19]Van den Heede P. Course transcript. Hamburg: German Osteopathy College; 5/2003.

23

Hyoid bone and anterior midline

Patrick van den Heede and Anne Jäkel

Introduction

Different structures appear in the early cranial-facial region of an approximately 30 days old embryo[1]:

- a large neural tube

- the notochord and the prechordal mesoderm

- the proenteron which is located ventrally

- aortic arches which surround the proenteron

- large masses of neural crest and mesenchyme

A primary important impulse that needs to be taken into consideration may be the interference of a genetically programmed patterning within all three of the original germ layers during the triblastic period of the embryo. All tissue layers in this region are dependent on Hox gene patterning. Hox genes interfere with specific receptors on the three germ layers in a colinear way (colinear Hox gene expression patterns). Each of the three layers depends on specific Hox gene information for its further differentiation and specification.

The visceral mesoderm is also dependent on Hox gene patterning in a co-linear way, together with the ecto- and entoderm. This visceral mesoderm is attached to the endoderm, later forming the circulatory, respiratory, and digestive systems.

The patterning follows an anterior to posterior progression and starts at the pharyngeal endoderm which functions as an inductive plateau for the early differentiation of the adjacent ectoderm. It also interferes with the definitive closure of the lateral mesoderm layers at the level of the future anterior midline.[2]

A specific part of the mesenchyme at the anterior midline seems to be informed by the Hox genes in a different way than the mesenchymal anlagen localized in the lateral mesodermal areas.[3] Hence, the anterior midline mesenchyme serves as an attractor for segmentally informed mesenchyme that is laid down in an **anterior-posterior** (a-p) **pattern** by Hox-gene information.

This Hox gene patterning displays the same a-p patterning at the level of the rhombomer formation as it does at the level of the corresponding pharyngeal arches. An intimate interference exists between Hox gene patterning and the concentration of cellular retinoic acid binding protein (CRAB) and retinoic acid receptors (RAR) in the different cell levels of the three distinct tissue layers.

An early and intimate relationship is established by the Hox gene patterning and initiates common time related inductive properties. The first relation between the anlagen of the rhombomeres and the formation of the branchiomeric segments is already apparent by colinear information of the Hox genes at the three tissue levels.

Cranial sensory ganglia and placodal precursors are generated, depending on these specific receptors for Hox gene information (CRAB and RAR) and their respective concentration gradient along the a-p axis of the triblastic embryo[4].

A second important event in the organization of the different midlines of the embryonic body is 'the *dorsal-ventral* emplacement' of the lateral plate mesoderm (LPM).[3]

Both the LPM and the surface ectoderm grow ventrally and meet at the anterior midline to form a closed body. The visceral mesoderm seems to play an inhibitory role by restricting the growth of somatic mesoderm during the development of the lateral body walls.

At the level of the anterior region of the embryo this anterior midline functions as an attraction for convergence and interaction of different cell types of different origin.

The ventral midline fulfills an analogous function similar to the apical ectodermal ring (AER) at the dorsolateral side of the embryo, by organizing and concentrating mesenchymal cell masses (for example pre-placodal material) and initiating differentiation and interference with cell-anlagen further away (interference between rhombomeres and branchial anlagen).

At the level of the early branchial arches there is a strong interaction between descending neural crest cells (NCCs), myocytes of the corresponding somitomeres and differentiating chondrocytes in situ.

NCC's segregated during the early rhombomeric segmentation transmit morphogenetic instructions during their migration to the connective tissue of the respective arches, which are formed by a simultaneous bending of the embryonic head region. The hotspot of interaction, differentiation and specification of the bilateral branchiomeric cell masses is found in the local mesenchyme that is located in between the different constituent layers of the already modified triblastic embryo.

This mesenchyme serves as an attraction pole for migrating cells and growth factors and possesses its own complex information dependent on gene patterning and NCC information.

The cell population at the level of the future anterior midline expresses a mixed pattern of NCC modulation and specific Hox gene information, together with a myogenic/osteogenic potential.

Globally it can be assumed that the connective tissue of the pharyngeal arches is informed by neural crest cells and by migrating cells, differentiating them from the first somitomeres and somites but also from the rhombomeres. Different space/time schedules seem to be integrated in the same tissue level.

It is important to understand that tissue memory is built by an aggregate of different developmental schedules that are not necessarily related to any anatomical or physiological properties of the tissue rather than to the constitutional history of the field energy. Change in function may express a disturbance in integrity of anatomy but could also be the hotspot for the emergence of hidden memory linked to other space/time units.

The morphogenetic control of tissue transformation of the anterior midline to its definite function preferentially resides in the connective tissue elements rather than in the osteogenic or myogenic cells.[2] Inhibition of chondrogenesis, on the other hand, is related to the surrounding ectoderm[1]. These facts are relevant to understand the importance of the epigenetic information as a contributor to adapted morphogenesis.

The tissues (muscles, cartilage, bone, and their anatomical relationships) of this particular level of morphogenesis express the capacity of having a dual function: they partly appear as biomechanical support for laryngeal and pharyngeal physiology, but they also seem to be related to more sensitive or even sensorial properties by being related to their tissues of origin. In the case of the secondary arch mesenchyme, there exists a direct continuity between the subhyoidal mesenchyme that connects the base of the heart with the hyoid bone (NCC information related to rhombomeric information and cardiac NCCs) and the styloid process and stapes of the middle ear bone structure. This type of development suggests that the hyoid bone is informed at an early stage during morphogenesis to becoming an important balance point between different types of origin and function of the tissues involved at that specific level.

A third important event should be considered. So far, the molecular properties of the hyoid bone formation and its related morphological fields have been described. One should not forget that the occurrence of genetic patterning is supported and probably guided by biodynamical events in conjunction with genetic information. In case of the hyoid bone, the epigenetic field determines and qualifies the final outcome of the pharyngeal arch morphogenesis.

To understand the importance of the biodynamic induction as an epigenetic field for hyoid bone formation and the generation of its interrelationship with adjacent structures or functions at 'distance', one has to go back to the early stages of embryogenesis.

During the early embryonic period one can already see an intense bending of the neural groove/tube (4th - 5th week). This bending facilitates a transverse alignment of the mesenchyme at the base of the mesencephalon. This is the initiating stage for the formation of the *septum submesencephalicum*. The notochord lies at the base of this septum and activates the mesoderm that will form the notochordal mesoderm. At the same time, the notochordal top is inducing the overlying ectoderm to differentiate into a region specific neurectoderm (neurulation). Rhombomeres are formed

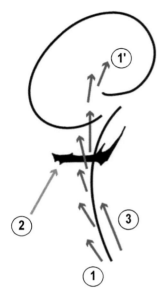

1   Prevertebral fasciae
2   Pretracheal and visceral fasciae of the mediastinum
3   Posterior dorsolumbar and cervicothoraic fasciae
1' Converging fasciae to the occipital and temporal areas

Figure 23.1
Os hyoideum and anterior cervical fasciae

in relationship with a shortening of the notochord during curving and folding of the base of the brain folds. This is due to the restraining action of the dorsal aorta in relation with the development of the heart. Surface enlargement of the ectoderm and endoderm at the level of bending provides space in the stroma of the different arches and concentrates different amounts of mesenchyme in these spaces.

The branchial space formation is the result of cranial-caudal progression of the folding brain. It is in these spaces that the arterial branchial arches are generated. The mesenchyme in these folds is stretched, becoming a restraining apparatus.[5] The head enlargement due to the broadening of the brain also widens the entodermal foregut transversely. Cerebralization further stretches the dural girdles and finishes with elevating the brain (erection of the brain with the mesencephalon being placed on top of the brain).

During that period the heart descends and an increasing amount of tension is imposed onto the stretched ventral mesenchyme. This creates a tension field that runs from crista galli to the ventrally positioned mesenchymal fascias that span the space between the erecting brain and the descending heart. The supranasal sulcus, which forms a transverse bridge between the frontal lobes and the nasal placode, becomes more tensed and centralized and is supporting a transverse folding by which the zygomatic arches are built. They, in turn, form the eye hammock and the major part of the floor of the orbits. The descent of the heart and the ascent of the brain have important influences on the mesenchymal structures that are located in between. A medial pathway for NCC migration directs towards the thymus primordium and thyroid follicles (C-cells). Additionally, a pathway for NCC is organized towards the heartanlage and most of the bilateral mesenchymal densities that serve the structural support of the branchial arches and the thorax, such as the branchiomeric mesenchyme and the sternal bars, fuse at midline level.

The mandible as well as the hyoid bone, are constituted at their central part by a **copula**: a centrally lying mesenchymal primordium that represents the midline part of these viscero-cranial ossicles. This centrally lying mesenchyme appears to function as an *attractor field* for genetically informed and segmented mesenchyme compartments that converge at this level. The mesenchyme of the copulae seems not to be informed by the same segmental information as the lateral mesoderm formation. This constitutes a *'neutral balance'* for integration and organization of lateral mesoderm compartments. The sternal bars also fuse in the same manner to form one single sternal body.

If the **functional, biomechanical and biodynamical aspects** of the hyoid bone in its myofascial environment are taken into account, then one can discover multiple relationships and interferences that are related to its actual position and function as well as to its morphological origin (Figure 23.1):

• The *subhyoidal muscles* are intimately related to the base of the heart and the great vascular trees arising from it alongside the *pretracheal fascia* and its extension, the *lamina thyro-thymopericardiaca*

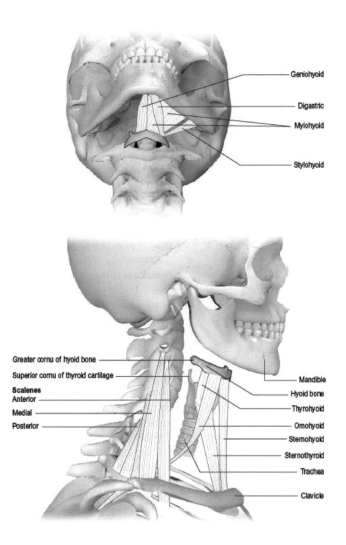

Figure 23.2
Hyoid and surrounding tissues

- The hyoid bone is linked to the mandible by the *suprahyoidal muscles* and their related fascia, the *superficial fascia* that envelops the complete neck region, comprising the occipital, the cervico-thoracic and mandibular-sternal spaces (Figure 23.2)

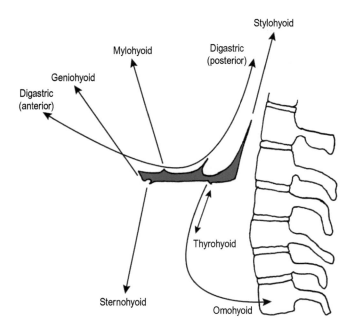

Figure 23.3
Muscular links of the hyoid bone

- The hyoid is also linked to the temporal bone by the *digastric muscle* and the *stylohyoid ligament*, being part of the *intermediate neck fascia*

- The hyoid interferes with the mobility of the scapular region by directly relating to the *omohyoid muscle* (Figure 23.3)

- At a more profound level, it builds an intimate relationship with the deep fascias of the laryngeal and tracheal spaces and with the fascias wrapped around the endocrine and neuro-endocrine organs: parotid gland, thymus, parathyroid and thyroid glands

It is evident that the hyoid integrates *different kinds of motion* and interferes at that level with *different types of mobility*:

- Arm and trunk movements are interfering with hyoid strength and position. Fixation or torque on the level of this tiny bone could interfere with the balance and coordination expressed at the biomechanical level of limb/trunk movements and at the level of the psychomotoric expression related to it

- The hyoid bone represents the mechanical fulcrum for swallowing, consciously and automatically, providing stability, motility and orientation at the same time to the laryngeal and pharyngeal spaces

- It offers stability to the tongue, supporting its compressive, protruding and retracting motion that serves swallowing, breathing and speaking. The vocal cords together with the subhyoidal muscles are all linked to verbal expression and the hyoid bone should be considered the mechanical fulcrum for the 'spoken word'

Imagine how much of the somatic sensory, viscerosensory, autonomic and branchiomeric motor information of the lower brainstem is related to this little bone by superficial and deep muscle compartments, peripheral sensory ganglia and endocrine glands!

Motion and mobility are intimately linked at the level of the hyoid and support different functions ranging

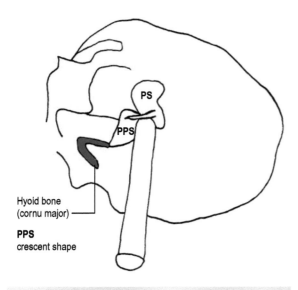

Hyoid bone
(cornu major)

PPS
crescent shape

Figure 23.4
Hyoid bone: balance of peripharyngeal space (PPS)/Parotid space (PS)/submandibular space (adapted from Harnsberger[6])

from biomechanical support to hemodynamic and endocrine integrity (Figure 23.4).

When we consider a more subtle function of the hyoid that relates to **interferences between fields of expression and integration**, then one can enumerate a completely different array of subtleness. Imagine how sophisticated its interaction could be as a leverage system for tension exchanged between the sternal manubrium and body and the viscerosensory-cranium. It represents a mobile balance between the intra-thoracic activity (heart/lungs/digestive system) and the viscero-cranial compartments. Once again, one has to consider the hyoid as an integrative tool for external mechanical and vibratory tension, but it also can be considered a dispatching center for tension and forces that relate to organs at distance. In other words, it could transmit part of the 'mechanical' environment of the body to organ level. In contrast, it is also worth to take into consideration that subtle disturbances at organ level are dispatched

by the hyoid bone to different parts of the body, independent of their possible function. Taking the anatomical relationships of the hyoid into account with the heart, thymus, thyroid gland, vocal cords, middle ear etc., one can conceive *the hyoid bone as a mechanical and fascial balance for integration and dispatch of different kinds of mechanical (mobility/motion and fascial drags) and functional properties of the cranial-sternal-sacral unit* (Figure 23.5).

On an even subtler level it should be remembered that the hyoid bone is related to distinct **vibratory levels** by its morphodynamic relationships during embryology and fetal development:

- Its branchiomeric origin displays a direct relationship with the middle ear bone (stapes) and its branchiomeric components organized by Hox gene expression and NCC patterning. The mesenchyme at the midline of the body that also contains the substrate for the hyoid body is related to lateral mesenchymal, branchiomeric levels of tissue information that link the midline to segmentation and level specific inductive moments.

- There exists not only level specific (segmental) information but also a wide variety of inter-branchiomeric exchange of tissue differentiation at other branchiomeric levels.

- The stylohyoid ligament links the hyoid bone to the maturation of the stylohyoid process of the mastoid bone and to the integrity of the mastoid cells.

One has to remember the following events to understand the complexity of the interrelationships of the hyoid bone at distance: an airy/bony skull in relation to airspaces of the cranium, erection of the skull/brain and maturation of the vocal apparatus/consciousness.

The osteopathic armamentarium has to integrate different kinds of palpatory information and skills at the level of the hyoid bone to be capable of interpreting the integrity of the anterior midline function. Simultaneously, it will guide the palpating fingers of the osteopath in the complex field of interference of the space/time relationship of the body.

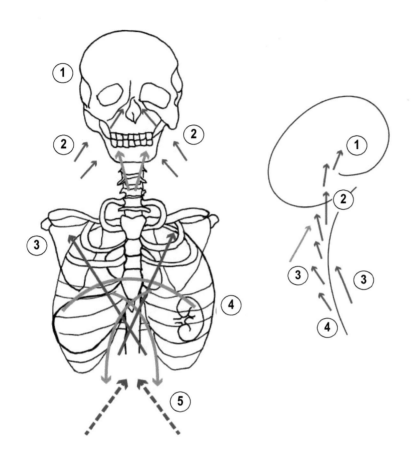

Figure 23.5
Gateways to midline function: the hyoid bone as a fulcrum

1. Epi/pericranial gateway
2. Cervico-cranial gateway
3. Mediastinal-thoracic gateway
4. Visceral-diaphragmatic gateway
5. Abdominal-pelvic gateway

References

[1]B.M. Carlson., Human embryology and developmental biology., pp.,278-279, Mosby Year Book, 1994.

[2]L.N. de la Rosa et al., The lateral mesodermal divide: an epigenetic model of the origin of paired fins. 16:1, 38-48, 2014.

[3]J.F. Rodriguez-Vàzquez et al., Human fetal hyoid body origin revisited. J. Anat, 219, pp., 143-149, 2011.

[4]E. Saliba et al., Médicine et biologie du développement., pp., 15-39, éd. Masson, 2001.

[5]E. Blechschmidt & R.F. Gasser., Biokinetics and biodynamics of human differentiation., 125-127, Charles C Thomas Publishers, 1978.

[6]Harnsberger., Handbook of head and neck imaging, Mosby Year Book, 1990 2nd ed.

24

The fluid body

Torsten Liem

The tactile movement begins by drawing near out of the void and ends by reaching further into the void.

Erwin Straus[1]

Introduction

In the course of its development every living creature and each of its organs passes through a liquid phase. The fertilized ovum consists of about 95% liquid. The embryo lives and grows in a liquid milieu and consists of over 90% liquid. The liquids are not merely already flowing before the vessels and heart are formed: they actually induce vessel formation. Even the fully-grown human still consists of about 70% liquid (as does the earth, the environment in which we live). Health cannot develop in an organism independently of the milieu in which it lives. For example, if water is contaminated then all living things are affected in the long term. It is therefore necessary that our conscious awareness of health extends beyond the body. Water as an information medium has already been used for therapy in the setting of homeopathy (e.g., in dilutions [potentiations] that go beyond the detectable level of active ingredient molecules). Similarly, the crystal photographs taken by Masaru Emoto have impressively helped us to see and experience the many different "faces of water."[2] According to Emoto, water has the capacity to react to the vibrations of music, speech, written words, emotions, and thoughts, and is able to reflect and store them. These altered material arrangements in liquids can be made visible by crystallization. In osteopathy too there are procedures designed to promote the fluid qualities of the organism. In employing these procedures osteopaths use not only their hands but their whole being to synchronize with the different fluid elements in the organism.

While still inside the uterus, the embryo – surrounded by a protective spherical envelope of water – molds its as yet almost liquid form, which gradually becomes more condensed.[3] Regions of more rapid growth protrude, while regions of slower growth are held back through a suspension of growth or are even dissolved again. Thus the fertilized ovum initially displays swelling enlargement with subsequent in-tucking in gastrulation.[4] Out of the complex interplay of fluid movements the material condensations finally attain their visible shape.

On being born the child enters into a relationship with the directional gravitational forces of the earth. As it interacts with these forces there is further densification and solidification of its structures. The spiraling shapes of the bones and muscles of the extremities in particular bear witness to the interplay between their fluid origin and directional gravitational forces and to a purposeful aim toward mastery of the solid.

For example, the bones of the extremities are permeated by tiny fissured systems that reflect the laws governing the flow of water and point to the flowing movement from which they originate. These current systems can be followed right into the interior of the bones where they end in the spongy bone structures (trabeculae). The trabecular structures then extend to the articulated surfaces and are continued in the neighboring bone.

Muscles and vessels also speak of the same streamlined systems seen in bone. This streaming movement in spiraling forms runs through the tendons into the muscles. Bones, muscles, tendons, ligaments, and vessels are all together an expression of the same underlying flowing movement. The overlapping of currents and rhythms – a characteristic feature of bodies of water – is also seen in the circulation of the blood.

Overlapping waveforms give rise to hollow spaces in which, for instance, air is enclosed. In precisely the same way, hollow spaces of this kind can be formed between two different media, or even different qualities within the same medium, for example, cold and warm water. This shape-forming principle is also found in living creatures. The hollowing out of inner spaces is the archetypal form–gesture in all organic creation and is seen, for example, in the invaginating processes of the gastrulation phase.[5] Here the differences in speed of the fluid flow correspond to the different rates of growth or development, i.e., slower and more rapid, and of neighboring tissue layers.

Vortex dynamics manifest themselves as specific rhythmic movements: in the course of organ development these form their own inner surfaces, which separate one layer from another. Like vortices in water, organs have their own life and autonomy: they are distinct forms within the organism as a whole and are yet in constant flowing interplay with it![6] In this sense, boundary surfaces may be regarded as the birthplaces of dynamic processes; one example of this is the cell membrane that separates the cytoplasm from the extracellular substance.

In the paired arrangement of the vortices in a vortex train we have a principle of construction that occurs in the formation of paired organs. The movement potentialities of the living creative force are already laid down in the fluid archetype. The completely developed organ, for example the organ of hearing in humans, appears as a movement that has come to rest; the still invisible fluid dynamic archetype becomes visible as a pattern in the fully developed organ.

James Jealous's concept of the fluid body

The fluid body is characterized by specific dynamics. It is believed that during the inhalation and exhalation phases of the primary respiration a dynamic is triggered in the fluid, which potentiates it. However, this process is not synonymous with the formation of hydraulic waves but is thought rather to be the expression of a kind of metabolic dynamic. The primary respiration causes a rhythmic transmutation, an inherent disengagement, and a synchronization to occur in the fluid. This fluid body is not limited by tissue barriers. During embryonic development, in particular, it becomes clear how fluid dynamics shape their environment.

According to Jealous,[7] the fluid body does not act as a fluid but as a living continuum with its own intelligence, the internal forces of which are specifically involved in therapeutic interactions. In this process its therapeutic interactions are specifically tailored to the particular states, requirements, and needs of the organism.

Parts of the effects of the fluid body may go into dysfunction. In this case various irregular lateral fluctuations arise. According to Jealous, dysfunctions and dysfunctional forces may be reflected in the fluid body, as in a footprint.

In order to be able to palpate and assess the presence of the fluid body, it is necessary to wait until the organism finds its point of balance and enters the neutral state. Only in the neutral state can the practitioner sense how the fluid body responds uniformly, i.e., simultaneously in all its dimensions – to the primary respiration with a constant rhythm of about 2.5 cycles (or slower) per minute. Jealous asserts that if the neutral state is not present, it is virtually impossible to make a diagnosis via the fluid body.

Fluid dynamics can be palpated in all regions of the body. Gentle touch is the prerequisite that enables the quality of these dynamics to be assessed and estimated. It is important to note that no hydraulic forces are produced, guided, or amplified in the fluid body; instead, in contrast, the practitioner should go with the automatic shifting and the fluid drive generated by the primary respiration. The activity of the primary respiration should not be impaired by palpation and the gentle fluid dynamics should not be hindered.

Palpation

- Establish the neutral state.

- For Jealous, it is important to focus palpatory sensing directly on the fluid body and not to confuse sensing of the fluid body with transitional tissue zones or with the interactions of the fluid body.

- Sense the presence of the primary respiration in the fluid body, i.e., you will sense an alteration in your consciousness.

- Sense the automatic shifting in the fluid body in the neutral state.

- The fluid body may possibly transmute into a more potent fluid function that is less influenced by circumstances and conditioning.

- Diagnosis is possible using an automatic shifting fulcrum.

Box 24.1

Diagnostic questions to ask when palpating the fluid body

- What is the frequency and amplitude of the rhythmic expression?

- Are frequency and amplitude constant?

- How is the end-feel of the amplitudes in the inhalation and exhalation phase?

- Are the rhythmic phenomena symmetrical?

- How easy and unforced is the rhythmic expression?

- Is there a perceptible spontaneous disengagement at the end of the inhalation phase?

- What is the fluid drive like and where does its potency come from?

- Does the fluid drive have direction, and if so, where to?

- Where is the fulcrum of the fluid body and fluid drive located?

- Are there any additional, asymmetric, and irregular fluctuations?

- Does the rhythmic quality appear simultaneously in all the dimensions of the fluid body?

- How clearly perceptible is the presence of the primary respiration?

- Is longitudinal fluctuation present and what are its characteristic qualities?

- Is any lateral fluctuation present (type, strength, and regularity)?

- Are there any perceptible dysfunctions?

Box 24.2

Dysfunctional patterns of the fluid body, according to Jealous

- Reduced amplitude at the coccyx as a result of general fatigue, acute illness, over-medication, excessive alcohol consumption, and compression of the long axis during the birth process

- Obstruction of longitudinal fluctuation in the course of its ascent (e.g., at the level of the respiratory diaphragm or cervicothoracic junction) as a result of long-term illness, worry, and rigid psychological attitudes

- Absence of longitudinal fluctuation, but awareness of an energy-rich state at the level of the coccyx, as a result of sexual or emotional rape or dissociated psyche

- Absence of longitudinal fluctuation and awareness of an energy-less state at the level of the coccyx, as a result of cocaine consumption, chemotherapy or radiotherapy, long-term steroid medication, or addiction denial

- Excessive lateral fluctuation as a result of burn-out syndrome, and as compensation where longitudinal fluctuation is no longer present

- In addition, the fluid body or the expression of the primary respiration in the fluid body is then best capable of reflecting the pattern of health and of setting healing reactions in motion.

A brief tour of the minnow and into the fluid developmental dynamics of the eyeball

On various occasions at the end of a course on the cranial concept, Sutherland liked to hold a lecture entitled "A tour of the minnow."[8] The underlying idea was to illustrate insights into and about the living brain. We will adopt Sutherland's idea, but we will accompany the minnow on a sightseeing tour to the period when the eye is being formed. This description will serve as an example of fluid developmental dynamics. By palpation using gentle and meaningful hand contact, you can attempt to follow these developmental dynamics:

- The minnow finds itself in the primary forebrain.

- It observes how the primordium of the eye appears on day 25/26 (at a time when the neural tube has not yet closed) as a small groove (the optic sulcus) on the forebrain.

- It accompanies this development further and notes how this groove rapidly deepens and how, following closure of the neural tube, the tiny optic vesicle appears as a projection of the primary forebrain.

- The minnow attentively observes how the optic vesicle in its further growth dynamics reaches toward the external boundary of the body on about day 32 and finally touches it.

- As soon as it touches the epidermis, the optic vesicle flattens and undergoes indentation to form the optic cup. The minnow witnesses a repeat of developmental dynamic movements similar to those leading to the formation of the neural tube.

- At this point of contact with the outer body surface something else occurs. The minnow again notices how the initially flat epidermal cells become columnar, and undergo condensation and invagination. This developmental dynamic is similar to gastrulation and neurulation. The optic vesicle is pressed in by the future lens material and yields around it.

- The minnow accompanies the lens on its inward migration until this finally detaches from the skin surface. (The process is similar to the formation of the neural tube from the neural plate, except that in this instance a circular rather than a cylindrical basic form develops.)

- On about day 40 the lens is surrounded by the optic cup that has formed.

- On the inner surface of the retina the cell layer has developed to form neurons, the axons of which grow across the inner surface of the retina and finally into the optic stalk. The minnow allows itself to be carried to an outlet for the stream carrying it, to the exit point for the optic nerve, and reaches the midbrain where the axons spread into the midbrain roof.

- Finally, the minnow emerges in the central fovea, as if carried along by the current of a stream.

Treatment principles underpinning the fluid variant of the EV-4 and CV-4 technique

The CV-4 technique and the EV-4 technique, in the narrower sense, are performed in the cranial region in the vicinity of the fourth ventricle. However, both the CV-4 and the EV-4 technique are simultaneously also general treatment principles for approaching the fluid body. In this sense they are by no means limited to the cranial region. Hand contact may be established at any point on the body.

For James Jealous, correct application to the fluid body or an appropriate approach to the fluid body presupposes the realization that the fluid body goes beyond the simple boundary of the skin and also extends to the field surrounding the body.

Hand contact

The ideal is for bilateral, symmetrical hand contact in one body region, e.g., in the shoulder-blade region, at the level of the developmental dynamic fulcrum of the fluid body.

Method

- Adopting a neutral, non-invasive, and empathic attitude, establish hand contact with the patient.

- Synchronize yourself with the fluid field.

- Sense any dysfunctional dynamics in this fluid body.

- The inherent forces will decide whether a CV-4 or an EV-4 technique is to be performed. The responsibility of the osteopath is to sense the dynamics that are unfolding in the dysfunctional fluid body and to go with them in their dominant direction: either toward the midline (CV-4) or toward the periphery (EV-4).

- Go with the potency to its fulcrum.

- The onset of palpatory rest/stillness signals the approach to a state of balance in the fulcrum of the potency. Simultaneously, you will notice a change in your consciousness.

- Therapeutic interaction consists of maintaining palpatory contact with this fulcrum.

- At the same time establish contact with the health in the patient, with the fluid body that cannot go into dysfunction. (There exist two fluid bodies: one can go into lesion, the other cannot.)

- Sense how the health in the patient interacts with the dysfunctional fluid body: automatic shifting occurs. The osteopath functions as a kind of fulcrum or support for this process.

- In the treatment it is important to sense the process of the "mutual seeing" of health and of the dysfunctional fluid pattern and to allow this to happen.

- The dysfunctional fluid body gradually re-orients itself toward the midline and toward health and develops symmetry. (This process generally also continues for days after treatment.)

- Maintain this therapeutic process until you sense a change that also includes the body as a whole and the region surrounding the patient.

- Sometimes you may sense a longitudinal fluctuation ascending from the coccyx and cascading to spread in the cranial interior.

- Constant longitudinal fluctuation lasting for at least 3 cycles indicates the endpoint of treatment.

Note

Under no circumstances should the osteopath alter the speed of rhythmic phenomena.

For details on treating the third ventricle (CV-3) and the ignition system see Torsten Liem: *Cranial Osteopathy – A Practical Textbook* (Seattle: Eastland Press; 2009:470).

Box 24.3

Questions to ask when evaluating findings made during the CV-4 and EV-4 techniques

- Which dynamics are perceptible in the fluid body?

- Are the patient's therapeutic forces or vital forces oriented toward the midline or away from it?

- Which intra-osseous and inter-osseous dynamics are perceptible during inhalation and exhalation?

- Which dynamics are perceptible at the reciprocal tension membrane during inhalation and exhalation?

- Which dynamics are perceptible in the longitudinal fluctuation during inhalation and exhalation?

- Which dynamics are perceptible in the "potency" during inhalation and exhalation?

- What are the features of the autonomic activity state?

Phenomenological approaches to the cerebrospinal fluid (CSF) in osteopathy

In osteopathy it is important that the rhythmic fluctuations of the CSF are distributed in the cranium and throughout the body without impediment. According to Sutherland, impaired activity of the CSF may be caused by a wide variety of dysfunction, for example those involving the intracranial membranes.[9] In osteopathy in the cranial field it is believed that restrictions that impede the free flow of the CSF may provoke disturbances and dysfunctions in the cranial sphere and even in the body as a whole. In Sutherland's terminology, the movement of the CSF within its natural cavity is called fluctuation.[10] In adopting this usage, Sutherland was following the views of A.T. Still, who regarded the CSF as the highest known element in the human body. For Sutherland, there resides in the CSF an invisible element, which he called the Breath of Life, or the "fluid within this fluid, something that does not mix, something that has potency as the thing that makes it move."[11] This potency has intelligence which, according to Sutherland, has the capacity to do the therapeutic work and which should not be driven by external forces. All that the practitioner is required to do is to give a small "kick-off" impetus in a given direction.

Sutherland described the potency of the CSF as being like an electrical potential, which continually builds up and discharges through its substance and its sphere of influence.[12]

Using osteopathic treatments, Magoun tried to alter the pattern, speed, amplitude, and direction of the CSF fluctuation.[13]

In cranial osteopathy a palpatory distinction is drawn between the longitudinal and the transverse or lateral fluctuation of the CSF. These palpatory experiences are defined and interpreted slightly differently by some osteopaths. Perronneaud-Ferré, a French osteopath, defines transverse/lateral fluctuation as CSF flow in the cranium, whereas longitudinal fluctuation is extracranial CSF flow in the spinal canal.[14] Perronneaud-Ferré suspects that longitudinal fluctuation occurs to a greater extent in the waking state and is dependent on the activity of the sympathetic nervous system, whereas transverse fluctuation predominates during sleep and is dependent on the parasympathetic nervous system.[14]

According to Magoun, the ideal normal fluctuation is oriented in the longitudinal axis of the body, with waves equal in length and amplitude.[15] By contrast, transverse fluctuation arises as a result of dysfunctions, e.g., of membranous origin, or as a possible reaction to manual therapy. Furthermore, Magoun held that for therapeutic reasons it might be necessary to deliberately initiate a transverse wave so as to bring the fluid to a state of equilibrium for the particular dysfunctional pattern present; to incite more activity when fluctuation is weak or uneven; or to calm and palliate excessive activity in the fluid.[16]

Via manual contact on the temporal bones, for example, Sutherland used the "father Tom" technique to induce lateral fluctuation of the CSF and to urge the fluctuation into activity, whereas the palliation of "mother puss" was used to accompany a smaller, more rapid excursion that approaches a still point.[17]

Jealous defines longitudinal fluctuation (in agreement with Sutherland) as CSF fluctuation along a longitudinal axis, which is oriented spatially toward a bioelectric midline,[18] while lateral fluctuation occurs lateral to the midline. He comments that small lateral fluctuations out of synchrony with the "intelligence of the tide" are frequently encountered during motion testing. Lateral fluctuation with high amplitude may even mask the absence of longitudinal fluctuation.

Similarities between the ideas of Sutherland and Swedenborg

- To some extent, early osteopathic ideas relating to the cranial sphere show remarkable parallels with theories elaborated by Emanuel Swedenborg in the early to middle years of the 18th century. Both Still and Sutherland were familiar with at least some aspects of Swedenborg's teachings, as confirmed, for example, by the fact that Sutherland quoted Swedenborg.[19]

- Exactly like Sutherland after him, Swedenborg referred to rhythmic phenomena – albeit with a much faster rhythmicity – to which he gave the name "tremulation." He believed this tremulation to be important for the body as a whole. Anticipating Sutherland, Swedenborg already attributed to the brain a "reciprocal and undulatory motion," which causes fluid to be continually pressed in and out, propelling it to the extremities and thence back to its "original fountain."[20]

- For Swedenborg and in line with views held in osteopathy, obstruction of motion was like life that had been deprived of a spark of its proper nature. As soon as something more moving is added, the liveliness is seen to be increased.[21]

- It is also notable that for Swedenborg and for Sutherland the CSF and the dural membranes played an important role for the body as a whole, far more so than can be accounted for on the basis of current knowledge in mainstream medicine. Thus Swedenborg considered the entire membrane system of the body to be nothing but a continuous extension of the dura mater.[22] He believed that tremulation, which begins in the nervous system, was transmitted from the dural membranes throughout the entire membrane and nervous system of the body and even as far as the bones, like the oscillations in fluids or in the atmosphere.[23] Swedenborg held that the degree of fullness of life was related to the degree of tension in the meninges,[24] and that the CSF flowed into all the membranes and all the finest and most remote expanses of the body.[25]

- It appears highly likely that Sutherland, in his descriptions of palpatory findings at the cranium, was also basing his ideas on views elaborated by Swedenborg at the start of the 18th century[26, 27] and on Still's hypotheses at the end of the 19th century. With regard to the CSF, these views are based on pre-modern principles of Galenism (and dating back as far as 3500 BC): namely that the soul or anima resides in fluid, i.e., in the CSF.

- As early as 3500 BC two Egyptian physicians were the first to describe the presence of fluid in the cranium.[28]

- Terms such as "vital spirits" and "animal spirits" were first introduced between about 130 and 200 AD.

Following the demystification of CSF physiology during the 20th century, further discussion and clarification are needed to determine whether some of Sutherland's palpation descriptions may need to be qualified in the light of modern-day knowledge, and perhaps be replaced or supplemented by better validated and more up-to-date descriptions or palpation models that take account of recent discoveries in CSF physiology. On the other hand, it seems clear that Sutherland – at least in his later years – shifted his focus in treatment more toward bioelectrical phenomena in the fluid (see above). These phenomena find their parallels in modern-day energy medicine models of the human body.

References

[1]Straus E. Vom Sinn der Sinne. Ein Beitrag zur Grundlegung der Psychologie. 2nd ed. Berlin: Springer; 1956:407.

[2]Emoto M. Messages from Water. Los Angeles: Hado Publishing: 1999.

[3]Schwenk T. Sensitive Chaos: The Creation of Flowing Forms in Water and Air. Forest Row, East Sussex: Rudolf Steiner Press; 2004:24.

[4]Schwenk T. Sensitive Chaos: The Creation of Flowing Forms in Water and Air. Forest Row, East Sussex: Rudolf Steiner Press; 2004:61.

[5]Schwenk T. Sensitive Chaos: The Creation of Flowing Forms in Water and Air. Forest Row, East Sussex: Rudolf Steiner Press; 2004:41.

[6]Schwenk T. Sensitive Chaos: The Creation of Flowing Forms in Water and Air. Forest Row, East Sussex: Rudolf Steiner Press; 2004:41.

[7]Jealous J. The Biodynamics of Osteopathy. Fluid body (audio CD series). 2001. Marnee Jealous Long, 6501 Blackfin Way, Apollo Beach, FL 33572, mjlong@ tampabay.rr.com.

[8]Sutherland WG. Contributions of Thought. 2nd edn. Portland: Rudra Press; 1998:334f.

[9]Sutherland AS, Wales AL (eds). Contributions of Thought. The Collected Writings of William Garner Sutherland, D.O. 2nd edn. Portland: Rudra Press; 1998:75f., 94f., 99, 119, 194.

[10]Sutherland WG. Teachings in the Science of Osteopathy. Sutherland Cranial Teaching Foundation; 1991:13.

[11]Sutherland WG. Teachings in the Science of Osteopathy. Sutherland Cranial Teaching Foundation; 1991:14.

[12]Magoun HI. Osteopathy in the Cranial Field. 1st edn. Kirksville: Journal Printing Company; 1951:72.

[13]Magoun HI. Osteopathy in the Cranial Field. 1st edn. Kirksville: Journal Printing Company; 1951:81.

[14]Perronneaud-Ferré R. Ostéopathie crânio-pelvienne. Aix en Provence: Verlaque; 1989:31.

[15]Magoun HI. Osteopathy in the Cranial Field. 3rd edn. Kirksville: Journal Printing Company; 1976:108.

[16]Magoun HI. Osteopathy in the Cranial Field. 3rd edn. Kirksville: Journal Printing Company; 1976:115.

[17]Sutherland WG. Contributions of Thought. 2nd edn. Portland: Rudra Press; 1998:174f.

[18]Jealous J. Biodynamic course script: CSF activity. 1997. Marnee Jealous Long, 6501 Blackfin Way, Apollo Beach, FL 33572.

[19]Sutherland AS, Wales AL (eds). Contributions of Thought. The Collected Writings of William Garner

Sutherland, D.O. 2nd edn. Portland: Rudra Press; 1998:163f.

[20]Swedenborg E. On Tremulation. Boston: Massachusetts New-Church Union; 1899:36.

[21]Swedenborg E. On Tremulation. Boston: Massachusetts New-Church Union; 1899:10.

[22]Swedenborg E. On Tremulation. Boston: Massachusetts New-Church Union; 1899:29f.

[23]Swedenborg E. On Tremulation. Boston: Massachusetts New-Church Union; 1899:32.

[24]Swedenborg E. On Tremulation. Boston: Massachusetts New-Church Union; 1899:35.

[25]Swedenborg E. On Tremulation. Boston: Massachusetts New-Church Union; 1899:39.

[26]Swedenborg E. On Tremulation. Boston: Massachusetts New-Church Union; 1899:37.

[27]Swedenborg E. Dynamics of the Soul's Domain. Boston: Massachusetts New-Church Union; 1899:270f. (vol. 1), 245 (vol. 2).

[28]Schiller F. The cerebral ventricles: from soul to sink. Arch Neurol 1997;54:1158–1162.

Energy bodies

Torsten Liem

Introduction

The contents of this chapter as a whole are highly controversial because at present their corroboration by objective investigation is less than adequate. It is not the purpose of this chapter to demonstrate the ontological existence of energy bodies or to discuss the arguments "for" and "against," but merely to outline the potential importance of these models and phenomena in osteopathic treatment.

Body–sheath–consciousness model in the Vedanta/Vajrayana tradition

Vedanta psychology distinguishes three bodies and five sheaths ("koshas") or layers of spirit. These are to be understood as phenomenological realities that have their origin in the philosophical systems of Vedanta and Vajrayana. They refer to different specific aspects of the subjective experience of being alive. The gross body, which forms the densest manifestation, is associated in particular with sensorimotor and physical sensations. The subtle body comprises vital, emotional, and sexual energy, the mental and higher-mental body, and the body of light. Finally, the causal body is the vehicle for sensing potent emptiness and formless reality. Even though these bodies, sheaths and their associated consciousness states are present and accessible from birth (and even before), the gross, subtle, and causal expressions of consciousness evolve simultaneously during the course of life (Table 25.1).

Each sheath must be cleansed and transcended. Unconscious, conditioned identification exclusively with the sheaths ("upadhis" or limiting conditions) needs to be differentiated, relativized, and transcended if a person is to identify with the self (atman) and be able to recognize the inner self. This occurs via a stepwise development of consciousness to the transcendent, ever-present self or witness (turiya), ultimately leading to the non-dual state (turiyatita).

The analogy of a glass container and the space inside can be used to illustrate the relationship between upadhis and atman: the glass container represents the obscuring force of the sheaths. The space stands for atman. The glass appears to separate and divide the spaces inside and outside the glass. However, this division is merely illusory because the space remains one and indivisible.

Further refinement of the Vedanta model – matter/energy as exterior and consciousness as interior

The model of inner growth stages of consciousness used by these early mystics remains unsurpassed in its topical relevance. However, Ken Wilber has further refined this pre-modern Vedanta/Vajrayana model by relating the increasing complexity of matter that occurs during the evolution of consciousness to an increase in the degree of consciousness. Because of their introspective mystical focus and understanding, the ancient seers and sages were denied this insight – with the result that they understood all subtle and causal consciousness states as existing beyond matter. It was only with the more sophisticated understanding brought by science with its outward-looking focus that it became clear, in terms of phylogenetic as well as ontogenetic dynamics, that matter (including the energy fields bound to matter) appears as externally objective right through to the ultimate, internal subjective level, the highest possible level of consciousness. In this process Wilber leaves it open whether a subtle and causal body simultaneously exists that even after death might permit a non-material continuation of emotional, mental, and spiritual experiences.

In Indian and Chinese medicine human beings are viewed as manifestations of a universal continuum of energy and consciousness, with neither aspect being reduced to the other. The energy bodies become

Body	Sheath ("kosha")	State	Possibly influenced by
Gross physical body; stula sharira	Annamaya kosha; food sheath	Waking	Asana, food, healthy lifestyle
Subtle body; linga/ sukshma sharira	Pranayama kosha; vital sheath, prana-emotional-sexual Manomaya kosha; mental sheath Vijnanamaya kosha; intellect sheath	Dreaming	Pranayama, psychotherapy Mantra, ritual, withdrawal of senses, concentration, selfless service Study of sacred writings, formal questioning, meditation
Causal body; karana sharira	Anandamaya kosha; overmental or blissful sheath	Dreamless deep sleep	Samadhi

TABLE 25.1: Taxonomy of bodies, sheaths, and consciousness in the Vedanta/Vajrayana model

manifest as a specific frequency type in a specific time interval. Energy and energy patterns or signatures are therefore assigned to the exterior, in exactly the same way as the physical body is. The increase in the complexity of material form (i.e., exterior) is associated with an increase in the refinement of energies (i.e., exterior) and an increase in inner consciousness (i.e., interior): the more complex the gross forms, the more subtle the accompanying energy patterns/fields and the greater the inner consciousness.

The complexification of gross form is the "vehicle" of manifestation for both subtler energies, as well as for greater consciousness. In ontological terms, therefore, matter, energy, and consciousness are not completely independent of and separate from each other; instead mutual correlations exist.

The Vedanta models and their further refinement are of major usefulness for osteopathy in that they have elaborated differentiated paradigms of tissue (matter) energy and consciousness. Without the differentiation, integration, and methodological implementation of the energy aspects and consciousness aspects in our palpatory approach to tissues, there is a danger that osteopathic treatment will become reductionist and potentially dissociative, regardless of the theoretical superstructure.

Energy fields

Each level of energy surrounds the body with a field, and these energy fields are organized as a holarchy (nested hierarchy). Each field that arises later in evolutionary terms envelops the previous field and transcends it (Figure 25.1).

An infant already possesses a gross, a subtle, and a causal energy field because it has access to all three major states of consciousness (waking, dreaming, and dreamless deep sleep) but not to all the subspecies and further differentiations of these energy fields. The latter emerge only as the child matures and develops and they are associated with the developmental stages of consciousness.

Our energy fields are constantly changing – usually without us being aware of this. Change depends on the strength of our vitality, the emotions unfolding and stirring within us, and the type of consciousness that is currently the main focus of our personality, etc. Many people are unaware that they can also influence these energy fields subconsciously. Energy follows thought, intention, and purpose.

Knowledge of these interactions is essential for the successful treatment of dysfunctional tissue–energy–consciousness complexes. Somatic dysfunctions are associated with specific energy manifestations, physical experiences, emotional stirrings, and cognitive interpretations.

Evolutionary development of energy families

The different energy families have emerged or manifested successively over the course of evolution.

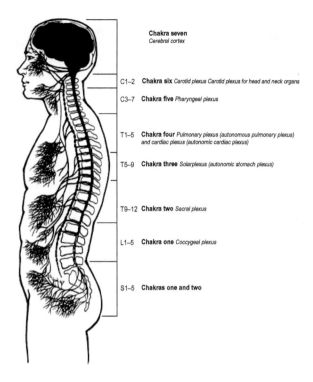

Chakra seven
Cerebral cortex

C1–2   **Chakra six** *Carotid plexus Carotid plexus for head and neck organs*

C3–7   **Chakra five** *Pharyngeal plexus*

T1–5   **Chakra four** *Pulmonary plexus (autonomous pulmonary plexus) and cardiac plexus (autonomic cardiac plexus)*

T5–9   **Chakra three** *Solarplexus (autonomic stomach plexus)*

T9–12 **Chakra two** *Sacral plexus*

L1–5   **Chakra one** *Coccygeal plexus*

S1–5   **Chakras one and two**

Figure 25.1
Energy fields.

Causal field, Mental field, Astral (emotional-sexual) field, Etheric (vital) field

The gross energy forces came into being with the Big Bang, the subtle energy forces emerged with living cells, and causal energy forces evolved with the appearance of the triune brain. All three energy families are intrinsic to a human holon and are already present at the time of conception.

Energy and consciousness

Gross bodies/energies support waking consciousness; subtle bodies/energies support the dreaming state, intermediate-level consciousness, and meditative states; and causal bodies/energies support formless states of consciousness associated with dreamless deep sleep (Table 25.2). At birth every individual has access to the three main realms of consciousness (waking, dreaming, and dreamless deep sleep), and to the three major energy families.

However, the "content" of these realms (what a person "sees" there and how that person interprets it) only fills, so to speak, as the individual develops and matures (Table 25.3). Consequently, thoughts emerge only on entry into the noosphere, both in the waking state and in the dreaming state. Furthermore, it is a characteristic of this development that "temporary states" can be converted into "permanent traits." Thus, in the course of development, the three great states come increasingly to the fore: the waking state becomes more lucid, more visionary, more creative; the dreaming state becomes more wakeful and dreams are experienced more consciously; and finally – with sufficient enlightenment – the person achieves the witness state, in which they can permanently access the whole range of consciousness states.[1]

The taxonomy of energy fields

There exist various taxonomies of the energy fields surrounding the human body and of the energies operating within it. One proposed taxonomy describes gross energies (electromagnetic, gravitational, and strong and weak nuclear), subtle energy fields (etheric/vital, astral/emotional, mental, and higher mental), and a causal (or overmental) energy field (see Table 25.3). They all surround and permeate the body and mutually influence each other.

Individual energy patterns arise not only in one field, but are dependent on specific interacting dynamics and mechanisms. Simultaneously, the individual fields in turn are involved in the more global, more universal fields.

In the ideal state the energy bodies and fields repel what is harmful and unnecessary for them and attract or absorb what they need; thus, they stand in a balanced relationship to the exterior world. Disturbance of this balance provides the platform for ill health to emerge.

The following sections outline a possible taxonomy of energy fields (see also Table 25.3, Chapters 4 and 25). A description of gross energies has been omitted deliberately because these are already adequately covered in the scientific literature.

Body/energy	Gross	Subtle	Causal	Non-dual
Consciousness	Waking	Dreaming: - Dreaming state - Meditative states - Unusual states, etc	Dreamless* deep sleep	Outside – permeating/ experiencing everything, but also transcending it

TABLE 25.2: Realms/states*

*The term "states" in this context must not be confused with developmental stages. Dreamless deep sleep is assigned to the causal state. The capacity for dreamless deep sleep emerges with the development of the triune brain, whereas conscious access becomes possible only with the development of the complex neocortex.

Each of the three major realms of consciousness (waking, dreaming, dreamless deep sleep) is available at birth. In the dreaming state, for example, a person is aware of images, visions, and archetypes. The content of this phase also occurs naturally in the waking state, but it is designated as the dreaming state because nothing apart from this content occurs in the dreaming state. The number of levels in this classification scheme is relatively arbitrary (rather in the same way that temperature can be measured on either the Fahrenheit or the Celsius scale), and if required, far more elaborate taxonomies can be proposed.

Matter	Energy	Consciousness
Atoms, molecules	Electromagnetism Gravitation Strong nuclear energy Weak nuclear energy	Sensorimotor (physiosphere)
Biological life: beginning with prokaryotes, eukaryotes, neuronal organisms	Etheric: L-field 1; biological life	Vital, biofield 1 (emergence of the biosphere)
Brain stem, limbic system	Astral, L-field 2	Emotional-sexual, biofield 2
Triune brain (neocortex)	Psychic-1, T-field 1; (emergence of causal energies)	Mental (emergence of the noosphere)
Complex neocortex	Psychic-2, T-field 2	Higher mental
Complex neocortex	Causal or C-field Non-dual	Overmental (emergence of the theosphere) Supermental

TABLE 25.3: Ken Wilber's taxonomy of matter, energy, and consciousness

L-field = life field; T-field = thought field. The increasing complexification of matter is associated with an increase in consciousness and, as the exterior objective dimension, it correlates with the interior subjective development of consciousness. The right-hand column is intended to illustrate that each developmental stage of consciousness (the interior subjective dimension) is associated with a particular mode of seeing or experiencing the world. Accordingly, in holarchic terms, sensorimotor (physical) consciousness represents a lower level than mental consciousness.

Subtle fields

The subtle category comprises the vital, emotional–sexual, and mental (higher mental) fields.

- Etheric (vital) field:
  - The most important function of the etheric field is the transfer of life energy or vitality from the universal field to the individual field and thence to the physical body. It extends for about 5–7 cm beyond the surface of the physical body.

    The etheric field, which is more subtle than gross energy, is believed to be the energy system that acts as the connecting link between the gross and the astral fields.[2]

    The etheric field extends for 5–7 cm (Gelder-Kunz) or for 0.5 cm (Pierrakos) beyond the periphery of the physical body and is almost transparent.

- Astral (emotional–sexual) field:
  - This is the seat of strong desires and emotions.[2] It extends for 38–45 cm (Gelder-Kunz) or for 7–10 cm (Pierrakos) beyond the periphery of the physical body and is shimmering blue.

- Mental field (including the higher mental field):
  - This extends for 90 cm (Gelder-Kunz) or for 15–20 cm (Pierrakos) beyond the periphery of the physical body (in the open air these distances may increase to several meters). It is an almost transparent sky blue.

Causal field

This is the seat of dreamless deep sleep and the vehicle for sensing potent emptiness and formless reality. According to Gelder-Kunz, it extends for 90–110 cm beyond the periphery of the physical body.

The chakra system

"Chakra" is a Sanskrit word meaning "wheel" and refers to the energy vortices that permeate the different gross, subtle, and causal bodies and form part of the exchange of energy with the universal energy field. The chakra system is very helpful for the treatment of energy bodies. Each chakra represents gross, subtle, and causal energies. At the same time each chakra represents a specific developmental stage of consciousness.[3]

In the gross dimension the chakras are associated with bodily organs and systems. In the subtle dimensions the chakras appear as they are most often depicted, that is as subtle centers of energy, aligned along the spine, with some secondary chakras (some of which are aligned lateral to the spine) and the energy channels (nadis) which, according to Motoyama,[2] are identical with the meridian system. In the causal dimension the chakras exist as archetypes or as the causal ground and support of the subtle and gross dimensions.

Function of the chakras

The chakras operate centripetally and represent the "portals" for drawing in energies from the surrounding atmosphere into the body.[4] Via the chakras the energies enter the other layers or they are converted into low-dimensional energy in order to act, for example, in the gross body.

The principal function of the chakras is to synchronize energies from the different levels. In the etheric field they serve primarily to help regulate the orientation of energy in the body. Chakras are believed to function as transmitters and transformers of energy from field to field, thus synchronizing gross, subtle (etheric, emotional, etc.), and causal energies and coordinating the dynamic interactions between the different fields. The fulcrum of the chakra is a type of interaction point at which energy flows from field to field and/or from level to level. Like breathing, this is a continuous process of taking in and giving out.

Energy is thought to be drawn-in and collected centripetally in the fulcrum of the chakra. From there the energy reaches the spinal column, and then circulates in the tiny pathways of the etheric body (nadis), which have been suggested as being connected to the nervous system of the physical body. Finally, the energy returns to the fulcrums of the chakras before being distributed centrifugally in spirals through the periphery. The spiraling vortex pattern of spread becomes wider and wider, gradually blending and fading into the entire field of the etheric body.

Chakras here are not separate from the fields themselves; instead they resemble vortices that concentrate the energy within the fields (just as whirlpools are formations in and of water).[5]

The chakras simultaneously represent seven levels of consciousness (Table 25.4). The chakra that is the principal focus of the individual's mind determines

Chakra	Gross	Subtle (vital and emotional body)
#1 Muladhara chakra Color: red	Legs, feet, bones, colon, teeth; blood and the building of cells; adrenals; coccygeal plexus	Survival, grounding
#2 Svadhisthana chakra* Color: orange	Uterus, genitals, kidneys, bladder, circulatory system (blood, lymph, digestive juice, sperm), instinctive drives; ovaries, prostate, testicles; sacral plexus	Desire, pleasure, sexuality, reproduction (expansion and letting go of self in sexual union); link between pelvis and heart
#3 Manipura chakra Color: yellow	Digestive system, muscles, autonomic nervous system; pancreas; celiac ganglion	Will, power, assertiveness, projection of personal energy (emotions, individual unconscious, according to Motoyama); joie de vivre; astral energy penetrates the etheric field here
#4 Anahata chakra Color: emerald-green	Heart, lungs, pericardium, thoracic region; thymus gland; cardiac plexus	Empathy, love, integration and general balancing function,*** emotional openness
#5 Vishuddha chakra Color: blue or turquoise	Neck, upper extremities, thyroid; laryngeal plexus	Communication, creativity****
#6 Ajna chakra Color: purple or deep blue	Face, eyes, nose, ears, cerebellum, central nervous system; pituitary; carotid sinus/body	Clairvoyance, intuition, intellectual clarity, visualization (extrasensory perception)
#7 Sahasrara chakra Color: white	Cerebral cortex; pineal gland	Thinking, information, understanding, synthesis

TABLE 25.4A: The dimensions and seven developmental stages of the chakra system

*According to Leadbeater (p. 7),[8] arousing the Svadhisthana chakra is a misfortune to be avoided. When activated, it not only produces more energy, but may also result in an increase in sexual lust and negative emotions, such as hatred and jealousy. Instead, Leadbeater refers to the spleen chakra (not indicated in Indian writings), which is located over the spleen lateral to the spine. The spleen chakra is principally responsible for taking in vital energy from the general field, modifying it and distributing it further, for example, in the physical body. According to Pierrakos, the first chakra has more to do with receiving, and the second chakra has more to do with giving.
**According to Motoyama.[2]
***If this has developed, then sense-dependent distinctions and the resultant egotistical desires have been transcended.
****If the lesson of this chakra has been mastered, then "truth" can be heard and communicated without prejudice and with great inner spaciousness.

particular modes of seeing or particular conditionings of perception. For example, if the mind is centered in the three lower centers, it is attached to worldliness.

According to Pierrakos, the first four chakras at the front of the body are primarily feeling centers. At the back of the body, again according to Pierrakos, there are five further centers that are the will centers: one over the sacral region acts in conjunction with the front pubic chakra, and another between the shoulder-blades regulates two sub-regions (one in the neck and another at

Chakra	Location	Causal	Associated characteristics
#1 Muladhara chakra Color: red	Perineum, at the level of the tip of the coccyx; opens downward	Stillness, security, stability, rootedness, (physical) will to be	Material world
#2 Svadhisthana chakra* Color: orange	About 3 cm below the navel,** lower abdomen, genitals, uterus; opens forward	"I feel," creative reproduction of being	Sexuality and physical desire
#3 Manipura chakra Color: yellow	Between navel and solar plexus; opens forward	"I can," shaping of being	Ego, personality, attainment of realistic self-esteem; trust, fear
#4 Anahata chakra Color: emerald-green	Cardiac region at the level of the sternum; opens forward	Devotion, self-abandon	Love, hate, resentment, devotion, empathy
#5 Vishuddha chakra Color: blue or turquoise	Neck; opens forward	Synthesis of ideas into symbols, resonance of being	Self-expression, deceit, ignorance
#6 Ajna chakra Color: purple or deep blue	Central location between the eyebrows; opens forward	Knowledge of being	Intellect, intuition, knowledge, wisdom
#7 Sahasrara chakra Color: white	Highest point on the head; opens upward	Bliss, pure seeing	Spirituality, trust in God

TABLE 25.4B: The dimensions and seven developmental stages of the chakra system

the posterior attachment of the respiratory diaphragm) and is associated with the will toward the outer world. Another at the level of the occiput possesses both a will function and a mind function. By contrast, the sixth and seventh chakras are mind centers (Figure 25.2).

The chakras and health

Depending on state of health, vitality, state of consciousness, and individual circumstances, the chakras in the etheric body differ markedly in terms of rhythm, size, speed of movement, rotational direction and form, brightness and color, etc. (see pp 288ff., 378ff.).

Development of the chakras

At birth the neonate possesses all seven chakras, but primarily in the gross form. In the etheric body the chakras are generally thought to have a diameter of about 3 cm in the neonate. However, like the subtle and causal dimensions, the higher chakras – especially in their subtle form – are present initially as potential blueprints that reveal themselves and evolve as the individual matures and develops.

Each chakra expresses itself accordingly in the waking state (gross), dreaming state (subtle), and dreamless

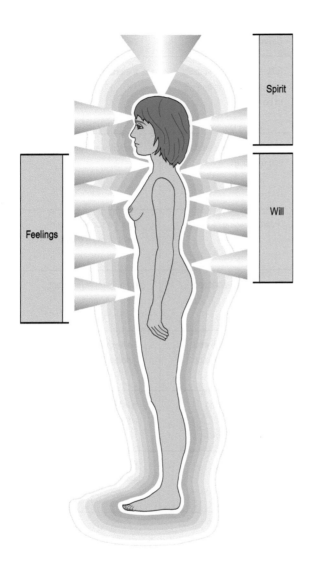

Spirit

Will

Feelings

Figure 25.2
Energy fields and centers (chakras), according to Pierrakos.[14]

deep sleep state (causal). The non-dual state is, as it were, the ground for all of them. The higher chakras become accessible during the course of development. However, development in the different dimensions (gross, subtle, and causal) generally follows a heterogeneous pattern, i.e., it is possible and indeed quite common for there to be advanced development in the gross dimension, whereas development lags behind in the subtle and causal dimensions.

Exercise to develop sensitivity for the intention of touch[15]

When treating the energy body it is important first to be able to differentiate the various basic forms of energy exchange in palpation: giving, taking, neutral, and merging.

Carry out this exercise with a partner. One of you plays the active role, and the other is passive. Assuming that you begin by playing the passive role, you should stand with your back to your partner. Your partner now tries to concentrate on each of the four following intentions of touch:

1 A giving touch, for example, giving energy, strength, or support.

2 A taking touch, for example, drawing out or leading away an excess of energy or any congestion that may be present.

3 A merging touch between two persons.

4 A neutral touch, containing as far as possible no intention of giving, taking, or merging.

Your partner should perform each of these intentions of touch in an arbitrary sequence using the touch of the hands on your shoulders. Your task is to identify which intention your partner is using. Write down on a piece of paper the intention of touch that you detect on each occasion, and compare results at the end of the exercise. Where your results disagree, you should repeat that particular intention of touch. Such disagreements may be attributable equally to a lack of clarity in the touch of the person doing the touching and to the perception of the person being touched. You do not necessarily have to achieve 100% agreement, but you do need to develop a consciousness and sensitivity for the intention of touch you are using in your approach to your patients. Most of the time we are not conscious of the way we touch others. This exercise teaches us a great deal about ourselves and our needs. It also develops our sensitivity toward other people, their needs, and the unconscious, unspoken messages that their bodies and tissues can nevertheless communicate to us.

For further details on the diagnosis and treatment of energy fields and chakras, see pp. 288ff., 378ff. and Chapter 26.

References

[1]Comment from M. Habecker: Personal correspondence, 6/2005.

[2]Motoyama H, Brown R. Chakra-Physiologie. Freiburg im Breisgau: Aurum; 1990:116 ff., 124.

[3]Wilber K. Toward a Comprehensive Theory of Subtle Energies. Excerpt G.

[4]Pierrakos J. Core Energetics. Developing the Capacity to Love and Heal. Mendocino, CA: Life Rhythm; 1987.

[5]Van Gelder-Kunz D, Karagulla S. The Chakras and the Human Energy Fields. Wheaton, IL: The Theosophical Publishing House; 1989: 35.

[6]Sharamon S, Baginski BJ. The Chakra Handbook. Wilmot, WI: Lotus Light Publications; 1996.

[7]Anodea J. Wheels of Life. 2nd edition. St. Paul, MN: Llewellyn Publications; 1999.

[8]Leadbeater CW. The Chakras. 9th printing. Wheaton, IL; The Theosophical Publishing House: 2001.

[9]Motoyama H, Brown R. Chakra-Physiologie. Freiburg im Breisgau: Aurum; 1990.

[10]Brennan BA. Hands of Light. A Guide to Healing through the Human Energy Field. New York; Bantam New Age; 1988.

[11]Myss C. Anatomy of the Spirit: The Seven Stages of Power and Healing. New York; Three Rivers Press; 1996.

[12]Prabhavananda SW, Isherwood C. How to Know God: The Yoga Aphorisms of Patanjali. Hollywood, CA; Vedanta Press; 1996.

[13]Van Gelder-Kunz D, Karagulla S. The Chakras and the Human Energy Fields. Wheaton, IL: The Theosophical Publishing House; 1989.

[14]Pierrakos J. Core Energetics. Developing the Capacity to Love and Heal. Mendocino, CA: Life Rhythm; 1987.

[15]Liem T. Cranial Osteopathy. A Practical Textbook. Seattle: Eastland Press; 2009:359.

26

Chakra system related to pre- and perinatal dynamics

Terence Dowling

Introduction

The ancient Indian teaching about the chakra system goes back at least as far as the later Upanishads, which appeared sometime before 200 BC. Although the idea of chakras is now comparatively widespread and popular in many circles in the West, the original concept is still not very accessible to our modern Western mentality.

The chakra tradition is rooted in a very subtle awareness and understanding of the human being in the world. The radical divergence between our modern, primarily materialistic, scientific worldview and the cosmology and comprehensive anthropology, which is to be found in the Upanishads, should not be underestimated. This disparity becomes clear when we realize that there is not as yet the slightest scientific evidence for the existence of the chakras. Perhaps, however, with a deeper understanding of their nature, empirical evidence may be forthcoming. The insights presented below hope to support such a development.

Chakras are traditionally envisaged in India as wheel-like vortices of subtle energy, mysterious force-centres, which are connected to specific areas of the body and emanate from there out into the invisible layers of human manifestation. They are considered to be special points or "organs" for the reception and transmission of subtle energies between our physical body and the subtle, invisible energy systems, which surround, envelop and maintain us. Ultimately, they are believed to resonate with cosmic forces, well beyond our present scientific understanding.

One modern interpreter gives the following description:

A chakra is believed to be a centre of activity that receives, assimilates and expresses life-force energy. The word chakra literally translates as wheel or disk and refers to a spinning sphere of bioenergetic activity, emanating from the major nerve ganglia branching forward from the spinal column. Generally, six of these wheels are described, stacked in a column of energy that spans from the base of the spine to the middle of the forehead, the seventh lying beyond the physical world ...[1]

In order to make the idea more accessible, several other modern authors suggest, like Judith, that there is a relationship between the major nerve ganglia, which branch forward from the spinal column and the chakra system (see Figure 26.1). Each chakra along the spinal column is believed to influence or even govern the bodily functions related to that region of the spine.

However, it must not be forgotten that autopsies do not reveal chakras. They simply reveal nerve plexuses and the chakra tradition is a very distinctive, non-European way of seeing significance in these empirical features of our anatomy.[2]

The real problem of interpreting the chakras becomes apparent when it is remembered that in the original early sources and right up until the present day, there is a huge discrepancy concerning their exact number. Different systems posit various numbers. Many authors also speak of a number of subsidiary, supplementary or minor chakras.

It is also important to remember that it was only in 1927 that the now dominant theory of seven main chakras was introduced to the West. Sir John Woodroffe (1865–1936), a British Orientalist, who is better known under his pseudonym as Arthur Avalon, was deeply interested in Hindu philosophy and Yogic practices, especially in Hindu Tantra. He published the remarkable book, *The Serpent Power – The Secrets of Tantric and Shaktic Yoga* in 1918. This became the most important source of our modern Western understanding of Kundalini Yoga.

In this book, Woodroffe translated two important Indian texts and provided a sophisticated philosophical commentary: the *Satcakra-Nirupana* ("Description of and Investigation into the Six Bodily Centres") written in AD 1577 by the pundit Purnananda, a yogi from

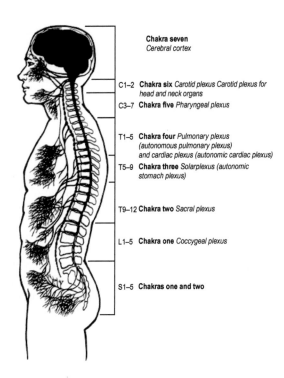

Chakra seven
Cerebral cortex

C1–2 **Chakra six** *Carotid plexus Carotid plexus for head and neck organs*

C3–7 **Chakra five** *Pharyngeal plexus*

T1–5 **Chakra four** *Pulmonary plexus (autonomous pulmonary plexus) and cardiac plexus (autonomic cardiac plexus)*

T5–9 **Chakra three** *Solarplexus (autonomic stomach plexus)*

T9–12 **Chakra two** *Sacral plexus*

L1–5 **Chakra one** *Coccygeal plexus*

S1–5 **Chakras one and two**

Figure 26.1

Energy fields

Bengal; and the *Padaka-Pancaka* ("Five-fold Footstool of the Guru") probably dating from the tenth century AD and written by the guru Goraknath for his disciples. The ideas in this complex work were eventually simplified and made more accessible by Charles Webster Leadbeater (1854–1934) in his well-known book *The Chakras* (1927). Leadbeater was a clergyman in the Church of England but his interest in spiritualism led him to leave that church to become an eminent member of the Theosophical Society. It was an explicit aim of this society "to investigate the unexplained laws of Nature and the powers latent in man."[3]

Several of the sources, which directly inspired Leadbeater's particular exposé of the chakra system, the view, which has become the dominant understanding of the chakras in the West, do not come from India or the Far East at all. They are to be found in European occultism and in certain Christian mystics. For example, Leadbeater was deeply interested in Johann Georg Gichtel (1638–1710), a German mystic, who explicitly refers to inner force centres in his *Theosophia Practica* (1696), an idea very much reflected in Leadbeater's depiction of the chakras. The illustration on the front cover of the book Leadbeater published in 1927 was taken directly from Gichtel's work (Figure 26.2).

More recently, there have been several attempts to revise and extend Leadbeater's interpretation. Elias Wolf, for example, claims that there are in total twenty-eight chakras.[4] Almut Klöpfer[5] and Jude Currivan and Wulfing von Rohr[6] claim that there are eight main chakras. Yet other interpretations describe one or more so-called transpersonal chakras, located above the crown chakra and an Earth-Star chakra posited to be beneath the soles of the feet.

Perhaps these authors have been influenced by an acquaintance with the Tibetan Buddhist theory of the chakras in which there are ten main chakras to be found along a central channel. This channel is believed to begin at the so-called third eye, curve up to the crown of the head and then to descend down through the body to the tip of the sexual organ. However, only four or five of these ten chakras are considered in Tibet to be of any real importance.

Thus, it is clear that the tradition of the chakras is not at all fixed and never has been. Even the basic concept itself remains speculative and open to further research. Whatever the chakras may or may not be, there is room for new interpretations. The chakra teachings must be permanently questioned and reinterpreted if they are going to have any real meaning for us today and help us in our pursuit of health and happiness.

Perhaps the chakras are simply very open metaphors, unique symbols related to specific regions of the body and which can be used in abundant ways to connect our bodily experience with our more subtle, mental insights and our cosmological beliefs and speculation.

The problem with metaphors is that they cannot be tested. They can only be transmitted and received, felt and appreciated or rejected as personally unhelpful or even untrue.

Perhaps everything in life can be related to the chakras and every experience can be believed to be influenced by them. Thus it is possible to create all sorts of statements about the chakras, which sound quite plausible to one person but are felt to be ridiculous humbug by another. It appears from a close study of the

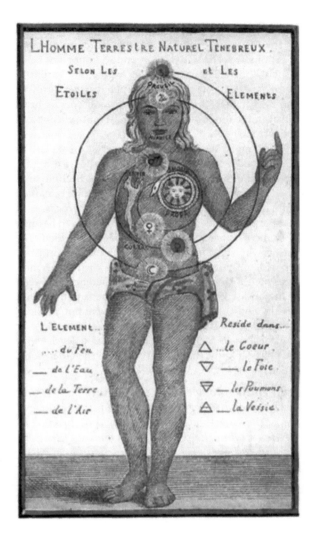

Figure 26.2
This picture appears on the front cover of Charles W. Leadbeater's book *The Chakras* (1927). He took it directly from *Theosophia Practica* (1696) by the German mystic, Johann Georg Gichtel (1638-1710).

literature that energies, experiences and ideas, which are, for example, explicitly connected by one author to Muladhara, the Root chakra might easily be attributed by another to Manipura, the Solar Plexus.

It is thus not at all surprising when a modern teacher, Tenzin Wangyal Rinpoche, even introduces a computer analogy. For him, the main chakras – of which in his view there are six – are like hard drives. Perhaps the hardware in question is indeed the nerve plexuses, the existence of which is known to every anatomist. However, what is of importance is the information, which is stored in the hard drive, and the way in which this information can be accessed and used. Tenzin teaches that each chakra contains much information, stored in many files. He considers that at least one of the files in each chakra is always open and in use, no matter how closed, hidden, protected, and inaccessible the rest of the information might be.

Furthermore, it is the specific information stored in each chakra, which forms and shapes our experience on many levels. The chakra information, which is actually accessible, determines what we can see, what we can experience, as well as that which remains hidden to our perception and awareness. Yoga is one way, according to Tenzin, in which to clear files and open others in any given chakra.[7]

The ether-body according to Rudolf Steiner

Because Rudolf Steiner rejected Charles Leadbeater's promulgation that the then sixteen-year-old Krishnamurti was a new Messiah, he and practically all German-speaking members separated from the Theosophical Society in 1911. One year later they founded the Anthroposophical Society. Steiner's own esoteric ideas became seminal for this new movement. One of these ideas was his concept of the four bodies or levels of manifestation in human beings.

According to Steiner, four levels of manifestation can be distinguished in the human being: (1) the physical, material body, (2) the ether body, (3) the astral body, and (4) the I (ger. Ich). (The latter two levels will not be discussed here.) In 1910 Steiner wrote:

In our 20th century a part of humanity will gradually develop a new human spiritual faculty. For example, before the 20th century is over, it will be possible to perceive the human ether-body.[8]

The physical body is the level of manifestation, which can easily be perceived empirically. It is quite obviously materially present. Any scientific method, which is able to observe and measure matter and the phenomena related to matter and energy transformation, can also

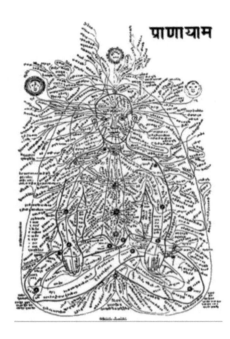

Figure 26.3

The Nadis - variously translated as 'conduits', 'nerves', 'veins', 'vessels' or 'arteries' - constitute the subtle or Yogic body in Tantra. Like the Chinese meridians, they are channels of vital force *(prana)* between the so-called **nadichakras** of which there are thousands

reveal structures and functions of the human body. At this level, the level at which traditional Western medicine still exclusively operates, linear chains of cause and effect can be deciphered. Medical research in the West aims to elucidate such causal chains in ever more microscopic detail and understands illness as a disruption of the smooth working of these chains. The various techniques of Western medicine are aimed at re-establishing homeostasis within these individual physical systems, especially within the organs and cells, when necessary by radical modification (e.g., surgery) and physical or chemical intervention (e.g., the use of radiation or pharmacological agents). By this quite narrow approach, medicine in the West has achieved remarkable insights and can produce impressive results.

However, every relationship within the human body and any function beyond the physical interaction of organs and cells remain uninteresting and neglected in the Western empirical approach. Many sorts of questions are censored *a priori* and so important fields of new knowledge are stifled at source. For example, many aspects of the processes, which maintain growth and health, also those involved in spontaneous healing or in the onset of disease, remain quite elusive and mysterious.

For example, Western medical experts can explain in great detail how a person has become ill with a viral infection but not why just this person has become so ill when others equally exposed to the virus have remained quite healthy. The initial causes of many processes of chronic physical degeneration – the decision to become ill in the first place, so to speak – remain hidden. The reason why someone remains healthy in the midst of illness is unknown. This is one reason why epidemics pose such a threat. Fundamental differences between health and sickness, between the propensity to remain healthy and the tendency to get ill, have not yet been fully understood.

According to Steiner's view, there is a level above the physical body, that which he called the ether-body, which:

is the entity through which the physical body is preserved from disintegration throughout the course of life… The ether-body is not simply a by-product of the material of the physical body and its functioning, but rather is an independent, real force, which awakens the so-called physical material to life in the first place… In every plant and animal, apart from the physical form there is also the life-fulfilling spirit-form… This life-giving force infuses the physical body and connects it with its ancestors and descendants and places it within a pattern of relationships, with which the bare material level is not in itself engaged.[9]

In modern terms, we can understand that the so-called ether-body exists at the level of information, which informs the physical body and allows and maintains certain life functions, which otherwise would not occur. To use a computer analogy, the ether-body corresponds to the software, which informs the physical, anatomical hardware. Just as with a computer, this information is stored within the hardware. Special parts of the body – and not just the cerebral cortex – are dedicated as "memory." In fact, all living units must have a memory function and must contain information in order to perform correctly within the environment in which they live.

At this "memory" level, the simple laws of cause and effect are no longer adequate to understand all the observable phenomena. Western medical research, for example, has at last arrived at the new science of epigenetics. Genetics was primarily interested in the building blocks and especially in hardware failure within the genes. Now epigenetics has realized that genetic defects and mutations in the genes at their chemical level do not explain the observable phenomena of inheritance or of human biological resilience. The genes are far more intelligent and respond quickly to new environmental demands. Our genome resonates with changes in our surroundings and life style and prepares us to meet new environmental challenges. Information is stored without change in the genetic hardware but through change in genetic function. Which genes are active, which genes have been deactivated and which genes can be reactivated, determines our ability to remain healthy and deal with the demands of life.

Information transfer in general does not take place through simple linear chains of cause-and-effect but through the subtle phenomena of resonance. Learning, for example, is not simply a question of exchange at a material, physical level. Whatever changes might be microscopically observable at that level, learning, imitation, empathy, and indeed all processes involving the transfer and acquisition of information cannot be understood as relatively passive processes of material transmission – like being poisoned or infected. There is rather a subtle transmission and transfer of energy. This energy-transfer produces resonance phenomena in order to influence the receiver and is usually open to feedback, which modulates the exact flow of information from the transmitter.

The chakras can thus be best understood not as the anatomical nerve plexuses themselves, situated at particular places within the human body (the hardware), but as the information, both the transgenerational and the personally unique information (the software), which is stored at these specific bodily locations and which can decisively influence the course of an individual human life. The nerve plexuses may indeed be the gross hardware involved in chakra memory. However, more subtle forms of cellular memory – for example, epigenetic modulation – should not to be discounted.

Four levels of awareness: Otto Scharmer's Theory U

It is impossible to "see" pure information. Information can only be observed in action, in the movements of the structures, which it informs and affects. However, this observation always involves special skill for it is all too easy just to see the parts in motion and not have a feel for the information, which alone fully explains the particular action taking place and which indeed makes that unique action possible in the first place.

How might the information contained in the chakras be perceived? It is obvious that the yogis, who first observed them, were most likely in a state of altered consciousness. A subtle form of perception is therefore probably required in order to perceive the chakras and their influence upon a person's life – the form of perception, which Rudolf Steiner hoped would become more common as we progress into the 21st century.

In Theory U (2009) by Otto Scharmer,[10] he describes four fundamentally different ways of perception, four ways that open us to distinct aspects of reality (Figure 26.4). Scharmer calls Level 1 perception downloading (p.119 f.). By this is meant that a person's primary concern is to seek acknowledgment for and approval of longstanding beliefs and well-established attitudes in whatever is experienced. The observer is anchored in routine and patterns from their restricted, individual past. The person is conventional, attempts to hold on to traditional views at all costs and seeks confirmation for tried-and-tested ways of behaving. There is little room for experiment and novelty, little room for learning. These people say what they want to hear and only see what they have seen before.

Level 2 is termed simply seeing (p.129 f.). In this position, a person is basically open and inquisitive. He is prepared to go to the edge of his personal boundaries and limitations in order to learn something new. This is what is generally meant by the phrase open-minded. Novelty and divergent points of view are accepted as potentially enriching. However, the personal point of view maintains priority and when it comes to disagreement, also claims authority. The person tries to be objective. Perception is focussed on dissonance and on non-conforming information. There is a change from conforming (Level 1) to confronting (Level 2).

Level 3 is termed sensing (p.143 f.). Here a person begins to perceive not only differences and unique qualities because they are interesting and provide for cognitive enrichment. The observer at Level 3 moves out of his own limited frame of reference and attempts to see the world from the point of view of another person. This is the beginning of empathy, the opening not only of the mind but also of the heart. With an open-heart, a process of personal decentralization begins to take place. We begin to see and feel the world from a point of view other than our own. This can bring with it radically new insights. We begin to go beyond ourselves. We begin to see ourselves as part of a much greater whole. Truth becomes intrinsically dialogical.

At Level 4, this process is intensified. Scharmer calls it presencing (p.163 f.) and speaks of open-will and deep listening. It is at this level that we begin to perceive the fullness of information, which is present in each moment of perception. This level opens us to a timeless perspective, which can see and value past realization in the same way as future possibility. This way of perception allows for evolution, for handling out of the future. It enables innovation at all levels. It is the mental attitude, which relies upon and trusts intuition. It is the source of true creativity.

It is exactly this sort of perception, Level 4 intuition, which is required if we wish to perceive the subtle biographical information stored in any individual person's chakra system.

The chakra system as meta-theory

From the above introduction and basic observations, it is clear that it is all too easy to make very general statements about the chakras, statements, which appear to have said something quite meaningful but which in the last analysis either say nothing specific at all or remain rather incomprehensible and non-verifiable. Many books about the chakras provide nothing more than a sweeping introduction into a meta-theory through an accumulation of miscellaneous and fanciful correlations.

The chakra symbols, each ultimately related to a specific part of the human body, can be imagined as connected through all manner of resonances to an infinite number of other phenomena. Thus, it is very easy to use chakra symbolism and terminology to say something suggestive of deep insight but at the same time to remain unspecific. Here are some typical statements taken from the Internet, which illustrate this problem:

- Each chakra develops in cycles at particular times in life, beginning in the womb.

- Childhood up to the age of seven years is a very formative period for the chakras.

- Traumatic experiences, lack of love, parental indifference, all negative influences and the suppression of natural desires during the critical time of childhood can cause an individual chakra or even several chakras to develop inadequately or not at all.

- The first year of life is especially important for the Muladhara or Root chakra, which is responsible among other things for basic trust. If an infant is separated from its mother or primary caregiver during this time and its need for human contact, warmth and nourishment are not met, this can cause an adult to suffer from lack of trust in life and carry within himself a deep-seated fear.

- Experiences later in life or a false lifestyle can cause a well-developed chakra to become blocked.

- Feelings such as fear, envy, jealousy, and hate can lead to obstruction of the chakras.

- Exaggerated adjustment to parental demands with accompanying emotional restraint can cause an unhealthy accumulation of energy, energy congestion in a particular chakra with the possibility of a dangerous discharge – for example, an explosion of anger.

In her compendium about the chakras, *The Wheels of Life* (1987),[11] Anodea Judith has collected together an enormous amount of information about the chakra system. For each chakra, she lists every conceivable connection. Practically all books about the chakras tend to be very eclectic. Towards the end of the book, however, she states the following details concerning the development of the chakras from the womb, through childhood, and up until early adulthood:

- Muladhara, the Root chakra, is influenced by very early events from the womb and into the first year of life.

- Svadhisthana, the Sacral or Sexual chakra, is influenced by events that occur between 6 and 18 months after birth.

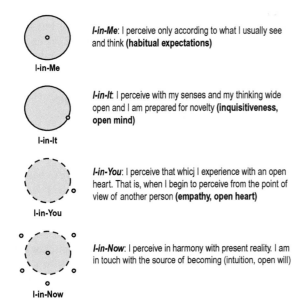

I-in-Me: I perceive only according to what I usually see and think **(habitual expectations)**

I-in-Me

I-in-It: I perceive with my senses and my thinking wide open and I am prepared for novelty **(inquisitiveness, open mind)**

I-in-It

I-in-You: I perceive that whicj I experience with an open heart. That is, when I begin to perceive from the point of view of another person **(empathy, open heart)**

I-in-You

I-in-Now: I perceive in harmony with present reality. I am in touch with the source of becoming **(intuition, open will)**

I-in-Now

Figure 26.4

Four perceptual positions: four qualities of attention according to Otto Scharmer.

- Manipura, the Solar Plexus, is influenced by events that occur between 18 months and 3 years

- Anahata, the Heart chakra, is influenced by the years of childhood between 4 and 7.

- Vishuddha, the Throat chakra, is influenced by the last years of childhood, 7 to 12 years old.

- Ajna, the Brow chakra or Third Eye, is influenced by puberty.

- Sahasrara, the Crown chakra, is influenced by the first years of adulthood.

For each of these periods, she gives general, good advice to parents and others about how to look after the children in our care. However, she does not develop her basic assertion that the chakras develop through the years of childhood in the way she proposes. Nor does she hint at any supporting evidence or corroborative observations. The schema she proposes is quite suggestive of truth and might indeed be factual and prove to be in some way useful. In the last analysis, however, it remains as yet unfounded and unconfirmed.

Methodology: corroboration of new insights into the chakra system

Any theory about the chakras, which attempts to deepen our insight in more than an evocative manner, must do so by elaborating the traditional information and insights that we have at our disposal and do so in such a way that new and interesting hypotheses are generated, propositions, which can be empirically tested and discarded if unconfirmed.

The chakras, as powerful symbols of subtle aspects of human life and consciousness, must be elaborated in such a way that our knowledge about these various aspects of life is shown to be a synthetic whole with practical consequences for our way of living. Any new insights must lead to a unifying theory, which in turn generates further insights and inspires further research.

If there is any truth in the chakra teaching for us today, it must be shown to be in itself completely coherent and to be congruent with modern scientific knowledge. Any new insight into the chakras must open the whole ancient teaching up to us. Any new insight must show us the beauty of the chakra system, the deep wisdom which it contains, and help us to use this ancient knowledge in our present day systems of healing.

The chakra system must be revealed to be congruent with other subtle insights into human nature, which are similar and which are taught in other ancient esoteric traditions. For example, the Lataif teaching of the Sufis, which has obvious parallels with the chakra tradition but also subtle differences, must also be illuminated by any new insight. Any new insight must show that the two systems, the chakra and the Lataif, are not contradictory but rather that they complement each other.

Pre- and perinatal psychology and medicine

At least since the publication of Otto Rank's book, *The Trauma of Birth* in 1924,[12] there has been a steady increase in our knowledge and understanding of the roots of human consciousness within prenatal life and our experience of birth. Otto Rank's student, Nandor Fodor, was the first to dedicate a book (*The Search for the Beloved*, 1940)[13] to the exploration of the prenatal roots of our deep unconscious structures.

Since then, countless researchers and authors have drawn attention to the importance of prenatal experience for the health and well-being of human beings. Peter Nathanielsz, for example, details in *Life in the Womb, The Origin of Health and Disease* (1999),[14] how the behaviour and life experiences of the mother during pregnancy determine many aspects of our future health. Her lifestyle during those nine months determines the health prospects of her child for life. Whether a mother smokes, drinks alcohol, takes drugs or medication, nourishes herself healthily, and is happy, safe, and secure, all these factors and more determine the basic psychosomatic health of her baby in later life. Early experience from the womb onwards influences not our genetic makeup but our epigenetic profile, that is, which of our 30,000 genes have been activated or deactivated. This determines much more of our health potential, our phenotype, than the genomic structure itself.

Empirical scientific research is revealing in ever more detail the primal aspects of human health. (See, for example, the websites run by Michel Odent: www.primalhealthresearch.com and www.wombecology.com)

Old dogmas about the overpowering influence of the genes and genetic disorder as the root-cause of disease must now be abandoned. The new science of epigenetics has demonstrated that it is not simply crude genetic defects that determine our illnesses. Rather our health is a question of which of our genes are operative and which are not.

Early experience from conception onwards is registered and expressed in our epigenetic makeup. Which genes in our genome are activated decides most of our health potential as well as any predisposition to disease and disorder.

Any successful healing – no matter how it is brought about – must result in a permanent change of lifestyle and an accompanying and permanent change in our epigenetic profile. This fact encourages us to understand that all alternative approaches to health, no matter how apparently spiritual and unempirical, can have a deep and lasting effect upon us – provided that our epigenetic constitution is touched by the healing experience.

Thus, modern science has revealed that much of our human misery is rooted in early experience but that healing is possible through strong, new experiences, which help us to change our lifestyle in an enduring way.

The primal programming of the chakras and Lataif

Waiting for birth – dreaming of being born

From the middle of the pregnancy onwards, babies begin to turn and rest their head in the pelvis of the mother. According to my own observation over many years, which is backed up by Nicette Sergueef in *Die Kraniosakrale Osteopathie bei Kindern*,[15] about 70% of babies choose the so-called first anterior occipital or left occipito-anterior (LOA) position. In this position, the crown of the baby's head is directed towards the pelvic floor and the impending birth canal with the left side of the baby's face snuggled up against the relatively flat surface of the mother's sacrum. The right side of occiput is tucked up against the mother's pubis. The left side of the baby's body rests against the posterior wall of the uterus towards the mother's relatively solid posterior abdominal wall and her spinal column. The right-hand side of the baby's body is held by the softer tissues of the mother's anterior abdominal wall. The baby's right shoulder lies above the mother's pubis and will later become the first shoulder to be born. The baby's left shoulder is folded down against the thorax. This gives the heart more room.

How long a baby experiences itself and the world around it in this position depends upon how early it turns – or indeed whether it turns into this position at all. Some babies remain in the breech position.

However, for most people (about 70%) the important developmental experiences towards the end of uterine life are experienced and recorded precisely in this special bodily position. In later life, when these same parts of the body are touched, when this unique position is reproduced, then we are in a position to remember the intrauterine time of waiting to enter into a world as yet not fully known to us – our postnatal family.

The crown of the head with its open fontanels, soft and relatively vulnerable, feels its way carefully into the pelvic floor – especially when the mother is standing upright and walking.

Furthermore, the upper entrance to the mother's pelvis, consisting of the os sacrum and ossa iliaca, form a relatively hard, bony ring around the baby's head, sitting like a prenatal tonsure or an organic halo. Some babies choose to remain in the breech position because this ring is too uncomfortable for them. During a difficult and painful birth, it is this ring, which can become a veritable crown of thorns for the child.

Before birth for most people (about 70%), the left side of the baby's body has a firm contact with the mother's posterior abdominal wall, where her spinal column lies. Especially when she is lying down, resting, or asleep while lying on her back, this becomes the baby's living mattress – with the prenate sleeping in the embryonic position on its left side and tummy.

Chakra Sahasrara

It is in this unique bodily position, with head bowed down and sheltered in the mother's pelvis, eyes closed, little hands often tucked up under the chin with little room to move, squatting and waiting for birth – or in some cases, perinatal death – that the prenatal baby learns that there is an extra-uterine world, another world outside and beyond the sacral room, the first soul chamber, which the baby has come to know so well in the first nine months of existence.

This prenatal knowledge or intuition of a beyond is not based upon sight. The rudimentary visual perceptions, which are possible at this stage of life, are related to the baby's own hands, to the placental tree, the serpentine umbilicus and the walls of its small, cave-like container. These visual experiences do occur at the same time as a sense of a beyond slowly dawns on the child and later can also be used to awaken this knowledge. However, the main messengers of this experience are tactile and acoustic (see the work of Alfred Tomatis, www.tomatis.de)

Our first knowledge of a beyond is more or less completely dependent upon a sort of prenatal hearsay, a rumour of a beyond, caused by the perception of sounds coming from the otherwise mysterious world outside and beyond the womb, the postnatal world in which the mother lives and moves. The baby usually hears that there is plenty of life going on beyond the small and intimate realm of its uterine existence – especially during the daytime, when the womb is generally visually brighter and the mother in her world more active than at night.

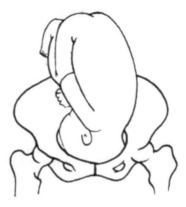

Figure 26.5
The birth position chosen by 70% of babies.

For all babies, who survive the challenge of birth, the prenatal rumour of a world beyond the womb proves to have been true.

Exactly which sounds and exactly how intense the baby's auditory experience is vary from pregnancy to pregnancy and differ markedly from person to person. However, that there is an acoustic world beyond the present one slowly dawns to consciousness and is registered in the child in precisely this distinctive bodily position with its corresponding tactile stimuli. It is a complex world of multifarious sounds beyond the relative monotonous din of the tight womb and the familiar tones of the mother's voice, a wide-open world beyond the baby's present state of veiled and constricted existence.

Varying and various experiences of touch and pressure on the crown of the head and on the left side of the baby's body (at least in the 70% majority of people) correspond to and become correlated to the messages coming to the as-yet-unborn child from the world beyond.

In most traditional interpretations, the Sahasrara chakra is related to our awareness of the Beyond – every form of a beyond that postnatal life might reveal to us. It is related to our ability to anticipate and to open ourselves and prepare ourselves to participate in as-yet-unseen possibilities. The Crown chakra is that which has most directly to do with our so-called spiritual perception and awareness. This chakra is the door in our consciousness to new and unknown worlds. When it is opened, it is possible for us to see the light in full blaze – to become enlightened. We can begin to intuit our future and live according to it already now in the present.

It is claimed that when Sahasrara is free from all disturbance and obstruction, that a person has access to a deep feeling of inner peace and to a spiritual understanding of life. The tradition teaches that if the Sahasrara has been opened and remains so, then the person has in some special way realized the point of existence, has attained enlightenment on Earth before death.

If this chakra is blocked or disturbed, then a person is caught up in a world, full of fetters. The person is beset by a gnawing feeling of deprivation, emptiness, and dissatisfaction. He is weary of the world and feels trapped within it. He lives in a gloom, is depressed, dispirited, and despondent, mentally and spiritually exhausted. There is no belief in a happy future or in a life after death. There is no expectation that there might be meaning to be found in life. Existence here on Earth appears to be a drudge, the world nothing but a valley of tears, a torment, a Gethsemane full of impossible challenges with no way out and no way ahead, no way of knowing what an uncertain future might hold in store for us.

The Yellow Latifa, also known as Qalb

According to the Sufis, the Lataif are understood to be holy impulses, holy dynamisms or even divine emotions, seated deep within us and supporting healthy movement through life. They remain hidden and unconscious to most people. However, a conscious knowledge and dedicated employment of the Lataif in life is a most important part of becoming a fully realized human being, in tune with the Cosmos and the Divine.

Each of the five Lataif is an important aspect of the whole-human state. We need each of them to inform our daily living in order to live in harmony with ourselves, with others and the world around us.

The Yellow Latifa, also known as Qalb, is to be experienced in most people on the left side of the body, the side where the heart lies. Qalb is Arabic for heart. However, the Sufi masters are observant and know that it can also reside in some people on the right side of the body. In yet others, it is extremely difficult, if not com-

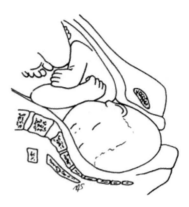

Figure 26.6
The fetal resting position before birth. The baby lies with its left cheek upon the mother's pelvis in about 70% of cases.

pletely impossible, to locate this Latifa in any particular part of the body. However, the Sufi masters do not know why this is so. They simply respect what they see and do not attempt to simplify or change the truth of their perceptions to fit a theory.

The fact is that about 10% of people are born from the so-called second anterior occipital or right-occipito-anterior (ROA) position. This is a mirror image of the first position with the baby placing its right cheek on the mother's sacrum, lying before birth with its right side against the posterior wall of the abdomen and with the left shoulder waiting to be born first.

This position is chosen by so few because it is not an easy position from which to be born. When the baby pulls up its left shoulder in order to fit diagonally into the pelvic opening in this position, this automatically compresses the heart in the thorax against the left arm. Thus when a baby chooses to lie in the second position during labour, the baby's heart has less room and freedom and therefore less possibility to do its vital work efficiently. The second position often leads to a more complicated birth.

The remaining 20% of babies chose even more difficult positions in which to lie in the womb, for example, posterior occipital presentations and breech.

For various reasons, often known only to the baby itself, they experience the last weeks of their prenatal life being kinesthetically stimulated on quite atypical parts of their body, often not involving the crown of the head or predominantly one side of the body as opposed to the other as primary focuses of prenatal experience.

No matter how it is lying before birth, whether on the left (70%) or on the right side (10%) of its body or in a very uncommon position (20%), the Yellow Latifa is always located in that part of the body where physical contact later in life reminds the person of their own specific origin in the womb of their mother preceding birth.

Above all, the womb before birth is a place and time where the parasympathetic nervous system should reign over the child and the mother – and in most cases it does. The weeks before birth in a happy and healthy pregnancy tend to be a time of tranquillity, an experience of very special expectant awareness in mother and in child, a time of waiting, in which not much else happens. All are awaiting the disclosure, the unveiling and the revealing of the child to the world.

The Yellow Latifa is exactly this joy, this confidence. It is a joy caused by the prospect and inner certainty of discovering something, which has not yet been, which has not yet been seen or experienced by anyone else – but by me right now! It is a childlike inquisitiveness, an openness for and expectation of that which is not-yet.

The Yellow Latifa is absolutely essential to healthy human living. It blesses us with light-heartedness, with a playful nosiness, which ensures that we move through life, from stage to stage, from experience to experience, from wish to wish, like a child playing at being a great adventurer, all the while knowing that we are still small and growing and learning all along the way. It is the eager awaiting, the ardent yearning, which causes us to nurture all our dreams – but especially the deep desire to live in light, peace, and harmony. The Yellow Latifa keeps us happily on the road of time but always moving in the direction of eternity. Many children nowadays manage to keep it alive and active in themselves well into puberty.

The internal rotation

In comparison to the human pelvis, that of the chimpanzee is relatively long so that it might be expected that birth for our closest primate relatives might be quite difficult. However, the cranial and caudal orifices of the

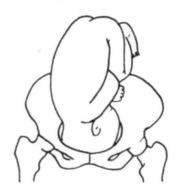

Figure 26.7
Baby in the second birth position, right cheek to mother's sacrum.

chimpanzee pelvis have more or less the same diameter in the same axis. Their pelvis is like a straightforward tunnel or tube. Thus, most chimpanzee babies have a very easy passage. They are born in the so-called brow or straight occipito-posterior (SOP) position. They do not need to rotate within the pelvis during the process of birth. Human babies, on the other hand, no matter whether they are lying in the left or right occipito-anterior position, have to make a rotation of 45 degrees in order to attain a position in which they can flex their neck muscles and deliver their face.

The so-called internal rotation takes place during the first phase of labour as the contractions are increasing in strength and duration. For the first time in his life, the unborn child in the ROA position (70%) feels pressure on the right side of his body. In the LOA position (10%), this pressure is felt on the left side of the body. The mother's diaphragm and the uterine muscles begin to push the baby down into the pelvis. The baby must maneuvre his head against all obstacles deeper and deeper into the narrow pelvic opening. The left side of the face (in ROA) or the right side (in LOA) is slid against the mother's sacrum until the coccyx sits like a claw between the eyebrows and just above the bridge of the nose.

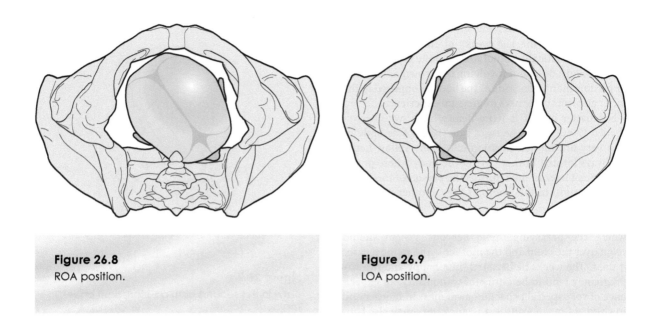

Figure 26.8
ROA position.

Figure 26.9
LOA position.

Once in this position, the child is then able to flex his neck muscles, push his occiput hard against the mother's pubic bone and thereby lever his face through the tissues of the pelvic floor. This is a much more complicated and dangerous process than the simple birth experienced by a chimpanzee. Above all, it involves pressure being exerted on the facial bones asymmetrically. In ROA, the left side of the face experiences forces, which lengthen it in comparison to the right side. In LOA, a similar deformation occurs on the right side of the face.

The Red Latifa, also known as Ruh

According to Sufi teaching, the Red Latifa is located in most people on the right side of the body. In a minority, it is to be found on the left. In yet others, it has a bodily location, which is difficult or even impossible to determine.

The Arabic word Ruh used to describe this essential energy means spirit or soul. This is a fiery force in us, which makes us courageous and adventurous. It is the feeling of true physical, mental, and spiritual power. It endows us with a sense of innate ability. It is this energy, which enables us to achieve what we desire. It enables us to strive. It is inspired, resourceful and brave – in the sense of spirited. It strengthens us to overcome whatever

obstacles we encounter so that we can persevere and continue on life's journey. It is this force, which upholds in the face of difficulties.

The Red Latifa is an energy, which enables us to be true to ourselves, even at the cost of comfort. It enables us to discern what is truly good for us and what is not. It is the strength, which we continuously need in order to set ourselves apart from anything that would constrict or sully our true identity.

The death of the fetus, the birth of the child

The zenith of the birth has been reached when the broadest part of the child's head is trapped in the narrowest part of the mother's pelvis. In most cases, this is when the mother's coccyx is pressing into the child's forehead and the child's occiput is squarely situated against her pubis.

This unique position marks the moment when the child must realize that its fetal existence has come to an irreversible end. There is now no going back into the womb and the way forward into life is fraught with danger and uncertainty. There is no other moment in human life – apart possibly from the moment of death itself – that is so overwhelming, so crushing and so devastating. Our uterine past has been forever

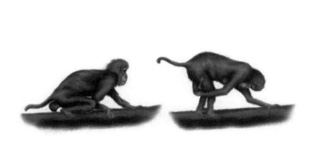

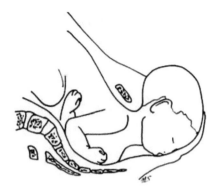

Figure 26.10
Brow (SOP) presentation in chimpanzees.

Figure 26.11
Birth of the face after the internal rotation.

extinguished. Every baby finds itself on the brink of a completely new form of existence – if it survives the crossing into the postnatal world.

This journey can only be completed if and when the child decides to force itself against all odds through the massive pelvic constriction and over the threshold. This can only be achieved by the exertion of brute force, especially in the baby's trunk and legs. Concern now for the safety and even the shape of the skull become secondary. The head must be used like a ram to penetrate and break a way free for the whole child. As every mother and midwife knows who has experienced it, when the child now refuses to cooperate, thus endangering its own and possibly also the mother's life, brute force from outside must be used to push and/or pull the child into the world.

Chakra Ajna

The so-called third eye or Ajna chakra is traditionally considered to be intimately involved with perception – more specifically with our personal perception of truth. (In Sanskrit Ajna means knowledge or knowing.) Nowadays truth is a very difficult concept for many people in the West. We are so used to believing that there is only subjective or relative truth. It is believed that this belief alone can save us from all sorts of imperialism

and authoritarianism. There is a legitimate fear of the concept of objective truth. For even in our recent past, this concept has been used to suppress the freedom and rights not only of certain types of individual but of whole nations and cultures.

The Ajna chakra has to do with the profound distinction between truth and illusion, between perceiving what is there and what we expect to be there. This chakra has to do with the ability to distance ourselves from our subjective and narrow expectations, which are all too often founded on fear and past frustration. That is why this chakra is intimately involved with memory and the healing of memories. Ultimately it can be claimed that there can be no real sense of lasting healing without the activation of this chakra. It is the activation of this chakra that frees us from our past and allows us to enter into the present. Whoever manages to achieve a healthy distance to the voices from the past within the mind – especially the voices of criticism, inhibition, and intimidation – is rewarded with a self-esteem and strength, which are so stable and unconditional, that negative external forces from the world around us – even the recognition of our own natural inadequacies – can no longer influence our self-confidence. This process does not lead to pride but, on the contrary, to a deep and lasting humility. We learn to bow before the truth of the moment, which we

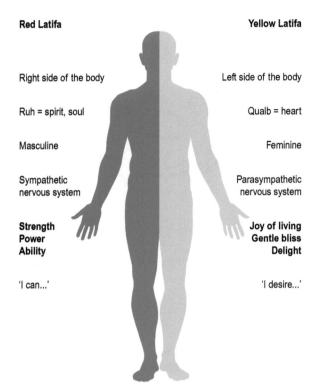

Red Latifa

Right side of the body

Ruh = spirit, soul

Masculine

Sympathetic
nervous system

**Strength
Power
Ability**

'I can...'

Yellow Latifa

Left side of the body

Qualb = heart

Feminine

Parasympathetic
nervous system

**Joy of living
Gentle bliss
Delight**

'I desire...'

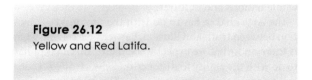

Figure 26.12
Yellow and Red Latifa.

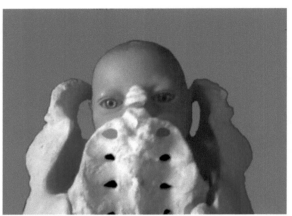

Figure 26.13
The zenith of birth coccyx pressing into the child's forehead.

ourselves do not control. We no longer take anything personally – not even ourselves. For we have realized that personhood has got absolutely nothing to do with the past. Personhood is a present moment, which opens itself to an unknown and unconditional future. The future is, of course, knowable. But only in so far as we abandon the past, remain in the present, refrain from fear and do that very, very little, which is in the present moment necessary. That very little, which is necessary is usually described in spiritual literature as non-doing, because it is indeed very little in comparison to what people normally feel forced to do.

The Ajna chakra is intimately involved with devotion to the truth and self-abandonment. The German word here is better and clearer. Self-abandonment does not involve any form of self-neglect or hatred, as some spiritual traditions would teach us and have us practice. It has to do with the state of pristine presence in the here-and-now through a radical Selbstvergessenheit (a forgetting or gentle disregard of the old self, that is, ego death). It involves a radically new evaluation of our past, which in most cases leads eventually to its complete eradication.

All of the above can be experienced and stored in the Ajna chakra. That is, in that position in which the head of the soon-to-be-transformed fetus is compressed within the mother's pelvis and feels the spur of her coccyx in the middle of the brow. For the very first time in life during a natural, spontaneous birth, the fetus is called to abandon its prenatal existence in its uterine abode, accept this "death," this perinatal passage, and enter into a completely new life as a liberated, breathing, and active being in a postnatal world.

Of course, the "hardware" which constitutes the Ajna chakra is not simply the so-called third eye, the point where, for example, Hindu women paint a red Bindi spot to show that they are married. The hardware involved is the whole of the base of the skull through which not only the spinal cord passes but also the cranial nerves

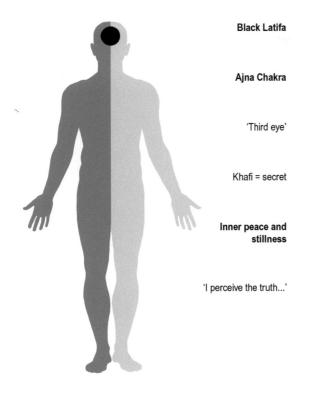

Black Latifa

Ajna Chakra

'Third eye'

Khafi = secret

Inner peace and stillness

'I perceive the truth...'

Figure 26.14

belonging to the vegetative nervous system. The motility of the sphenoid bone and its relationship to the occiput as seen in the state of the synchondrosis sphenobasilaris (SSB) are the unique anatomical structures involved in the subtle functioning of the Ajna chakra. As such, the Ajna chakra has much to do with the interrelationship between brain as main seat of the mind and body. It influences the subtle and empirically observable communication between our mind and the biophysical energies and events, which are revealed in our personal presence in the world.

The Black Latifa, also known as Khafi

The Black Latifa in the Sufi tradition is the homologue of the Ajna chakra in the Indian tradition. It also is understood to be located in the middle of the forehead just above the bridge of the nose. It is known as Khafi, which means hidden or secret. It is characterized not only by a sense of deep inner peace and stillness but also by an unshakable certainty that one can perceive the truth, that one can be real. When we are in touch with this essential quality, we ourselves become unflinching, resolute, and determined. We become single-minded and strong-minded.

When this Latifa is active in us, we are capable of subtle perception of what really is there to be perceived. We are able to perceive the unique newness, the freshness of each new moment in life. We no longer hang onto expectations, which are fed on past experience. Our perception becomes free of habit and routine. We expect change. We expect to be confronted by novelty. We look forward to it. We are not afraid that the old will have to be extinguished in our onward journey towards the new. We know that what is real is to be experienced only in each moment.

With the black Latifa active within us, we can abide in the present moment in deep tranquillity. We are no longer hectic and driven. We no longer search beyond our means and beyond our present horizon. We no longer strive for what we know is unattainable at present. We know what power and presence are involved in not doing. We have a deep certainty that we will know exactly what to do exactly when we have to do it – and not before.

References

[1] Judith Anodea, *Eastern Body Western Mind: Psychology And The Chakra System As A Path To The Self*, 1996, p.5.

[2] Susan G. Shumsky, *Exploring Chakras*, 2003, p.37.

[3] *The Theosophist*, Vol. 75, No. 6, p. ii.

[4] Elias Wolf, *Das Buch der 28 Chakren – Ein Handbuch zu den wichtigsten Energiezentren unseres Körpers*, 2006.

[5] Almut Klöpfer, *Das achte Chakra: Die Verbindung zum höheren Selbst*, 2007.

[6] Jude Currivan, Wulfing von Rohr, *Das Geheimnis des 8. Chakras*, 2008.

[7] Tenzin Wangyal Rinpoche, *Awakening the Sacred Body, Tibetan Yogas of Breath and Movement*, 2011.

[8] Rudolf Steiner, *Das Ereignis der Christus-Erscheinung*

in der ätherischen Welt, GA 118, 18 April 1910, S. 156 f.

[9]Steiner Rudolf, *Theosophie. Einführung in über-sinnliche Welterkenntnis und Menschenbesinnung.* Dornach 1986. Taschenbuchausgabe 6150, p. 30–35.

[10] Otto Scharmer, *Theory U*, 2009.

[11]Judith Anodea, *The Wheels of Life*, 1987.

[12]Otto Rank, *The Trauma of Birth*, 1924.

[13]Nandor Fodor, *The Search for the Beloved*, 1940.

[14]Nathanielsz, *Life in the Womb, The Origin of Health and Disease*, 1999.

[15]Nicette Sergueef, *Die Kraniosakrale Osteopathie bei Kindern*, 1995, p.19

27

Development of the cranium and an outline of the growth dynamics of cranial bones

Torsten Liem

Contributions from Marie-Odile Fessenmeyer

But as you descend into that domain, the domain of the cells … this sort of heaviness of Matter disappears – it begins again to be fluid, vibrant. This would tend to prove that the heaviness, thickness, inertia, immobility, is something added … It is the false Matter, that which we think and feel, but not Matter itself, as it is.

Sri Aurobindo[1]

Embryology describes the evolution of forms, the interrelationships of the resulting structures, the growth movements of structures, and the morphogenetic fields that underpin these developments. A knowledge of embryology in general and of the development of the cranium, in particular, provides the foundation for understanding many structural, physiological, functional, and dysfunctional relationships that are of major importance for palpation and therapy. From embryology the osteopath gains insight into the inherent dynamics of tissue growth and into the developmental dynamics of the particular tissue in interaction with the developmental dynamics of other tissue structures. As well as seeing any structural dysfunctions present at the time of examination in relation to the overall picture, the osteopath who is well versed in embryology will also be able to sense, palpate, understand, and treat by factoring in the temporal dynamics of prenatal and postnatal relationships and formative processes.

The present structuring of the organism and of each individual tissue is simultaneously also the expression of its development and of the emergence of its individual equilibrium. Many osteopaths believe that, even after the growth process is complete, the embryological growth movements of the structures persist as extremely delicate, inherent rhythmic movements and that these offer an insight into the fine morphogenetic structure of the tissues. Knowledge of embryological growth movements provides the osteopath with an indication as to how the inherent movements of the individual structures feel in their ideal state.

Embryological dynamic movement axes co-exist alongside biomechanical movement axes in joints and other structures. These are based on the particular growth processes and formative processes of the structures in question.

In psychotherapy it has long been suspected that traumatic experiences – especially in the early years of life – can influence further personality development even into old age, and that consciousness-awakening processes can be used to resolve or constructively integrate problems and psychological disturbances caused by past experiences.

A similar hypothetical approach can also be used as a basis for working with the tissues. By focusing attention on the inherent tensions and tissue movements, the osteopath will be able to palpate and resolve tissue tensions caused by prenatal or postnatal factors or trauma.

Phylogenesis

According to Portmann,[2] the primitive vertebrate cranium can be subdivided into three relatively autonomous segments:

- The CNS and sensory organs surrounded by the neurocranium: here the cranial base as far as the region of the pituitary (and the anterior end of the notochord) has come into being through the transformation of vertebrae.

- The foregut together with the branchial region: at an early stage the four pharyngeal arches presumably already show a relatively constant relationship with the four pharyngeal nerves (CN V, VII, IX, and X).

- The lateral line organs of the skin and the dermatocranium.

Humankind's evolution to assume an upright gait has given rise to certain structural changes in the body: the emergence of the clavicle, the take-over of the defensive and prehensile functions of the jaw by the upper extremities, and the development of the orolarynx into a highly specific organ of phonation, etc.

For Delattre and Fenart[3] the most important cranial change associated with hominization was the posterior rotation of the occiput. This completely altered the volume of the intracranial space and led to further changes, such as outward and downward rotation of the outer part of the petrous bone (mastoid process), extension of the pterygoid processes, and increased height of the maxillae and the mandibular rami, associated with a lowering of the hard palate and horizontal mandibular body, etc. The recession of the face is a further important phylogenetic change.

Ossification of the neurocranium and viscerocranium

Bone differentiation is one of the last tissue differentiation steps to occur in humans. To understand the development of the cranial bones it is imperative to have some knowledge of the underlying positional development of the organ systems before birth.

The cranium develops from the mesenchyme that envelops the cerebral vesicles, and may be subdivided into the neurocranium (brain case) and the viscerocranium (facial bones of the skull). The neurocranium in turn comprises the cranial base and the cranial vault. The cranial base is formed by endochondral ossification, i.e., it develops first as cartilaginous tissue. The cranial vault and the facial bones of the skull are formed by desmal ossification, i.e., the bones develop directly from the mesenchymal connective tissue. Some bones that form part of both the cranial base and the cranial vault ossify simultaneously by both mechanisms (Tables 27.1 and 27.2). While the adult cranium consists of 22 bones, the cranium of a neonate still has 45 bones. The cranium of a human embryo actually has between 110 and 120 ossification centers.

Appositional periosteal growth at the surface of the bone following the appearance of ossification centers

After the appearance of the ossification centers and the increase in bone formation, the growth of the cranial bones inside the ossification centers comes to a halt, with the result that further growth is possible only at the periphery of the bones in question.

At the surface of the bone by appositional, periosteal growth

Here bone is laid down on one periosteal surface of the bone, and is partly resorbed again on the other periosteal surface of the bone. In this process the entire surface of the bone acts as a more or less powerful growth field. Alongside the growth of the bone in its totality there is also a continuous process of intra-osseous remodeling and movement of individual bone regions in relation to other bone regions.

According to Delaire, periosteal growth is dependent on the tissues and visceral structures that have attachment to and surround the particular cranial bone in question. Bone growth is not merely induced by the soft-tissue matrix but is also determined by it. "The 'blueprint' for the design, construction, and growth of a bone lies in the composite of the muscles, tongue, lips, cheeks, integument,

Cranial vault	Desmal ossification
Cranial base	Endochondral ossification
Viscerocranium (facial bones)	Desmal ossification

TABLE 27.1: Ossification of the cranium

Endochondral ossification	Desmal ossification
Neurocranium Chondrocranium, cranial base:	**Desmocranium, cranial vault:**
- Occipital bone, below the superior nuchal line	- Occipital bone, supra-occiput
- Sphenoid bone, except for the vertical part of the greater wing	- Greater wing of the sphenoid bone
- Ethmoid bone	- Parietal bone
- Petrous portion of the temporal bone	- Frontal bone
	- Squama of the temporal bone
Viscerocranium	
- Nasal septum	- Maxilla
- Inferior nasal concha	- Mandible (except for the mental region and the condylar process)
- Body of the hyoid bone and the greater horns of the hyoid bone	- Zygomatic bone
	- Palatine bone
	- Nasal bone
	- Lacrimal bone

TABLE 27.2: Classification of individual bones of the neurocranium and viscerocranium in terms of their ossification mechanism (see also Fig. 27.8)

Synchondrosis formed from the perichondrium of cartilaginous tissue	Synfibrosis formed from the periosteum of membranous tissue
Compression-adaptive growth	Tension-adaptive growth
Growth adaptation Morphogenetic fields Result of past and current epigenetic factors	

Figure 27.1

Sutural growth (according to Fessenmeyer).[5]

mucosae, connective tissue, nerves, blood vessels, airway, pharynx, the brain as an organ mass, tonsils, adenoids, and so forth, etc."[4] The growth of these functional factors moves the bone and regulates its growth so that it can fulfill its function through its specific shape and size.

Growth in the cranial sutures (the seams filled with fibrous connective tissue between the margins of adjoining cranial bones)

Synchondroses – the cartilaginous joints between the cranial bones – create the conditions for sutural bone formation. Cartilage is the only tissue that retains its growth capacity even when exposed to pressure forces (compression-adaptive growth zone), by contrast with the sutures, which are inhibited in their growth when exposed to pressure (tension-adaptive growth zone). The cranial bones are moved apart by the growth of the synchondroses and soft tissue. This produces tension on the cranial sutures. As a result the sutural tissue is stimulated to preserve bone-to-bone contact and to form new bone, with the result that the bones grow by a secondary mechanism (Figure 27.1).

While the cranial bones move apart as they develop, the fibrous connective tissue grows centrifugally. The growth process is characterized by equilibrium between the distraction of the cranial bones, the growth of the fibrous connective tissue in the sutures, and the desmal ossification.

Embryological growth dynamics of the cranial bones unfold as a result of different and to some extent simultaneous mechanisms:

1 Movement of individual bone areas due to irregular deposition and resorption processes.

2 Movement of the entire bone as a result of its own increase in size; due to its expansive growth the soft tissue first creates space between adjoining bones, thus permitting bone growth. While the bone is growing in one direction, it is displaced in the opposite direction; for example, the maxilla is moved anteriorly while it lays down bone and grows posteriorly (Figure 27.2).

3 Movement of the entire bone due to an increase in the size of an adjoining or other more remote bone, e.g., the movement of the maxilla due to growth of the adjacent nasal septum or, further away, of the cranial base.

In studies of the influence of hemodynamics on bone growth in young tracker dog pups a movement at the frontal suture and sagittal suture of 5–10 μm was recorded in synchronicity with aortic flow and the electrocardiogram.[6]

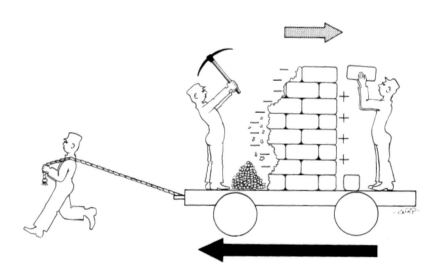

Figure 27.2
Bone growth and bone displacement (from D.H. Enlow: *Handbook of Facial Growth*).[4]

According to Dambricourt-Malassé,[6] the staged rotation of the basisphenoid during phylogenesis is a characteristic feature of humankind's evolutionary development. Ontogenetically, this corresponds with the rotation of the basisphenoid during week 7 of embryonic development, followed by the posterior rotation of the basiocciput (posterior-most blastema) during week 8. This development is the consequence of the dynamics of the neural plate, centered at the tip of the notochord. The vertical dimension of the cranial base and the verticalization of the craniosacral axis, associated with shortening of the cranium, therefore appear at a very early stage in ontogenesis.

In phylogenetic terms, the very recent contraction of the cranial base is accompanied by an improvement in locomotor balance, the development of bipedal stance, and telencephalization (thus ensuring psychomotor control).

The neurocranium

During the fourth intrauterine week, from the capsular mesenchymal membrane that forms around the evolving brain, the endomeninx develops on the inside and the ectomeninx on the outside. The endomeninx consists of neural crest material whereas the ectomeninx develops both from neural crest material and from paraxial mesoderm. The pia mater and arachnoid membrane arise from the endomeninx. The ectomeninx continues developing inwardly to form the dura mater. Outside, on the surface of the ectomeninx, the neurocranium is formed from the membranous cranial vault (desmocranium) surrounding the brain and from the cartilaginous cranial base (chondrocranium) at its floor (Figure 27.3).

It is the growing brain that exerts the greatest influence on the shape of the neurocranium. Without the development of the brain, neither the dura mater nor the cranial vault would be formed. On the other hand, the growth of the brain is limited in turn by the dural bands or girdles, with the result that the connective tissue dura also exerts a shaping influence on the brain as well as on the cranial vault. Figures 27.4–27.6 illustrate the interplay between the growing brain and the development of the dura and neurocranium, according to Blechschmidt.[8]

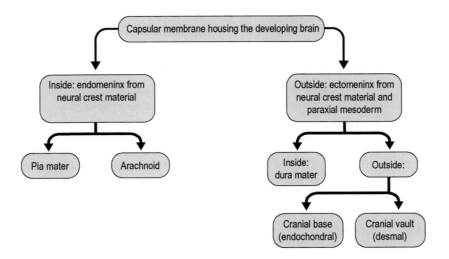

Figure 27.3

Schematic diagram illustrating the development of the neurocranium.

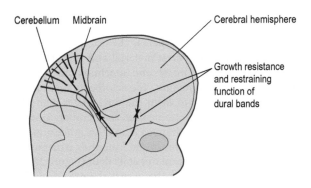

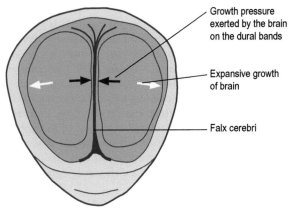

Figure 27.4

Influence of the brain on cranial development in a 29 mm embryo. Formation of connective tissue dural bands between the cerebrum and the cerebellum, and between the frontal and the temporal lobes.[9]

Figure 27.5

Anterior view of left and right dural bands in the frontal region of a 29 mm embryo.[9]

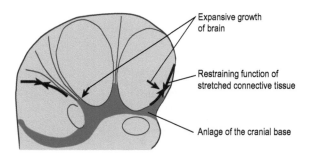

Figure 27.6

Lateral view of the dural bands in a 29 mm embryo. The cartilaginous cranial base develops from a densation field at the base of the dural bands.[9]

Due to the growth of the brain the stroma in the hollows between contiguous, expanding segments of the brain is hindered in its growth and so becomes compressed and stretched, thus forming a system of anchoring dural bands. A paired dural band gives rise to the falx cerebri between the two cerebral hemispheres, and an unpaired dural band helps to form the tentorium (awning) separating the cerebellum and the cerebrum. According to Blechschmidt, the dural anchoring bands rather resemble window-frames around the cerebellum and parts of each cerebral hemisphere.[9] Bulging through the "windows" the brain arches outward between the stretched dural bands toward the skin: paired brain bulges therefore arise in each of the frontal and temporal regions, and an unpaired bulge in the occipital region of the future cerebellum. The dural bands of each side are interwoven at the base of the brain in the connective tissue of the cranial base.

Development of the chondrocranium (cranial base)

As a result of the increasing longitudinal growth of the neural tube coupled simultaneously with the relative growth lag (restraining function) of the accompanying neural tube vessels, the brain is bridled and displays ventral, concave flexion over the heart swelling. During the initial flexion process the submesencephalic mesenchyme is oriented transversely to its longitudinal axis, between the forebrain and the hindbrain, and forms the transverse mesencephalic septum. At the base of the septum the notochord adapts to the transverse broadening of the tissue during the flexion of the embryo by bending to the side and thus becoming shortened in its principal orientation.

The cranial part of the notochord (= central axial skeleton of the embryo) is located at the level of the buccopharyngeal membrane, which surrounds the stomodeum. The hypophyseal pouch (Rathke's pouch) is situated in front of the buccopharyngeal membrane. It is formed from the ectodermal roof portion of the stomodeum and eventually gives rise to the anterior lobe of the pituitary.

The parachordal cartilage develops from the embryonic connective tissue (mesenchyme) on either side of the cranial end of the notochord. Caudal to the parachordal cartilage are four sclerotomes (i.e., anlagen of skeletal elements) of the occipital somites (primitive segments from the mesoderm). While the topmost sclerotome disappears, the remaining three sclerotomes fuse with the parachordal cartilage and together form the anlage for the future basilar portion of the occipital bone. Later the cartilage becomes more extensive and surrounds the spinal cord, thus forming the boundaries of the foramen magnum.

The hypophyseal cartilage is located rostral to the parachordal cartilage. It forms on both sides of the pituitary stalk, around Rathke's pouch. The hypophyseal cartilage eventually develops into the body of the sphenoid bone. The two trabeculae cranii are located anterior to the hypophyseal cartilage. They fuse to form the body of the ethmoid bone.

On both sides of the median line there are further cartilaginous foci. The most rostral, the ala orbitalis, forms the lesser wing (ala minor) of the sphenoid bone. Caudally it is followed by the ala temporalis, which gives rise to the greater wing (ala major) of the sphenoid bone. Posterior to the ala temporalis, on both sides of the parachordal plate, are the otic capsules. These develop to become the petrous portion of the temporal bones.

The nasal capsule becomes chondrified during the second intrauterine month and forms a cavity that is bounded on the outside, inside, and above by walls of cartilage. From the lateral wall arises the lateral mass of the ethmoid bone and the inferior nasal concha. From the medial wall develops the cartilaginous nasal septum; the exception here is its posterior, inferior part, which ossifies and forms the anlage for the vomer. The vomer wings extend as far as the sphenoid bone and form the roof of the nasopharynx. The cartilaginous nasal septum in the fetus intervenes between the cranial base above and the pre-maxilla, the palatal processes of the maxilla, and the vomer below. Its growth exerts a force that is directed downward and forward on the growth of the maxilla and it is supported in this by the appositional growth of the posterosuperior margins of the vomer.

These developmental stages are illustrated in Figures 27.7–27.10.

The initially separate centers of cranial base chondrification fuse into a single, elongated, and much-perforated cartilage plate, known as the basal plate, which extends from the nasal region as far as the foramen magnum.[10,11]

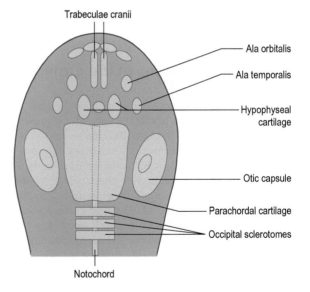

Figure 27.7
Six-week-old embryo (viewed from above).

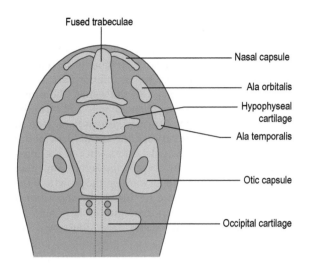

Figure 27.8
Seven-week-old embryo (viewed from above).

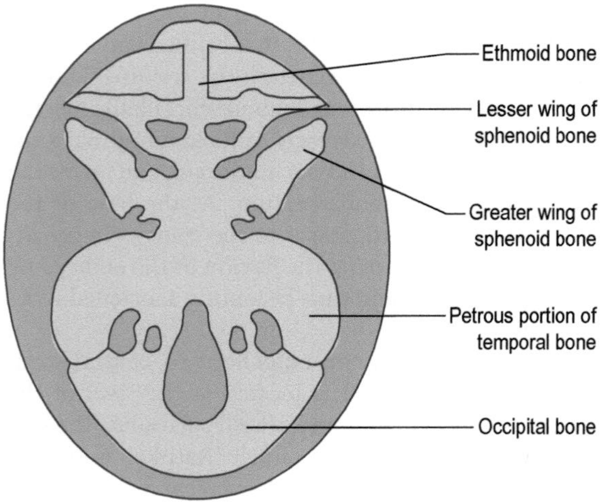

Figure 27.9
Twelve-week-old embryo (viewed from above).

Formative processes at the cranial base (Figure 27.11)

After the cranial base has been formed by the dura at the basal surface of the brain, the continuing growth of the brain there leads to closer packing or consolidation of the tissue (a phenomenon known as a densation field). The resultant loss of intercellular fluid leads to thickening with the formation of pre-cartilage, which continues to develop into cartilage by the time the embryo is about 40 days old. The first cranial bones are formed from the third fetal month onward at the margin of the cartilaginous cranial base. According to Blechschmidt,[12] detraction fields arise there in tissue zones where water is expressed due to viscous gliding movements in opposite directions. The tissue loses water and consolidates so extremely that small ossification centers are formed.

The bones at the cranial base are connected to each other by cartilaginous articulations, known as synchondroses (Figure 27.12). The timing of ossification of the different synchondroses at the cranial base varies markedly, depending on the stimuli to which they are exposed by the continuing growth of the soft tissues. While some become ossified even during the fetal period, others ossify only in old age. These synchondroses are of major importance for the development of the cranial base. The bones are pushed apart by the interstitial growth of the synchondroses, with the result that they are able to increase in size by appositional growth at the margins of the cranial sutures.

While there are no hard-and-fast rules concerning the timing and extent of ossification of the cranial base, this process always occurs according to a fixed pattern: ossification always commences in areas of the frontal bone, followed in posterior-to-anterior sequence by the occipital, the basisphenoid, the presphenoid, and finally the ethmoid bone.[13–15] Ossification of the occipital, sphenoid, and temporal bones is endochondral and membranous, whereas that of the ethmoid bone and the inferior nasal concha is completely endochondral.

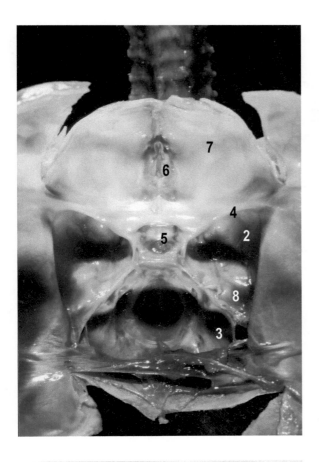

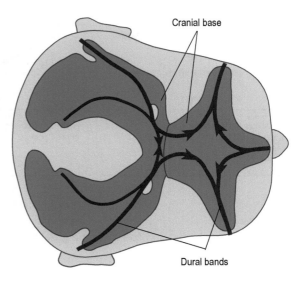

Figure 27.11

Cartilaginous cranial base of a 29 mm embryo seen from above. Black lines: stretched connective tissue of dural bands.

Figure 27.10

Neonatal cranial base (from L.P. Dombard). (2) Middle cranial fossa; (3) Posterior cranial fossa; (4) Foramen magnum; (5) Sella turcica; (6) Cribriform plate; (7) Lesser wing of sphenoid bone; (8) Petrous portion of temporal bone.

Development of the intersphenoidal synchondrosis[6]

Marie-Odile Fessenmeyer

This suture forms the articulation between the posterior and the anterior parts of the body of the sphenoid bone.[16] Our remarks here are based on the research conducted by Delattre and Fenart on the hominization of the cranium and published in 1954 by the Centre National de Recherche Scientifique (CNRS).[3]

Following orientation of the cranium according to the "vestibian axis" proposed by Perez, the rotation dynamics of the occipital compartment (i.e., the cartilaginous part of the occipital bone, the petrous portions of the two temporal bones, and the posterior part of the sphenoid body) were defined.

The concept of the positive rotation of the occipital compartment is added to the phylogenetic development of posture. (We are not concerned here with the relationship between the development of the neural tube, circulatory system, and cranial position, but merely point out that these connections are indissolubly linked.)[17] The following comments refer to the exocranium (Figures 27.13 and 27.14).

Due to positive rotation, which is the result of cervical lordosis, the development of the entire cranial base is altered as follows:

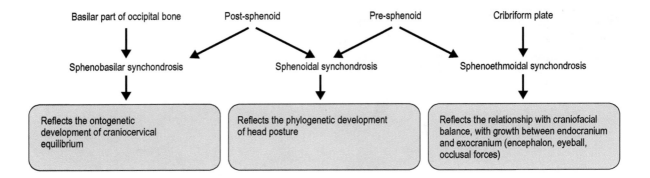

Figure 27.12
Morphogenetic factors influencing the growth of the synchondroses at the cranial base (according to Fessenmeyer, modified).[6]

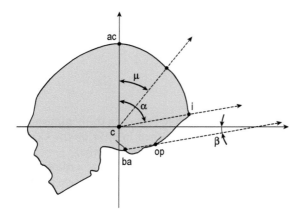

Figure 27.13
Sagittal profile of a human cranium in vestibular orientation. C = axis intersection; ba, op = orientation of the foramen characterized by the straight line from the basion to the opisthion; i = inion; ac = acrion; α = hiatus angle; μ = lambda angle; β = foramen angle.

4 Upward displacement of the basiocciput and consequent lifting of the posterior part of the sphenoid body.

5 Lifting of the apex of the petrous portion of the temporal bone, which moves with the body of the occipital bone, with an increase in the angle described by the two petrous portions.

6 Reduction of the sphenoidal angle, combined with a backward gliding of this angle into a vertico-frontal vestibular plane, associated with recession of the viscerocranium. Delattre and Fenart describe this dynamic as "fracture of the cranium."

7 "Stretching" of the greater wings of the sphenoid:
   a The posteroinferior part of the greater wing, which moves with the body of the sphenoid bone, is drawn inward and forward.
   b The anterosuperior part, which moves with pterion and thus moves backward with the viscerocranium, is drawn outward and downward. These forces operating in opposite directions also act on the petrous portion of the temporal bone, firstly via the petrosquamous suture and secondly via the sphenosquamous suture, while

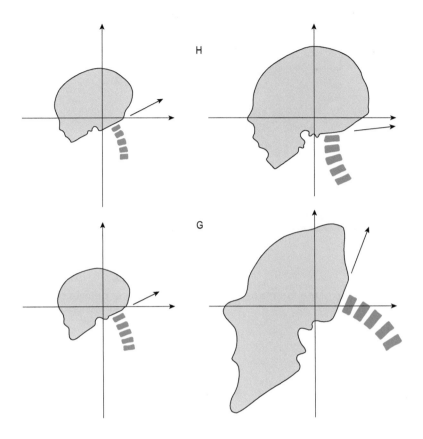

Figure 27.14

Top: Development of a human (H) cranium from birth to adulthood. Note the position of the cervical spine in relation to the orientation of the foramen magnum (arrowed). Bottom: Development of a gorilla (G) cranium from birth to adulthood. Note that the starting position of the cervical spine is the same as in humans, whereas the end position is distinctly different.

the reciprocal relationship of the petrojugular suture remains constant. As a result the petrous portion undergoes torsion (Figures 27.15 and 27.16).

Cranial base angle (Figure 27.17)

The inferior angle of the cranial base is formed by the intersection of the line from nasion to the sella turcica of the sphenoid bone and the line from the sella to basion. This angle is initially fairly flat (approximately 150° in intrauterine week 4) and becomes increasingly acute during the course of development (approximately 120° by week 10). Between intrauterine weeks 10 and 20 the angle again becomes more obtuse (125°–130°) and this angulation is also retained after birth.

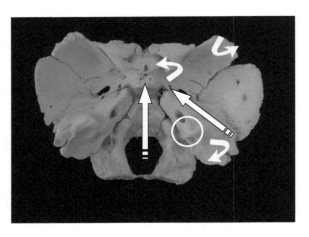

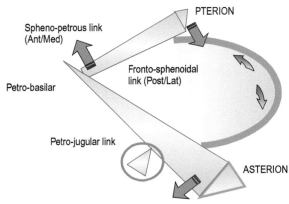

Figure 27.15

Torsion of the petrous portion of the temporal bone.

Figure 27.16

Torsion of the petrous portion of the temporal bone and its local adaptations.

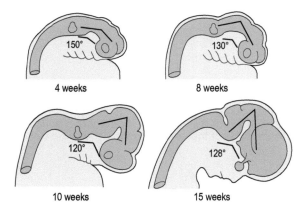

Figure 27.17

Changes in the cranial base angle during embryological development (from Sperber: *Craniofacial Development*).[10]

Growth dynamics and factors influencing the growth of the cranial base

- The occipital and sphenoid bones move apart (Figure 27.18). Explanation: growth of residual cartilage in the synchondroses, particularly in the sphenobasilar synchondrosis (SBS), is due to the growth and the weight of the brain and face. Genetic growth factors of the SBS have also been discussed, but in any case its further growth can be achieved only with mutual dependence on the growth of the brain.

- The inferior angle of the cranial base becomes increasingly acute over time (approximately 120° in week 10 of fetal development). This phenomenon corresponds to the flexion movement of the cranial base. Explanation: pressure exerted by the expansive growth of the brain on the cranial base.

- The foramen magnum moves downward and backward (Figure 27.19). Explanation: there is endocranial resorption and exocranial deposition at the occipital bone.

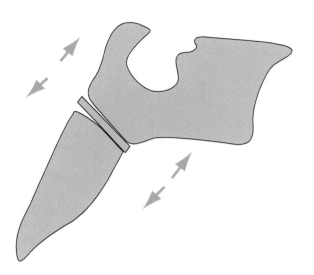

Figure 27.18
Separation of the sphenoid and occipital bones.

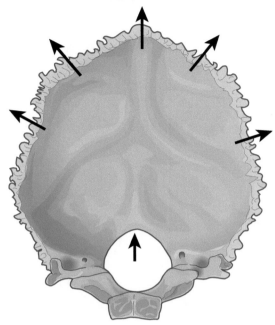

Figure 27.19
Inferoposterior growth movement of the foramen magnum and enlargement of the occipital squama.

- The occipital squama shows a greater size increase than the foramen magnum (Figure 27.19). Explanation: more expansive growth of the occipital lobe compared with the spinal cord.

- The anterior cranial fossa migrates forward. Explanation: sutural growth. The anterior cranial fossa becomes larger as a function of the growth of the frontal lobe. The vomer and the perpendicular plate of the ethmoid bone (which participates in forming the nasal septum) show vertical elongation in their sutures.

- Centrifugal growth of the bones of the cranial base (Figure 27.20). Explanation: the increasing size of the brain and the growth occurring at the SBS exert tensile forces on the sutures of the cranial base, with the result that the bones of the cranial base grow and are displaced along the length of their sutures.

- The region around the SBS shows less growth than the peripherally located cranial fossae. Explanation: the structures above the SBS (such as the medulla

oblongata, pituitary, and hypothalamus) show a lesser size increase than the cerebral lobes in the other cranial fossae.

- The structure of the interior surface of the cranial base develops as a function of the shape of the brain. The structure of the outer surface of the cranial base is adapted more to the fascial, cervical, and pharyngeal structures.

The influence of sutures and synchondroses on cranial growth (Figure 27.21)

- The SBS is important for the anteroposterior and vertical growth of the cranial base. The middle cranial fossa pushes forward the anterior cranial fossa, the

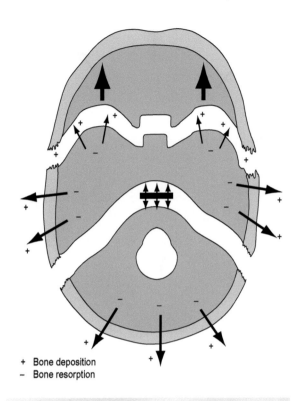

Median palatine suture

Transverse palatine suture

Sphenobasilar synchondrosis

Petrobasilar suture

Occipitomastoid suture

↕ Predominantly anteroposterior growth

↗↙ Predominantly lateral growth

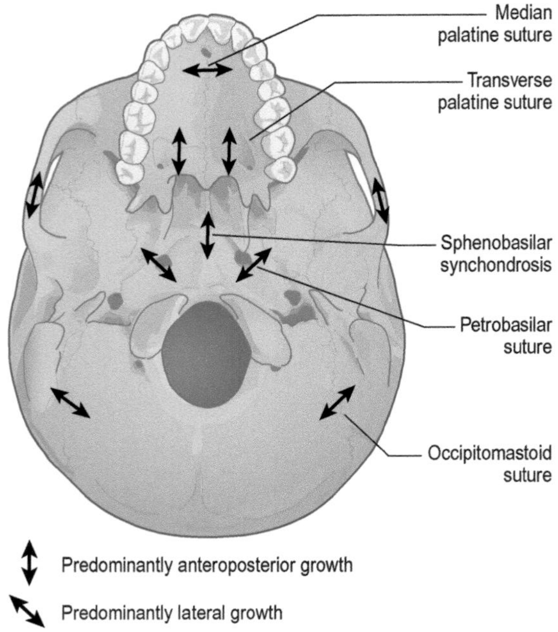

Figure 27.21
Directions of sutural bone growth at the cranial base.

+ Bone deposition
− Bone resorption

Figure 27.20
Centrifugal growth of the bones of the cranial base illustrating sutural and periosteal bone deposition and resorption.

mid-facial region with the maxillae, as well as the mandible. After birth the SBS is the structure that participates most in the growth of the cranial base. Its premature ossification leads to a "dished" face and a "saddle nose," such as are encountered in many craniofacial malformations.

- The intra-osseous synchondrotic articulations of the sphenoid bone are important for the transverse growth of the cranial base and face.

- The nasal septum, described by Couly[18] as the anterior synchondrosis of the ethmoid bone, regulates the sagittal and vertical growth of the maxillae.

- The tension-adaptive sphenofrontal, sphenoethmoidal, and frontoethmoidal sutures regulate the sagittal growth of the anterior cranial fossa.

- The occipitomastoid suture participates in the longitudinal growth of the posterior cranial fossa.

Numerous factors therefore regulate the growth of the cranial base. The form of the cranial base in turn is responsible for the spatial development of the cranial vault. Thus, for example, the endochondral ossification of the otic capsule regulates the position of the intramembranously ossifying temporal squama and of the bony wall of the auditory canal, as well as the position of the mandibular fossa and hence the mandible. The cranial base determines whether the developing cranial shape is rounded (brachycephalic), intermediate (mesocephalic), or elongated (dolichocephalic). In addition, it is the foundation for the expression of the nasomaxillary complex and is one of the factors responsible for the shape of the viscerocranium. The maxillae are displaced forward and downward due to the growth of the cranial base. As a result the maxillae are able to increase in size more posteriorly, thus creating space for the wisdom teeth. Space is also created for the growing nasopharyngeal complex.

Pneumatization of the sphenoid and ethmoid bones coincides with the ossification of certain components of these bones between the third and the fifth months of fetal development. Secondary pneumatization is also dependent on the fusion of the ossification centers and the fusion of the interosseous synchondroses.[19] Thus, for example, the anterior-to-posterior conversion of red to yellow bone marrow in the sphenoid bone precedes the start of secondary pneumatization in the third or fourth year of life.[20–22] During intrauterine development the spheno-occipital synchondrosis forms an antero-posterior axis of the cranial base which, according to Lee et al., is part of a spheno-occipito-vertebral axis. The occipital component here functions as a pressure-transmitting structure at the craniocervical junction.[23]

Etiopathogenesis and dysfunction of the cranial base

Marie-Odile Fessenmeyer

Analysis of the development of the cranial base is linked with:

- The morphogenetic concept[24] of the development of the skeleton, both in a phylogenetic and an ontogenetic sense. (Morphogenesis = a process by which the organism adapts its forms and inner structures in the best possible way to the world around it and which lasts from the time when the ovum is fertilized right through until death.)

- The concept of the skeletal unit, as defined by Moss:

A portion of a skeletal part, which is impossible to separate from it but which possesses true morphological and functional individuality. This is susceptible to palpation and enables us to reduce the bone or skeletal part into its individual components.[25]

- For example, if we consider the temporal bone as a skeletal element, it seems to be of major importance that analysis of the temporal squama in terms of the cranial vault is separate from analysis of the petrous portion in terms of the cranial base and from analysis of the zygomatic process in terms of the viscerocranium. Each individual component part of this bone is associated with a different functional unit and is consequently exposed to mutually opposing forces and orientations.[6]

- The concept of the plasticity and tensegrity of bone.[26]

Finally, analytical study of the bony development of the cranial base permits definition of etiopathogenesis. As a result the intention of the osteopathic intervention can be tailored more precisely. Definition of the etiopathogenesis of the dysfunction takes account of both trauma and function:

1 Bone "absorbs trauma." If it is not accepted and adapted to, trauma alters the morphogenetic development of the bone or, more accurately, of a component part of the bone and thus of the skeletal unit. The bone adapts, its structure is altered, and it undergoes consolidation. This information relates to both the bone as well as its associated function(s) (Figure 27.22).

2 Function is analyzed in its temporal sequence, i.e.:
   a In regard to its own phylogenetic and ontogenetic development.
   b In regard to the development of other functions.

Tele-radiographic analysis of the cranium by Delaire confirms the usefulness of this type of study.[27] When monitoring the growth of the infant and child the osteopath is thus able to determine quite precisely whether involvement is appropriate or not.

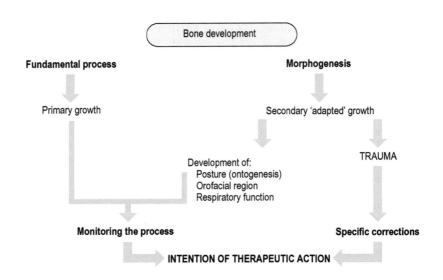

Figure 27.22
Bone development.

Postnatal growth dynamics

Occipital bone

- The foramen magnum expands primarily throughout the first six years of life.

- Bony tuberosities arise with the development of muscular attachments to the occipital bone, e.g., as a result of maintaining a vertical posture of the head against gravity.

At birth

Sphenoid bone

- According to Sperber, the cranial base angle is approximately 128°; by the age of six years there is increasing flexion movement of the cranial base due to upright posture.

- The greater-wing/pterygoid process complex and the lesser wing/body complex articulate with each other through a mixture of cartilage and ligaments.[28]

- The pterygoid process is short with a somewhat horizontal orientation; this drops down into a U-shape, thus further opening up the space for the pharynx.

- The lesser wings fuse during the first year of life; they are pulled laterally by the anterior transverse septum.

- As the sphenoid bone grows, its rostral caudal axis expands.

Ethmoid bone

- Still cartilaginous and incomplete; therefore, according to Carreiro, the ethmoid bone is a vulnerable point for strains of a compressive or torsional nature.[29]

- The cribriform plate in infants is clearly shorter than in adults, i.e., the crista galli lies on the same plane as the lesser wings of the sphenoid bone, while in adults it is anterior to them.

- The medial portion of the orbital wall formed by the ethmoid bone is still not fully established at birth and in early childhood and is therefore extremely sensitive. It is not until about the age of seven years that the area becomes more stable due to the complete growth of the upper nasal cavity.

- The ethmoid bone undergoes extensive remodeling as the nasal passages widen and the conchae develop.

- In the course of development the conchae erode through the orbital plate of the ethmoid bone.

Temporal bone

- At about two years of life the mastoid process is formed due to the tension of the sternocleidomastoid muscle.

- In the first 6 years of life numerous changes take place: the flared, trumpet-like shape of the external auditory meatus develops; its position shifts from facing inferiorly to a more sagittal plane. As this happens, the position of the mandibular fossa changes from an anterior to an inferior orientation.

- The petrous portion becomes elongated.

- The styloid process is elongated as the muscles attaching to it increase in strength.

- The carotid canal develops postnatally; its initial, relatively vertical orientation changes to having a 90° bend in it.

- The Eustachian tubes are tipped out of their initially horizontal plane and become obliquely angled.

Development of the desmocranium (cranial vault)

The bony cranial vault develops directly from the mesenchymal connective tissue that envelops the anlage of the brain. At birth the cranial sutures are 1–10 mm wide. At those sites where more than two bones meet, the cranial sutures become wider. These sites, numbering six in total, are called fontanelles (Figure 27.23A,B). They do not close completely until early childhood.

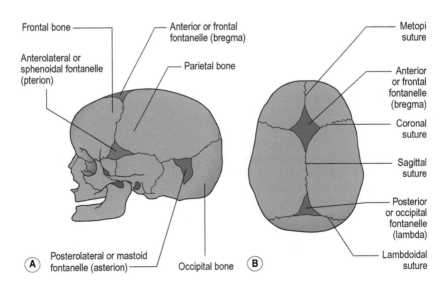

Figure 27.23
Cranium of a neonate viewed from the side (A) and from above (B).

Fontanelles

The following are typically found:

- Fonticulus anterior (located at bregma, the junction of the frontal, coronal, and sagittal sutures): anterior or frontal fontanelle (single). Bounded by the frontal bone and the two parietal bones. Closure: during first to second year of life.

- Fonticulus posterior (located at lambda, the junction of the sagittal and lambdoidal sutures): posterior or occipital fontanelle (single). Bounded by the occipital bone and the two parietal bones. Closure: during first to third month of life.

- Fonticulus anterolateralis (located at pterion, the junction of the parietal and frontal bones): anterolateral or sphenoidal fontanelle (paired). Each is bounded by the parietal bone, frontal bone, temporal squama, and the greater wing of the sphenoid bone. Closure: during sixth to twelfth month of life.

- Fonticulus posterolateralis (located at asterion, the junction of the lambdoidal, parietomastoid, and occipitomastoid sutures): posterolateral or mastoid fontanelle (paired). Each is bounded by the parietal bone, occipital bone, and temporal bone. Closure: during sixth to twelfth month of life.

After the dural bands have formed structures resembling window-frames for the cerebellum and cerebrum, the growing brain bulges outward through the "windows" between the stretched dural bands toward the skin. Paired bulges arise in the frontal and temporal regions, produced by the frontal and temporal lobes of the cerebrum, and an unpaired bulge arises in the occipital region to accommodate the future cerebellum. The tissue at these areas of bulging undergoes densation. According to Blechschmidt,[30] this densation is caused by viscous gliding movements in opposite directions, in the course of which water is expressed, causing extreme dehydration in the "window areas" (detraction fields).

The detraction fields cause five foci of ossification to arise and these enlarge to become the bones of the cranial vault: they are the anlagen of the left and right frontal bones, the left and right parietal bones, and the broad unpaired occipital bone (Figure 27.24).

Growth movements and factors influencing the growth of the cranial vault

- The bones of the cranial vault move centrifugally (Figure 27.25). Explanation: expansive growth of the brain.

- The frontal and parietal bones and the squama of the occipital and temporal bones move apart (Figure 27.26). Explanation: centrifugal movement of the cranial vault bones due to the expansion of the brain, which produces stretching or tension at the sutures. This leads to sutural bone growth. In addition, new bone is deposited at the internal and external surfaces of the bones.

- The convexity of the cranial bones decreases and the bones become flatter (Figure 27.27). Explanation: centrifugal movement of the bones of the cranial vault due to expansion of the brain and specific bone deposition and resorption processes on the external and internal surfaces of the cranial vault bones close to the sutures.

Influence of the cranial sutures

- The cranial sutures along the sagittal midline, e.g., the sagittal suture, facilitate the transverse growth of the neurocranium and viscerocranium.

- The transverse sutures, e.g., the coronal suture, facilitate the anteroposterior growth of the neurocranium and viscerocranium.

Compact bone layers

Whereas the cranial vault of a newborn consists of just one single lamella, an inner and an outer compact bone layer develop from the fourth year of life onward:

- The structure of the inner layer of compact bone is determined principally by the development of the brain and by intracranial pressure.

- The outer layer of compact bone is influenced more by the tension of the external musculature and by supporting forces.

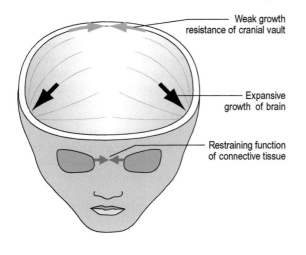

Figure 27.24

Anterior view of the frontal bones of a 50 mm fetus. The foci of the two frontal bones move away from each other and there is radial deposition of new bone due to the expansive growth of the brain.

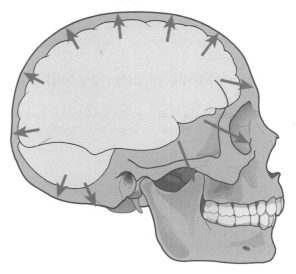

Figure 27.25

Passive centrifugal growth of the cranial vault bones due to the expansive growth of the brain, which generates tensile forces at the sutures.

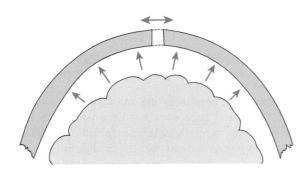

Figure 27.26

The cranial vault bones move apart.

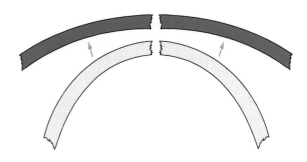

Figure 27.27

Growth movements lessen the convexity of the cranial vault.

According to Delaire,[31] the development of the cranial vault is also influenced to a lesser extent by the endochondrally ossifying cranial base and the viscerocranium.

The importance of asterion and pterion

For Fessenmeyer, the craniometric landmarks of asterion and pterion are of special importance in the cranial vault.[32]

Asterion

Delattre and Fenart[33] compare the asterion with the mechanical model of a mortise and tenon that is primarily intended to promote mobility. In this model the mortise is represented by the chondral part of the occipital bone and by the mastoid part of the temporal bone. The tenon is formed by the parietal bone.

The mobile zones of the head form a functional unit and articulate at the asterion:

- The petrous portion of the temporal bone.

- The petrojugular synchondrosis.

- The horizontal part of the greater wing of the sphenoid bone (inferior to the future sphenosquamous pivot point).

- The posterior part of the squama of the temporal bone.

This functional unit stands in relationship with the mandibular ramus and the alar ligament.

Pterion

The fixed pterion stands in contrast to the mobile asterion. The functional unit of pterion is formed by:

- The zygomatic process of the frontal bone.

- The vertical part of the greater wing of the sphenoid bone (superior to the future sphenosquamous pivot point)

- The anterior part of the squama of the temporal bone.

This functional unit stands in relationship with the pterygoid process and the face.

The pterion appears as a fixed zone that arises when the craniofacial bones are rolled up due to flexion of the cranium (causing the cranial base angle to become more acute). This cornerstone seems to be essential for maintaining craniofacial–cervical equilibrium because it preserves the virtual space that comprises the oropharyngeal canal and connects the cranial base with the funnel-shaped thoraco-mandibular space.

This is the result of two opposing phylogenetic (and ontogenetic) movements: posterior rotation of the occipital compartment (similar to flexion movement of the occipital bone) and recession of the face.

Development of the viscerocranium (Figure 27.28)

The viscerocranium arises from the single frontonasal prominence and the paired maxillary and mandibular prominences. These form around the anlage of the future oral cavity (stomodeum). The maxillary and mandibular prominences originate in the cartilage of the first pharyngeal arch, which is a kind of blueprint containing the information for the later formation of the maxillae and mandible. All the facial prominences and the six pharyngeal arches derive from the ectomesenchyme of the neural crest.

The viscerocranium is formed by desmal ossification. The essential prerequisite for the formation of the facial bones is an interaction between the ectomesenchyme of the pharyngeal arches and the ectodermal epithelium located above it. If this interaction is prevented, the facial bones cannot develop.

Development of the pharyngeal arches and pharyngeal pouches

- Because the growth of the accompanying vessels of the neural tube does not keep pace with the longitudinal growth of the neural tube itself, the brain is forced to bend over the cardiac bulge. The result of this first bending process of the embryo is the formation of endodermal and ectodermal "bending folds" on the ventral aspect of the lower head region (by day 26), features that are known as pharyngeal arches.

- This increasing curvature causes the embryonic face to broaden between the heart and the brain.

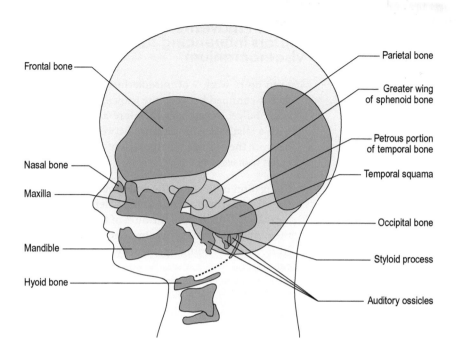

Figure 27.28
Embryonic cranium at 20 weeks (lateral view).

- The embryonic mouth at this stage shows characteristic transverse alignment, causing the connective tissue stroma lateral to the mouth to be stretched, almost parallel to the first pharyngeal arch.

- This stretching causes resistance to the longitudinal surface growth of the first pharyngeal arch. Consequently, ectoderm and endoderm growth is circular to the direction of the stretch, causing the first pharyngeal arch to thicken and bulge. Caudally, this may lead to the appearance of the first pharyngeal pouch on the inside of the adjoining walls.

- Surface enlargement of the ectoderm and endoderm provides space in the stroma in the interior of the pharyngeal arch for the anastomosis of the paired dorsal aorta and the unpaired ventral aorta. Associated with this, the space necessary for mesenchyme disappears in the pharyngeal pouches.

Pharyngeal arches

The pharyngeal arches come into being during week 4 of embryonic development and surround the primitive foregut. Their formation begins with the migration of cells from the neural crest.

Each pharyngeal arch consists of a mesodermal core covered externally by ectoderm cells and internally by endoderm cells. In addition, each pharyngeal arch possesses a cartilage component, a muscle component, a pharyngeal arch artery, and a pharyngeal arch nerve (sensory and visceromotor), which corresponds to a particular cranial nerve.

The first pharyngeal arch

- Muscles: muscles of mastication, the mylohyoid, the anterior belly of the digastric, the tensor veli palatini, and the tensor tympani.
- Nerve: mandibular division of the trigeminal nerve (CN V).
- Artery: involvement in the maxillary artery and external carotid artery.

The first pharyngeal arch cartilage/Meckel's cartilage/hyaline arch forms two of the auditory ossicles (the malleus and the incus), the sphenomandibular ligament, and the anterior ligament of the malleus.

The mandible is formed by desmal ossification from the mesenchymal tissue surrounding Meckel's cartilage. (The ossicula mentalia at the tip of the chin on the mandible arise directly from the pharyngeal arch cartilage and ossify endochondrally.) The maxillae, the zygomatic bones, and the squama of the temporal bones are formed by desmal ossification from the mesenchymal maxillary process of the first pharyngeal arch.

The second pharyngeal arch

- Muscles: stapedius, stylohyoid, the posterior belly of the digastric, and the muscles of facial expression.
- Nerve: facial nerve (CN VII).
- Artery: stapedial artery (disappears during the fetal period).

The second pharyngeal arch cartilage/Reichert's cartilage forms the stapes, the superior part of the body of the hyoid bone, and the lesser horn of the hyoid bone, the styloid process of the temporal bone, and the stylohyoid ligament.

On practical grounds Sperber[11] divides the face into upper, middle, and lower thirds, corresponding approximately to the embryonic single frontonasal prominence, and the paired maxillary and mandibular prominences, respectively.

The maxillary and mandibular bones arise from neural crest cells that originate in the mid- and hindbrain regions of the neural folds. The further development of the viscerocranium is characterized by merging of the facial prominences and by fusion of the maxillonasal components.

Growth movements and general factors influencing the growth of the viscerocranium

- Even up to week 7 of intrauterine development the face is confined between the growing brain and the heart bulge; the embryo therefore has a broad face, with a relatively wide distance between the eyes and between the nostrils, and the cleft of the mouth is oriented transversely.

- Elongation of the face: the embryonic heart follows the diaphragm in its descent, whereas the brain ascends as it grows and the dura of the upper part of the head with the falx becomes increasingly distant from the descending ligament system of the cervical viscera. This causes the connective tissue deep within the face to become stretched like a "muzzle" between the falx above and the hyoid arch below, thus creating space for the longitudinal growth of the face.

- The bilateral facial structures move closer together. The floors of the orbits – the anlagen for the palatine processes – are also involved, move closer together, and finally have contact medially.

- It is not until the late embryonic period that the dorsoventral dimension of the face (i.e., its depth) also increases. This process is related to growth of the cartilaginous mandible (Meckel's cartilage) which is directed ventrally.

- The stroma of the palatine processes is stretched by these dorsoventral growth phenomena, with the result that the palatine processes – which initially have a convex border with the convexity directed medially and caudally – become progressively straightened and the interpalatine space closes.

- As the tissue in the region of the nasal capsules is stretched, the mucosal lining epithelium becomes so compressed that it bends into folds forming the initially membranous nasal conchae.[34]

- The elongated face develops. According to Blechschmidt,[35] the connective tissue deep within the face is stretched into a "muzzle" by the growth of

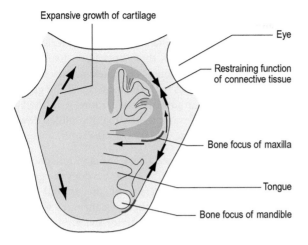

Expansive growth of cartilage

Eye

Restraining function of connective tissue

Bone focus of maxilla

Tongue

Bone focus of mandible

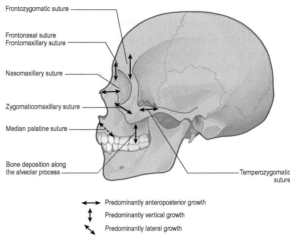

Frontozygomatic suture

Frontonasal suture
Frontomaxillary suture

Nasomaxillary suture

Zygomaticomaxillary suture

Median palatine suture

Bone deposition along the alveolar process

Temperozygomatic suture

←→ Predominantly anteroposterior growth
↕ Predominantly vertical growth
⤡ Predominantly lateral growth

Figure 27.29

Frontal section through the facial region of a 37 mm embryo. Formation of the elongated face. Convergent arrows: restraining function of the connective tissue. Diverging arrows: growth expansion of nasal cartilage.[36]

Figure 27.30

Directions of sutural bone growth in the viscerocranium.

the nasal cartilage. This tissue also has attachment to the cartilaginous cranial base and to the future mandible and hyoid arch. As the "muzzle" becomes more tightly stretched, so the cartilaginous skeleton of the nose enclosed within becomes more elongated (Figure 27.29).

• Growth of the zygomaticomaxillary suture and intermaxillary suture results in a broadening of the face.

• According to Delaire,[37] the cranial sutures surrounding the maxillae and the cranial sutures between the cranial base and cranial vault as well as the SBS regulate the vertical and anteroposterior growth of the viscerocranium. The development of the ethmoid bone and of the other components of the nasal septum acts as a stimulus in this process (Figure 27.30).

• The growth of the nasal septum transmits a downward and forward force to the maxilla; the further consequence of this thrust and pull of nasal septal growth is to separate the frontomaxillary, frontozygomatic, frontonasal, and zygomaticomaxillary sutures. The thrust exerted on the maxilla by the ethmoid bone and the other components of the nasal septum in the course of their pre- and postnatal growth positions the viscerocranium in relation to the cranial base and provides stimuli to the development of the viscerocranium.

• The eye, the nasal cavity, and the external ear also determine certain aspects of the growth of the facial bones. For example, the growth of the eye provides an expanding force separating the neurocranium and the viscerocranium, particularly at the frontomaxillary and frontozygomatic sutures.

• The growth of the alveolar process of the maxilla and mandible produces an increase in the vertical height of the face and permits enlargement of the maxillary sinus.

- After birth the development of the viscerocranium is also dependent on four further factors: the growth of the paranasal sinuses, the growth and suckling action of the tongue, the development of the teeth, and the action of the oromasticatory muscles (Figure 27.31).

Upper third of the face

The nasal placodes, development of which is induced by the olfactory nerves, are formed at the inferolateral corners of the frontonasal prominence. At about 8 weeks after conception ossification centers for the nasal and lacrimal bones appear in the frontonasal prominence (in the membrane covering the nasal capsule). The following growth movements and factors influencing the growth of the upper third of the face are observed:

- The upper third (frontal bone) moves outward and forward. Explanation (Figure 27.32): expansive growth of the frontal lobe of the brain; the frontal bone initially shows the most rapid development; and its growth is largely completed by the age of 12 years.

- Enlargement of the frontal bone by sutural growth.

- The orbit rotates so that the axis of the eye lies horizontally. Explanation: rotation of the frontal lobe.

- The orbits rotate to the midline (Figure 27.33). Explanation: expansive growth of the frontal and temporal lobes.

- The medial walls of the orbits grow laterally, and the ethmoidal air cells become larger.

- The roof of the orbit grows forward and downward. Explanation: forward and downward growth of the frontal lobe of the brain.

- The orbits are pushed forward.

- The orbits become larger. Explanation: growth in the sutures participating in the orbit.

- Rotation of the lacrimal bone, causing its inferior part to move laterally (Figure 27.34). Explanation: expansion of the ethmoid air cells and bone growth processes. The lacrimal bone plays a particularly important role in the growth of the orbit: it articulates with many other orbital bones, with the maxilla, the ethmoid, and the frontal bones and the inferior nasal concha. As they grow, these bones are displaced in very different directions. Nevertheless, they are able to maintain contact with the orbital wall by gliding movements at the sutural articulations with the lacrimal bone. For example, the maxilla glides downward without losing contact with the orbit.

- Formation of the frontal sinus. Explanation: once the growth of the frontal lobe ceases, so does the growth of the endocranial surface of the frontal bone; however, its exocranial surface continues to move forward, thus creating an interior space.

Middle third of the face

The middle third of the face is the most complex in terms of its skeletal development. It incorporates the nasal extension of the upper third, part of the cranial base, and part of the masticatory apparatus. During week 8 after conception, ossification centers for the palatine bones and the vomer arise in the maxillary mesenchyme surrounding the nasal capsule.

The medial lamina of the pterygoid process of the sphenoid bone is also formed from the maxillary prominence. (Further ossification centers arise for the greater wing of the sphenoid and the lateral lamina of the pterygoid process of the sphenoid. The medial and lateral laminae unite by bony fusion in month 5 of fetal development.)

As early as week 7 after conception, a primary ossification center for the maxilla arises at the end of the infraorbital nerve. Further ossification sites come into being; for example, the premaxilla (incisive bone), which fuses with the rest of the maxilla during the first year of life, forms from intermaxillary ossification centers. In addition, one ossification center each arises for the zygomatic bone and the temporal squama. The growth movements and factors influencing the growth of the middle third of the face are as follows:

- The zygomatic bone together with the maxilla is displaced forward due to growth in the temporozygomatic suture and downward due to growth in the frontozygomatic suture (Figure 27.35). Explanation: forward and downward growth of the nasal septum.

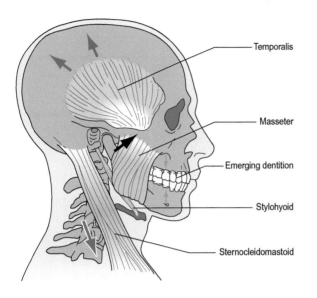

Figure 27.31
Postnatal factors influencing the growth of the viscerocranium.

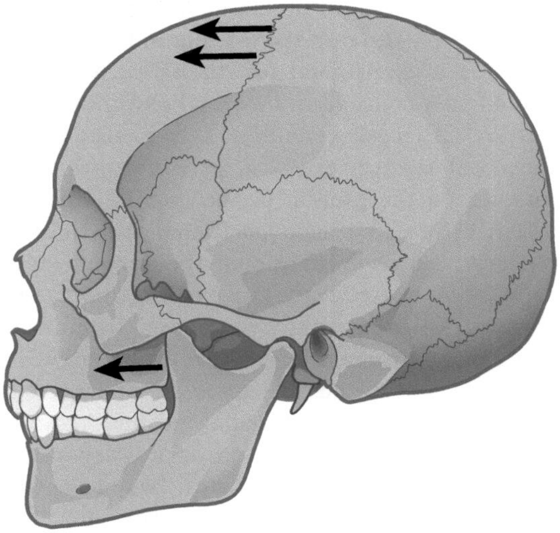

Figure 27.32
Enlargement of the frontal bone by sutural growth.

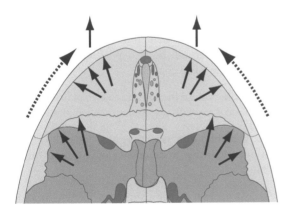

Figure 27.33
Rotation of the orbit toward the midline.

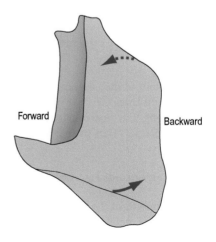

Figure 27.34
Growth rotation of the lacrimal bone.

- According to Delaire,[38] the ethmoid bone and the other components of the nasal septum transmit a thrusting pressure on the maxilla in the course of their pre- and postnatal growth. Between weeks 10 and 40 post-conception the nasal septum expands its vertical length sevenfold. Due to this growth the nasal septum exerts a force downward and forward on the growth of the maxilla, and it is assisted in this by the appositional growth of the posterior superior margin of the vomer (Figure 27.36). The consequence is a pushing apart of the frontomaxillary, frontozygomatic, frontonasal, and zygomaticomaxillary sutures. The growth of the nasal septum has the most direct impact on the nasal part of the maxilla and on the anteroposterior growth of the nasomaxillary suture. The growth of the SBS regulates the anteroposterior growth of the maxilla. Fatty tissue, interposed between the posterosuperior surfaces of the maxilla and the cranial base, provides a compression-resisting structure. The expansively growing maxilla is displaced downward and slightly forward by the resistance of the fatty tissue pad and the cranial base.

- The zygomatic arch moves laterally.

- The floor of the orbit, together with the nasomaxillary complex, moves downward, forward, and laterally. Explanation: intra-osseous transformation processes.

- The nasal cavity and the orbit move downward with the maxilla.

- However, the floor of the nasal cavity is lowered to a far greater extent than the floor of the orbit. Explanation: opposing intra-osseous processes of bone deposition and resorption in the floor of the orbit and nasal cavity.

- The nasal region expands anteriorly.

- Longitudinal growth of the nasomaxillary complex. Explanation: bone deposition and resorption processes and displacement.

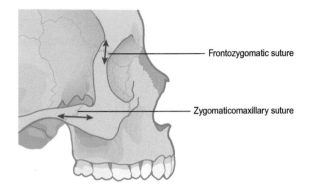

Figure 27.35
Displacement of the zygomatic bone with the maxilla due to sutural growth.

- The nasal space expands laterally, forward, and downward. Explanation: bone resorption in the nasal walls and floor, but not in the roof.

- Downward movement of the palate. Explanation: bone resorption at the nasal floor and displacement of the maxilla.

- The inferior nasal concha moves downward and laterally. Explanation: bone deposition beneath and lateral to the nasal concha.

- The maxillary sinus increases in size. Explanation: bone resorption at its walls (except for the medial wall).

- Enlargement of the nasal part of the maxilla. Explanation: expansive force due to enlargement of the orbit.

- Vertical growth at the frontomaxillary, ethmoido-maxillary, frontoethmoidal, frontonasal, and frontozygomatic sutures. Explanation: eyeball and nasal septal expansion.

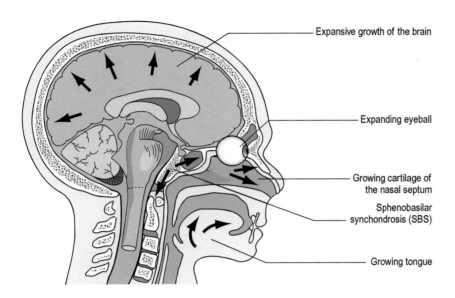

Expansive growth of the brain

Expanding eyeball

Growing cartilage of the nasal septum

Sphenobasilar synchondrosis (SBS)

Growing tongue

Figure 27.36
Factors influencing cranial growth: the growth of the nasal septum exerts a force downward and forward on the growth of the maxillary complex.

- Anteroposterior growth at the temporozygomatic suture. Explanation: anteroposterior growth of the brain and cranial base.

Other growth factors

- The tooth buds form the basis for the development of the alveolar process of the maxilla.

- The alveolar process in turn permits the expansion of the maxillary sinus.

- The teeth and the alveolar process participate in the downward growth movement of the maxilla.

- The anterior cranial fossa is in equilibrium with the maxilla, with the result that both structures usually experience equivalent expansive growth.

- The body of the maxilla forms below the infraorbital nerve.

Lower third of the face

The lower third of the face is composed skeletally of the mandible with its masticatory apparatus. The mandibular prominences develop intramembranous ossification centers for the mandible and the tympanic ring of the temporal bone. Growth movements and factors influencing the growth of the lower third of the face are as follows:

- Growth of the mandibular ramus backward and upward (Figure 27.37). Explanation: bone formation in the mandibular condyles.

- Downward and forward displacement of the mandible as a whole. Explanation: backward and upward growth of the mandibular ramus.

- Posterior divergence of the two halves of the body of the mandible (Figure 27.38). Explanation: posterior growth of the condylar heads.

Other factors influencing the growth of the mandible

- The mandibular nerve is the first structure to form in the territory of the mandible. It probably induces the formation of the mandibular prominence from a membranous condensation of ectomesenchyme. In week 6 after conception a single ossification center arises for each mandibular half (in the vicinity of the bifurcation of the inferior alveolar nerve and the inferior alveolar artery). Ossification continues along the alveolar nerve and its branches while the cartilage of the pharyngeal arch is almost totally lost.

- As a reaction to the early swallowing and suckling activity of the fetus, the transformation from woven bone to lamellar bone occurs earlier in the mandible than in other bones (month 5 of embryonic development).

- In week 12 after conception, independently of pharyngeal arch cartilage, secondary cartilage arises as a precursor for part of the condylar process, for the head of the mandible, and the mental protuberance.

- Whereas the secondary cartilage of the condyle is replaced by bone, the upper part remains as articular cartilage and a growth center. This growth center is particularly important for the further shaping of the mandible.

- The activity of the lateral pterygoid muscle regulates the development of the condylar process.

- The activity of the temporalis muscle influences the development of the coronoid process.

- The activity of the masseter and pterygoid muscles has an influence on the development of the angle and the ramus of the mandible. The tooth buds form the basis for the development of the pars alveolaris of the mandible.

- Vertical growth movement of the teeth.

- The growth and movement of the tongue also influence the development of the maxilla.

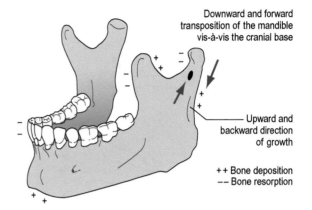

Downward and forward transposition of the mandible vis-à-vis the cranial base

Upward and backward direction of growth

++ Bone deposition
−− Bone resorption

Figure 27.37
Growth movement of the mandible.

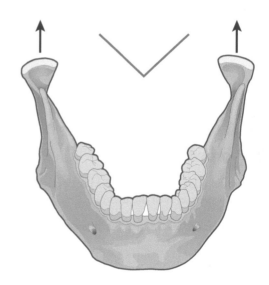

Figure 27.38
Lateral divergence of the mandibular ramus.

At birth

Maxilla

- Short and broad, the transverse and anteroposterior diameters being greater than the vertical; and increases in length in the early years of life.

- The alveolar process and, in particular, the maxillary sinus are very small initially; it is only later that they dramatically increase in size.

Palatine bones

- The orbital and sphenoidal processes are made of cancellous bone.

- The dimensions of the horizontal and perpendicular plates are almost equal (in adults the length of the perpendicular plate is twice that of the horizontal plate).

Lacrimal bones

- Meeting point of conflicting stresses arising from the cranial base and the face (pressure from the ethmoid bone in an anterior direction or from the frontal process of the maxilla in a posterior direction).

- Commonest problem: dacrostenosis (blockage of the lacrimal duct, e.g., due to facial presentation at term).

Summary

There is a close interplay between the development of the neurocranium – and to a lesser extent of the viscerocranium – and the development of the brain. The development of the neural tube is induced by the notochord from the chordomesoblast. Neural tube development in turn induces the development of the vertebral arches and the neurocranium. The emergence of the viscerocranium depends on the growth of the cranial base and of the brain and it is formed as a function of the local soft tissues. The bones arise, as it were, in an adaptive process and in a functional relationship with the development of the visceral structures. In this process, the development of the cranial base is characterized by greater independence than that of the other cranial bones.

Other local and more remote factors influencing the development of the cranial and facial bones include: the surrounding cranial sutures, gravitational forces, static and dynamic forces (locomotion, masticatory processes, development of the paranasal sinuses, and teeth, etc.), as well as genetic influences.

The hyoid bone arises from the cartilages of the second and third pharyngeal arches. Two ossification centers each form the greater horn (week 38 of fetal development), the body (at term), and the lesser horn (2 years after birth) of the hyoid bone (Figure 27.8).

The sacrum consists of five modified vertebrae, the prenatal development of which is consistent with that of the other vertebrae. Ossification of the sacral segments is complete by about the age of 25 years. The sacrum follows the overall flexion of the embryo, with the result that its base undergoes posterior or backward motion, a phenomenon known as counternutation.

References

[1]Aurobindo S. The Mother. Notes on the Way. 2nd edn. Pondicherry: Sri Aurobindo Ashram Press; 2002:5.

[2]Portmann A. Einführung in die vergleichende Morphologie der Wirbeltiere. 6th edn. Basel: Schwabe & Co.; 1983:175.

[3]Delattre A, Fenart R. L'hominisation du crâne étudiée par la méthode vestibulaire. Centre National de Recherche Scientifique: Paris; 1960.

[4]Enlow DH. Handbook of Facial Growth. Philadelphia: W.B. Saunders; 1982:26.

[5]Fessenmeyer MO. A propos du développement de la base du crâne. ApoStill 2001;8:82–84.

[6]Oudhof HA, van Doorenmaalen WJ. Skull morphogenesis and growth: hemodynamic influence. Acta Anat 1983;117:181–186.

[7]Dambricourt-Malassé A, Palevol CR. Evolution du chondrocrâne et de la face des grands anthropoïds miocènes jusqu'à Homo sapiens, continuités et discontinuités. Académies des sciences 5 (2006).

[8]Blechschmidt E. The Ontogenetic Basis of Human Anatomy. Berkeley, CA: North Atlantic Books; 2004:140–141.

[9]Blechschmidt E. The Ontogenetic Basis of Human Anatomy. Berkeley, CA: North Atlantic Books; 2004:141.

[10]Sperber GH. Craniofacial development. Hamilton, Ontario: BC Decker Inc.; 2001:91.

[11]Belden CJ, Mancuso AA, Kotzur IM. The developing anterior skull base: CT appearance from birth to 2 years of age. Am J Neuroradiol 1997; 18:811–818.

[12]Blechschmidt E. The Ontogenetic Basis of Human Anatomy. Berkeley, CA: North Atlantic Books; 2004:86.

[13]Kjaer I. Ossification of the human fetal basicranium. J Craniofac Genet Develop Bio 1990;10:29–38.

[14]Nemzek WR, Brodie HA, Hecht ST et al. MR, CT and plain film imaging of the developing skull base in fetal specimens. AJNR Am J Neuroradiol 2000;21:1699–1706.

[15]Ricciardelli EJ. Embryology and anatomy of the cranial base. Clin Plast Surg 1995;22:361–372.

[16]Rouvière H. Anatomie humaine: tête et cou. Volume 1. Paris: Masson; 1981.

[17]Couly G. Développement céphalique. Edition CCP; 1991.

[18]Couly G. La dynamique de croissance céphalique. Le principe de conformation organofonctionelle. Actualités Odonto Stom 1977; 117:63–69.

[19]Mann SS, Naidich TP, Towbin RB, Doundoulakis SH. Imaging of postnatal maturation of the skull base. Neuroimaging Clin North Am 2000;10:1–21.

[20]Aoki S, Dillon WP, Barkovich AJ, Norman D. Marrow conversion before pneumatization of the sphenoid sinus: assessment with MR imaging. Radiology 1989;172:373–375.

[21]Scuderi AJ, Harnsberger HR, Boyer RS. Pneumatization of the paranasal sinuses: normal features of importance to the accurate interpretation of CT scans and MR images. AJR Am J Roentgenol 1993;160:1101–1104.

[22]Kuzma BB, Goodman JM. Presphenoidal marrow changes in the pediatric skull base. Surg Neurol 2000;53:91.

[23]Lee SK, Kim YS, Jo YA, Seo JW, Chi JG. Development of cranial base in normal Korean foetuses. Anat Rec 1996;246:524–534.

[24]Delaire J. L'harmonie céphalique. Conférence Paris, 1999.

[25]Moss ML. Ontogenetic Aspects of Cranio-Facial Growth. Pergamon Press; 1971.

[26]Belet R. Systèmes de tenségrité dysfunction sacro-occipitale intra-osseuse et test de flexion assis. Mémoire en vue de l'obtention du diplôme en ostéopathie; 2002

[27]Delaire J. L'harmonie céphalique. Conférence Paris, 1999.

[28]Bosma JF. Postnatal ontogeny of performances of the pharynx, larynx and mouth. Am Rev Respir Dis 1985;131:10–15.

[29]Carreiro JE. An Osteopathic Approach to Children. Edinburgh: Churchill Livingstone; 2003:144.

[30]Blechschmidt E. The Ontogenetic Basis of Human Anatomy. Berkeley, CA: North Atlantic Books; 2004:142–143.

[31]Delaire J.

[32]Fessenmeyer MO. Personal communication with Torsten Liem, 2004.

[33]Delattre A, Fenart R. L'hominisation du crâne étudiée par la méthode vestibulaire. Centre National de Recherche Scientifique: Paris; 1960.

[34]Blechschmidt E, Gasser RF. Biokinetics and Biodynamics of Human Differentiation: Principles and Applications. Springfield, Illinois: Charles C. Thomas; 1978:136.

[35]Blechschmidt E. The Ontogenetic Basis of Human Anatomy. Berkeley, CA: North Atlantic Books; 2004:130.

[36]Blechschmidt E. The Ontogenetic Basis of Human Anatomy. Berkeley, CA: North Atlantic Books; 2004:132.

[37]Delaire J. Considérations de la croissance faciale. Rev Stomatol 1971;72:59–60.

[38]Delaire J. L'articulatio fronto-maxillaire. Rev Stomatol 1976;77:922.

28

Intraosseous techniques

Torsten Liem

Form is always the outline of a movement.

Henri Bergson[1]

Introduction

Any bone may be susceptible to abnormal tension patterns and to limitations in its adaptation to tension – phenomena that are referred to as intraosseous dysfunctions – and any bone can be treated specifically (see also Chapter 20). Knowledge of the developmental dynamics of the structures involved is a prerequisite for a successful treatment outcome in this context. The treatment of a number of structures will be presented below as illustrative examples.

However, note that, these techniques may also be used in adults. While the ossification of the bone is still incomplete, the morphology of the bone can be influenced far more distinctly. For didactic reasons, this chapter will focus primarily on the structural approach.

Vitalistic approaches differ principally in that the practitioner does not address any physiological tissue barriers either when testing or treating. The general vitalistic approach can be used, as appropriate, for the techniques described below:

- Synchronize yourself with the primary respiration.

- Listen, and establish a resonance with the tissue.

- Establish balanced tension (without addressing any tissue barriers).

- Achieve disengagement or compression as an invitation to the tissue or to move the tissue gently out of the tension range (without confronting any tissue barriers) or else actively "wait" for spontaneous disengagement. (Disengagement or compression should be performed before establishing balanced tension if inherent resolution of tension is prevented by the presence of excessive dysfunctional or rigidified biokinetic forces.)

- Establish balanced tension (without addressing any tissue barriers).

- Focus your attention on the activity of the inherent homeodynamic forces.

- Sense any change in consciousness that occurs during the therapeutic interaction.

- Sense any automatic shifting.

Occipital bone

Cranial base–occiput–foramen magnum technique in young children (Figure 28.1)

Practitioner: take up a position at the head of the patient.

- Hand position:
  - Place your index and middle fingers of one hand on the occipital squama and between the atlas and occipital bone. Your thumb should be placed a little higher on the occipital squama.
  - Place your other hand on the frontal bone, with your index finger lying along the metopic suture.

- Method:
  - Anterior–posterior decompression of the SBS and anterior intraoccipital synchondrosis between the

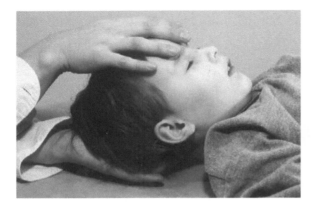

Figure 28.1
Cranial base–occiput–foramen magnum
technique in young children.

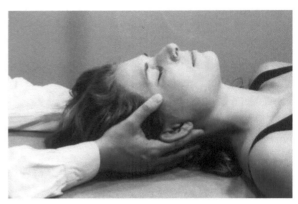

Figure 28.2
Platybasia technique.

lateral and basilar parts of the occipital bone: use
your hand on the frontal bone to apply traction in
an anterior direction.
- Posterior–anterior decompression of the posterior intraoccipital synchondrosis between the
squama and the lateral parts of the occipital
bone (and of the anterior intraoccipital synchondrosis): use your index and middle fingers
to apply traction in a posterior direction to the
occipital squama.
- Lateral decompression of the lateral parts of the
occipital bone: spread your index and middle fingers, while focusing your attention on the lateral
parts of the occipital bone.
- Rotation of the occipital squama: use your
thumb placed on the occipital squama to rotate
the squama against the restriction (direct
technique).
- Establish the PBMT: use your other hand placed
on the frontal bone to direct a fluctuation wave in
the direction of the restriction.

Platybasia technique (Figure 28.2)

- Practitioner: take up a position at the head of the
patient.

- Hand position:
  - Place your thumbs on the greater wings of the
  sphenoid.
  - Position your index fingers on the temporal bones
  anterior to the occipitomastoid suture.
  - Place your middle, ring, and little fingers on the
  occiput.

- Method:
  - Anterior-posterior decompression of the SBS: use
  your thumbs on the greater wings of the sphenoid
  to apply traction in an anterior direction.
  - Decompression of the occipitomastoid suture:
  move your index and middle fingers apart.
  - Posterior–anterior decompression: with your
  middle, ring, and little fingers apply traction
  to the occiput in a posterior direction so as to
  decompress the squama from the lateral parts, the

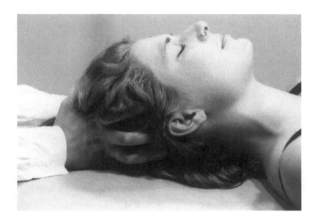

Figure 28.3
Occipital squama technique.

lateral from the basilar parts, and the basilar parts of the occipital bone from the sphenoid.

- Establish the PBMT and PBFT.

Occipital squama technique (Figure 28.3)

- Practitioner: take up a position at the head of the patient.

- Hand position:
  - Place your hands symmetrically on either side of the patient's head.
  - Position your little fingers bilaterally on the inter-parietal occiput.
  - Position your ring fingers posterior to the lambdoid suture.
  - Position your middle fingers anterior to the lambdoid suture.
  - Let your index fingers rest lightly on the parietal bones, without exerting any pressure.
  - Your thumbs should be touching each other above the vertex, but not in contact with the patient's head.

- Method:
  - Decompress the lambdoid suture by spreading your middle and ring fingers.
  - Harmonize intraosseous tensions using your little and ring fingers.
  - Treat the occipital squama.

- Testing: perform passive palpation or actively test the motion of the squama in rotation, flexion, extension, and side bending. Use your little fingers and ring fingers to encourage the particular motion that you are testing, and compare the amplitude, ease, and symmetry of this motion.

- Treatment:
  - Use your little fingers and ring fingers to guide the squama in the direction of the motion restriction and wait for the release of the tissue (direct technique).
  - Alternatively, guide the squama in the direction of ease (indirect technique).
  - Establish the PBMT and PBFT.

Sphenoid bone (Figure 28.4)

Technique to release tensions between the pre- and post-sphenoid

Note, this technique is indicated particularly in newborn babies and infants.

- Patient: supine.

- Practitioner: take up a position at the head of the patient.

- Hand position:
  - Cranial vault hold.
  - Place your hands on either side of the patient's head.
  - Position your index fingers on the greater wings of the sphenoid, behind the lateral corners of the eyes.
  - Position your middle fingers on the temporal bones, in front of the ears.
  - Position your ring fingers on the temporal bones, behind the ears.
  - Position your little fingers on the sides of the occiput.

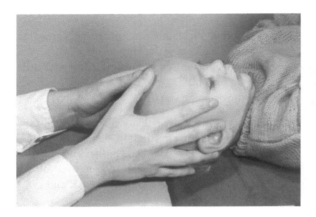

Figure 28.4
Technique for relieving tensions between the pre- and post-sphenoid.

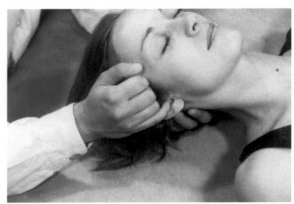

Figure 28.5
Petromastoid part/tympanic part (right side).

- If possible, your thumbs should meet and touch on top of the patient's head to act as a fulcrum or fixed point.

- Method:
  - Begin by sensing the tissue tension between the pre- and post-sphenoid.
  - Move both parts of the bone in the direction of their motion restriction.
  - Establish the PBMT and PBFT between the pre- and the post-sphenoid.
  - Maintain this position until you sense a release of tension between the pre- and the post-sphenoid.

Temporal bones

Primary intraosseous dysfunctions may be the result of direct force to the temporal bones, especially during birth and in early infancy.

Secondary dysfunctions may occur as a result of dysfunctions involving other bones (occipital bone, sphenoid). To ensure the success of intraosseous techniques it is important that all the sutural articulations of the temporal bones have free mobility.

The following articulations are treated:

- Petromastoid part/tympanic part

- Petromastoid part/squamous part

- Squamous part/tympanic part.

Petromastoid part/tympanic part (right side illustrated) (Figure 28.5)

- Hand position:
  - Hold the patient's occiput in your left hand, with your fingertips resting on the mastoid part and mastoid process.
  - Place the little finger of your right hand in the external auditory canal.

- Alternative hand position (Figure 28.6):
  - Turn the patient's head to the left.
  - Place the thumb of your right hand on the mastoid process.
  - Place the thenar eminence of your right hand on the mastoid part of the temporal bone.
  - Hold the occiput with the remaining fingers of your right hand.

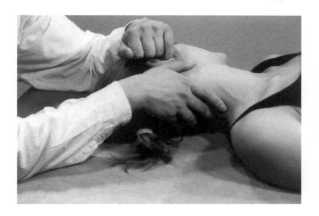

Figure 28.6
Petromastoid part/tympanic part, alternative hand position.

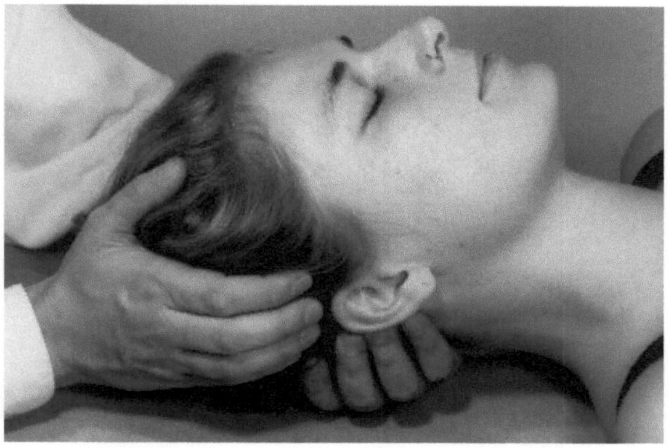

Figure 28.7
Petromastoid part/squamous part (right side).

- Place the little finger of your left hand in the external auditory canal.

Petromastoid part/squamous part (right side illustrated) (Figure 28.7)

- Hand position:
  - Hold the patient's occiput in your left hand, with your fingertips resting on the mastoid part and mastoid process.
  - Rest the index and middle fingers of your right hand, and your ring finger if necessary, on the squamous part.

- Alternative hand position (Figure 28.8):
  - Turn the patient's head to the left.
  - Place the thumb of your right hand on the mastoid process.
  - Place the thenar eminence of your right hand on the mastoid part of the temporal bone.
  - Hold the occiput with the remaining fingers of your right hand.
  - Rest the index and middle fingers of your left hand, and your ring finger if necessary, on the squamous part.

Squamous part/tympanic part (right side illustrated) (Figure 28.9)

- Hand position:
  - Rest the index and middle fingers of your left hand, and your ring finger if necessary, on the squamous part.
  - Place the little finger of your right hand in the external auditory canal.

- Method – direct technique:
  - Guide both portions of the bone in the direction of their restricted motion until you reach the motion barrier.
  - Hold this position until a tissue release or a still point occurs.

- Method – indirect technique:
  - Move both portions of the bone in the direction of the dysfunction, in the direction of greater motion (direction of ease).
  - Establish the PBMT and PBFT (the position that achieves the best possible balance between these two portions of the bone).

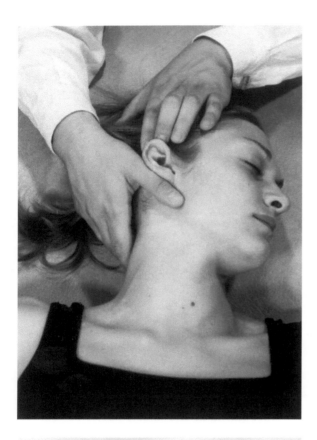

Figure 28.8
Petromastoid part/squamous part, alternative hand position.

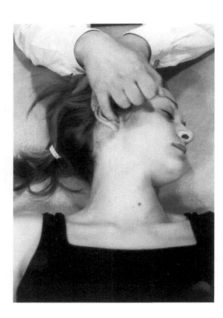

Figure 28.9
Squamous part/tympanic part (right side).

- Maintain this position until the tissues relax and mobility improves.

Technique for the auditory ossicles (Figure 28.10)

- Indications: tinnitus, deafness, and syringitis.

- Patient: jaw relaxed; masticatory surfaces of the teeth not in contact.

- Practitioner: take up a position at the head of the patient.

- Hand position: place the tip of your index finger on the tragus.

- Method – indirect technique:
  - With your index finger, administer pressure on the tragus in the direction of the external acoustic meatus.
  - Without reducing the gentle pressure, rotate your index finger in an anterior or posterior direction and establish the PBMT.
  - Direct your attention to the tympanic membrane, to the tissue tension of the tympanic cavity in the middle ear, and to the auditory ossicles.
  - You may also go with the rotating motions/tissue unwinding that may arise.
  - A fluid impulse may be directed from the pterion on the opposite side.

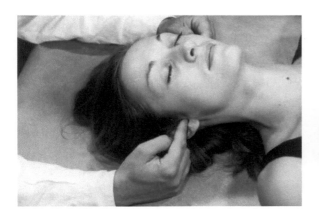

Figure 28.10
Technique for the auditory ossicles.

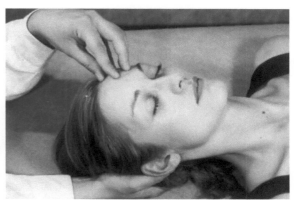

Figure 28.11
Molding the frontal tuberosity.

Molding

- Indications: asymmetrical convexity or flattening at the ossification centers.

- Hand position:
  - Draw the fingertips of one hand close together.
  - Place them on the squama.

- Method – to treat convexity:
  - Administer centrifugal impulses with your fingers, to flatten the site of the convexity.
  - You may augment this by inducing a fluid impulse directed toward the borders of the temporal bone.
  - Important note: before starting this technique, gently release the adjacent bones from the temporal bone.

- Method – to treat flattening of the bone:
  - Administer centripetal impulses with your fingers, aimed at making the flattened site more prominent.
  - You may augment this by inducing a fluid impulse toward the ossification center from the occipito-mastoid suture on the opposite side.

- Method – to treat torsion tensions:
  - Administer an impulse with your fingers in the direction of the restricted motion.
  - Establish the PBMT and PBFT.

Frontal bone

Molding (Figure 28.11)

- Indications: asymmetrical convexity or flattening, and torsion tensions at the ossification centers, usually as a result of birth trauma or a fall in early childhood.

- Hand position:
  - Draw the fingertips of one hand close together.
  - Place them on the frontal tuberosity.

- Method – to treat convexity:
  - Administer centrifugal impulses with your fingers, to flatten the site of the convexity.
  - You may augment this by inducing a fluid impulse directed toward the borders of the frontal bone.
  - Important note: before starting this technique, gently release the adjacent bones from the frontal bone.

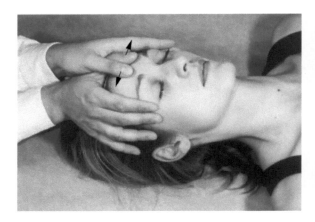

Figure 28.12
Spreading the metopic suture.

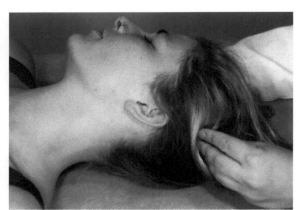

Figure 28.13
Molding the parietal bone.

- Method – to treat flattening of the bone:
  - Administer centripetal impulses with your fingers, aimed at making the flattened site more prominent.
  - You may augment this by inducing a fluid impulse toward the center of the frontal tuberosity from the occipitomastoid suture on the opposite side.

- Method – to treat torsion tensions:
  - Administer an impulse with your fingers in the direction of the restricted motion.
  - Establish the PBMT and PBFT.

Spreading the metopic suture (Figure 28.12)

- Indication: to correct compression of the metopic suture by transverse forces during the birth process.

- Practitioner: take up a position at the head of the patient.

- Hand position:
  - Cross your thumbs over the metopic suture so that they rest next to the suture on the opposite side of the frontal bone.

- Position the palms of your hands on the ipsilateral cranial vault on each side.
- With your thumbs, administer diverging lateral traction so as to spread the metopic suture.
- Permit all motions/tissue unwinding that may arise.
- Establish the PBMT and PBFT.
- Maintain PBMT until correction of the abnormal tension pattern has been achieved and stabilized by the inherent homeostatic forces (PRM rhythm, etc.).
- This treatment may be augmented by delivering a fluid impulse from the inion.

Parietal bones

The SBS, occiput, and temporal bones and the atlanto-occipital junction should also be examined, and treated as necessary.

Molding (Figure 28.13)

- Indications: asymmetrical convexity or flattening, and torsion tensions at the ossification centers.

- Hand position:
  - Draw the fingertips of one hand close together.
  - Place them on the parietal tuberosity.

- Method – to treat convexity:
  - Administer centrifugal impulses with your fingers, to flatten the site of the convexity.
  - You may augment this by inducing a fluid impulse directed toward the borders of the parietal bone.
  - Important note: before starting this technique, gently release the adjacent bones from the parietal bone.

- Method – to treat flattening of the bone:
  - Administer centripetal impulses with your fingers, aimed at making the flattened site more prominent.
  - You may augment this by inducing a fluid impulse toward the center of the parietal tuberosity from the opposite lateral border of the occiput.

- Method – to treat torsion tensions:
  - Administer an impulse with your fingers in the direction of the restricted motion.
  - Establish the PBMT and PBFT.

Intraosseous lines of force

The pressures associated with chewing combined with the pull of the muscles of mastication are responsible for the most powerful mechanical forces at work in the cranium. Special constructional features enable these forces to be dissipated in ways that are largely devoid of jarring or impact. The design of these constructional features is the main factor responsible for the efficient absorption of forces and is simultaneously an expression of the forces that are being generated (Figure 28.14).[2]

Mandible

Treating dysfunctional compressive trajectories running from the head to the body of the mandible

Compressive trajectories travel from the head of the mandible along the posterior segment of the ramus and then in a postero-inferior to antero-superior arc in the body of the mandible (Figure 28.15).

- Practitioner: take up a position beside the patient's head on the side opposite the dysfunction.

- Hand contact:
  - Place the thumb of your cranial hand on the head and neck of the patient's mandible on the side away from you.

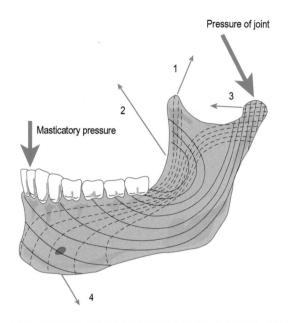

Figure 28.14
Influence of forces on trajectory lines:
(1) Postero-superior pull of the temporalis muscle; (2) Antero-superior force direction of the masseter and medial pterygoid muscles; (3) Antero-inferior pull of the lateral pterygoid muscle as it interacts with the (posterior part of) the masseter muscle; and (4) Force directions of the suprahyoid and infrahyoid muscles. Broken lines: tensile trajectories; solid lines: compressive trajectories.

- Rest your other fingers passively beneath the patient's neck and occiput.
- Position the index, middle, ring, and little fingers of your caudal hand on the alveolar part of the patient's mandible (approximately along the course of the compressive trajectories) on the side away from you.

- Method: compress the head and alveolar part of the mandible and establish a point of balance.

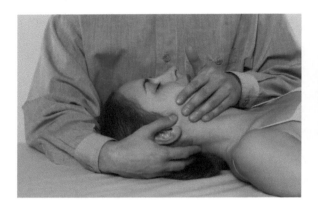

Figure 28.15
Treating dysfunctional compressive trajectories running from the head to the body of the mandible.

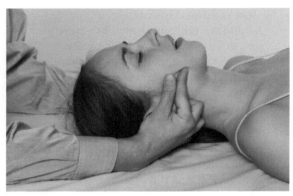

Figure 28.16
Treating dysfunctional compressive trajectories running from the coronoid process to the body of the mandible.

Treating dysfunctional compressive trajectories running from the coronoid process to the body of the mandible

The compressive trajectories at the anterior margin of the coronoid process travel in an arc to the body of the mandible (Figure 28.16).

- Practitioner: take up a position at the patient's head.

- Hand contact: place your index fingers and thumbs on the ramus of the mandible on both sides, approximately along the course of the compressive trajectories.

- Patient: the patient's mouth should be slightly open.

- Method: press your index fingers and thumbs together on both sides and establish a point of balance.

Treating dysfunctional tensile trajectories running from the head/ neck of the mandible

Tensile trajectories travel from the posterior region of the head and neck of the mandible to the anterior part of the mandibular angle and the alveolar part of the mandible. Some of the tensile trajectories travel caudally to the inferior border of the body of the mandible and therefore cross the compressive trajectories at right angles.

At the coronoid process the tensile trajectories run parallel to the path taken by the muscles and in the alveolar part they reach as far as the inner angle of the mandible (Figures 28.14 and 28.17).

- Practitioner: take up a position beside the patient's head on the side opposite the dysfunction.

- Hand contact:
  - Place the thumb of your cranial hand on the coronoid process, with your index finger on the posterior border of the head and neck of the mandible.
  - With the index, middle, and ring fingers of your caudal hand span the inferior border of the body of the mandible and cover the inner angle of the mandible. Your fingers should be aligned toward the head of the mandible.

- Method: use both hands to apply divergent traction and establish a point of balance.

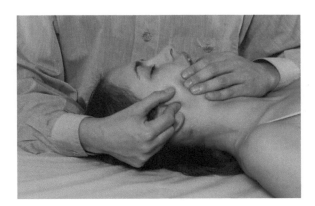

Figure 28.17
Treating dysfunctional tensile trajectories
running from the head/neck of the mandible.

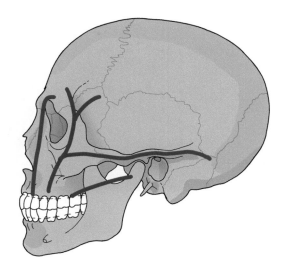

Figure 28.18
Viscerocranium with reinforcing buttresses.

Viscerocranium

The viscerocranium is characterized by its buttressed structure: the nasomaxillary (or canine) buttress transmits the forces from the alveoli of the canine teeth along the piriform aperture via the frontal process of the maxilla to the medial superior orbital rim.

The zygomaticomaxillary buttress distributes the forces from the alveoli of the molars to the zygomatic bone. From there the buttress divides into two: one part extends posteriorly to the inferior temporal line and anteriorly to the lateral part of the superior rim of the orbit. The second part extends along the temporozygomatic arch to the articular tubercle and the supramastoid crest.

The less robustly developed pterygomaxillary buttress transmits the pressure from the rear molars to the middle region of the cranial base.

Transverse horizontal buttresses are formed by the inferior and superior margins of the nasal cavity, the paranasal sinuses, and the orbits, with the superior orbital rim being the most pronounced (Figure 28.18).

Treating the nasomaxillary buttress (Figure 28.19)

- Practitioner: take up a position to one side of the patient's head.

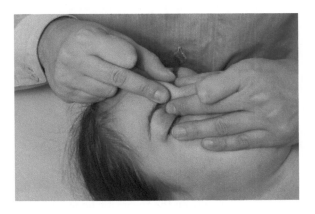

Figure 28.19
Treating the nasomaxillary buttress.

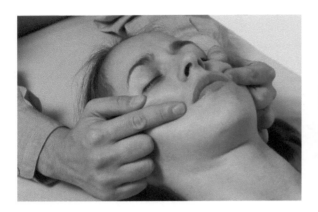

Figure 28.20
Treating the zygomaticomaxillary buttress.

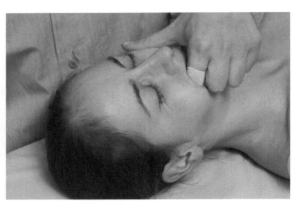

Figure 28.21
Treating the pterygomaxillary buttress.

- Hand contact:
  - Place the middle finger and thumb of your caudal hand bilaterally on the alveolar part of the canines over the frontal processes.
  - Position the middle finger and thumb of your cranial hand bilaterally on the medial superior margins of the orbits.

- Method: press your cranial and caudal hands toward each other and establish a point of balance.

Treating the zygomaticomaxillary buttress (Figure 28.20)

- Practitioner: take up a position at the patient's head.

- Hand contact: place your index fingers bilaterally on the molar alveoli of the maxillae, with your thumbs bilaterally on the zygomatic bone (the anterior convex surface and the orbital margin), and your thenar eminences on the inferior temporal line of the parietal bones.

- Method: press your index fingers and thumbs toward each other and establish a point of balance.

Treating the pterygomaxillary buttress (Figure 28.21)

- Practitioner: take up a position beside the patient's head on the side opposite the dysfunction.

- Hand contact: place the index finger of your caudal hand directly on the alveolar part of the patient's maxilla, with your finger pad on the lateral lamina of the pterygoid process.

- Method: press the pterygoid process and the posterior molar alveoli toward each other and establish a point of balance.

Treating the transverse horizontal buttresses (Figure 28.22)

- Take up a position at the head of the patient.
- With their tips touching, place your ring fingers bilaterally over the alveolar part of the maxillae.
- With their tips touching, place your middle fingers bilaterally over the inferior margins of the orbits.
- With their tips touching, place your index fingers bilaterally over the superior margins of the orbits.

- Method: using all fingers, direct compression medially and establish a point of balance.

Neurocranium

The structure of the neurocranium is reinforced by one median longitudinal pillar and by two transverse pillars that correspond to the boundaries of the cranial fossae (Figure 28.23).

The median longitudinal pillar runs from the sella turcica caudally down over the clivus, around the foramen magnum, and passes via the groove for the superior sagittal sinus to the frontal crest and crista galli. In this system the strong arched span of the falx cerebri acts as a type of reinforcing tension band.

The anterior transverse pillar forms the boundary between the anterior and the middle cranial fossae and has connections with the zygomaticomaxillary and pterygomaxillary buttresses of the viscerocranium.

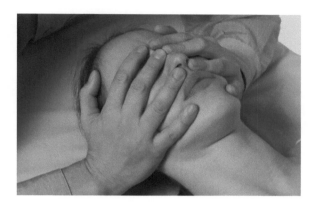

Figure 28.22

Treating the transverse horizontal buttresses.

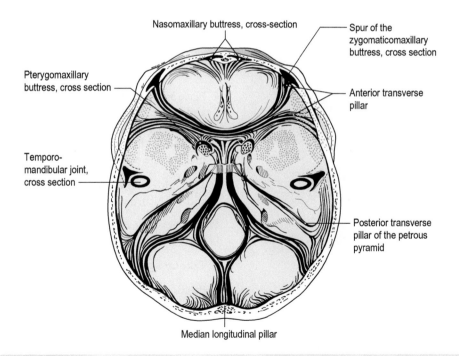

Figure 28.23

Cranial base with its system of reinforcing buttresses and pillars. The origins of the masticatory muscles are shown as areas of stippling.

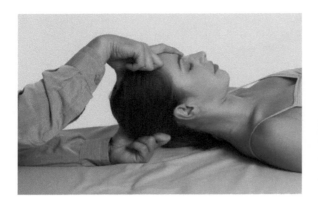

Figure 28.24
Treating the median longitudinal pillar.

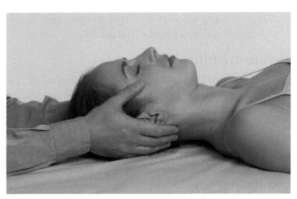

Figure 28.25
Treating the anterior transverse pillar.

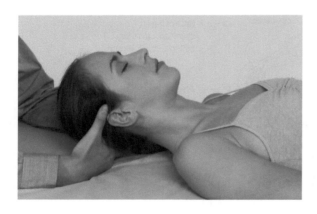

Figure 28.26
Treating the posterior transverse pillar.

The posterior transverse pillar is formed by the petrous portions of the temporal bones, which are connected to one another via the grooves for the transverse sinuses. The tentorium cerebelli roofs the posterior cranial fossa and acts as a reinforcing element in that region.

Treating the median longitudinal pillar (Figure 28.24)

- Take up a position at the head of the patient.

- Place one index finger at the nasion, with your thumb and index finger along the median line of the cranial vault. Position your other index finger as close as possible to the opisthion, with your thumb along the median line of the cranial vault.

- Method: compress the median longitudinal pillar and establish a point of balance.

Treating the anterior transverse pillar (Figure 28.25)

- Take up a position at the head of the patient.

- Position your thumbs bilaterally on and over the pterion and on the zygomatic bones.

- Method: compress the anterior transverse pillar and establish a point of balance.

Treating the posterior transverse pillar (Figure 28.26)

- Take up a position at the head of the patient.

- Position your index fingers one on top of the other along the path of the grooves for the transverse sinuses. Place your thumbs on and anterior to the supramastoid crest.

- Method: compress the posterior transverse pillar and establish a point of balance.

References

[1]Bergson H. Laughter: An Essay on the Meaning of the Comic. Rockville/Maryland: Arc Manor Publishers; 2008:20.

[2]Chauffour P, Prat E. Mechanical Link: Fundamental Principles, Theory and Practice Following an Osteopathic Approach. Berkeley/CA: North Atlantic Books; 2002:94f.

29

Developmental dynamic approaches to treating the head, dura, diaphragm, neck, and pharyngeal arches

Torsten Liem

God manifests Himself in matter, motion and mind. Study well His manifestations.

A.T. Still[1]

Developmental dynamic treatment of the cranial base

According to van den Heede, the region around the asterion is commonly a fulcrum/mechanical point of balance that has been exposed to compressive forces at birth. If light compression is exerted on the cranium, it reacts again by adopting its original rotation pattern and indicates this balance point where the original rotation "waits" for the reorganization of energy (Figure 29.1A,B).[2]

- Practitioner: take up a position to one side of the head of the patient.

- Hand position:
  - Place your cranial hand so that it spans the patient's cranial vault. (Alternative hand position: use your cranial hand to cradle the patient's occiput, with your thumb and little finger on or close to the asterion, your middle finger on the median line close to the opisthion, and your ring and index fingers in-between.)
  - Position your caudal hand gently round the patient's throat.

- Method:
  - Allow resonance with the developmental dynamic force vectors to arise by exerting

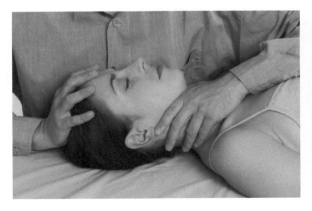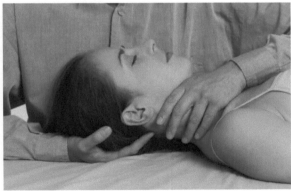

Figure 29.1
(A) Developmental dynamic treatment of the cranial base. (B) Alternative hand position.

gentle pressure from the brain caudally (using your hand on the cranial vault) and from the heart/diaphragm cranially (using your hand at the throat region). Permit the unfolding of the developmental dynamic relationship between brain and heart/diaphragm vis-à-vis the cranial base.

- A fulcrum will be established in the relational pattern between brain and heart/diaphragm.
- After the fulcrum has become established, you will sense a disengagement and flexion motion of the cranial base due to the caudal and cranial pressure on the cranial base, accompanied by a resolution of tension patterns in the cranial base.
- Support the resolution process by allowing it to unfold in a gentle compression field.

Viscerocranium (van den Heede's method I)

- Practitioner: take up a position at the head of the patient.

- Hand position (Figure 29.2A):
  - With one hand spanning the cerebellum, pons, and occipital lobe, cradle the patient's occiput.

- The heel of your palm should be at the lambda, your thumb and little finger at the asterion, and your middle finger as close as possible to the basion.
- With your other hand, span the front of the cerebrum. Position the heel of your palm at the bregma, your thumb and little finger as close as possible to the greater wings of the sphenoid, and your middle finger on the nasion and ophryon.

- Findings:
  - Has the brain been able to develop posteriorly?
  - Has a midline formed between the nasion and basion?
  - Where is the electrophysiological point?
  - Can you sense a cephalad dynamic of the occiput and the interparietal occiput, and a caudad dynamic of the frontal bone and frontoparietal region?

Technique

- Practitioner: take up a position to one side of the patient.

- Hand position (Figure 29.2B):

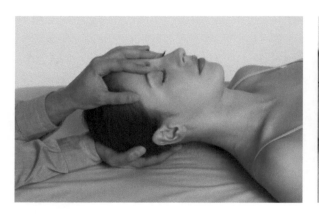

Figure 29.2A
Testing the viscerocranium.

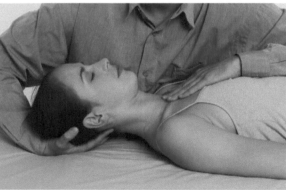

Figure 29.2B
Treating the viscerocranium (van den Heede's method I).

- With your cranial hand, span the cerebellum, pons, occipital lobe, and medulla oblongata. Position your hand under the patient's occiput, with your fingers directed caudally.
- Place the heel of your palm at the lambda, your thumb and little finger at the asterion, and your middle finger as close as possible to the basion.
- Place your caudal hand on the patient's thorax, with your fingers directed cranially. Position the palm of your hand on the sternum, with your fingertips touching the clavicles.

- Method:
  - Move the cranial base and the cardiac region toward each other and compress gently so as to produce a resonance with the embryonic growth dynamics.
  - While applying gentle compression, sense all the tissue dynamics but do not actively intervene.
  - As a rule you will sense the formation of a fulcrum between the two regions.
  - Once the fulcrum has established itself, you will sense the two structures moving apart (spontaneous disengagement).
  - Maintain gentle compression between the cranial base and the heart (or remain in resonance with the spontaneous disengagement of the two structures) and go with the decompression of the two structures – of the cardiac region in a caudal direction and of the cranial base in a cranial direction.

Viscerocranium (van den Heede's method II)

- Practitioner: take up a position to one side of the patient's head.

- Hand position (Figure 29.3):
  - Take hold of the patient's chin in the palm of your caudal hand. Position your index and middle fingers on the frontal processes of the maxilla, and your ring finger and thumb on the zygomatic bones.
  - Position the palm of your cranial hand over the bregma, with your middle finger on the median line. Place your index and ring fingers on the superciliary arches, and your thumb and little finger as close as possible to the greater wings of the sphenoid.

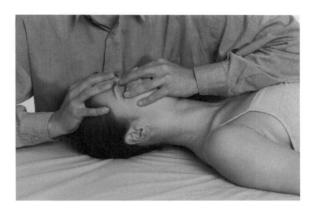

Figure 29.3
Treating the viscerocranium (van den Heede's method II).

- Method:
  - Gently move both hands toward each other and, in so doing, gently compress the ectomesenchymal facial tissue.
  - As a rule, you will sense the development of a fulcrum and, as this happens, there will be craniocaudal distraction or disengagement of the two structures. Encourage this process by maintaining gentle compression and going with the disengagement.

Growth dynamics of the dura (according to Blechschmidt)[3]

As early as week 4 of embryonic development, at the time of somite formation, the dura already ventrally encloses the neural tube relatively firmly and, as it develops, it displays far greater thickening ventrally than dorsally (Figure 29.4A–C).

The dura tightens ventrally to such an extreme degree that it becomes highly inelastic there, and thus functions as a restraining apparatus. As a result of its growth pull, it triggers the formation of the large sensory ganglia and nerve roots dorsally on the neural tube (Fig. 29.4C).

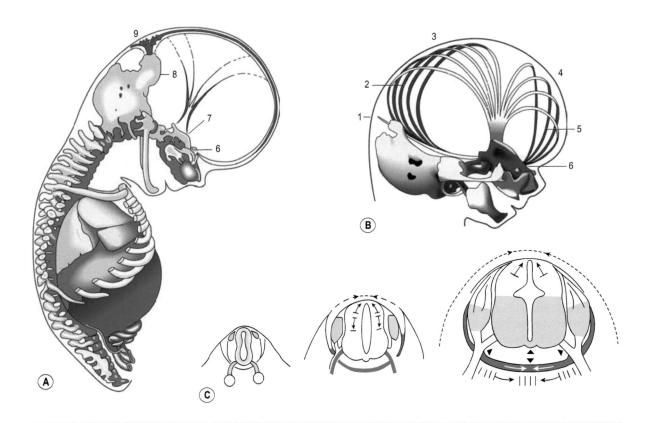

Figure 29.4A–C

Dural bands, 40 mm fetus, third month (Blechschmidt, Carnegie Coll. no. 10317); section series constructions of the desmal and chondral skeleton.[4] 1–5 Dural bands, main features of the desmal cranial skeleton, taut connective tissue in the large cerebral sulci: (1) tentorium cerebelli; (2) falx cerebri (posterior part); (3) parietal dural band; (4) frontal dural band; and (5) falx cerebri (anterior part). The arms of the dural bands in the basal region are tilted laterally. On the outer surface of these arms the mesenchyme has thickened and condensed, while in the interior it has become cartilaginous: (6) crista galli; (7) orbital ala; (8) otic ala of chondrocranium; and (9) confluence of sinuses.

By week 8 the brain has become enlarged eccentrically at the site of least resistance, particularly in the area opposite the basal region, known as the antibasal region, where the inelastic dura has not yet developed.

An inelastic and strong dura has developed only in the basal region (Fig. 29.4A,B). The basal dura is flattened due to the increasing growth of the brain. As a result, the mesenchyme attached to the basal aspect of the dura becomes condensed. This constitutes a contusion field for the pre-cartilaginous cranial base. Simultaneously, the tightened basal dura exercises a certain restraining function vis-à-vis the brain.

As a result of the continuing eccentric growth of the brain, growth resistances also gradually increase in the antibasal and laterodorsal walls of the cranial cavity to such an extent that the brain regions fold against each other.

The resulting fissures contain the taut structures known as the falx cerebri and the tentorium cerebelli. During the course of embryonic cerebral growth, the falx cerebri and the tentorium cerebelli are formed as mesenchymal tissue is pressed flat between the two cerebral hemispheres and between the cerebrum and the cerebellum.

The dura finally becomes consolidated between the varyingly bulging parts of the brain to form the dural band system (Fig. 29.4A).

Thereafter, surface growth of the brain is possible only in the windows between the dural bands. Spaces in the antibasal regions between the dural bands become fontanelles; in other words, the anlagen of the fontanelles already become apparent before the osseous tissue of the cranium starts to form (Fig. 29.4A,B). Figure 29.5 illustrates the relations of the dural band system to the cranial base in the neonatal cranium.

Counter-pull of the dura against the descent of the viscera (see also Fig. 29.4)

- Development of facial elongation: the embryonic heart follows the diaphragm in a descending movement whereas the growth process of the brain is characterized by an increasing ascent. During the ascending growth movement of the brain, the dura in the upper part of the head, together with the falx, moves away from the descending ligament system of the cervical viscera. As a result, the facial connective tissue between the falx and the hyoid tightens to form a muzzle-like structure, and the elongated face is finally formed.

- Dura acts to hold the crista galli in position: due to the restraining function of the falx cerebri and due to the antibasal dura, the crista galli remains anchored to the squamous mesenchyme of the cranial base during the uneven embryonic growth of the cerebral hemispheres.

- Dynamics in the nasal capsule: by contrast – via the continuity between the stroma of the cheeks and the sturdy conduction pathways of the cervical visceral structures – the connective tissue floor of the nasal capsule descends with the laryngopharyngeal tract. The dura exerts a counter-pull against this descending movement.

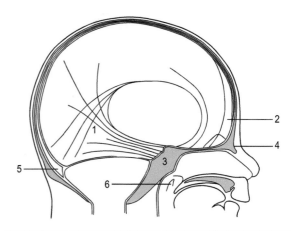

Figure 29.5
Neonatal cranium; schematic diagram illustrating the restraining bands at the cranial base.[4] (1) Tentorium cerebelli; (2) falx cerebri; (3) ossification in the cartilaginous cranial base (in this case, the region of origin of the sphenoidal sinus); (4) bony tissue in the region of origin of the frontal sinus; (5) confluence of the sinuses; and (6) auditory tube (entrance to the pharyngeal sinus pre-developed as the first pharyngeal recess). Due to the dural bands, the desmal skeleton of the cranial vault now contains several defined fields in which individual ossification centers are differentiating as flat "connective tissue bones." In the desmal skeleton of the cranial base the cartilaginous (chondral) part of the head also contains several ossification centers. The traction systems of the desmocranium in the facial region are not yet sufficiently powerful for paranasal sinuses to develop in response to their biomechanical growth pull.

- Development of the olfactory nerve fibers as tension structures: due to the separation of the upper face and the floor of the mouth, the olfactory nerve fibers develop as tension structures. These act as a restraining structure for the nasal capsule that has tightened like a muzzle as a result of the growth of the epithelial nasal meatus.

Dynamic developmental approach to the falx and tentorium

Step 1

- Practitioner: take up a position to one side of the patient's head.

- Hand position:
  - Use your caudal hand to span the cranial vault, with your palm over one side and your fingers over the other side of the cranial vault.
  - Your cranial hand should be beneath the inion, spanning the cerebellar region.

- Method:
  - Begin at the cranial vault and cerebrum by exerting gentle medial compression on the falx cerebri.
  - In this process your hand on the cranial vault projects itself to the median line in the region of the falx cerebri and establishes a resonance with the condensation of the mesenchyme along the course of the falx.
  - Then exert gentle compression between your cranial and caudal hands, so that the cerebrum and cerebellum are moved gently toward each other. Direct attention here to the region of the tentorium cerebelli. Establish a resonance with the condensation of the mesenchyme along the course of the tentorium

Step 2

- Practitioner: take up a position to one side of the patient's head.

- Hand position:
  - Place the palm and fingers of your cranial hand over the patient's cranial vault, with your middle finger on the median line.
  - The pad of your middle finger should be directly above the nasion, approximately in the region of the crista galli.
  - Position your caudal hand over the patient's face, with your middle finger directly beneath the nasion.

- Method: apply gentle compression until you sense a reaction in the form of ascending tension in the falx.

Step 3

- Practitioner: take up a position at the head of the patient.

- Hand position:
  - Position one hand on the cranial vault with your wrist immediately above the inion, and your middle finger along the course of the median line. Use this hand to take up contact with the falx cerebri.
  - Position the thumb and middle finger of your other hand along the line of the transverse sinus and take up contact with the tentorium cerebelli.

- Method: gently establish a balance of tension between the falx and tentorium.

Anterior dural band (according to James Jealous)

The anterior dural band runs along the posterior margin of the lesser wings and along the posterior part of the coronal suture as far as the greater wings of the sphenoid. (The term "anterior dural band" is generally used only during the early phase of embryonic development.)

Its function is unclear. It has been postulated that, as a fluid membrane structure, it is intended to exert an integrating function on the anterior cranial structures and may play a part, for example, in dysfunctions at the sphenosquamous pivot point and the pterion.

Anterior dural band: mandibular ramus

- Practitioner: take up a position at the head of the patient.

- Hand position:
  - Span the patient's coronal suture with the thumb and index finger of your cranial hand.
  - Span the mandible with your caudal hand.

- Method:
  - Establish resonance with the fluid and membranous matrix of the mandible.
  - Direct your attention to the inter-relationship between the anterior dural band and the mandible.

- Sense any possible forces of a rotational, translational, compressive, and decompressive character that may be acting in an anterior, posterior, superior, and inferior direction.
- Bring these into balance in a dynamic fulcrum between the anterior dural band and the membranous ring of the mandible.
- This will encourage the flow of potency in these regions.
- The resolution of abnormal tensions is generally associated with expansion of the structures involved.

Anterior dural band: maxillary arch

- Practitioner: take up a position to one side of the patient's head. In general, stand in such a way that your fingers are as relaxed as possible.

- Hand position:
  - Span the coronal suture with the thumb and index finger of your cranial hand.
  - Position the middle and index fingers of your caudal hand inside the patient's mouth on the palatine process of the maxilla.
  - If there is insufficient space on the palate, your middle and index fingers may also be positioned on the superior dental arches.

- Method: use the technique described above for the ramus of the mandible.

Anterior dural band: tentorium cerebelli

- Practitioner: take up a position slightly off center at the head of the patient.

- Hand position:
  - Span the coronal suture with the thumb and index finger of one hand.
  - Position your other hand on the inion, at the level of the transverse sinus and corresponding to the posterior attachment surface of the tentorium cerebelli.

- Method:
  - Use the technique described above for the ramus of the mandible.

- Important: avoid all pressure on the occipitomastoid suture.

Anterior dural band: sphenoid bone

- Indication: dysfunction at the sphenosquamous pivot point and the pterion.

- Practitioner: take up a position to one side of the patient's head.

- Hand position:
  - Span the coronal suture with the thumb and index finger of your cranial hand.
  - With the index and middle fingers of your caudal hand, span the greater wings of the sphenoid.

- Method: use the technique described above for the ramus of the mandible.

Growth dynamics of the descent of the diaphragm and viscera[5]

The growth of the embryonic liver on the underside of the diaphragm is involved as an initiating biodynamic factor in the descent of the viscera. This in turn is possible only as a result of the earlier development of the brain and heart:

- The intense growth of the brain is necessarily accompanied by intense vascularization.

- This causes the heart to enlarge, which in turn encourages blood flow to the heart to increase.

- The result is the growth of the liver as the collecting point for venous blood.

The stroma between the heart and the liver becomes compressed into a flat plate of tissue. As a result of these compressive growth forces the diaphragm is so intensely thinned and devoid of blood that the anlage of the central tendon of the diaphragm is already apparent at the beginning of the second month and only the more peripheral parts of the diaphragm dilate to form muscle fiber bundles.

The enlargement of the liver exerts a pull toward the umbilical area (caudally and ventrally), causing the dome of the diaphragm anlage to flatten. In this way the diaphragm anlage gives up its original position behind the heart and detaches from the cervical portion of the embryonic vertebral column, from the thoracic portion of the vertebral column and the adjoining ribs. Finally, the diaphragm remains in contact with the developing skeleton only in the region of the lumbar vertebral column and the inferior thoracic aperture.

These growth dynamics provide space for the expanding pleural sacs and the development of the lungs. The pericardium and heart move caudally, following the descent of the diaphragm. (As an extension of this process, the descent of the heart continues into old age.)

All of the cervical viscera in turn move caudally with the pericardium and heart. The supra- and infra-hyoid structures in the neck region are a particularly clear reflection of the polar developmental gestures of the ascending brain and descending viscera.

The development of the pituitary and thyroid glands is a further expression of this polar growth dynamic.

Treating the diaphragm: dynamic developmental approach (Figure 29.6)

- Practitioner: take up a position at the patient's right side at the level of the diaphragm.

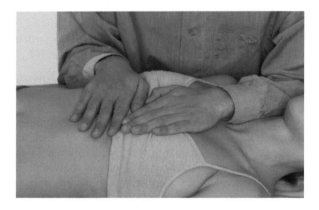

Figure 29.6
Developmental dynamic approach to treating the diaphragm.

- Hand position:
  - With your fingers pointing caudally, position your cranial hand slightly obliquely, from right cranial to left caudal, to cover the patient's heart and pericardium.
  - Rest your wrist cranially on the superior margin of the third chondrocostal joint and extending slightly into the second intercostal space on the left side.
  - Position your little finger and ring finger obliquely from the first to third intercostal space at the left border of the sternum to about the fifth intercostal space medial to the mammillary line (apex of the heart).
  - Place your thumb at the right border of the sternum.
  - Position your fingers approximately at the upper edge of the sixth rib on the left side.
  - Place your caudal hand over the patient's liver.
  - Position the radial edge of your hand approximately over the fifth intercostal space on the right side and the sixth intercostal space on the left side.
  - Locate the ulnar edge of your hand approximately over the costal arch.

- Method:
  - Palpate the mobility of the diaphragm.
  - Allow resonance to become established with the developmental dynamic force vectors by exerting gentle compression on the heart and liver, and permit the relationship to the diaphragm to unfold.
  - In addition, you may exert gentle pressure from the heart caudally and from the liver cranially.
  - Sense the inhalation and exhalation phases within the compression field.
  - A fulcrum will establish itself in the relational pattern between liver, heart, and diaphragm.
  - After the fulcrum has become established, you will not infrequently sense a descent of the liver and diaphragm, associated with resolution of tension patterns.
  - Encourage the resolution process by allowing it to unfold in a gentle compression field.

Neck area: dynamic developmental approach (Figure 29.7)

- Practitioner: take up a position to one side of the patient's head.

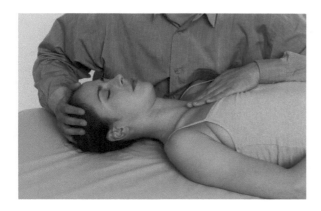

Figure 29.7
Developmental dynamic approach to treating the neck area.

- Hand position:
  - Span the cranial vault with your cranial hand. (Alternative hand position: use your cranial hand to cradle the patient's occiput with your thumb and little finger on or close to the asterion, your middle finger on the median line close to opisthion, and your ring and index fingers in-between.)
  - With your fingers pointing cranially, place your caudal hand over the cardiac region slightly obliquely, from left caudal to right cranial.
  - Rest your wrist on the upper edge of the sixth rib on the left side.
  - Place your little finger at the right border of the sternum.
  - Position your thumb obliquely from about the fifth intercostal space medial to the mammillary line (apex of the heart) to the level of the first to third intercostal space at the left border of the sternum.
  - Place your fingers cranially on the superior margin of the third chondrocostal joint on the right side and extending slightly into the second intercostal space on the left side.
  - Your caudal arm is an extension of the longitudinal axis of the patient's body.

- Method:
  - Allow resonance to become established with the developmental dynamic force vectors by exerting gentle pressure from the brain caudally (using your hand on the cranial vault) and from the heart/diaphragm cranially, and permit the developmental dynamic relationship between the two to unfold.
  - A fulcrum will establish itself in the relational pattern between the brain and the heart/diaphragm.
  - After the fulcrum has become established, you will not infrequently sense an ascent of the brain and a descent of the heart, liver, and diaphragm, with a resolution of tension patterns in the cervical viscera.
  - Encourage the resolution process by allowing it to unfold in a gentle compression field.

Treatment of the structures deriving from the pharyngeal arches and pharyngeal recesses

First pharyngeal arch (Figure 29.8)

- Practitioner: take up a position at the head of the patient.

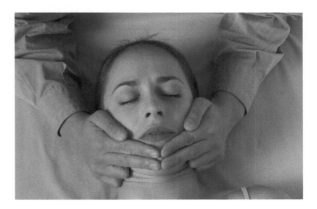

Figure 29.8
Treating the first pharyngeal arch.

- Hand position:
  - The wrists of both your hands are touching the tragus and the external auditory meatus.
  - Span the patient's mandible on both sides with your index and middle fingers.

- Method:
  - By flexion of the patient's head exert gentle compression – taking account of the developmental dynamic force vectors – in the region of the structures derived from the first pharyngeal arch and pharyngeal recess.
  - At the same time use your hands on the tragus and mandible to exert gentle compression against head flexion.
  - Establish a PBT.
  - Sense how an inherent disengagement spreads increasingly in the region of the first pharyngeal arch. This is generally oriented in line with the embryological growth dynamics.
  - Sense the inhalation and exhalation phases.

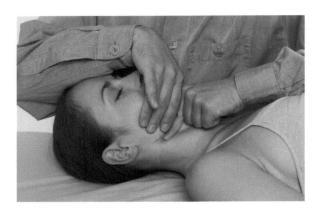

Figure 29.9
Treating the second and third pharyngeal arches.

Second and third pharyngeal arches (Figure 29.9)

- Practitioner: take up a position to one side of the patient's head.

- Hand position:
  - Using the index, middle, and ring fingers and the thumb of your cranial hand, span the patient's mandible on both sides.
  - Span the hyoid bone with the thumb and index finger of your caudal hand.

- Method:
  - By flexion of the patient's head exert gentle compression – taking account of the developmental dynamic force vectors – in the region of the hyoid bone (second and third pharyngeal arches).
  - At the same time use your hand spanning the hyoid to exert gentle compression against head flexion.
  - In addition, you may treat the relationship with the first pharyngeal arch by producing gentle compression between the mandible and the hyoid.
  - Establish a PBT.

- Sense how an inherent disengagement spreads increasingly in the region of the pharyngeal arches. This is generally oriented in line with the embryological growth dynamics.
- Sense the inhalation and exhalation phases.

References

[1]Still AT. Autobiography of Andrew T. Still. Published by the author. Kirksville, Mo.; 1908:188.

[2]Van den Heede P. Der natürliche Geburtsvorgang. Osteopath. Med. 2001;4:10–12.

[3]Blechschmidt E. Humanembryologie, Prinzipien und Grundbegriffe. Stuttgart: Hippokrates; 1974; 66f.

[4]Blechschmidt E. Die pränatalen Organsysteme des Menschen. Stuttgart: Hippokrates; 1973; 112, 120.

[5]Blechschmidt E, Gasser RF. Biokinetics and Biodynamics of Human Differentiation: Principles and Applications. Springfield, Illinois: Charles C. Thomas; 1978:137–142.

30

Development of the senses: a biodynamic perspective

Brian Freeman

Introduction

The material for this chapter is derived mainly from the embryological studies of Erich Blechschmidt (1904–1992), including his 1948 monograph[1] and an English edition of one of his last books.[2] Following some general remarks, the ontogeny of tissues associated with the five classic senses will be described in the following order: skin, eye, nose, ear, and tongue. This reason for treating skin first is simply that ectoderm and the associated sense of touch provides an opportunity to introduce some biodynamic principles concerning the growth of dendrites (sensory nerves); these principles apply to all sensory organs. Naturally the above order is arbitrary because it is impossible to specify a temporal sequence for the development of different senses. As discussed below, the origin of all organs can be traced sequentially back to fertilization, their growth depends on metabolic interactions with other growing parts, and different senses "mature" at different rates and stages. This also means that no particular sense can be considered to be more important or critical for life than another.

Design and function

First we must dispense with the notion that a sensory organ is something that is designed for a particular function. The claim that the eye is designed for seeing is teleological and therefore outside the realm of scientific investigation: there is simply no way to prove or disprove such a claim using rational methods. In embryology and anatomy, teleological thinking (i.e., the notion that outcomes guide development) leads to many paradoxes. One example is Helmholtz's remark to the effect that one could hardly find a more poorly designed optical instrument than the human eye. Another "design" paradox, described below, concerns the structure of the ear and the threshold for human hearing. In general, one cannot comprehend the development, the anatomy, or the function, of any sense organ at all by making a

claim about why the organ developed, based on how the organ happens to be used once it has developed.[a]

The reality of sensory development is more like this: a tiny structure, epithelial fold, thickening, or other feature (let us call it organ "X" to avoid any preconceptions) arises gradually in some region of the human embryo. As it grows, this dynamic organ comes into metabolic relationship with other, usually nearby, parts of the embryo. This mutual interaction has biodynamic components that are associated with vectors of biomechanical forces having magnitudes and directions. These are forces generated by living structures, so they are neither purely mechanical nor purely chemical; they lead, in turn, to new structures arising as a reaction or counter-balance. The sequence of alternating developmental actions and reactions starting from "X" results in an ensemble of organs known, say, as an eye with its surrounding components such as nerves, vessels, eyelids, glands, muscles, bones of the orbit, fat, etc. – the so-called adnexa of the orbit.

During normal development by definition, at all stages, all components of the ensemble "X" must be totally integrated and functioning harmoniously; the slightest discord would produce an abnormal eye. Naturally the embryo has no prior knowledge of how this ensemble will be used after birth. The only accurate claim is that, as a result of its development, this coordinated group of cells and tissues has some parts more-or-less transparent, has some parts movable at will, has parts that allow the external world to be imaged, parts with much black pigment (melanin) that absorb stray light, parts that are excited by electromagnetic radiation of certain wavelengths, and so on.

In other words, eyes do not develop in order to see. Rather, sight is one of the consequences of the

---

[a]Teleological ideas still pervade contemporary developmental biology and the discipline called "functional" anatomy.

development of an eye; the ability to cry is another, winking at friends yet another – some frogs even sink their eyes into the oral region to help in swallowing food! Nothing in the ensemble of structures associated with the act of seeing should be dismissed as being of "secondary" importance compared to a presumed "primary" role of seeing, as implied by the term adnexa. For example, eyes lacking eyelids or tear glands would soon become useless because of ulcerating corneas; in stationary eyes, without eye-muscles, the stabilized images formed on the retina would fade quickly from consciousness.

The misconception that a sense is associated with a "system"

The human body arises by subdivision of a single entity in a normal reproductive environment; the entity is the fertilized ovum or conceptus. The human being is never an ensemble of separate, or separable, cells and organs that are somehow "integrated" to work as a whole. Similarly we are never a concatenation of "systems" at any stage of our life. Systems, say sensory systems, do not exist as delimited or functional entities in the human body: this concept is a trite heuristic abstraction that has caused conflict and harm in our attempts to understand the body. Invariably it is impossible to specify where one "system" ends and the next one starts. One should therefore dispense with the notion that the body consists of anatomical–physiological systems; to retain such terminology clouds our thinking.

Outside–inside differentiation

The capacity to sense starts with fertilization. The first molecular signals that arise from the boundary (periphery) of the conceptus and alter the activity of a more central structure (nucleus) can be interpreted as afferent or sensory signals. The ovum is markedly responsive to mechanical, thermal, and chemical stimuli; it may also react to electromagnetic radiation and gravitational fields. This sensitivity, present from the start, continues and becomes more refined as the conceptus develops. The ability to sense is therefore a consequence of differentiation that starts on the outside and continues to the inside – all sensation is a recognition of something external to the body, possibly even a sense of time. Mature cells that convey information to the brain or spinal cord are described as sensory neurons and their signaling from periphery to center,

as afferent. The maturation and harmony of all human motor actions (i.e., the products of efferent signals) depends on the development of afferent organs.

Temporal sequence

It will be seen that the organs concerned with the five traditional senses do not develop independently of each other. For example, the development of the olfactory apparatus is predisposed by the location and form of two growing eyes – there could not be two nostrils and two regions of olfactory epithelium unless there were two eyes that had started their development slightly earlier than the nose. Similarly the two internal ears could not develop unless they were preceded by a single brain groove growing and flexing in a longitudinal arc around an embryonic heart. And the sensation of touch arises initially at certain parts of the skin that become relatively thicker because they are not stretched thin by the growing brain, heart, and liver.

The organs associated with each sense develop in particular positions (topogenesis) according to different local dynamics; thus the organs of sensation acquire unique forms (morphogenesis) and unique internal structures (tectogenesis). The head end of the embryo and the cranial nerves develop faster than other regions with spinal nerves; the head therefore is linked with the "special" senses of sight, hearing–balance, smell, and taste.

Since the human body is bounded topologically by a single surface, one must include signals from anywhere on this boundary as belonging to the gamut of human senses, even if we remain initially less conscious of some of them. Thus we develop sensory pathways from the gastrointestinal tract with its associated glandular organs (liver, pancreas, etc.), whose origin is driven initially by the growth dynamics of the single topological boundary of the body. The sensations arising in the viscera are mainly from chemical and mechanical stimuli. The same holds true for all organs and surfaces that arise within the inner tissue of the embryo, such as the pericardium, pleura, peritoneum, synovial membranes of joints, bursae, tendon sheaths, and their adjacent tissues. In this respect, there is little value in making the artificial distinction between visceral and somatic sensations. Similarly, there is nothing unique about interactions between the so-called viscera and the rest of the body: somatovisceral and viscerosomatic reflexes are essentially similar to any other kind of reflex with afferent and efferent components.

All senses initially involve a transfer of chemical information and so could be described as chemoreceptive. Later, on account of structural specializations in the organs, the chemical transfers become stimulated by different types of energy, e.g., mechanical or electromagnetic vibrations.

Skin senses

Most spinal and cranial nerves are present by the time the human embryo is 28 days old[b] and about 4.2 mm long,[c] described as Carnegie Stage[d] 13 (Figure 30.1).[3] These nerves develop according to the general rule that for a particular differentiation to take place, there must exist not only a spatial opportunity but also a direct biodynamic cause for that differentiation.

Blechschmidt's investigations of young human embryos show that the spinal sensory nerves appear regularly for the first time after the dorsal branches of the paired aortae (dorsal aortic rami) have already reached the flanks of the neural tube. Although they are just like capillaries, these dorsal branches of the aortae function as restraining structures. They hold on to the growing neural tube just as though they were cords under tension, so that the embryo flexes forward as it grows. Dorsal tributaries of the cardinal veins accompanying the arterial rami also act as anchoring structures. All embryonic vessels, tiny and capillary-like as they are, behave as gentle reins that tether the territories they supply or drain.[1,2]

Sensory ganglia of the spinal cord

The neural tube (anlage of the spinal cord and brain) of the embryo is enlarging by continual cell division and growth. When transverse sections from a series of growing embryos are examined at the same scale, the neural tube is found to be moving in a dorsal direction relative to the notochord (Figure 30.2B). Conversely, parts of the lateral walls of the neural tube remain attached metabolically to the ends of the segmental dorsal rami

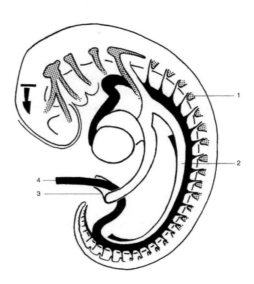

Figure 30.1

Cranial and spinal nerves of 4.2 mm long human embryo (Carnegie Stage 13), lateral view. Veins white, arteries black, and nerves stippled. Single arrow: growth flexion of the brain. Converging half-headed arrows: restraining function of large ventral blood vessels (aortae, inferior cardinal veins). 1, spinal (sensory) ganglion; 2, inferior cardinal vein; 3, umbilical vein; 4, umbilical artery.

of the aorta (Figure 30.1). As these vessels are tense and exchange nutrients at their tips, clusters of nerve cells tend to remain close to this nutrient supply; these cells become drawn out of the dorsolateral margins of the neural tube as the latter glides dorsally past the vessels. The cells that are dragged from the neural tube in this way are known collectively as neural crest. Many neural crest cells are the anlagen of spinal (sensory) ganglia, which arise sequentially (metamerically) along the back of the embryo (stipple, Figure 30.1). The concept that neural crest cells "migrate" of their own accord from the neural tube is incorrect; it ignores the anchoring role of the blood vessels and the dorsal growth and displacement of the remainder of the neural tube.

[b]Ovulational age, or theoretical age since fertilization, is estimated by subtracting 14 days from the end of the last menstrual period. The time from the end of the last menstrual period is known as the gestational age (of a conceptus, an embryo, or a fetus).

[c]Crown–rump (CR) length, usually measured in millimeters using calipers with the embryo immersed in fluid.

[d]International system for specifying the stage of development of conceptuses and embryos based on their anatomy; not applicable to the fetal period of development from 3rd lunar month onwards.[3]

Since cells are leaving the dorsal parts of the neural tube from the earliest stages onwards, cross sections of the spinal cord at later stages will obviously exhibit large ventral horns and smaller dorsal horns (Figure 30.2B). The number of spinal ganglia and sensory nerves is therefore determined by the number of vascular "guy-ropes" (connections) that anchor the sides of the neural tube (Figure 30.1).

Innervation

In young embryos, the most striking innervation by the developing nerves is twofold: (i) thickening epidermis and (ii) muscles arising in dilation fields. Both the thickening epidermis and the developing musculature are regions with special demands for growth. Thickened epidermis arises from the ectoderm of the young embryo, initially only in a zone that extends across the face and downwards over both flanks of the body wall to the lower end of the trunk, then across the groin region. This zone, where the skin is restricted in surface growth and so thickens, has the form of a folded ring or annulus – the ectodermal ring[4] (Figures 30.2A and 30.3); the ring is composed of tall, wedge-shaped cells.[e] Conversely, the skin of the embryo's back (covering the neural tube) and on the embryo's belly (covering the heart–liver mass) is scarcely restricted in its surface growth and so becomes thinner in these regions. The topology of the ectodermal ring determines the first sensory innervation in the human embryo, i.e., initially only the ring is innervated. This innervation, which is a consequence of the formation of dendrites of sensory ganglion cells, already designates those skin regions that later retain an especially rich sensory nerve supply. The branching of the spinal nerves to the back and to the ventral body wall (ramus dorsalis, ramus ventralis) occurs only as a secondary event following the innervation of the ectodermal ring.

Everywhere that the embryo has a greater degree of longitudinal curvature (that is, in the neck region and in the vicinity of the limb anlagen), the nerves that arise at successive distances from each other (metamerically) must converge as they lengthen. In all regions of convergence, the nerves merge together at a very early stage to form a network, a so-called plexus (cervical, brachial, and lumbosacral plexus; Figure 30.4). Conversely, in the thoracic region where the embryo's curvature is less, the convergence of the nerves is less and no significant plexus formation can arise.

A brief digression is now required to describe the second tissue that becomes innervated in the embryo, namely the musculature with its efferent or motor nerves. Unlike the ganglion cells for sensory innervation, the cell bodies for motor innervation develop within the densely packed ventral region of the neural tube or young spinal cord (Figure 30.2). Neurites of motor neurons grow out of the neural tube into the first muscle fields, which are initially found immediately adjacent to the ventrolateral aspect of the neural tube.[5] The growth-elongation of a somite is a dilation field with a material demand for nutrients.[2] The cytoplasm of every elongating muscle cell is a suction zone that induces an influx from any local "supplier," i.e., substances flow from the terminals of neurites into the growing muscle cells that are only one to two cell diameters away from the surface of the neural tube. Thus the nerve endings in muscle fibers become motor nerves only on account of their position and prior growth functions, not because these nerves are useful for initiating movement.

Similarly, neurites of sensory neurons grow in the opposite direction to their dendrites, namely from the spinal ganglia into the neural tube (Figure 30.2B); these ganglion cells are already connected to the skin of the ectodermal ring by means of their dendrites.[f] The membranes of neurites and dendrites, and especially their growing tips, are permeable to molecules, thereby enabling an intracellular and intercellular conduction of chemicals. One can anticipate that in a growing spinal cord, there is already the substrate for a reflex arc that is closed by metabolic movements between sensory and motor neurons (Figure 30.2A). In all probability, the developing brain and spinal cord already constitute a powerful reflex linkage, for which the periphery has sensory, i.e., regulatory, significance. Experiments on animal embryos might not be able to prove this interpretation conclusively; they do however support it.

Neural pathways

Blechschmidt's studies established several general propositions, one of which is that organs differentiate

---

[e]Columnar cells do not exist in the human body – all surfaces have varying curvature, so tall epithelial cells must possess a converging or diverging wedge shape.

[f]The term "axon" has been avoided because its use obscures the basic developmental and functional difference between dendrites (afferent) and neurites (efferent).

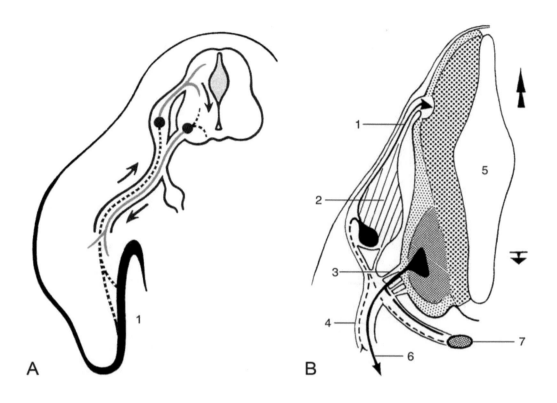

Figure 30.2
(A) Schema of spinal connections and reflex arc in ca. 8 mm embryo, transverse section, dorsal to top of figure. Afferent cell processes (dendrites), dashed black; efferent cell processes (neurites), grey. Arrows signify directions of 'information' (metabolic) transfer. Black circles at changeover from black dashes to grey represent intracellular transfer of information at cell bodies. Note the especially thick epithelium of the ectodermal ring in axilla and on flexor surface of upper limb fold (1). Cerebrospinal fluid in lumen of spinal cord, grey. (B) Nerve cells in spinal cord of 8 mm embryo, same orientation as A. Diverging arrows on right represent growth expansion of spinal cord, more in the dorsal direction than ventrally where greater resistance is encountered. Simple arrows at 1 and 6: growth directions of neurites (sensory and motor, respectively) as part of a reflex arc. Dashed lines: growth directions of dendrites from soma of spinal ganglion cell. 1, dorsal root fiber; 2, spinal ganglion; 3, ventral rootlet; 4, spinal (mixed) nerve; 5, spinal canal; 6, motor neurite; 7, sympathetic trunk.

wherever there exist both a spatial opportunity and a metabolic occasion, that is, in a biodynamic field. In the case of nerves, this does not mean that developmental dynamics alone is sufficient to provide the nerves with a pathway, but rather, that the path-finding of nerves has developmentally dynamic properties. The older concept that nerves "find" their innervation territories of their own accord, by some sort of blueprint or map, is incorrect because it ignores the role of developmental dynamics. In tissue culture experiments, it has never been possible to obtain a normal branching pattern of nerves. The pathway for nerve fibers is normally

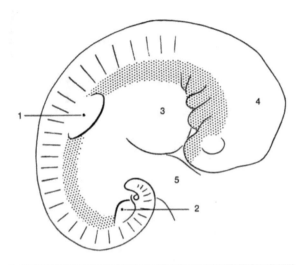

Figure 30.3

Human embryo, 4.2 mm long, age 28 days (Carnegie Stage 13). Ectodermal ring (thickened skin of lateral body wall) stippled. 1, anlage of upper limb; 2, anlage of lower limb; 3, heart bulge; 4, hindbrain region; 5, umbilical cord.

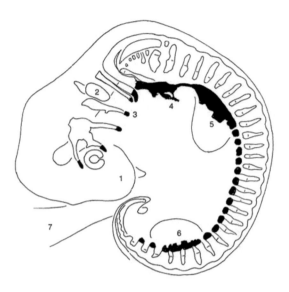

Figure 30.4

Lateral view of 6.3 mm human embryo (Carnegie Stage 14) showing early nerve plexus formation. Black: first sites of contact between (sensory) dendrites and overlying skin, which is the thickened epithelium of the ectodermal ring (stippled in Fig. 30.3). 1, forebrain; 2, otic vesicle with its dorsomedial endolymphatic sac; 3, complex of facial and vestibulocochlear nerves; 4, cervical plexus; 5, brachial plexus; 6, lumbar plexus; 7, umbilical cord.

prescribed by the organs to-be-innervated and is therefore laid down from the periphery, i.e., from without. It can be assumed that submicroscopic material (i.e., molecular) movements are decisive for this process. Stated in another way, ordered metabolic movements work in a manner that determines the form of the incipient innervation pattern.

The following analogy elucidates the argument. The course of a river cannot be explained on the basis of the development of its shipping, nor by a knowledge of its sources, its tributaries, or the specific locations of the harbors at its mouth. It is only the totality of topographical, geographical, and environmental factors that determine the course of a river. Similarly, the directions of growth flows (fluxes) within nerves cannot be explained on the basis of their subsequent use or significance for human behavior patterns.

As is true for all organs including peripheral sensory nerves, their 'design' is a consequence of local differences in their location and growth. The metabolic movements and metabolism in the vicinity of growing dendrites is certainly quite different from that of grow-

ing neurites, otherwise they would not appear so different by light and electron microscopy.[6] As a sign of their structural dissimilarity, one finds that dendrites and neurites grow into different regions of innervation. One therefore assumes that these regions contain metabolic fields with correspondingly different metabolic movements. As stated above, peripheral dendrites invariably arise in connection with an epithelium that has thickened due to a restriction in its surface growth. On the other hand, motor neurites arise in connection with fields of embryonic muscle cells that become slender as they are extended. It cannot be claimed, say, that skin acquires its dendritic (nerve) supply because such a supply is useful for the transfer of sensory information. Rather, skin becomes innervated in the embryo because there is both the spatial opportunity and the dynamic occasion for its innervation.

The significance of this is seen particularly well in the head region of a young embryo (Carnegie Stage 11; Figure 30.5). With growth flexion of the head, the body wall (ectoderm plus inner tissue) in the vicinity of the pharyngeal flexion folds[g] is restricted in surface growth and so thickens to become the facial part of the ectodermal ring. The tall wedge-shaped cells covering the flexion folds press laterally against one another and so probably release some of their fluid contents. A portion of these fluids, which passes into the inner tissue beneath the ectodermal ring, contains substances (probably polar) that can be taken up by the growing dendrites. Thus, as with sensory nerves of the trunk described above, there must already exist material connections (in the sense of pathways) between the innervation area of the growing face and the tips of the dendrites, well before the dendrites themselves have reached the actual base of the epithelium. The substances released by the ectoderm (catabolites) are used for synthesis (anabolism); by means of this absorption of substances, the dendrites elongate by apical appositional growth.

According to this interpretation, the lips, palms of hands, soles of feet, digital pads, and external genitalia are well supplied with sensory nerves, not because these cutaneous regions must subsequently acquire specially differentiated capacities for touch, but because during embryonic development, the nerve endings are responding to special growth stimuli on the part of a thickened epithelium.

In summary, there is much evidence for (and none against) the views that: (i) a developing dendrite sucks itself towards its innervation territory by material absorption and elongation of its apical region (growth cone), and (ii) growing muscle fibers on their part exert suction forces and so draw neurites into the muscle field. Morphological studies indicate that the growth cones of young (sensory) dendrites are initially large, pale-staining, metabolic workhouses whereas the tips of mature dendrites are especially delicate and pointed.[6] Conversely for the efferent neurites – these have delicate

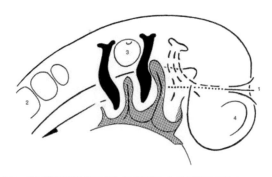

Figure 30.5

First sensory nerves in head region of 2.57 mm long human embryo (Carnegie Stage 11), lateral view. The trigeminal nerve is indicated by dashes. Nerves of second and third pharyngeal arches (facial and glossopharyngeal nerves, respectively) black. Their dendrites are in metabolic relation with the thickened ectoderm of the pharyngeal arches (stippled) that are part of the ectodermal ring. Half-headed arrow: restraining function of the dorsal aorta. 1, stretched connective tissue (nasal gubernaculum) extending from dorsal aorta towards ectoderm that thickens and becomes slightly depressed (nasal placode); 2, somite; 3, otic vesicle; 4, optic vesicle. Note that the nasal placode is located initially dorsal to the optic vesicle.

tips initially but later develop into broader contact zones (the so-called end-plates on muscle cells, or terminal boutons on dendrites).

This interpretation is so fundamental for understanding the integration of sensory and motor functions that it is worth expressing in a rubric: Dendrites suck themselves towards their source of supply; neurites are sucked by the living cells they will innervate (Figure 30.6).[7] In either case, the direction of growth of the nerves appears to be programmed by the metabolic field of their environment and not, say, through genetic information or "encoding." As far as touch is concerned, the skin and its growth determine topodynamically the pattern of its sensory (dendritic) nerve supply. Thus the differentiation of sensory nerves to the skin is something driven from the outside, namely the skin, and not something that is "programmed" from inside the nerves; it is another example of outside–inside differentiation.

---

[g]These folds in the human embryo used to be called branchial (gill) arches until it was appreciated that fish gills do not explain why folds arise in the human embryo.

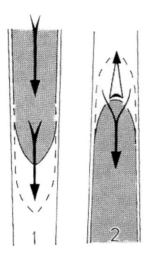

Figure 30.6

Left: growth dynamics in a neurite; tailed arrows indicate growth with metabolic movements and release of substances into an interstice (1). Right: growth dynamics in a dendrite; tailed arrow indicates appositional growth with uptake of substances into the cytoplasm (2); outlined arrow indicates direction of dendritic growth. Dotted lines represent subsequent elongation of each structure.

Similar considerations apply to neural growth anywhere in the body, including in the wall of the brain or spinal cord where dendrites and neurites are always morphological expressions of material fluxes, towards the cell body and away from the cell body, respectively. Blechschmidt proposed the following working hypothesis: the very growth of neuronal pathways is determined by outside–inside differentiation and is already an early nervous activity.

Specialized organs of somatic sensation

Although sensory dendrites innervate thick epithelium from Carnegie Stage 13 (4.2 mm, 28–32 days) onwards, Merkel cells and other specialized sensory organs associated with skin and touch (e.g., corpuscles of Meissner, Krause, and Vater–Pacini) are identified only at later stages, long after dendrites have grown appositionally closer to epithelial and other cells that contribute to the ending.

In different animals Merkel cells may arise from neural crest[8] or differentiate directly in the epidermis.[9,20] Merkel cells arise earlier than the corpuscular receptors described below and are a feature in humans of both hairy and smooth (glabrous) skin, where they form specialized Merkel cell–dendritic complexes in the basal layer of the epidermis. In human glabrous digital skin, Merkel cells could not be identified at 6–8 weeks estimated gestational age, but were obvious at 8–9 weeks when they play a role in finger print formation (dermatoglyphics).[10] Merkel cells are identified at 9 weeks in young human fingernail folds.[11]

With respect to the innervation of Merkel cells, it must be stressed that just because dendritic endings are not seen in the same field of view as their presumed target (especially using electron microscopy), it does not mean that there is no material transfer (i.e., signaling). As described above with the ectodermal ring, material transfers occur over distances of several cell diameters. Indeed wherever dendritic growth cones subsequently contact Merkel cells, the basement membrane of the epidermis is found to be discontinuous, suggesting a very efficient type of "signaling" that had developed from a much earlier stage between the Merkel cell and the growth cone. In animals it has been proposed that Merkel cells play a role in the development of epidermal pegs and papillary ridges[12] and that they may respond to electromagnetic radiation.[13] In humans, Blechschmidt and his students have provided a comprehensive description of the biodynamic events of skin development and the formation of papillary ridges.[14–17]

The development of Meissner corpuscles is a rather late event linked to the formation of dermal papillae in the digits; these corpuscles are also found in the tongue where connective tissue papillae abound. Only scant information is accessible about the fetal development of Meissner corpuscles in humans[18] but the corpuscles have been studied extensively in mice and monkeys, where they are recognized late in development when dermal papillae are distinct and dendrites lie immediately adjacent to the epidermis at the apex of each papilla.[19, 20] The lamellar cells that stack vertically in the mature corpuscle are derived from local connective tissue cells in the dermis.

A most exquisite lamellated corpuscle is known as the Vater–Pacini corpuscle. It is distributed widely in the body and may be found in retroperitoneal tissue, around joints, alongside limb vessels, in interosseous membranes, as well deep in the dermis of the sensitive skin of the digits, and in the less sensitive interdigital webbing. Many Vater–Pacini corpuscles are found along the splenic vein in its groove at the posterior aspect of the pancreas. In addition to its afferent nerve ending, each corpuscle has a remarkable vascular and lymphatic supply as well as an efferent (sympathetic) innervation. These corpuscles respond to vibrations, both internally from the movement of blood[21] and from external mechanical stimuli.[22]

The retroperitoneal Vater–Pacini corpuscles are particularly complex in structure[23] and are first recognized when the fetus is about 13–14 cm in length (towards the end of the fifth lunar month).[24] In the dermis of the hand, the corpuscles appear earlier and are recognizable in 7–9 cm fetuses, acquiring "adult" morphology when the fetus is about 20 cm long.[25] Unfortunately most reports on corpuscular development do not describe their topogenesis but rather are directed to details of structural development (tectogenesis) as revealed by light and electron microscopy. Such "close-up" examination often precludes an elucidation of possible influences from surrounding structures.

Fortunately some biodynamic conditions for the development of Vater–Pacini corpuscles in the human hand and foot during the second trimester have been established.[26] Lydecken found that in the digits of the hand, the corpuscles develop first in deep regions close to the skeleton. In particular, corpuscles arise in enlarging wedge-shaped regions vololateral to the digital skeleton where the first-order retension fields of the deep flexor tendons cross at right angles to the second-order, deeper, transverse retension fields that are stretched around the growing skeleton (Figure 30.7A). The enlargement of this wedge between two retension fields cannot be comprehended without understanding that the ectoderm, subcutaneous tissue, and deep flexor tendons of the digits of the hand are growth flexing during elongation of the finger and lifting, in a volar direction, off the skeletal substrate that lags behind.[2,4] Each wedge region is a kind of loosening zone that already contains sensory dendrites whose ends may then become encapsulated with Schwann-like cells. By the 7th month of

development, the size of a digital corpuscle is about half its adult size.

Conversely in the heel, Vater–Pacini corpuscles appear first in the more superficial dermis between the first-order retension fields of the dermis and deeper second-order retension fields around the anlage of the heel cushion (septa of fat lobules; Figure 30.7B). In the foot, the major growth movement that precedes the appearance of these corpuscles in the 4th–5th month is a flattening of the first-order retension field of the dermis in a dorsal direction against the heel cushion. As the heel widens and the dermis flattens, wedge-shaped zones loosen laterally between the septa (retinacula) of the adipose tissue and the dermis; this is one precondition for corpuscle formation. As in the fingers, the different orientation of the collagenous tissue on each side of the wedge is another important biodynamic condition. In the foot the retension fields of the deep flexor tendons do not loosen from the skeletal anlage but remain pressed against it; thus, unlike the hand, the initial Vater–Pacini corpuscles of the foot cannot develop close to the skeleton.

There may be analogous biodynamic circumstances that lead to the development of Vater–Pacini corpuscles in non-cutaneous regions. For example, in the retroperitoneum, the angled retension fields and loosening wedge-shaped zones might be associated with tension in blood vessels and nerve trunks, as well as local collagenous tissue. What is essential for an understanding of the topogenesis of a corpuscle in a particular location, is an anatomical analysis of the architecture of the surrounding tissue and the growth movements of major local organs before the corpuscle arises. Similar considerations apply to the development of other cutaneous receptors, such as corpuscles of Krause in the conjunctiva.

Eye: neural groove and optic groove

The development of the eye depends on the fate of the superior (cranial) end of the neural groove, which remains open to the amniotic fluid until closure of the superior (anterior, cranial) neuropore about 23–26 days after fertilization (Carnegie Stage 11). Initially, when the embryo is less than 2 mm long, a midline groove (neural groove) arises in the skin (ectoderm) of its back. The whole back of the embryo, including the groove, is bathed by amniotic fluid. Amniotic fluid is contained in a sac bounded above by a tense membrane (amnion)

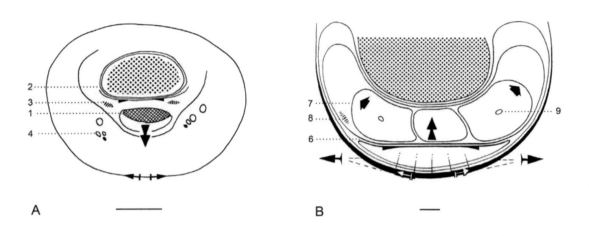

Figure 30.7

(A) Cross section of index finger at distal end of middle phalanx of a 7-month-old fetus (ca. 25 cm CR), palmar (volar) direction is to bottom. Phalanx stippled. 1, first-order retension field of tendon (cross-hatched) of flexor digitorum profundus muscle; 2, second-order retension field (converging half arrows) of periosteum aligned mainly at right angles to deep flexor tendon; 3, Vater–Pacini corpuscles developing in loosening wedge between first- and second-order orthogonal retension fields; 4, digital nerves and vessels. Large arrow: direction of volar displacement of flexor tendon (and skin) during growth flexion of finger: the tendon lifts away from its slower growing skeletal substrate. (B) Retension fields in cross section of heel-cushion of a 5-month-old fetus (ca. 18 cm CR), plantar director is to bottom. Heel cartilage and bone (calcaneus) stippled. Arrows with cross-tails: surface growth of epidermis and transverse widening of heel-cushion. 6, first-order retension field (converging half arrows) of connective tissue that becomes stretched, splitting off from the dermis as the heel-cushion widens transversely. Simple vertical arrow: approximation of the deeper stretched connective tissue to the heel bone. 7, second-order retension field around anlage of fat lobule. 8, Vater–Pacini corpuscles developing in the loosening wedge between first- and second-order retension fields. 9, central blood vessel of fat lobule. Broad arrows: fluid pressure in the lobules of fat tissue. Scale bars: 1 mm.

and below by the ectoderm of the embryo; embryonic ectoderm becomes amniotic ectoderm at the perimeter of the embryo. The neural groove arises partly from a longitudinal buckling that takes place as the ectodermal sheet of embryonic skin expands in surface area against the resistance of the tenser amnion. Either side of the midline, the walls of the neural groove rise up with surface growth to make two neural crests. The tall, wedge-shaped cells comprising the walls of the neural groove (neurectoderm) multiply faster than other cells in the embryo and so the walls thicken, as well as increase in surface area.

On the side of the neural groove that faces the vascularized bed of connective tissue, the surface growth of the neurectoderm is faster than on the side facing the amniotic fluid.[2] It is this asymmetry in areal growth between the two sides of the neurectoderm (i.e., the amniotic side and the tissue side) that soon forces the groove to close to a tube, initially in the region of the embryo's neck.[h] The neural tube itself is now covered by skin along the embryo's back; the cells in the wall of the tube become the neurons and glial cells of the spinal cord, and the former amniotic fluid contained in the lumen of the tube becomes the precursor of cerebrospinal fluid.

---

[h]The cause of neural tube closure is revealed by combining an examination of its cells with an awareness of their position and different metabolism in relation to neighboring cells and fluids, i.e., at each end of the cell as well as laterally.

At the cranial end of the embryo, the walls of the neural groove do not close for several days; the longitudinal slit-like opening seen here is called the superior (cranial) neuropore. Long before the superior neuropore closes, the anlage of the eye (the eye field) can be identified on each side as a shallow dimple or depression in the inner aspect of the right and left walls of the neural groove (1, Figure 30.8A). Each dimple could be considered to be the equivalent of the organ "X" for the eye. The wall of the depression thickens so that the shallow concavity (as seen looking laterally from the midline of the embryo) becomes squeezed into a groove, the optic groove or sulcus. Viewed from the amniotic sac and looking at the anterior end of the embryo, each optic groove appears like a crease caused by a local, lateral buckling of each wall of the still-open neural groove (2, Figure 30.8B and 5, Figure 30.9).[27]

The optic groove projects laterally and the outer aspect of its wall lies directly below the skin (ectoderm) of the embryo's head (Figure 30.9B and Figure 30.10).

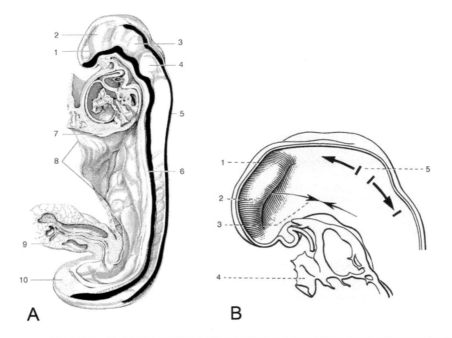

Figure 30.8

(A) Human embryo ca. 2 mm long (Carnegie Stage 10) sectioned in median plane (overview for B). Lumen of the neural tube lies between the two thick black lines; the tube is still open above and below (superior, inferior neuropore). 1, entrance to right optic vesicle (optic sulcus). 2, 3, 4 parts of wall of right brain; 5, roof of neural tube; 6, notochord; 7, anlage of liver; 8, cut edge of wall of yolk sac (yolk sac duct or vitelline duct); 9, body stalk; 10, undifferentiated tissue of rump bud (former primitive streak region). (B) Head region of same 2 mm long embryo viewed from left side, with ectoderm and underlying stroma removed revealing the left half of the neural tube and the anlage of the left optic vesicle (entrance to optic vesicle lies beneath plane of diagram). 1, cut edge of surface ectoderm; 2, anlage of optic vesicle (region of wall adjacent to surface ectoderm); 3, restraining function of inner tissue (anlage of nasal gubernaculum); 4, stem of aorta near heart (truncus arteriosus); 5, diverging arrows with cross-tails indicate growth elongation of neural tube.

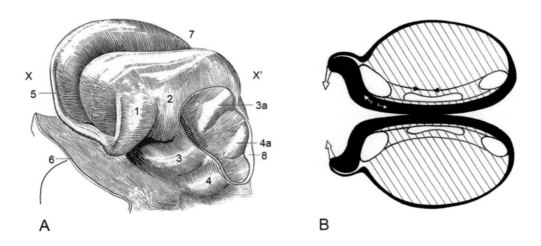

Figure 30.9

(A) Three-quarter left view of head region of 3.1 mm human embryo (Carnegie Stage 11) with window cut in ectoderm in ear region. 1, future lens region; 2, maxillary part of first pharyngeal arch; 3, mandibular part of first pharyngeal arch; 3a, trigeminal ganglion of first arch; 4, second pharyngeal (hyoid) arch; 4a, facial ganglion of second arch; 5, entrance to optic sulcus; 6, amnion (cut edge); 7, superior neuropore; 8, otic placode (in section). X–X' refers to plane of section for Figure 30.9B. (B) Horizontal section through head of 3.1 mm embryo, approximately in plane X–X' in A, showing superior neuropore on both sides. Black: wall of neural groove and ectoderm. Hatched, inner tissue of head with outlines of vessels. Outlined arrows near optic sulcus indicate growth movements during closure of superior neuropore. Diverging white arrows with cross-tails represent areal growth of wall of neural groove. Converging black arrows represent growth resistance of adjacent blood vessels.

The two optic grooves will cease to be visible from outside the embryo after the superior neuropore closes (Figure 30.11). Following neuropore closure, the precursor of each eye changes to a kind of cul-de-sac of the fluid-filled brain tube (strictly, a diverticulum of the lumen of the forebrain). This bubble-like sac is called the optic vesicle (Figures 30.5 and 30.11).[28,29] The optic vesicle remains joined to the wall of the neural tube by a tubular stalk (optic stalk) and it encloses a fluid-filled lumen (optic ventricle), which is continuous with the ventricle of the brain.

The optic vesicle grows in surface area and pushes outwards beneath the embryo's skin. The surface growth of the wall of the optic vesicle is not uniform in all regions; for example, the optic stalk grows less rapidly and remains relatively narrow. Also initially, the part of the optic vesicle wall lying directly under the skin tends to thicken more than grow in surface area, whereas the wall lying further from the skin remains thin and displays greater areal growth. Where the wall of the optic vesicle changes from thick to thin, especially dorsally, many cells are squeezed out to become future connective tissue, etc. around the eyeball (Figure 30.11). These displaced cells are known as optic mesectoderm: they are the precursors of components of the uvea, cornea, sclera, extra-ocular muscles, etc. The external surface of the optic vesicle sheds so many cells in such a short time, that it takes on a spiky, hedgehog-like appearance. Blechschmidt demonstrated that the optic vesicle is held in a bed of inner tissue (Halter der Augenanlage[24] or optic gubernaculum[i]), which aids the shedding of cells from the vesicle's wall.

---

[i]Gubernaculum is a generic term for a band of aligned tissue (e.g., an embryonic ligament) that "guides" the development of nearby structures; Blechschmidt stressed the biodynamic roles of gubernacula in many regions of the embryo.

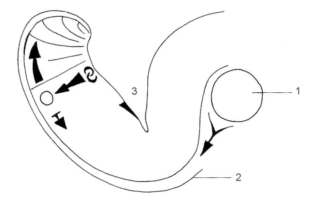

Figure 30.10

Drawing from horizontal hemisection through developing left eye of embryo, about 2 mm long; midline at top; superior neuropore at top left. Broad straight black arrow: displacement (not "migration") of daughter cells towards outer surface of neural epithelium following cell division in ventricular zone. Diverging arrows: surface growth, which, together with a similar contralateral growth, leads to closure of neural groove in forebrain region. Half-headed arrow near 3: site of little growth (growth pull) at inner surface of eye anlage. Tailed arrow: direction of nutrient movement in stroma. 1, blood vessel; 2, ectoderm covering the optic vesicle; 3, lumen of optic vesicle leading into lumen of neural groove (later, neural tube).

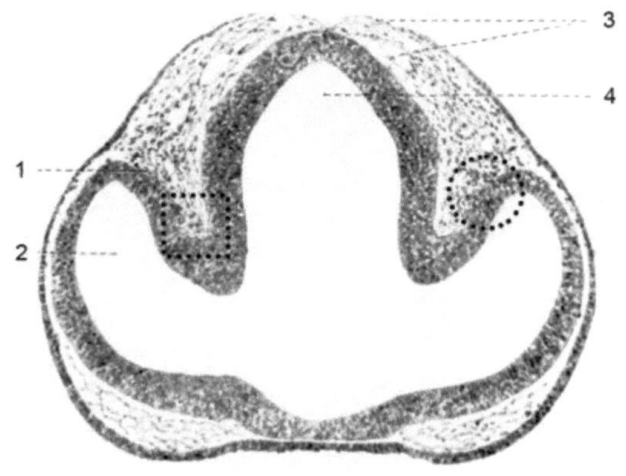

Figure 30.11

Transverse section through head of human embryo (28 somites, ca. 3.4 mm, Carnegie Stage 12). 1, optic neural crest; 2, optic vesicle; 3, ectoderm and inner tissue of head; 4, forebrain (prosencephalon). Dotted circle indicates optic neural crest being shed from dorsal region of wall of optic vesicle. Dotted box indicates nasal gubernaculum in transverse section.

Later the external contour of the optic vesicle wall will become smooth again.

A branch of the internal carotid artery in the embryo's head lies near the inferior surface of the optic stalk and supplies nutrients preferentially to that part of the wall of the optic vesicle directly under the skin. Biomechanically all embryonic vessels exert traction on their territories of supply and this means that the skin and the adjacent wall of the optic vesicle will grow less in area, thereby thickening and remaining anchored to the vessels. Thus blood vessels contribute to thickening growth more than areal growth and this asymmetry in the vesicle underlies its change of shape: the lumen of the vesicle narrows to a slit and the two walls approach. As it thickens, the wall that was ini- tially against the skin invaginates, so-to-speak, into the lumen of the optic vesicle – the resulting structure is now called the optic cup (Figures 30.12 and 30.13). Similar changes occur along the optic stalk, which thickens ventrally and stretches dorsally, developing a ventral groove.

Optic cup

From now on, the optic cup will comprise two con-cave walls or sheets of cells that grow in surface area at different rates, thereby continuing to approach one another. The thicker wall near the skin becomes the sensory (neural) retina, while the thinner, outer wall becomes the pigment epithelium of the retina. The outer wall is surrounded by embryonic connective tissue (optic mesectoderm), which provides a medium through which nutrients can percolate. This region is the precursor of the middle layer of the eye, called uvea. Later, blood vessels arise in this connective tissue bed

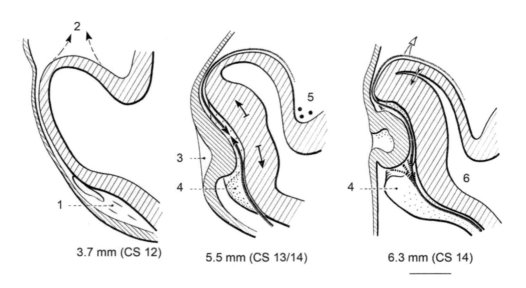

3.7 mm (CS 12)   5.5 mm (CS 13/14)   6.3 mm (CS 14)

Figure 30.12

Semi-schematic view of developmental movements in transformation of optic vesicle to optic cup in embryos 3.7 mm (Carnegie Stage 12), 5.5 mm (Carnegie Stage 13/14), 6.3 mm (Carnegie Stage 14). 1, vascularized connective tissue with an outline of capillary-like hyaloid artery; 2, displacement of cells from dorsal surface of optic vesicle (optic mesectoderm) assisted by optic gubernaculum (dashed arrows); 3, lens pit; 4, border of optic (choroidal) fissure; 5, dots indicate nasal gubernaculum in cross section, contributing to dorsal furrow between optic cup and optic stalk; 6, open connection between optic ventricle and third ventricle of brain. Converging arrows (5.5 mm): growth resistance due to hyaloid vessels. Diverging arrows (5.5 mm): areal expansion of sensory retina against resistance of hyaloid vessels, leading to concave thickening of the retina. Contoured arrow (6.3 mm): movement of optic cup relative to optic stalk. Tailed arrow (6.3 mm): start of nutrient uptake by sensory retina from outer wall of optic cup (pigment epithelium). Scale: 0.1 mm

(choriocapillaries) and supply nutrients directly to the pigment cells. The folded-over rim between the two walls of the optic cup will form the iris and the aperture within the rim, the pupil.

As the outer wall of pigment epithelium and the sensory retina approach one another, the lumen (optic ventricle) becomes obliterated and the pigment cells are able to nourish directly the sensory retina. This occurs because the pigment cells export nutrients absorbed from the neighboring uvea to meet the demands of the multiplying cells of the sensory retina. The unique feature of these movements of metabolites is that here, a single epithelium both imports nutrients from an underlying connective tissue bed and simultaneously exports a nutritional supply to a neighboring epithelium.

The hallmark of this intensive metabolic activity is that outer epithelial cells, initially transparent, soon accumulate a black pigment (melanin) to become the first non-transparent cells in the human embryo; hence the name pigment epithelium. The pigment arises first in an equatorial growth zone of the optic cup soon after the optic ventricle is obliterated, when the inner layer (sensory retina) flattens against the slower growing

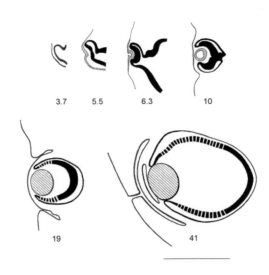

Figure 30.13
Drawings from sections showing growth movement from convex to concave retina with increasing retinal curvature (top row), then decreasing retinal curvature with flattening (bottom row). Length of embryos with Carnegie Stage (CS): 3.7 mm (CS 12), 5.5 mm (CS 13/14), 6.3 mm (CS 14), 10 mm (CS 16), 19 mm (CS 20), and fetus of 41 mm crown–rump length. Hatching represents the equatorial growth zone of sensory retina. Scale 1 mm.

choroid to match the demands of the sensory retina. One consequence of the enormous blood supply to the external aspect of the pigment epithelium is the efficient maintenance of retinal temperature within narrow limits. After birth, when ambient light is focused on the photoreceptors lying adjacent to the pigment cells, thermal equilibrium at the back of the eye prevents instantaneous coagulation of the photoreceptive proteins in the photosensitive cells of the retina. In addition, the metabolic connections between sensory retina and pigment epithelium continue throughout life: a detachment of the one from the other (no matter whether due to trauma or to a blister-like accumulation of fluid at the site of the original optic ventricle) may lead to a local blind spot or scotoma.

The optic cup, which has developed from the optic vesicle, behaves like a tiny hand by which the brain grasps, as it were, a piece of embryonic skin: this piece of skin is the precursor of the lens (Figures 30.12 and 30.13).[27] At first the lens is a placode[j] of thickening skin (ectodermal lens placode) confined within the rim of the optic cup. The thickening of lens epithelium is underpinned by a preferential supply of nutrients from the same branch of the internal carotid artery (hyaloid artery), which contributed previously to the thickening of the part of the vesicle wall that became the sensory retina. The cells in the lens placode prosper and multiply close to their nutrient supply, while the surrounding, thinner skin spreads away: the shape of the lens placode thereby transforms into a dimple called the lens pit. Eventually the pit closes over and becomes a vesicle that soon loses its connection with the skin; the ectoderm that seals over the lens vesicle becomes the external epithelium of the cornea. Only when the wall of the lens vesicle thickens, by virtue of an intensive uptake of nutrients and a simultaneous release of its watery by-products of metabolism, will the vesicle become the transparent lens of living cells that later regulates the refraction of light into the eye.

The watery by-products from the growth and multiplication of lens cells accumulate in the adjacent connective tissue under the curved ectoderm of the future cornea, giving rise to the anterior chamber of the eye containing aqueous humor. The connective tissue cells that remain between the pool of fluid and the corneal

pigment epithelium at Carnegie Stage 16 (8–11 mm, 4–6 weeks after fertilization). Blechschmidt used to comment poetically "the pigment cells work themselves black to supply the retina." Subsequently pigments arise in many inner tissues of the uvea derived from optic mesectoderm (choroidal melanocytes, iridial chromatophores, clump cells, etc.). Intracellular pigment is also a sign of intense metabolic exchange in other embryonic tissues, including the ear and brainstem.

By virtue of its areal growth, the sensory retina now becomes the "prime mover" or engine for the subsequent development of the eye and most of the extraocular structures. The abundant source of nutrients in the uvea enables this growth to accelerate, giving rise to a remarkable architecture of capillary vessels in the

---

[j]A patch of thickened epithelium, which can be compared to the more extensive ectodermal ring.

ectoderm, are stretched and flattened by the pressure of the accumulating aqueous humor on the one hand, and the tension and surface growth of the ectoderm on the other. This is the location of a series of powerful retension fields where collagen is "wrung out," so-to-speak, from the cytoplasm of these stressed connective tissue cells.[2] The layered sheets of collagen fibrils that align along the lines of tension contribute to the bulk of the cornea (substantia propria corneae).

The alignment and packing of the hydrated collagen fibrils in these curving sheets is so remarkably ordered that, collectively, the fibrils can transmit electromagnetic radiation of certain wavelengths and change its direction (refractive power of transparent cornea). Under conditions of insufficient hydration, the interspacing of collagen fibrils decreases, leading to a loss of corneal transparency. As the eyeball grows, other connective tissue cells lying external to the uvea also become simultaneously extended circumferentially and flattened in a radial direction. These are the biodynamic features of a retension field and sheets of collagen are also laid down here. However this collagen, with a different packing density of fibrils and possibly a different degree of hydration to that in the cornea, becomes the tough, opaque sclera (white of the eye) that serves to protect the uvea.

Retina, optic nerve

It is important to recall that the wall of the optic vesicle with its stalk is an extension of the neural tube and so part of the developing brain. The processes[k] of cells in the wall of the optic vesicle are aligned radially towards the nourishing connective tissue (optic mesectoderm), that is, towards the periphery of the vesicle. As the optic vesicle transforms into the double-walled cup, the cellular processes that were originally in the vicinity of the overlying skin now lie at the inner surface of the cup, directed radially towards the back of the lens. As the optic cup grows larger, its walls flatten, just like a re-opening of the little hand that previously grasped the vesicle of lens cells. An early optic cup in a 6 mm long embryo has a vertical diameter of, say, 0.4 mm, whereas the adult eye has a vertical diameter of about 24 mm. Over the course of its maturation, the retina flattens progressively and grows enormously in

surface area, but scarcely changes in thickness. The relative constancy of retinal thickness is a striking feature of ocular growth.

The radial flattening of the retina results in a change in the orientation of the fibrous processes of those cells at its inner surface. The bodies of these cells are dragged in the direction of retinal flattening, which is more-or-less at right angles to the processes of the deeper cells that retain a radial orientation (Figure 30.14). When the innermost cell bodies first become displaced, they leave a portion of their cytoplasm trailing behind; this portion becomes a neurite. At first glance, it appears as though the neurites are growing actively away from the cell bodies. However initially, the opposite is true; the tips of these neurites remain virtually fixed near that part of the optic cup where the rate of change of retinal curvature is least, while the bodies of the cells become displaced.[30] Initially, the region of minimal change in curvature corresponds to the place where the optic cup continues into the optic stalk. Thus, a layer of nerve fibers arises along the inner surface of the sensory retina, with tips remaining closer to the optic stalk and neurites being extended from here to their displaced cell bodies.

Soon the tips of these neurites will start to advance by appositional growth, according to rules for neuritic growth, along spatially ordered channels[31] that have arisen in the interstices of both the sensory retina[32] and the inner wall of the optic stalk (Fig. 30.14B). These channels contain fluids, which can be assumed to convey nutrients from the now actively growing tips of neurites in the optic nerve. The tips of optic nerve fibers are making metabolic connections with other cells in specific regions of the brain and are being sucked toward these regions as the embryo's head enlarges. Blechschmidt proposed that certain rapidly growing regions of the brain behave in an equivalent fashion to the dilation fields of muscles and suck in metabolites from the closest sources. At first the distances are small, e.g., in an embryo 13 mm long with many neurites in its optic nerve, the eye is only 1 mm or so away from one of the many "destinations" of its fibers. As the brain and head grow, the optic nerve connections simply elongate by interstitial growth of neurites, eventually reaching the typical adult distance of 9–11 cm between eyeball and terminals in the brainstem (superior colliculus) and thalamus (lateral geniculate nucleus).

---

[k]Generic term for neurites, dendrites, and fiber-like extensions of glial cells.

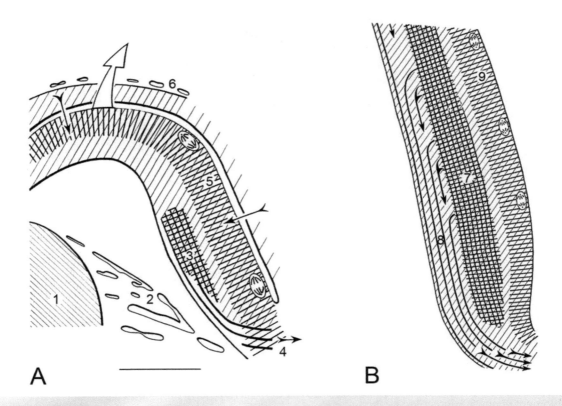

Figure 30.14
(A) Flattening of sensory retina and obliteration of optic ventricle in 15.5 mm long embryo (Carnegie Stage 18). 1, lens; 2, penicillar branching of capillary-like hyaloid vessels that supply lens fibers; 3, cluster of retinal ganglion somas; 4, neurites of retinal ganglion cells; 5, layer of ventricular mitoses; 6, choroid (uvea). Outlined arrow: growth direction of optic cup. Tailed arrows: nutrient movement from uvea via pigment epithelium to sensory retina; growth flux from neurites. Scale: 0.1 mm. (B) Later stage (29 mm embryo, Carnegie Stage 23) of retinal flattening with subsequent growth of neurites into optic stalk (anlage of optic nerve) interpreted as axoplasmic flow. 7, ganglion cell somas; 8, layer of ganglion cell neurites; 9, zone of ventricular mitoses (pigment epithelium not drawn).

In the retina, the first nerve cells to mature as retinal ganglion cells are found in the innermost layer (6, Figure 30.15). The ganglion cells represent a metabolic transfer station between sources in the uvea and sinks in the brainstem and thalamus. The photoreceptors, which arise in the deepest part of the sensory retina adjacent to the pigment epithelium, are the last cells to mature and also represent a kind of metabolic relay station. This sequence of development explains why a light-ray must first traverse layers of nerve fibers and

cell bodies before reaching the layer of rods and cones (outer segments of photoreceptors). The place where the nerve fibers pass from retina into optic stalk will have no photoreceptors, and so will correspond to the blind spot of the fundus.

Eye position, eyelids, and blinking

The eyes arise initially at the sides of the embryo's brain (i.e., facing laterally). After the superior neuropore closes, the growing brain pushes into the skin of the

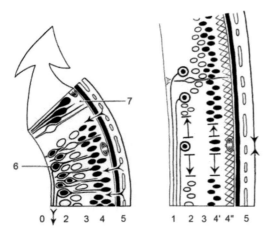

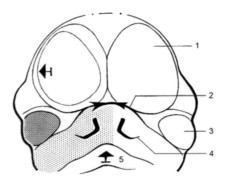

Figure 30.15

Schematic diagrams of retinal flattening during areal growth. Large outlined arrow: direction of retinal growth movement with little change in thickness. 0–5 direction from center of eye to periphery; 1, optic nerve fiber layer; 2, ganglion cell layer; 3, inner plexiform layer; 4, ventricular layer of nuclei (as yet unspecified); 4'–4", inner and outer nuclear layers separated by inner plexiform layer; 5, uvea (including pigment epithelium indicated by thick black line, choroidal vessels indicated by ellipses, and outermost anlage of sclera); 6, ganglion cell soma; 7, zone of wedge-shaped cells with geometry that predisposes a capacity for nutrient-uptake from pigment epithelium; 8, foot of radial glial (Müller) cell. Tailed arrows: main directions of nutrient flux across pigment epithelium and within neurites, respectively. Diverging arrows with cross-tails: growth pressure from cell division within sensory retina. Converging arrows: growth resistance from choroidal vessels (choriocapillaries) and anlage of sclera.

Figure 30.16

Forehead and face region of 16.2 mm long human embryo. Development of forward direction of gaze. Nose–cheek region stippled light gray; eye dark-gray. Lower arrow: direction of growth pressure from heart against the face during increasing flexion of embryo. Converging double arrow: restraining function of laterally compressed stroma between nose and forehead. Upper arrow: transverse widening of cerebral hemisphere above the eyes. 1, cerebral hemispheres; 2, tense connective tissue between left and right pairs of eyelids (interorbital ligament); 3, eye; 4, nostril (in process of temporary occlusion); 5, first pharyngeal arch (flexion fold of mandible).

forehead region and buckles at the sides to form two cerebral hemispheres each with a frontal lobe. The connective tissue below the forehead and above the nose, i.e., between the eyes, is compressed transversely and becomes taut, thereby tethering the eyes. This retension field is the basis for a ligament that is stretched across the face at the bridge of the nose, the interorbital

(palpebral) ligament[33,34] (Figure 30.16). The growth of the brain causes the forehead and mid-face to broaden. The widening mid-face in combination with the anchoring of the nasal aspect of the eyes, forces the eyes to a more frontal position. Eventually, the interorbital ligament will become the periosteum covering parts of the frontal and nasal bones of the skull.

Initially there are no eyelids: the ectoderm of the cornea continues directly into the skin of the face and the interorbital ligament fans out laterally either side of the bridge of the nose, splitting into smooth skin above and below each cornea. The slowly increasing tension in the interorbital ligament now causes skin folds to appear above and below the cornea, similar to tension-induced folds in cloth or rubber. These folds are the first hint of eyelids. Subsequently, the tension between the eyes becomes so great that the growing folds are dragged slowly across the cornea, so that the inside epithelium of the lid fuses with

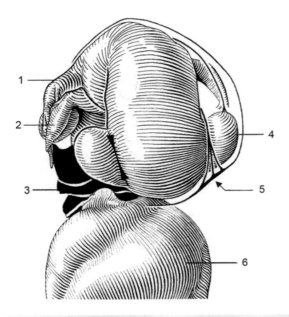

Figure 30.17
Cranial region drawn from a reconstruction of 3.4 mm long human embryo, viewed from front. Endoderm black. Converging double arrow (on right side of brain): restraining function of the inner tissue strand (nasal gubernaculum) between the optic vesicle and the forebrain. The nasal placode arises at the site where this strand merges with the ectoderm (5). 1, trigeminal ganglion; 2, facial and vestibulocochlear complex (with otocyst behind); 3, second pharyngeal pouch; 4, optic vesicle; 5, nasal placode (anlage of olfactory pit); 6, pericardium.

the corneal epithelium.[33] This fusion creates a temporary biodynamic fulcrum for further surface growth of the external aspect of the eyelid so that eventually the eyelids close together at the palpebral margin and, also temporarily, fuse here. A strong corrosion field[2] arises along the line of fusion of the eyelids and the palpebral fissure closes.[33] This event represents a non-muscular closure of the eyelids, due principally to the growth of the brain and the mutual tethering of the nasal aspect of the eyes.

As one skin fold is slowly transforming into an upper eyelid, the cells beneath the skin are stretched in a direction perpendicular to the edge of the fold, i.e., almost at right angles to the line of tension in the interorbital ligament. As a consequence of their extension, these cells are transformed into muscle cells, whose subsequent hardening ("contraction") during the continual growth of the head, will lead to a fixation of the upper eyelid. This is the action of the levator palpebrae superioris muscle. Further growth of the head enhances this fixation and the previously closed eyelids slowly "unfuse" in a process analogous to dehiscence. The closure and re-opening of the eyelids is the first blink: it is due to growth, not muscles. It is an exceedingly slow movement, taking days, and it is imperceptible except through an accurate analysis of successive stages of embryonic anatomy. Nonetheless it is a movement, with its own special dynamics: it could be called a growth blink.

The widening of the palpebral fissure slowly stretches other nearby cells beneath the skin into an annular muscle around the fissure; this is the dilation field for the orbicularis oculi muscle. When this muscle tenses, the eyelids will tend to close – this is the start of the second blink of the embryo, a movement now partly due to growth and partly due to muscular hardening. The sequence repeats itself, only faster, each time leading to the development of stronger muscles. Finally, these movements become so rapid that they can be detected as blinking during ultrasound scans of fetuses around the 26th week of pregnancy.

The development of the capacity to blink is one of many examples of what Blechschmidt described as the *reversal* between an embryonic function and an adult function: embryonic cells must first be stretched by the growth activity of surrounding cells and cellular ensembles before they can develop into muscle cells capable of shortening. Another example: embryonic cells must first be stretched in one axis and compressed from the sides before the collagen expressed from them is strong enough to resist the extension (development of cornea, sclera, ligaments, and tendons in retension fields).

At any stage, whether embryonic or adult, the capacities of a human organism are the direct consequences of the totality of prior development. Without a shallow depression "X" in the lateral wall of the tiny embryo's neural groove, there would be no optic sulcus, no optic vesicle, no optic cup, no eyeball, and no muscles for opening or closing the eyelids. It can be shown that most adult structures arise from the attempts of one part of the conceptus to counteract or balance the otherwise disruptive influences from another part: hence the frequent reversal of functions between embryonic life and maturity.[28]

Neural connections and visual field

As an extension of the brain, the optic nerve is a tract of the so-called central nervous "system" rather than a peripheral nerve. Therefore changes inside the skull (such as elevated intracranial pressure) and within the orbit, may cause changes along the optic nerve that manifest themselves at the site where the optic nerve emerges from the eyeball. For example, the presence of a tumor growing inside the skull and causing an increased amount of fluid to form at the optic nerve head (papilledema) might be revealed using an ophthalmoscope, the instrument invented by Babbage in 1847, and independently by Helmholtz in 1851, to examine the fundus.

Most nerve fibers from the eye relay to the visual part of the cerebral cortex via the thalamus. The visual cortex, located near the occiput of the skull, receives much of its oxygen and nutrients via the posterior cerebral artery, which is a continuation of the vertebral artery. On each side, the vertebral artery ascends to the brain through a series of transverse foramina in the upper six vertebrae of the neck. Thus changes in the alignment of neck vertebrae (through accidents or manipulation) can alter the blood supply to the visual cortex. Similarly, tension in muscles attached to the vertebrae of the neck may lead to changes in visual capacity. Furthermore, some optic fibers relay to parts of the brainstem (superior colliculus, etc.), which have connections to other parts of the brainstem that control eye movements, the position and thickness of the lens, and the diameter of the pupil. Most of these structures are also supplied by branches from the vertebral artery, so it is not surprising that how we use our necks may have widespread consequences for many aspects of vision, including the ability to focus and follow moving objects with the eyes.

The two optic nerves meet at the optic chiasm where more than half the nerve fibers from one eye cross to the opposite side of the brain, in such a way that the primary visual cortex in each hemisphere receives information from the opposite half of the visual world (visual hemifield). Much is written about how the cerebral cortex might "resynthesize" a single visual world (i.e., as seen by the "mind's eye") from these two hemifields. Here it is important to recall that the retinae are also part of the brain and that each retina is "seeing" almost the same visual world that the mind "sees."

Nose

Like the lens of the eye, the nose also first appears in the embryo as a left and right ectodermal placode that signifies a region of restricted areal growth in an epithelium. The nasal placode arises just where it does, initially above the eye on either side of the midline, because of preceding biodynamic circumstances in this region. Blechschmidt's histological sections demonstrate that the deep surface of the nasal placode lies adjacent to a confined bundle of inner tissue cells that seems to be aligned at an angle to the ectoderm. This bundle of oriented connective tissue cells together with their surrounding viscous matrix has the form of a loose strand or fascicle that is a continuation of the tension in the longitudinal vessels at the ventrolateral surface of the growing brain. The strand seems to radiate into the base of the ectoderm (Figures 30.5 and 30.17).[27,34] Blechschmidt's three-dimensional reconstructions show that the strand becomes narrower like a sheaf further from the placode, particularly where it is impeded in its growth between the wall of the brain and the wall of the optic vesicle. This cord-like arrangement of cells and matrix is an embryonic ligament called the nasal gubernaculum; like all embryonic ligaments, it arises in a retension field and acts as a restraining apparatus. The location and ligament-like nature of the gubernaculum is demonstrated by the profiles of its nuclei, which appear as circles when the ligament is cut in cross section above the optic stalk (nuclei in center of dotted box, Figure 30.11).[1]

Where the sheath-like gubernaculum ends at the base of the ectoderm, the connective tissue cells impede the surface growth of the ectoderm. This restriction of surface growth is the biodynamic cause of a local ectodermal thickening in the form of the nasal placode. As described above, placodes of ectoderm, just like the ectodermal ring, have a higher metabolic exchange of anabolites and catabolites per unit surface area than regions of thinner epithelium. These metabolic exchanges will take place with whatever tissues happen to lie nearby. In the case of the nasal placode, the wall of the highly metabolically active brain lies only a fraction of a millimeter away. Thus each

---

[1]The three-dimensional form of a nucleus of a cell in a retension field is a prolate ellipsoid or spindle, whose long axis is aligned in the direction of traction.

nasal placode comes into metabolic relationship with the brain, whereby the brain sucks in nutrients from the cells of the nasal placode. As the brain and placode grow apart, extensions of the placodal cells remain anchored metabolically near the surface of the brain. Some of these extensions (processes) are neurites of future olfactory cells; expressed another way: sensory neural pathways arise between the nasal placode and the brain and the placode becomes a specialized olfactory epithelium for the sense of smell.

These young neural connections anchor, biomechanically speaking, the placodal cells to the brain cells. With continual growth of the embryonic head, the nasal placode soon transforms into a pit-shaped structure with thickened epithelium at the base of the depression. The two pits, which are seen clearly when the embryo is about 7 mm long (Carnegie Stage 15), are the anlagen of the nostrils (Fig. 30.16). Since there are two eyes, two optic stalks, and two gubernacula, there must be two nasal placodes and so two nostrils. Initially both nasal placodes develop laterally, corresponding to the wide separation between the eyes. The nostril is therefore a developmental product of the eye and the brain.

Further growth of the relatively unanchored epithelium surrounding the nasal pits leads to a deepening of the nostril, as the olfactory epithelium remains anchored to the brain via olfactory nerve filaments. In a Carnegie Stage 18 embryo (ca. 13.5 mm long) the olfactory epithelium is less than 1 mm from the surface of the brain (Figure 30.18). Compared to the growth of the face, this distance will increase only slightly by "adult" maturity. It is often stated that the olfactory mucosa is "buried deep" in the face–nose region, whereas it is really the nose and face that has grown far beyond the anchored mucosa. Figure 30.18 also demonstrates the remarkable conformity in a sagittal plane between the shape of the olfactory epithelium and the shape of the olfactory part of the brain, reflecting their intimate metabolic relationship.[34]

At the beginning of the 2nd month the human nose appears wider than it is long; elongation of the nose does not occur until the fetal face starts to lengthen as the head lifts away from the heart. Elongation of the nose is driven by its initial midline densation field changing to a distusion field.[35] The swelling of cartilage cells is permitted more in the anterior direction than posteriorly where there is strong resistance to distusion from the firm cranial base.

Paranasal sinuses

The paranasal sinuses arise only after elongation of the fetal face. The sinuses develop from an actively growing limiting tissue, namely the superior and lateral nasal walls (Figure 30.19). Blechschmidt's investigations show that epithelial surface growth alone is insufficient to account for the formation of a sinus. The areal growth of the nasal epithelium must be accompanied by a kind of suction field in the connective tissue bed (stroma) of the epithelium, as is found in the formation of glands.[2] All incipient sinuses exhibit gland-like epithelial sprouts in their most rapidly growing regions; this is seen clearly in Broman's (1927) reconstruction of the lateral nasal wall of a 53.2 mm fetus where epithelial buds are found at the deepest, most lateral wall of the maxillary sinus.[36] The stroma loosens because it is biomechanically anisotropic, i.e., composed of firmer and weaker parts; the stronger parts consolidate as ligaments (retension fields) and/or osteoid (detraction fields) and the weaker parts loosen (suction fields). The loosening regions lie adjacent to the deep inner tissue of the nasal wall whereas the consolidating regions usually lie closer to the skin (ectoderm) of the head, which is growing more rapidly in surface area. An interesting feature of the epithelium of the nasal wall is that its cells, prior to being given the opportunity to spread out, pass through a phase of restricted surface growth, which results in them becoming temporarily taller and more wedge-shaped.

The stronger consolidating structures, being the perichondrial ligaments of the cranial base and the osseous foci of specific cranial bones (e.g., maxillae, nasal bones) are subject to continuously oscillating growth tractions. In the case of the maxillary sinus, laterally directed traction in the connective tissue of the zygomatic arch drags the firmer substrate of the nasal capsule (anlage of nasal skeleton) away from the nasal mucosa.[37] This is the cause of the suction field described above. Thus the tiny epithelial anlage of the maxillary sinus appears deep to the focus of chondrification of the nasal capsule; the positional relations are reminiscent of a bell-tent (nasal epithelium) covered by a fly (nasal capsule). A focus of bone arises in the external perichondrium of the cartilaginous nasal capsule, so that there is a precise sequence in the topography from nasal ectoderm, stroma, nasal capsule, external perichondrium, intramembranous ossification, stroma, and skin. Kallius' (1905) illustration of a frontal section through

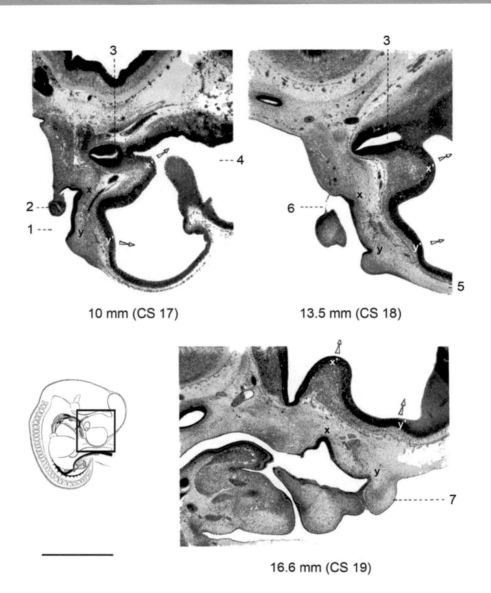

10 mm (CS 17)   13.5 mm (CS 18)

16.6 mm (CS 19)

Figure 30.18

Development of form of olfactory pit, based on sagittal sections of head region of embryos in same orientation (as indicated in inset of 10 mm embryo with box showing region of interest). In each embryo, the contour of thick epithelium of the nasal pit (between x and y) conforms to the contour of thick epithelium of the olfactory region of the forebrain (between x' and y'). 1, olfactory pit; 2, palate; 3, optic recess of third ventricle; 4, lumen of midbrain or mesencephalic (so-called cerebral) aqueduct; 5, dorsal meninx (thinner compared to basal meninx); 6, bucconasal membrane (region of choana); 7, tip of nose. Open arrows indicate growth elevation of brain. Scale: 1 mm.

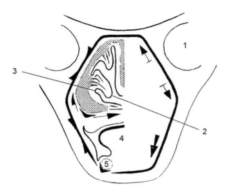

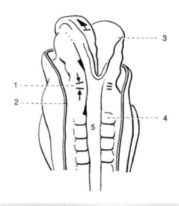

Figure 30.19

Frontal section through facial region of 37 mm long fetus. Formation of the long face with stretching of connective tissue of the nasal capsule ("muzzle"), thick black line external to the nasal cartilage (stippled). Converging half-headed arrows: restraining function of stretched connective tissue. Diverging arrows: piston-like growth and expansion of the nasal cartilage. 1, eye; 2, middle concha; 3, middle nasal meatus (site of growth of the maxillary sinus); 4, tongue; 5, Meckel's cartilage with bone formation on lateral aspect.

Figure 30.20

Head and neck region of human embryo about 2 mm long, dorsal view showing neural groove and superior neuropore. Upper arrow with cross-tail: longitudinal growth and flexion of head. Converging half-headed arrows: restraining function of left dorsal aorta. Converging arrows: restricted surface growth in region of anlage of the left otic placode. 1, ectoderm near otic placode; 2, cut edge of the amnion; 3, transition zone between ectoderm and neural epithelium at margin (neural crest) of neural groove at superior neuropore; 4, somite; 5, neural tube.

the head of a 15-week fetus (reproduced in reference 36, p. 90) shows this nicely. Subsequently, growth tractions are replaced by frank muscular traction as the skeletal muscles of the head, neck, and face start to oscillate in cycles of activity; these continue through puberty as the paranasal sinuses enlarge.

Ear

Some regard the ear as a precocious organ because its inner part achieves its adult form by the start of fetal life about 8–9 weeks after fertilization, and its adult size by the end of the 6th lunar month of development in utero (fetus ca. 22 cm). The ossicles of the middle ear achieve their final dimensions at about 22 weeks and are the first bones to fully ossify and achieve adult status in utero. The cochlea is fully coiled by 9 weeks and structurally mature in the fetus by about 24 weeks[38] when the fetus is

able to hear and respond to external sounds.[39] There are descriptions on the effects of music on the fetus, which influences are carried into childhood and beyond.[40]

In the 1940s the amplitude associated with the threshold for human hearing was calculated to be of the order of atomic dimensions.[41] It remains a puzzle that the energy associated with the threshold of hearing is comparable to the energy of molecular vibrations due to thermal (Brownian) motion at body temperature. If the ear obeyed the laws of inanimate physics and chemistry, then it is strange that one is not deafened by the "roar" of Brownian motion in one's hair cells, tectorial jelly, basilar membrane with blood vessels, etc. From the viewpoint of teleological design, one cannot comprehend why a hearing organ would be "constructed" with blood vessels so close to its sensory cells. However there are some simple features of the complex anatomy of the ear (with its inner, middle, and external parts) that can be revealed by starting with the development of its position (topogenesis) and the relations of the developing ear to neighboring embryonic structures.

Inner ear and nerves

A dorsal view of the head region of a young human embryo (ca. 2 mm long) shows the open superior neuropore between the walls of the neural groove (Fig. 30.9 and Figure 30.20). Here the width of the neuropore (i.e., the distance between the two neural folds) in the vicinity of the flexed head has actually widened compared to what it was earlier in the region of the neck. Blechschmidt's reconstructions of embryos of different ages show that the transient widening of the superior neuropore is associated with increasing flexion of the head around the heart. It can therefore be hypothesized (using Occam's razor) that the flexion of the head, being a preceding and thus more basic developmental movement, is the cause of this widening. The widening is reminiscent of a skin wound along the back of a finger that splits open when the finger is flexed.[2] Within about a day, the growth in the lateral walls of the cranial part of the neural groove overcomes the flexion-induced widening and the superior neuropore closes; yet the

consequences of the temporary widening remain throughout life!

As the neural tube gapes open, the dorsal neural folds incline markedly to each side and in a unique region (indicated in Fig. 30.20 by converging arrows), the surface growth of the ectoderm becomes constrained. In this zone the ectoderm thickens locally and becomes a placode (otic placode) composed of tall ectodermal cells. Located very close to the wall of the hindbrain, the otic placode comes into anchored metabolic exchange with the brain; the surrounding unanchored parts of the ectoderm continue to grow in surface area and move away. The otic placode then becomes a depression, the otic pit, and then a vesicle, the otocyst.

The events that underlie these transformations are the result of cell division occurring at the exposed surface of the placode adjacent to the (amniotic) fluid, as opposed to cell growth that occurs mainly at the base of the thickened ectoderm, adjacent to the nutrient-rich stroma.[1,42] The placodal cells are wedge-shaped and the biodynamic events here are similar to what occurs in other thick epithelia such as the wall of the neural groove. The greater growth at the base of the placode enables it to arch initially inwards and then finally close over as the otocyst (Figure 30.21).[43]

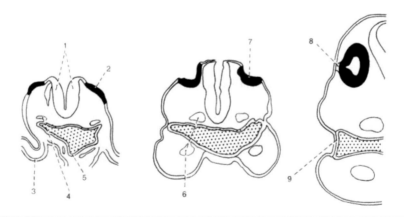

Figure 30.21

Three stages in the development of the ear anlage (black) in 2 mm, 2.6 mm, and 4.2 mm long human embryos. Left: stage of otic placode (2); middle: stage of otic pit (7); right: stage of otic vesicle (8). 1, neural groove; 3, rim of umbilicus; 4 and 6, aorta; 5, foregut endoderm (lumen stippled); 9, anlage of tympanic membrane (ectoderm of first pharyngeal groove in contact with endoderm of first pharyngeal pouch).

The development of the otocyst from a placode is a beautiful example for Blechschmidt's claim that the basis for an embryological feature is not to be sought solely in the cells of the feature itself but also in the surrounding cells and their growth movements. In fact, the otic placode itself is a consequence of brain and heart interaction, irrespective of how the tall wedge-shaped cells of the placode might subsequently multiply and press on one another laterally,

The wall of the otocyst has a varying thickness; its medial wall abuts the lateral surface of the hindbrain.[44] As with the optic vesicle, many cells are squeezed from the uneven wall of the otic vesicle to become inner tissue cells that surround the otocyst; this can occur anywhere over its surface but is particularly noticeable at its rostral (anterior) aspect where the emerging cells give rise to most of the vestibulocochlear ganglion.[45] Generally cells shed from the otocyst are described as otic neural crest or otic mesectoderm; the biomechanical features of their formation are no different to neural crest cells anywhere else in the embryo. Some of these shed mesectodermal cells become ganglion cells while others develop into the otic capsule and musculoskeletal elements etc. of other parts of the ear. Other cells that are squeezed from the wall of the adjacent hindbrain may also contribute to the vestibulocochlear ganglion.

As soon as the otic placode has a sufficient number of cells, dendrites from ganglion cells grow appositionally towards it. At Carnegie Stage 13, the otocyst and the ganglion cells are separated by less than 50 μm, a convenient distance for metabolic movements that occur regularly in the metabolic field of a thickened epithelium; these molecular movements represent incipient synaptic contacts between thick parts of the otic vesicle and dendrites of vestibulocochlear ganglion cells. This relationship is already obvious in a human embryo only 6 mm long (Carnegie Stage 14), when nerves to the anlage of a crista ampullaris have been identified among the tall epithelial cells long before semicircular ducts form.[46] Thus the otocyst is said to 'receive' an afferent or sensory innervation. As long as the adjacent ectoderm of the otocyst remains slightly thinner, it remains uninnervated. Ongoing anterior and dorsal growth of the brain, combined with traction via dendrites at the rostral aspect of the otocyst, causes the otocyst to grow even more asymmetrically and roll over its ganglion, which now becomes located more ventromedially.

At Carnegie Stage 14, the otic vesicle is slightly piriform (pear-shaped) and has a dorsomedial extension called the endolymphatic sac (Figure 30.4).[47] In a 10 mm long embryo viewed from the side (Figure 30.22), the otic vesicle consists of three parts: endolymphatic sac (dorsomedial), anlage of labyrinth (central), and anlage of cochlea (inferior). The overall shape of the central and inferior parts is like a comma. As the otic vesicle grows, the increase in surface area of the central part outstrips the capacity of the otocyst to increase in volume. The dorsolateral region of the otocyst starts to thin (i.e., tall cells become flatter) and the labyrinth begins to collapse. A topographical feature that may be associated with the failure of the volume of this part of the otic vesicle to keep pace with its surface growth, is the proximity of the endolymphatic

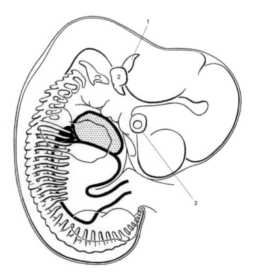

Figure 30.22

Serial section reconstruction of 10 mm long human embryo (Carnegie Stage 17). Skeleton outlined, heart stippled, lung black, and liver white. 1, endolymphatic sac; 2, labyrinth (part of otocyst) with anlage of cochlea below; 3, optic cup with lens vesicle. Thick black line indicates the serosa of the future pericardial and abdominal sacs.

sac to the developing meninges of the brain.[48] Later in embryonic and fetal life, the sac lies epidurally adjacent to a bend in the sigmoid sinus where it remains nestled.[49] The structure of the sac wall suggests that there is a continual leakage of fluid from the more "stagnant" otocyst via the endolymphatic sac into the nearby sigmoid sinus; this hypothesis is supported by studies in the mouse.[50] The phenomenon could be similar to the continual leakage of fluid that occurs from the allantois into the paired umbilical arteries in the embryo's connecting stalk.

During this period of otocyst growth with internal suction, parts of the opposite walls of the dorsal region of the otocyst gradually come into contact with each other. At these sites, according to the rules applying to corrosion fields,[2] the ectodermal cells die, leaving behind only the peripheral zones of the otic vesicle to continue further areal growth. Investigations in animals also demonstrate cell death in the central zone of the labyrinth.[51] In this way, three semicircular ducts arise at the perimeter of the wide part of the otocyst; the order of their appearance is: anterior, posterior, and lateral semicircular duct (Figure 30.23).[52]

In biodynamic embryology, the basis for the mutually perpendicular nature of the three semicircular ducts should be sought in the dynamics of surrounding structures. Blechschmidt's reconstructions of human embryos indicate that there are multiple, aligned

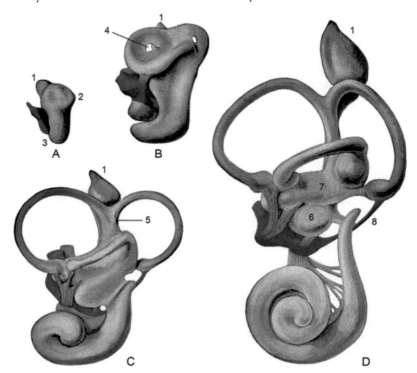

Figure 30.23
Development of left otocyst into membranous labyrinth as seen in lateral views of models, anterior to left of figure (adapted from Arey, 1947). Crown–rump lengths of embryos: A, 6.6 mm; B, 13 mm; C, 20 mm; D, 30 mm. 1, endolymphatic sac; 2, utricular portion of otocyst; 3, cochlear portion of otocyst; 4, corrosion field leading to formation of anterior semicircular duct and common crus; 5, common crus of anterior and posterior semicircular ducts; 6, saccule; 7, utricle; 8, dendrites to crista ampullaris of posterior semicircular duct.

pre-existing tensions in structures that "cradle" the growing otocyst.[1,53] These alignments are: (i) anteriorly, the vertically disposed facial nerve and its ganglion cells, (ii) posteriorly, the vertical glossopharyngeal nerve and its ganglion cells, and (iii) inferolaterally, the longitudinal superior cardinal vein (Figures 30.5 and 30.24). To these tensions one must add a pulsatile, laterally directed growth pressure from the widening brain. Already in embryonic stages, as the head changes position, fluid flows along the walls of the three mutually perpendicular ducts (similar to the movement of a liquid in a spirit-level) thereby leading to stimulation of the sensory nerve fibers. These early functions are a precondition for the subsequent ability of the labyrinth to function as an organ to assist in the maintenance of body equilibrium.

At the ventromedial edge of the otic vesicle (i.e., the sharp end of the comma), the epithelium is innervated by the cochlear nerve, that is, by dendrites of ganglion cells from otic mesectoderm. The tip of the comma has the tallest wedge-shaped cells and exhibits a high rate of surface growth. Nerves accompany this small portion of the otic vesicle as its epithelium grows in surface area and the tip of the comma elongates against the traction of the young dendrites. In comparison to the epithelial surface growth of this part of the otocyst, the dendrites lag a little behind. Due to the restraining action of the dendrites, the tip of the otic vesicle rolls inwards as it grows, so forming the initial coiling of the cochlear duct of the inner ear.[54] The duct spirals around the central axis of traction in the dendrites, called the modiolus. The part of the wall that is thickest becomes the organ of Corti, the thinnest part becomes the vestibular membrane (of Reissner) and the external part of the wall becomes the stria vascularis (Figure 30.25).

The young stria vascularis is a site of tall wedge-shaped epithelial cells with such intensive metabolic activity that the epithelial cells and loops of capillaries interdigitate as they grow, resulting in the development of the only vascularized epithelium in the body. As a sign of this intensive metabolism, melanin is found in deep parts of the epithelial cells of the stria vascularis and in adjacent connective tissue cells, as well as in the modiolus, ampullae, and saccule. In mid-fetal life (20 weeks) epithelial cells containing melanin and its precursors are found in the crista ampullaris, semicircular ducts, and endolymphatic sac;[55] essentially these cells are intra-epithelial melanocytes.

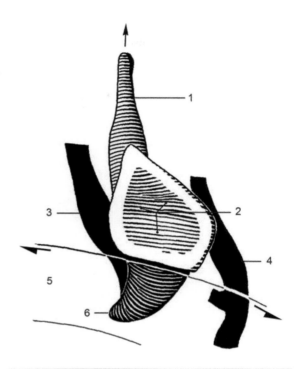

Figure 30.24
Lateral view of anlage of inner ear (left side) of 7.5 mm embryo (Carnegie Stage 16), superior (rostral) to left, dorsal to top. 1, endolymphatic duct; 2, region of flattening of the vestibular part of otocyst (location of future corrosion fields); 3, facial and vestibulocochlear ganglion–nerve complex; 4, glossopharyngeal ganglion and nerve with tympanic nerve (cut) emerging rostrally; 5, outline of superior cardinal vein (rendered transparent) with diverging arrows representing tension in wall; 6, growing apex of cochlear duct (medial to cardinal vein). Simple arrow above endolymphatic duct represents tension between duct and meninx.

At the end of the embryonic period (ca. 8 weeks after conception), the membranous ducts of the labyrinth and cochlea are surrounded by cartilage that is known as the otic capsule, which is derived from otic mesectoderm. From this time onwards the cartilage grows and maintains its external form while fluid spaces enlarge

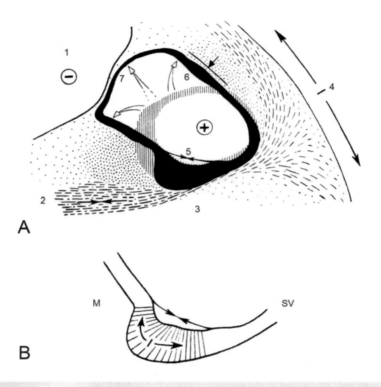

Figure 30.25

(A) Development of cochlea in superimposed drawings at same magnification from basal turn of cochlear duct (+) in 39 mm fetus (vertical lines) and 80 mm fetus (black). The two stages are superimposed with the anlage of the thickest part of each duct in register (this region exhibits greatest anchoring and serves as a reference). 1, scala vestibuli; 2, basilar membrane with dendrites of cochlear nerve; 3, scala tympani; 4, distusion of otic capsule (cartilage); 5, tectorial membrane; 6, stria vascularis; 7, vestibular (Reissner's) membrane. Contoured arrows show direction of growth movements of wall of younger cochlear duct. Simple arrow with cross-bar near 6 indicates growth resistance in vicinity of stria vascularis, resulting in intra-epithelial capillaries. Converging arrows near 2, 5: growth resistance in basilar membrane and tectorial membrane, respectively. The – sign indicates reduced osmotic pressure in scala vestibuli, a region of tissue loosening or cartilage deconsolidation; conversely, + sign in cochlear duct refers to higher osmotic pressure. (B) Schematic diagram of development of organ of Corti in a single turn of cochlear duct in fetuses between 39 mm and 64 mm crown–rump length. Diverging arrows: growth pressure in wall of cochlear duct from tall wedge-shaped cells. Converging arrows: growth resistance on the part of apical cytoplasm (ectoplasm) leading to tectorial jelly being dragged from the tall cells. M, direction of modiolus (central axis of cochlea). SV, direction of stria vascularis (outer wall of cochlear duct).

at the interface between the inner surface of the cartilage and the outer surface of the complex internal form, i.e., the membranous labyrinth. Streeter described this internal "excavation" as dedifferentiation of cartilage to form a watery reticulum and then a system of canals.[56]

The initial motor for the form and development of the capsule is found in the dynamics of growth of the epithelium of the labyrinth, which continues to increase until it achieves its adult dimensions at about 5–6 months in utero. Thus the inner dedifferentiation of otic capsular cartilage must be a consequence of surface growth of an epithelium and piston-like growth of cartilage, whose outer surface grows faster than its inner surface can sustain. Blechschmidt pointed out the similarity between (i) the dedifferentiation of cartilage during growth and remodeling of the otic capsule and (ii) the continual liquefaction of fluid under the parietal pleura during the growth and remodeling of a cartilaginous rib.[1]

In terms of metabolic fields, the formation of endolymph in the scala tympani, scala vestibuli, vestibule, periductal spaces, etc. is partly the consequence of a suction field that arises in the wake of a moving distusion field. The suction field is combined with multiple corrosion fields that destroy the strands of cells that traverse the watery spaces of the reticulum, resulting in canals filled with perilymph that surround the membranous labyrinth.

The ear is not purely sensory – the phenomenon of weak signals (oto-acoustic emissions) that can be recorded from the external auditory canal means that the ear has effector capacities.[57] As well as its afferent (sensory) nerve supply, the inner ear has an efferent nerve supply, the olivocochlear nerve (arising mainly from the contralateral brainstem) that has an inhibitory action on the activity of oto-acoustic emissions from outer hair cells in the organ of Corti. This motor nerve constitutes the basis for a simple clinical neural test in newborns and premature babies.[58,59]

Concerning efferent nerves to the inner ear, it seems logical that the structural and metabolic complexity of the wall of the otocyst could be associated with the capacity to suck up nutrients from the nearby brain, as well as release nutrients for dendrites from the ganglion cells. The metabolic needs of some cells of the otocyst would lead to the drawing in of neurites from the hindbrain, which neurites become the efferent fibers of the olivocochlear bundle. In fact such neurites are found crossing the midline close to the floor-plate of the hindbrain in an 8 mm human embryo (5–6 weeks).[60] The neurites enter the otocyst wall near the junction of its cochlear and utricular portions; they stain intensely in histological sections, suggesting they are sites of high metabolic transfer from the hindbrain to the otocyst. Windle believed that they represent the very first efferent fibers to develop in the human embryo but it is uncertain whether these neurites come into metabolic relation with the wall of the otocyst before, together with, or after the sensory dendrites. In animal studies

(mice and chicks), efferent neurites seem to develop only after afferent dendritic connections are made with the sensory cells of the inner ear.[61–63] However an important study in the chick finds an extremely early emergence of efferent neurites from the brainstem, just as the otic pit is closing at 2.5 days of incubation.[64] In light of the fact that metabolic transfers can occur over distances longer than one or two cell lengths (>50 µm), functional efferent connections could exist between brainstem and otic pit at the same time as afferent connections are forming.

External ear

The growth of the head in a longitudinal arc around the heart leads to compression of the first two pharyngeal folds (visceral arches) in the vicinity of the face. With transverse growth of the brain, the initially small face widens and the sides of the pharyngeal arches become tilted laterally at about 45 degrees to the median plane. The surface growth of the ectoderm of these pharyngeal arches is compromised dorsally by further growth and widening of the brain and ventrally by the enlargement of the heart. Both brain and heart exhibit oscillating, pulsatile growth. Compressed from above as well as below, the initially smooth surface of the first two arches becomes creased transversely, i.e., the transverse creases are compression folds caused by dorsolateral growth of the brain above and an ever-enlarging, beating heart below. These complex creases constitute the initial high and low relief-formation of the external ear, the anlage of the pinna,[65] which is initially just a partial relief of the whole lateral neck region (Figure 30.26). Isolated bumps or so-called auditory hillocks that are not related to any of the above dynamic factors are never observed in young human embryos.

Blechschmidt traced the growth dynamics for the densation field that leads to the helix of the pinna (Figure 30.27) as well as the antihelix.[28,65] The main events are extension of the head, formation of the neck, and traction between the head, face, and sternum. He also noted the formal similarity between the internal ear and the external ear.[1] The intricate folding of the external ear is no less striking in adults than its biodynamics are in the embryo.

The groove between the 1st and 2nd pharyngeal arches is very deep and the foregut endoderm of the 1st pharyngeal pouch lies so close to the ectoderm, that the ear drum (tympanic membrane) arises here as a thin

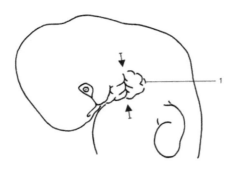

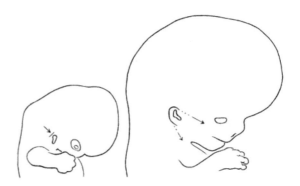

Figure 30.26
Head region of 11 mm human embryo (Carnegie Stage 17) already showing alternating high and low transverse reliefs, which represent collectively the anlage of auricle or pinna (1). Tailed arrows represent growth compression from hindbrain above and heart below.

Figure 30.27
External ear development in embryos 15.5 mm (Carnegie Stage 18) and 29.5 mm (Carnegie Stage 23) drawn at same scale. Left: arrow and line indicates direction of impediment to skin growth at posterior border of external ear, mainly due to widening of brain and head. Right: arrows indicate directions of traction from continuous collagen fibers into tendon of sternocleidomastoid muscle and periosteum of zygomatic bone, respectively; this traction changes the architecture of pinna. Note the elongation of neck and mandible in older embryo.

sheet of tissue that is the medial boundary of the external ear (Figure 30.21). As long as the face remains relatively small, the growth of the brain forces the side of the head to incline obliquely outwards. The tympanic membrane also conforms to this oblique inclination, just like the pinna.

Middle ear

The tympanic membrane, being the floor of the groove between the 1st and 2nd pharyngeal arches, is the boundary between the external auditory meatus and an internal passageway, the tubotympanic recess of the 1st pharyngeal pouch, which is the anlage of the Eustachian tube. This tube, which is initially a slit-like recess, remains throughout life as a deep diverticulum in the lateral wall of the pharynx. Infections may lead to swelling in the walls of this tube and its closure can temporarily impair hearing ability.

The dorsal, blind-ended part of this recess located deep to the tympanic membrane is called the middle ear. The inner tissue that underlies the endoderm lining the

middle ear is derived from the 1st and 2nd pharyngeal arches. During the embryonic period, the three auditory ossicles (malleus/hammer, incus/anvil, and stapes/stirrup) start to arise in the inner tissue here, each in a precise sequence of densation field, contusion field (precartilage), distusion field (cartilage), and detraction field (bone).[2,28] In principle, the dynamics of the sequence for the formation of an ossicle is no different to that occurring, say, in the terminal phalanx of a finger. In each case, the sequence is initiated by early changes in the contour of the local, adjacent limiting tissue, irrespective of whether it is ectoderm or endoderm. The origin of the unique form of each tiny middle ear bone must be sought in the form and surface growth of the endoderm in relation to the underlying inner tissue, adjacent nerves and vessels, i.e., the cause of the shape of the stirrup is not to be found solely in the anlage of the stirrup. As in limb development,[1,2,28,37] a subtle change in the external contour of the wedge-shaped cells of the epithelium is always the precondition for the position and form of a particular densation field. In the middle ear, the ossicles are always covered by a thin layer of endoderm and remain attached by ligaments to the endodermal walls where the undulations originally appeared. The auditory ossicles are the first bones in the body to attain their adult shape and size.

Mastoid air cells

In principle the future air cells of the middle ear arise in the same way as the paranasal sinuses, only later. In the case of the middle ear, a growing endodermal mucosa covers the bones, ligaments, nerves, tendons, and muscles that are often described (incorrectly) as lying inside the middle ear chamber. These elements are no more "inside" the middle ear than loops of gastro-intestinal tract are inside the peritoneal sac; topologically, the mucosa of the middle ear is no different to visceral and parietal peritoneum. The epithelium lining the air cells is strongly adherent to the bone and is known as mucoperiosteum.

After birth the fluid in the middle ear chamber is replaced by air. In response to traction in the sternocleidomastoid muscle, the mastoid process elongates and the endoderm grows in surface area internally forming an increasing number of diverticula (air cells). It may be anticipated that the deconsolidation and remodeling of connective tissue that accompanies the surface growth of the endoderm in forming the increasing number of air cells has similar biodynamics to the dedifferentiation of cartilage that occurs in the otic capsule and paranasal sinuses, as well as on the pleural side of the growing ribs as mentioned above.

Taste

Taste is a sense associated with tiny local thickenings of epithelium, taste buds, which can arise almost anywhere on the oronasolaryngeal surface. Taste buds are associated with various forms of inner tissue elevations or papillae. Of course the main organ associated with taste is the tongue, which itself starts life as a tiny epithelial papilla on the floor of the embryo's mouth. Since it is difficult to define the boundary between ectoderm and endoderm in the floor of the embryonic mouth,[66] it remains possible that part of the surface of the tongue is derived from ectoderm; some believe that most of the body of the

tongue anterior to its foramen cæcum and terminal sulcus is covered by ectoderm from the 1st and 2nd pharyngeal arches and innvervated by dendrites from their respective cranial nerves.[67] Irrespective of how much of the tongue's epithelium is from ectoderm or endoderm, we can envisage that its surface becomes innervated during embryonic life according to the growth rules for dendrites and tall, wedge-shaped cells described above.

Despite much work in animals (fish, chick, and rat) indicating the importance of nerve fibers for taste bud differentiation,[68] there is scant information about the development of taste buds in human embryos. It is known that initially taste buds are relatively more widespread in the fetal oral epithelium than in the mouth of the adult, possible due to an initial overproduction.[69] The number of taste buds decreases throughout life,[70] although the sense of taste may not necessarily diminish. On the other hand, taste buds can regenerate provided that sensory dendrites are nearby.[71]

Taste buds may be found almost anywhere in the stratified squamous oral epithelium, on the free edge of the soft palate, on both surfaces of the epiglottis, and even in the larynx; buds are also found in palatal ciliated epithelium that is characteristic of respiratory mucosa.[72] Indeed the actual taste bud is similar in structure to the neuro-epithelial body of bronchi, the development of which does not appear to have been studied in humans.[73–75]

Electron microscopical studies on human embryos and fetuses suggest that taste buds mature between the end of the embryonic period (ca. 8 weeks) and about week 14, when the buds have an "adult" morphology.[76] This study confirms that the origin of taste buds starts with a local thickening of the oral epithelium, whereby the basal cells become markedly elongated and a basement membrane soon condenses around the dendrites that then traverse it. At this stage the tall sensory cells remain covered by a single layer of flat cells (a kind of "periderm"); by week 9 or 10, the taste cells have apical microvilli that project directly to the oral surface and connective tissue papillae are distinct.[76] The anlage of the taste bud could be likened to a "mini" placode that acquires dendritic innervation from cells in ganglia of the 7th, 9th, and 10th cranial nerves.

As with Merkel cells described above, Arey's studies show that single taste buds are intimately associated with the development of lingual papillae. Epithelial thickening precedes the appearance of each fungiform papilla. With papillary growth a single bud occupies its top (oral) surface. Later several taste buds arise on the upper surface of the larger vallate papilla. The often-repeated claim that the buds on the top of a vallate papilla die before birth and are replaced by definitive buds in the inner and outer walls of the deeper "moat" of the vallate papilla ignores the local growth dynamics of the papilla. Any translational (planar) movement of the epithelium of a papilla, which is known to occur in skin in the creation of whorls, etc.[14,15], may simply carry the taste buds to the lateral walls.

Clearly the development of human taste buds needs to be re-investigated from a biodynamic viewpoint, with respect to the areal growth and surface contour of the wedge-shaped epithelial cells, the restraining action of dendrites and vessels, and the consolidation of the connective tissue into a papilla. The fact that taste buds are already contacted by dendrites in an 8-week-old embryo suggests that they must be defined long before this stage, at a time when the ends of the dendrites may not even be in the same field of view of the electron microscope as the cells of the future taste bud.

Similar considerations also apply to other aspects of human sensory development not covered in this chapter, including early dendritic innervation of the carotid body, teeth, and muscle spindles, the development of the terminal nerve and ganglion, efferent neurites to the retina, etc. Some information may be uncovered by a closer study of Blechschmidt's publications[77] (e.g., his papers on tooth development) but other data will require re-appraisal of "conventional" anatomical studies from a biodynamic perspective as well as completely new investigations. The vomeronasal organ (of Jacobson)[78] represents a particularly interesting case for a biodynamic study in human embryos: some authors have commented that the organ seems to arise by being "torn off from the nasal mucosa,"[79] suggesting a strong biomechanical tension between the brain and the mucosa.

To comprehend any sensory organ or ensemble of cells, future studies must: (i) examine the spatiotemporal growth of surrounding organs and structures, (ii) consider the local biomechanical forces at work, and (iii) avoid the prejudices of chemical thinking ("molecular biology") in embryology.[m]

---

[m]A more complete list of Blechschmidt's publications,

ACKNOWLEDGMENTS

The author is grateful for assistance from the publishers listed below.

Figures 30.1, 30.2B, 30.3–30.6, 30.7B, 30.8, 30.10, 30.16, 30.17, 30.19, 30.20–30.22, 30.26 are taken with permission of the publisher from *The Ontogenetic Basis of Human Anatomy: A Biodynamic Approach to Development from Conception to Birth* by Erich Blechschmidt, edited and translated by Brian Freeman, published by North Atlantic Books, copyright © 2004 by Traute Blechschmidt. Figure 30.2A is modified with permission from Muster-Schmidt Verlag, Göttingen. Figure 30.9 is reproduced with permission of C.M. Blechschmidt from *Humanembryologie. Prinzipien und Grundbegriffe* by Erich Blechschmidt, Stuttgart: Hippokrates, 1974 (Abb. 4/7, Abb. 4/8). Figures 30.11 and 30.12 are reproduced from reference 27, Figures 30.13, 30.14, 30.15 are from reference 30, and Figure 30.27 is from reference 60, all with permission of S. Karger AG, Basel. Figure 30.18 is reproduced from reference 34 with permission from Schweizerbart'sche Verlagsbuchhandlung (www.schweizerbart.de). Figure 30.23 is reproduced from reference 43 with permission of Elsevier. Figures 30.24 and 30.25 are modified from references 53 and 54, respectively, with permission of Springer Science+Business Media. Figure 30.7A is redrawn from reference 26.

References

[1]Blechschmidt E. (1948) Mechanische Genwirkungen. Göttingen: Musterschmidt

[2]Blechschmidt E. (2004) The Ontogenetic Basis of Human Anatomy. A Biodynamic Approach to Development from Conception to Birth. Berkeley: North Atlantic. (translation of Anatomie und Ontogenese des Menschen. Quelle u. Meyer, Heidelberg, 1978)

[3]O'Rahilly R, Müller F. (1987) Developmental Stages in Human Embryos. Washington: Carnegie Institution Publication 637

[4]Blechschmidt E (1951) Die frühembryonale Lageentwicklung der Gliedmaßen. Entwicklung der Extremitäten beim Menschen. Teil I). Z Anat Entwickl-Gesch 115: 529–540

---

including some from his students, etc. may be found at http://www.drawingonanatomy.com.au.

[5]Blechschmidt E (1969) Differenzierungen im kinetischen Feld (Entstehungsbedingungen der Metamerie). Acta Anat 73: 351–371

[6]Blechschmidt E, Daikoku S (1966) Die regionale Verschiedenheit embryonaler Dendriten und Neuriten (Elektronenmikroskopische Untersuchung). Acta Anat 65: 30–57

[7]Blechschmidt E (1977) The programming of afferent and efferent nervous fibers in man. Arch Psychiat Nervenkr 224: 259–272

[8]Szeder V, Grim M, Halata Z, Sieber-Blum M (2003) Neural crest origin of mammalian Merkel cells. Dev Biol 253: 258–63

[9]Pac L (1984) Contribution to ontogenesis of Merkel cells. Z Mikroskop-Anat Forsch 98: 36–48

[10]Moore SJ, Munger BL (1989) The early ontogeny of the afferent nerves and papillary ridges in human digital glabrous skin. Brain Res Dev Brain Res 48: 119–141

[11]Moll I, Moll R (1993) Merkel cells in ontogenesis of human nails. Arch Dermatol Res 285: 366–371

[12]Morohunfola KA, Jones TE, Munger BL (1992) The differentiation of the skin and its appendages. I. Normal development of papillary ridges. Anat Rec 232: 587–598

[13]Irmak MK (2010) Multifunctional Merkel cells: Their roles in electromagnetic reception, finger-print formation, Reiki, epigenetic inheritance and hair form. Med Hypoth 75: 162–168

[14]Blechschmidt E (1963) Die Gestaltungsfunktionen der menschlichen Oberhaut. I. Mitteilung. Die Schichtenbildung des Integuments. Arch klin exper Dermat 215: 567–578

[15]Blechschmidt E (1963) Die embryonalen Gestaltungsfunktionen der menschlichen Oberhaut. II. Mitteilung: Die Entstehung des Papillarkörpers in den proximalen und distalen Abschnitten der Fingerbeere. Z Morphol Anthrop 54: 163–172

[16]Schmidt SS (1964) Die Entstehung der digitalen Tastballen. Z Morph Anthrop 55: 1–10

[17]Riegel P (1965) Die Frühentwicklung der Ultrastruktur in der Epidermis menschlicher Embryonen. Z Morphol Anthrop 56: 195–205

[18]Djordjevic-Camba V, Unkovic N, Mrvaljevic D, Unkovic S, Bumbasirevic V (1980) [Morphologic study of Wagner-Meissner corpuscles in the skin of the right index finger during ontogenetic development]. [Serbian] Srpski Arhiv Za Celokupno Lekarstvo 108: 21–26

[19]Renehan WE, Munger BL (1990) The development of Meissner corpuscles in primate digital skin. Brain Res Dev Brain Res. 51: 35–44

[20]Saxod R (1996) Ontogeny of the cutaneous sensory organs. Microsc Res Tech 34: 313–333

[21]Gammon GD, Bronk DW (1935) The discharge of impulses from Pacinian corpuscles in the mesentery and its relation to vascular changes. Am J Physiol 114: 77–84

[22]Munger BL, Ide C (1987) The enigma of sensitivity in Pacinian corpuscles: a critical review and hypothesis of mechano-electric transduction. Neurosci Res 5: 1–15

[23]Takashi M, Sakai I, Usizima H (1955) On the terminal neural apparatus detectable in the retroperitoneum of man – a complex pattern of Pacinian corpuscle. Anat Rec 122: 17–38

[24]Takashi M (1957) On the development of the complex pattern of Pacinian corpuscle in the human retroperitoneum. Anat Rec 128: 665–678

[25]Cauna N, Mannan G (1959) Development and postnatal changes of digital Pacinian corpuscles (Corpuscula lamellosa) in the human hand. J Anat 93: 271–286

[26]Lydecken K (1966) Die foetale Entstehung der Lamellenkörperchen in den Extremitäten. Ann Acad Scien Fenn A 122: 1–24

[27]Blechschmidt E (1967) Die Entwicklungsbewegungen der menschlichen Augenblase. Ihre Bedeutung für die frühe Gesichtsbildung. Ophthalmol 153: 291–308

[28]Blechschmidt E. (1961) The Stages of Human Development Before Birth. Basel: Karger

[29]Bartelmez GW, Blount MP (1954) The formation of neural crest from the primary optic vesicle in man. Carnegie Institution of Washington Publication 603, Contributions to Embryology 35: 55–71

[30]Blechschmidt E (1967) Die Entwicklungsbewegungen der menschlichen Retina zur Zeit der Irisenentstehung. Die Entstehung des Ganglion opticum als Beispiel einer submikroskopisch untersuchbaren Entstehung einer Cytoarchitektonik. Ophthalmol 154: 531–550

[31]Blechschmidt E (1957) Vacuolisierungsvorgänge in den embryonalen Meningen und im Neuralrohr. (Be-

biodynamic perspective

iträge zur Entwicklungskinetik). Z Anat Entwickl-Gesch 120: 45–71

[32]Rhodes RH (1979) A light microscopic study of the developing human neural retina. Am J Anat 154: 195–210

[33]Blechschmidt E (1950) Über die Wachstumsbewegungen der Hautorgane bei menschlichen Embryonen. Z Anat Entwickl-Gesch 115: 224–248

[34]Blechschmidt E (1957) Die Differenzierungsbewegungen der menschlichen Nase. Z Morphol Anthrop 48: 213–226

[35]Blechschmidt M (1976) The Biokinetics of the Basicranium. In: Bosma JF (Ed) Symposium on Development of the Basicranium. DHEW Publ (NIH) 76-989, NIH, Bethesda, pp. 44–53

[36]Broman I. (1927) Die Entwicklung des Menschen vor der Geburt. München: Bergmann, p. 91

[37]Blechschmidt E, Gasser R. (1978) Biokinetics and Biodynamics of Human Differentiation. Principles and Applications. Thomas, Springfield, Illinois, p. 269

[38]Igarashi Y (1980) Cochlea of the human fetus: a scanning electron microscope study. Arch Histol Jap 43: 195–209

[39]Birnholz JC, Benacerraf BR (1983) The development of human fetal hearing. Science 222: 516–518

[40]Lind J (1980) Music and the small human being. Acta Pæd Scand 69: 131–136

[41]Bialek W (1987) Physical limits to sensation and perception. Ann Rev Biophys Biophys Chem 16: 455–478

[42]Blechschmidt E (1956) Entwicklungsfunktionelle Untersuchungen am embryonalen Eingeweidesystem. (Bauprinzipien der Eingeweide, Beobachtungen zur Frage der funktionellen Bedeutung des Keilepithels und der ventrikulären Mitosen). Morphol Jb 96: 393–416

[43]Arey LB. (1947) Developmental Anatomy. A Textbook and Laboratory Manual of Embryology. Philadelphia: Saunders

[44]Hinrichsen KV. (1990/1993) Humanembryologie. Berlin: Springer, p. 502

[45]Politzer G (1956) Die Entstehung des Ganglion Acusticum beim Menschen. Acta Anat 26: 1–13

[46]Yokoh Y (1971) Early formation of nerve fibers in the human otocyst. Acta Anat 80: 99–106

[47]O'Rahilly R (1963) The early development of the otic vesicle in staged human embryos. J Embryol exp Morph 11: 741–755

[48]Blechschmidt E. (1961) The Stages of Human Development Before Birth. Basel: Karger, p.310

[49]Lo WWM, Daniels DL, Chakeres DW, Linthicum FH Jr, Ulmer JL, Mark LP, Swartz JD (1997) The endolymphatic duct and sac. Am J Neuroradiol 18: 881–887

[50]Hultcrantz M, Bagger-Sjöbäck D, Rask-Andersen H (1987) The development of the endolymphatic sac and duct. Acta Otolaryngol 104: 406–416

[51]Fekete DM, Homburger SA, Waring MT, Riedl AE, Garcia LF (1997) Involvement of programmed cell death in morphogenesis of the vertebrate inner ear. Development 124: 2451–2461

[52]Streeter GL (1906) On the development of the membranous labyrinth and the acoustic and facial nerves in the human embryo. Am J Anat 6: 139–165

[53]Blechschmidt M (1982) Das frühembryonale Wachstum des Labyrinths. Arch Oto-Rhino-Laryngol 234: 293–303

[54]Blechschmidt E (1952) Funktionsentwicklung des Corti'schen Organs. Arch Ohr–, Nas–Kehlk–Heilk 162: 35–52

[55]Igarashi Y (1989) Submicroscopic study of the vestibular dark cell area in human fetuses. Acta Otolaryngol 107: 29–38

[56]Streeter GL (1917) The factors involved in the excavation of the cavities in the cartilaginous capsule of the ear in the human embryo. Am J Anat 22: 1–25

[57]Kemp DT (1978) Stimulated acoustic emissions from within the human auditory system. J Acoust Soc Am 64:1386–1391

[58]Di Girolamo S, Napolitano B, Alessandrini M, Bruno E (2007) Experimental and clinical aspects of the efferent auditory system. Acta Neurochir - Suppl 97: 419–424

[59]Gkoritsa E, Tsakanikos M, Korres S, Dellagrammaticas H, Apostolopoulos N, Ferekidis E (2006) Transient otoacoustic emissions in the detection of olivocochlear bundle maturation. Int J Ped Otorhinolaryngol 70: 671–676

[60]Windle WF (1970) Development of neural elements in human embryos of four to seven weeks gestation. Exp Neurol Suppl 5: 44–83

[61]Anniko M, Nordemar H, Sobin A (1983) Principles in embryonic development and differentiation of vestibular hair cells. Otolaryngol Head & Neck Surg 91: 540–549

[62]Whitehead MC, Morest DK (1985) The development of innervation patterns in the avian cochlea. Neuroscience 14: 255–276

[63]Fritzsch B, Nichols DH (1993) DiI reveals a prenatal arrival of efferents at the differentiating otocyst of mice. Hear Res 65: 51–60

[64]Fritzsch B, Christensen MA, Nichols DH (1993) Fiber pathways and positional changes in efferent perikarya of 2.5- to 7-day chick embryos as revealed with DiI and dextran amines. J Neurobiol 24: 1481–1499

[65]Blechschmidt E (1955) Entwicklungsfunktionelle Untersuchungen an der menschlichen Ohrmuschel. Acta Anat 25: 204–220

[66]Hinrichsen KV (1990/1993) Intestinaltrackt. In: Humanembryologie, ed. KV Hinrichsen. Berlin: Springer, p. 518

[67]Arey LB (1974) Developmental Anatomy. A Textbook and Laboratory Manual of Embryology. Philadelphia: Saunders, p. 233

[68]Oakley B (1998) Taste neurons have multiple inductive roles in mammalian gustatory development. Ann NY Acad Sci 855: 50–577

[69]Hinrichsen KV (1990/1993) Intestinaltrackt. In: Humanembryologie, ed. KV Hinrichsen. Berlin: Springer, p. 523

[70]Arey LB, Tremaine MJ, Monzingo FL (1935) The numerical and topographical relations of taste buds to human circumvallate papillae throughout the life span. Anat Rec 64: 9–25

[71]Arey LB, Monzingo FL (1942) Can hypoglossal nerve fibers induce the formation of taste buds? Quart Bull Northwestern Univ Med Sch 16: 170–178

[72]Lalonde ER, Eglitis JA (1961) Number and distribution of taste buds on the epiglottis, pharynx, larynx, soft palate and uvula in a human newborn. Anat Rec 140: 91–95

[73]Hoyt RF Jr, McNelly NA, Sorokin SP (1990) Dynamics of neuroepithelial body (NEB) formation in developing hamster lung: light microscopic autoradiography after 3H-thymidine labeling in vivo. Anat Rec 227: 340–350

[74]Haller CJ (1994) A scanning and transmission electron microscopic study of the development of the surface structure of neuroepithelial bodies in the mouse lung. Micron. 25: 527–538

[75]Van Lommel A (2001) Pulmonary neuroendocrine cells (PNEC) and neuroepithelial bodies (NEB): chemoreceptors and regulators of lung development. Paed Resp Rev 2: 171–176

[76]Witt M, Reutter K (1996) Embryonic and early fetal development of human taste buds: a transmission electron microscopical study. Anat Rec 246: 507–523

[77]In memoriam des Anatomen und Embryologen Erich Blechschmidt (1904–1992). Ann Anat 174: 479–484

[78]Blechschmidt E. (1961) The Stages of Human Development Before Birth. Basel: Karger, p. 168

[79]Kjær I, Keeling JW, Hansen BF. (1999) The Prenatal Human Cranium. Copenhagen: Munksgaard, p. 76

31

The brain as a morphogenetic field

Patrick van den Heede, Rüdiger Goldenstein and Torsten Liem

The brain is a constantly changing morphogenetic field. It uses the patterns of development as hinge points for the integration of past and future. In this process, references to the basic state are created via various neutral points. Information is transformed into energetic values, ranging from chemical-electrical through electrical to electromagnetic elements ('bits' of information).

By means of these processes, the brain creates memory as 'bits' of information are assembled. These processes help control actions and build up patterns of relationship in time. The body receives feedback information and organization is created through changes in tonicity, position and anatomical and physiological adaptation. Transitions between matter and energy are accompanied by the brain's developmental history – its molecular, neurochemical and electrochemical history in its various stages of development.

Biophysical components are a determining factor in organization and the development of structure. During the course of its development, each brain is to an extent supported and fixed in and through a development fulcrum (which is itself more or less fixed).

Structural and functional patterns of the brain

Vectorial patterns:

Myelin structure of the brain of varying densities. (Caudal – rostral, posterior – anterior, medial – lateral — capsules, corpus callosum and commissures)

Positional patterns:

Three main, developmentally determined, positional patterns can be distinguished:

- caudo-rostral development, brain stem (more or less stable).
- limbic; C - shaped (dynamic).
- cortical; internal – external and C – shaped (depending on the predominant developmental dynamics).

Positions and patterns of development:

The various parts of the body work together to create a defined functional structure. Flexures, ventricles, meninges and vascularization play an important role in shaping the adult brain.

Morphodynamic patterns create a primary space/time program for these processes of development. Electrochemical patterns for the development of the mature brain (determined by genes, neuromodulators and neuronal differentiation) also play a role in this, as do electrical frequencies, and wave patterns and rhythms. There is also a connection between structures and developmental fields of various kinds.

Integrative morphology

In integrative morphodynamic therapy, we follow the rhythms and relationships of the various developmental patterns in our palpation. The developmental dynamics of the nervous system are described in detail elsewhere and so do not need to be repeated here.

Just as happens in the rest of the body, the brain is formed by the developmental processes and in turn forms the bony cranium. Interrelationships are retained. Following the principles put forward by Blechschmidt, further molecular components are now known in addition to the morphomechanical components. Some of these are epigenetically or genetically determined. Other influences are also being considered, for example energetic effects.

The following two basic developmental patterns, summarized briefly here, provide the preparatory context for the practical section: the formation of the midline, and the development of further axes and symmetries in the developing system.

Axiality and symmetry of the neuroectoderm (the future brain)

These illustrations (Figures 31.1 and 31.2) show that basic patterns such as symmetry and axiality are present from the earliest stages of development. It is

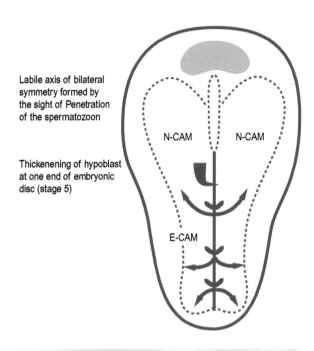

Labile axis of bilateral symmetry formed by the sight of Penetration of the spermatozoon

Thickenening of hypoblast at one end of embryonic disc (stage 5)

N-CAM   N-CAM

E-CAM

Figure 31.1
Development of axes and symmetries under the influence of molecules responsible for development (N-CAM, E.CAM: adhesion molecules, Neurothelial and Endothelial Cell Adhesion Molecules; SHH: Sonic HedgeHog: signal molecule.)

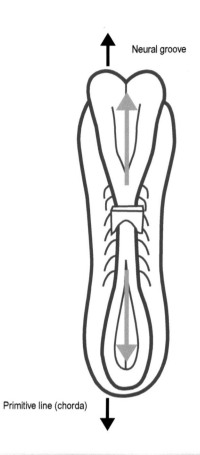

Neural groove

Primitive line (chorda)

Figure 31.2
Formation of the midline.

around these patterns that the body orients itself in the course of development, as the fully developed form takes shape. These two basic patterns provide the initial orientation for the practitioner.

Practical aspects

Basic considerations relating to all palpation of the brain:

Although we cannot contact the brain directly, we can receive the impression of palpation of the various levels, anatomical structures and functional and developmental motions using imagination of the anatomical structures. We can interpret these in accordance with embryological developmental patterns.

In the context of treatment, we follow the developmental patterns of the hinge points. Fulcrums are created here both in and between various tissues. This brings about a fresh balance, which usually involves less tension for the body, so reducing the amount of energy being expended.

Preparation:

For this type of palpation, it is important for practitioners to constantly refresh their awareness of their own position in the room, their own midlines and tensions. This ensures that they do not interpret their own patterns of tension as those of the client.

In practice, then, practitioners should center themselves before taking up the contact, so as to fine-tune their perception and become receptive. As soon as contact with the patient has been established, practitioners should check this centering of themselves once more.

In your role as practitioner you should ask yourself the following questions:

- Where do I, as the practitioner, sense the greatest stillness in myself?

- What is the most efficient way for me to sit or stand?

- How do I achieve the ideal degree of relaxation in myself for carrying out the palpation?

Road maps through the brain

1 Palpation of the depths of brain levels by palpation of growth dynamics of the brain.

2 Palpation of brain position and dynamics in relation to developmental dynamics.

3 Palpation of memories of hinge points of brain development. (Example: Zero point of motion).

Palpation of different depths of the brain

The sections illustrated in Figures 31.4–31.6 show three anatomical regions at different depths, which are differently perceived by palpation:

The cerebral cortex (pallium), region of the commissures, and central nuclei.

These three different levels represent parts of the brain that are different in terms of the evolutionary development. These are also reflected in ontogenesis. Hence we are able to 'grasp' not only developmental patterns that take place over time, but also the functions associated with these regions.

Palpation detects the following three growth movements:

1 <u>Dorsal growth:</u> It feels as if the brain is rising or descending in your palpating hands. This is the growth movement of the deepest level.

2 <u>Radial growth:</u> The brain expands in your palpating hands and there is a sense of distension. This is the middle level.

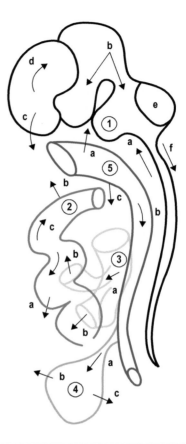

Figure 31.3
Illustrating developmental dynamics. Drawing by P van den Heede.

3 <u>Appositional growth:</u> It feels as if the brain is folding in your palpating hands, and the gyri are taking shape (like the growth of a cauliflower). This is the outermost level, the newest in terms of the developmental history.

Palpation of the different levels of the brain, described

As we practice and develop the capacity to palpate the different levels of the brain, this enables us to comprehend the first developmental patterns of the brain. As it

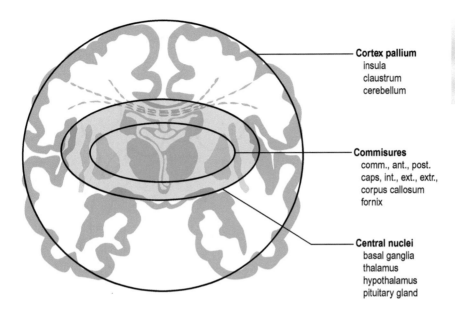

Cortex pallium
   insula
   claustrum
   cerebellum

Commisures
   comm., ant., post.
   caps, int., ext., extr.,
   corpus callosum
   fornix

Central nuclei
   basal ganglia
   thalamus
   hypothalamus
   pituitary gland

Figure 31.4
The three different depths of palpation: coronal section.

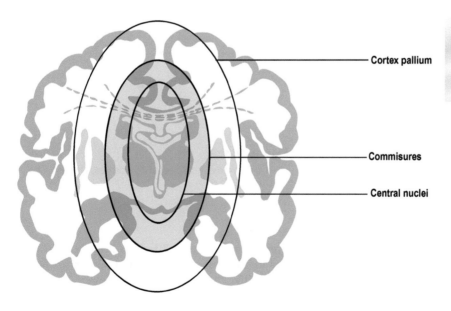

Cortex pallium

Commisures

Central nuclei

Figure 31.5
The three different depths of palpation: frontal section.

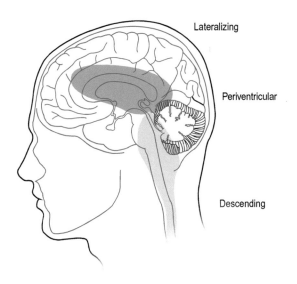

Figure 31.6
The three different depths of palpation: sagittal section.

Lateralizing

Periventricular

Descending

develops, the brain takes shape by performing various developmental movements. The levels represent different partial regions of the brain, each with different degrees of myelination, neuron density and structure.

The patient lies supine and relaxed, leaving sufficient space at the head end of the treatment table for the practitioner's forearms or elbows (depending on the particular hold being used for contact).

This enables the creation of the appropriate fulcrum without any further effort during the palpation itself. If wished, you can help the patient to achieve better relaxation by placing a support under the patient's knees, or by raising the patient's feet.

- Practitioner: Before taking up contact, center yourself as previously described (see 'Preparation' above).

- Hand position: Place the fingers of each hand gently on each side of the parietal bones with a gentle contact. Your thumbs should be touching, above the sagittal suture, so as to create a fulcrum. (See Figures 31.7-31.9)

Once you have taken up the contact, wait to discover what information on the individual developmental patterns reaches your hands. You use this as your guide

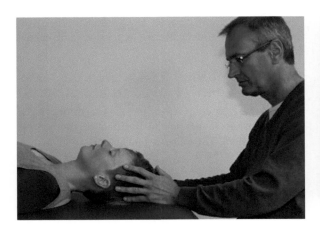

Figure 31.7
Palpation of different levels of the brain.

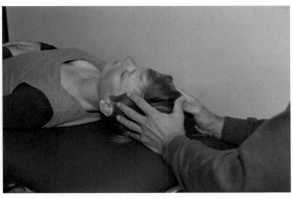

Figure 31.8
Palpation of the position of the central nervous system.

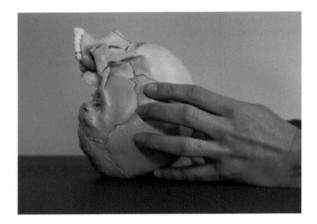

Figure 31.9
Palpation of the bony structures.

Growth of cortex

1	Dorsal growth 'The brain ascends/descends in the palpating hands'
2	Radial growth 'The brain expands in the palpating hands'
2	Appositional growth 'The brain bulges in the palpating hands'

Figure 31.10
The three different growth dynamics.

---

to help you perceive the different levels and their developmental dynamics.

This palpation exercise prepares you to assess the influences and pivot points of brain development, to assess different regions of the brain and the patterns of relationship to other organs and developments of organs.

The growth dynamics can be sensed not only at the brain, but also at the spinal cord (Figure 31.11)

It is also helpful to use this form of palpation following medullary contusion. The patterns of tension shown in Figure 31.12 should be assessed in this case.

You need to assess when and which region the compression occurred. The following causes may account for the compression:

- Prenatal compression (uterine, pelvis, umbilical cord?).
- Perinatal (forceps delivery/sacral compression).
- Postnatal manipulation.
- Postnatal trauma (blows/impact, contusion, surgical operations).
- Trauma affecting the adult (whiplash injury, emotional trauma).

The approach from here on is to balance the corresponding space-time patterns of tension and enable tissue release.

Palpation: position of the central nervous system (brain and spinal cord).

The task here, in contrast to the assessment of growth movements, is to assess the position of the central nervous system. The following positions can be distinguished:

1 "Ascended" – "descended" brain

2 Global retroposition

3 Global anteposition

Course of palpation:

The patient lies supine and relaxed, leaving sufficient space at the head end of the treatment table for the practitioner's forearms or elbows (depending on the particular hold being used for contact). This enables the creation of the appropriate fulcrum without any

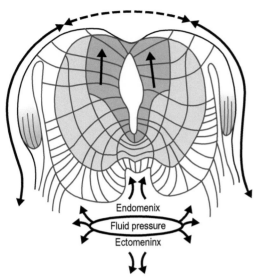

Dorsal appositional growth

Nervous system
(after Blechschmidt and Gasser)

Dorsal appositional growth is identical
for spinal cord as for brain development

The brain ascends/descends in the
palpating hands'

Parenchymal expansion field

Endomenix
Fluid pressure
Ectomeninx

Basal restraining function of ectomeninx

Figure 31.11
Growth dynamics in the
spinal cord.

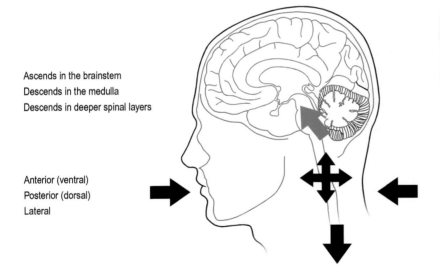

Ascends in the brainstem
Descends in the medulla
Descends in deeper spinal layers

Anterior (ventral)
Posterior (dorsal)
Lateral

Figure 31.12
Patterns of tension
appearing following
contusion.

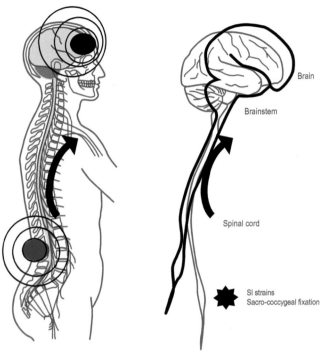

Brain

Brainstem

Spinal cord

SI strains
Sacro-coccygeal fixation

Global ascent or superior position of medullo-cortical unit

Figure 31.13
Palpatory impression of the global ascent of the central nervous system.

Brain

Brainstem

Foramen magnum:
brain stem

CO/C1 strains

Spinal cord

Fixation at filum terminale
Sacro-coccygeal fixation

Global descent or inferior position of medullo-cortical unit

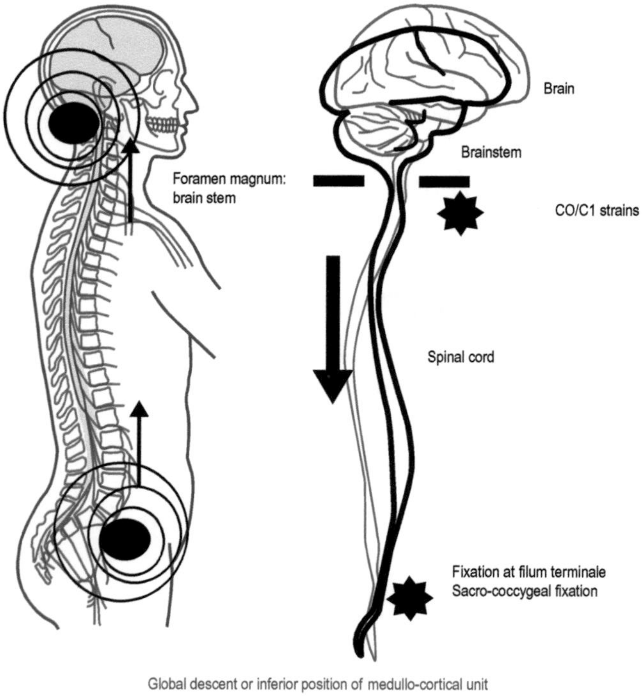

Figure 31.14
Palpatory impression of the global descent of the central nervous system.

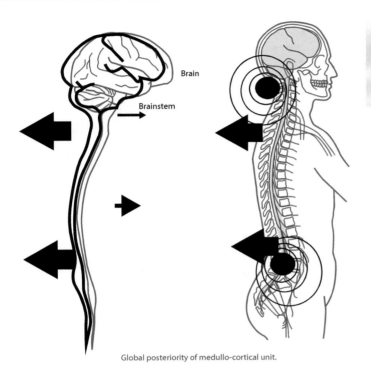

Brain

Brainstem

Global posteriority of medullo-cortical unit.

Figure 31.15
Palpatory impression of the global retroposition of the central nervous system.

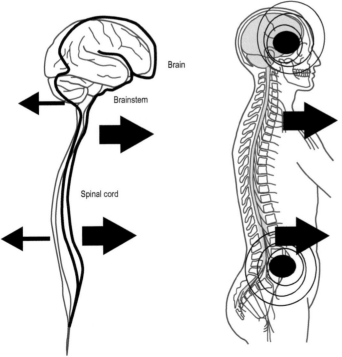

Brain

Brainstem

Spinal cord

Global anteriority of medullo-cortical unit

Figure 31.16
Palpatory impression of the global anteposition of the central nervous system.

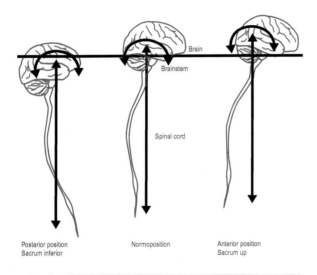

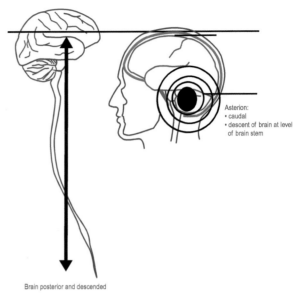

Figure 31.17
Relationships between the position of the central nervous system (brain and spinal cord) and that of the sacrum.

Figure 31.18
A posterior, descended position. Note the difference in the caudad perpendicular in comparison with the previous figures.

further effort during the palpation itself. If wished, you can help the patient to achieve better relaxation by placing a support under the patient's knees, or by raising the patient's feet.

- Practitioner: Before taking up contact, center yourself as previously described (see 'Preparation' above).

- Hand position: Place the fingers of each hand gently on each side of the parietal bones with a gentle contact. Your thumbs should be touching, above the sagittal suture, so as to create a fulcrum. (See Figures 31.7-31.9) Once you have taken up the particular contact, wait to discover what information on the position of the central nervous system reaches your hands.

The following positions – illustrated below – can be found. (The Figures represent an idealized form. Various kinds of rotation and lateral variation are also possible.)

In embryological development, the CNS executes developmental movements as demonstrated (for example) by Blechschmidt. Palpation should assess what information we receive about the brain and spinal cord regarding their position.

All these positions are associated with certain hinge points, around which developments of movement take place. As palpation proceeds, we can build up fulcrums relating to these points and establish relationships with other developments of organs within the body as well as with emotional states.

Palpation of the "zero point of motion"

There is a 'null point' in embryological developmental movements at the notochord (*chorda dorsalis*). What this means is that this is a point around which all developmental movements are organized, but which itself remains at rest. According to Freeman,

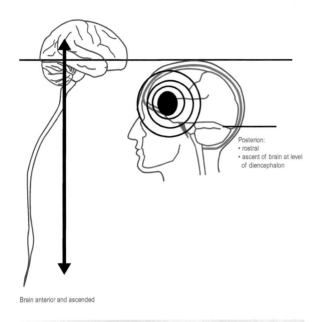

Brain anterior and ascended

Figure 31.19
Anterior, ascended position. Again note the
difference in the caudad perpendicular in
comparison with the previous figures.

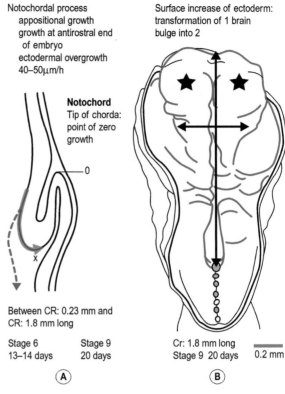

Notochordal process
appositional growth
growth at antirostral end
of embryo
ectodermal overgrowth
40–50μm/h

Notochord
Tip of chorda:
point of zero
growth

Surface increase of ectoderm:
transformation of 1 brain
bulge into 2

Between CR: 0.23 mm and
CR: 1.8 mm long

Stage 6   Stage 9
13–14 days   20 days
(A)

Cr: 1.8 mm long
Stage 9 20 days   0.2 mm
(B)

Figure 31.20
The point of zero growth in stages 6 and 9.

this point of zero growth is already evident in the
early stage of development, stage 9. (See Figures 31.20
and 31.21)

We can trace what happens to this point over the
further course of development.

When growth reaches its conclusion, this point lies at
or immediately above the tip of the dens.

Palpation

- <u>Practitioner:</u> Take up and check your position again,
  as previously. Palpation now continues as follows:

- <u>Hand position:</u> Place the tips of your two index
  fingers over the arch of the atlas, so that they meet
  near the spinous process of C1. The tips of your

middle fingers should be in the region between C1
and the occiput. Your fingers should be aligned perpendicularly to the sagittal plane.

The contact established is only very light. Place your
other fingers lightly on the table. Either hold your
thumb in the air, or, if this creates too much tension,
allow the thumb to touch the patient's head lightly.
(Figures 31.22 and 31.23) Wait for the information
coming from this region. The impression received
conveys the developmental movements around this
point. Because all the morphodynamic developments
of the body proceed from here, it is a point at which
relationships to a great variety of regions of the body
are detectable.

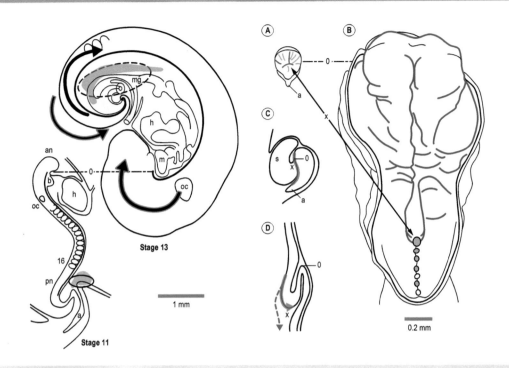

Figure 31.21
The point of zero motion in stage 11.

Key: **an** anterior node; **pn** posterior node; **oc** occiput; 16 numbers of somites; **h** heart; **a** allantois; **0** is the point of zero motion.

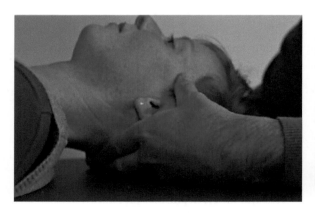

Figure 31.22
Palpation of the zero point of motion.

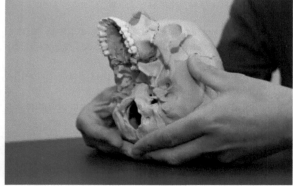

Figure 31.23
Palpation of the bony structure.

32

Osteopathic brain and spinal cord assessments

Bruno Chikly and Torsten Liem

General principles of diagnosis and treatment

Introduction Torsten Liem

The brain is not directly accessible to palpation. Just as attempts can be made, for diagnostic and therapeutic purposes, to palpate the heart or the lungs via the ribcage or the cerebral ventricles via the cranium, we can also seek to take up palpatory contact with specific cerebral tissues via the fluid, fascia, and osseous components of the cranial cavity. To date, these therapeutic approaches have not been objectively verified.

In this chapter, we are going to present different osteopathic diagnostic techniques employing a fluid or a more solid or mechanical approach to the nervous system.

Central nervous system motilities

Introduction: Torsten Liem

Motility is the property of a substance that involves the substance changing its shape, Numerous rhythms with specific frequencies have been described (see Chapter 3). The therapist synchronises with different aspects of these rhythms such as frequency and symmetry and may use them in assessment and treatment. This approach is noninvasive and 'soft'. However, no inter-rater reliability is proven for the brain.

Sutherland motility of the primary respiratory mechanism

Torsten Liem

The Primary Respiratory Mechanism (PRM) is a fundamental aspect of the classical cranial osteopathic model. According to Sutherland, the components of the PRM form the basis of an inherent rhythm that can be palpated on the cranium and the rest of the body. It is believed to occur independently of cardiac and respiratory activity and at a slightly slower rhythm than pulmonary breathing. Yet there is no adequate explanation for the differentiation and ontogenesis of these rhythms and their clinical significance (see also Chapter 3). While Sutherland himself never quoted a precise frequency, in his later years he did speak of using the motion of the tides to assist diagnosis and therapy and about the importance of slower rhythms in and around the body. According to William Garner Sutherland the first aspect of the PRM comprises the inherent motions of the brain and spinal cord. According to Magoun, there is a slow, rhythmic rolling and unrolling of the cerebral hemispheres. In one phase of this, the longitudinal diameter of the hemispheres is thought to decrease, while they broaden laterally. In the opposite phase their longitudinal diameter is thought to increase as they become narrower laterally. As this takes place, it is accompanied by a dilatation and contraction of the cerebral ventricles. Some osteopaths believe that this minute motion in a sense repeats the growth movement followed by the tissues and organs during embryonic development. During their development, they rolled up like a ram's horns. As they came into being, they first moved in a superior direction (frontal lobe), then posterior (parietal lobe), inferior (occipital lobe) and anterolateral (temporal lobe). This offers an explanation for the fine rolling and unrolling motion that follows a ram's horn pattern that some osteopaths believe to be sensed.

Ventricular system asynchronous motility

Bruno Chikly

Independently from Sutherland's motility, an asynchronous (but symmetrical) rhythm can be palpated in the ventricular system. The same type of asynchronous (but symmetrical) rhythm can be found in the lymphatic system and the venous system. This asynchronous cerebral motility could also follow a different type of embryologic development, reported by Blechschmidt.[6]

The conventional view is that the cerebral hemispheres grow symmetrically...in other words, what appears to be a symmetrical growth of the cerebral hemispheres is really an oscillating process between the right and left sides of the head.[6]

This motility is an easy and noninvasive approach to the cerebrum that can help with assessment at the beginning of treatment.

Palpation and diagnosis using the asynchronous motility of the ventricular system

- Patient's position: the patient is in supine position.

- Practitioner: contact the cranium with utmost respect and attention.

- Method: always use soft, flat hands and let the ventricular structure come to your hands. Do not press, in any way, on the cranium but let your hands synchronize very precisely with the structure you are attuning to. Feel the ventricles of the brain as two large fluid "lakes." You can spend some time following their contours and the fluid inside them.

Initial contact

Take time to appreciate the quality of the cerebrospinal fluid (CSF) inside each ventricle. It is a really wonderful fluid with a very expansive quality. Synchronize with it and expand. With time, you will eventually develop something like a "library of sensations" and you will be able to identify physiologic from dysfunctional or pathologic qualities and their presence in the intraventricular CSF.

Fluid model

Choose to follow precisely the ventricles' asynchronous motility – one ventricle starts a little bit before the other, but their overall range of motion is symmetrical. A regular, slight ventricular asynchrony with a regular delay of one ventricle in relation to the other (but with the same amplitude for each ventricle motility) is typical. This rhythm is not correlated with the cranial rhythmic impulse. Follow their fluid mechanics and specifically attune to their quality (observe the effect). The structures may simply readjust this way.

Solid model

In a second phase, you can now evaluate structures outside of the ventricular system. Use a high level of attention to check if a "solid" structure is possibly compressing the system or impeding natural intraventricular flow. Identify outside compression or external barriers to CSF flow inside the ventricle and, if possible, use your anatomic knowledge to identify a specific structure, for example, an intracranial nuclei, cortex, or white matter bundle (e.g., corpus callosum). For instance, if a structure is impeding CSF flow just above the lateral ventricles, it is most probably the corpus callosum or the indusium griseum. They constitute the "roof" of the cranial ventricles. If a structure is positioned laterally to the ventricle and protrudes on one side, it could be the head of the caudate nucleus and so on. The island of Reil or insular cortex, for example, is located too far laterally to impede the intraventricular flow and cannot be properly assessed with this approach.

Other motilities of the central nervous system
Bruno Chikly

Numerous other motilities can be palpated but we can only provide a few more examples in this limited chapter. It is possible to perceive, for example, another type of motility, a perfectly reciprocal motility (a symmetrical motility but in the opposite direction on each side of the midline), between the two brain hemispheres, the two brain ventricles, the two halves of the spinal cord, or within a specific structure. This perfectly reciprocal (opposite) motility can be perceived during nerve firing.

Other motilities could include the different cranial tides (middle tide, long tide, and very long tide) as well as the motility of the cerebrum in relation to the notochord or the motility reproducing cerebral development in relation to the embryologic lamina terminalis, and so forth. All these motilities seem to give different information about the tissue and suggest a different approach, diagnosis, and treatment of the patient.

Finding the lesion through palpation of the cranial rhythmic impulse

Central nervous system motilities
Torsten Liem

The practioner tunes in to the CRI. Mentally, he starts to go through the areas of the 1. Cortex, 2. Comissures, 3. Ventricles , 4. Basal nuclei.

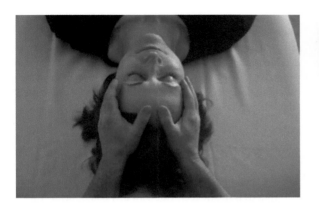

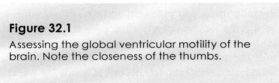

Figure 32.1
Assessing the global ventricular motility of the brain. Note the closeness of the thumbs.

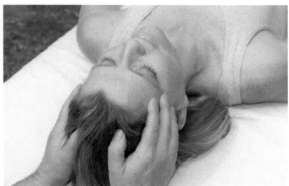

Figure 32.2
Brain mobility assessment.

Any perceived change in rhythm, e.g a brief interruption, a decreased amplitude etc., may indicate an osteopathic lesion of the respective region.

Subsequently, the particular region is examined more closely using the same method. E.g.

1 the cortical region:
- individual lobes
- insula
- claustrum
- cerebellum

2 in the area of the commisures:
- commissura anterior, commissura posterior
- capsula interna, externa, extrema
- corpus callosum
- fornix

3 in the area of the ventricles.
- the lateral ventricles, 3rd and 4th ventricle

4 in the area of the central nuclei
- basal ganglia
- thalamus
- hypothalamus
- hypophysis

Following the examination, the individual areas can be treated osteopathically.

Palpation of cerebrospinal fluid waves
Torsten Liem

1 Palpate CSF waves that originate from cardiac pulsations at around 60 cycles per minute, and that begin in peri-arterial regions and extend centrifugally to the brain

2 Palpate CSF waves that originate from respiration at approximately 18 cycles per minute; these occur in peri-venous areas with centripetal periodical pulsations towards the centre of the brain

3 Palpate slow CSF waves with about 1.5 to 4.5 cycles per minute, that are related to vasomotor tone. These waves originate from electrophysiological activity coupled with neurovascular activity and are related to autonomic regulation of brain circulation

4 Palpate very slow CSF waves with around 0.6 to 1.6 cycles per minute, related to vasomotor tone (parasympathetic and sympathetic activity).

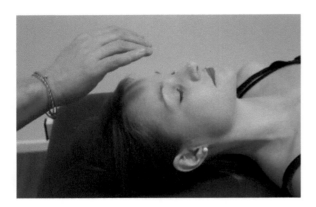

Figure 32.3
Assessment of off body projections.

Palpation of inherent rhythmic, adaptive variation of tension
Torsten Liem

The practitioner follows the dynamics of the cerebral tissue during breathing and/or primary respiration. A comparison is made of mobility, ease of mobility, extent of motion, and symmetry, as well as the quality of brain motion.

- To begin with, direct your attention to the reaction that breathing or primary respiration evokes in the cerebral tissue.

- Sense the structures that produce motion restriction in the cerebral tissue in question.

- It may also be possible to palpate embryologic force vectors.

- You can also actively test the mobility of the cerebral tissue. Sense the direction in which the cerebral tissue moves easily or where there are restrictions to movement. This testing can be done in harmony with the phases of breathing or primary respiration or independently of these. It is not performed up to the limit of motion but remains beneath the threshold of the limit of motion.

Gentle compression (or less commonly disengagement) makes the pattern of tissue relationships stronger and clearer. Compression may become necessary to establish contact with very early tissue dynamics. For example, the dynamics of embryologic tissue development, such as the birth process, are usually associated with compression. (see Chapter 20, page 367f)

Assessing CNS using "ease" or the "path of least resistance": the "tissue falls on its lesion"
Bruno Chikly

Another diagnostic technique for any osteopathic lesion is to "follow the ease," in other words, to let the tissue naturally bring you precisely, in three dimensions, to the specific location of a dysfunction. It is a very classic and old osteopathic technique that implies the tissue "falls on its lesion." The examiner contacts the brain tissue "as a whole" and lets his or her hands "be pulled" by the tissue. This diagnostic technique is fast but the authors assume it may only help identify fascia or fiber lesions and may miss some fluid lesions.

Testing elasticity
Torsten Liem

- Apply gentle pressure on the cerebral structure.

- Assess the way the tissue reacts to or resists this pressure, i.e., the ease and extent of deformation (resistance) and how the tissue reacts as you release the pressure (resilience). Reduced or increased tension is indicative of dysfunction.

Palpation of tissue density in the braintissue
Torsten Liem

Hardening can provide an indication of the severity of the dysfunction and can be due to previous posttraumatic injuries. A gentle pressure is applied with the fingers to assess the density/hardness of the tissue being examined. The expression of softness or hardness is found in the interaction of force between pressure and counter-pressure. Hardness produces increased resistance to palpation.

The examination is carried out first globally over a large area of the brain and then locally on specific brainareas.

Brain and spinal cord mobilities to assess brain nuclei

Bruno Chikly

This is another type of diagnostic process that may be just a little slower than previous techniques. This approach is not a technique where the practitioner typically follows the "ease" or the barrier of the tissue fibers as is usually done in manual therapy. This technique is a parenchyma method where the practitioner follows the movement (not the motility) of the brain parenchyma as it tries to go back to its (proper) place, to its "throne." In this approach, the practitioner does not need to pay much attention to the "ease" or the resistance of the surrounding fibers. (See Chapter 33.)

To use this approach, the practitioner needs to use the correct pressure and the precise depth needed to engage brain (or spinal cord) mobility. When the brain starts to move and tries to come back to the exact location of its optimum "seat," at some point, an obstruction to the free path of the brain can be felt. This barrier can, for example, be a specific location within the brain. In this case, these are usually nuclei that present a dominant osteopathic lesion and need to be released before the brain is able to come back to its optimal location.

Off-body projection

Torsten Liem

Speculative as this may be, the cranial sphere and brain tissue can also be assessed off-body. There exist various taxonomies of the energy fields surrounding the human body.

The osteopath can try to perceive parts of the electromagnetic spectrum in the form of radiation in the infrared or other wavelengths. Heat is one of the many ways in which energy is expressed. The osteopath can try to identify minor changes and variations in skin temperature and other electromagnetic waves.

Possible approaches and methods are Barral's manual thermal evaluation and Liem's palpation of energy fields (see Chapter 18).

Protocol for treating the central nervous system

Bruno Chikly

Manual therapy treatments should generally follow the practitioner's findings especially within the CNS. Here,

---

Box 32.1

Brain and spinal cord: basic protocol

- Phase 0: dominant or primary restrictions

- Phase 1: downregulation; neural motilities; tissue with cellular fear

- Phase 2: anatomic structures (nuclei, white substance, etc.)

- Phase 3A: brain mobility

- Phase 3B: spinal cord mobility

- Phase 4: other structures (peripheral nervous system, etc.)

- Phase 5: recheck compensations; address other structures as needed

---

we will dare to propose a basic protocol for starting work with the CNS. This protocol is just a suggestion but can be especially helpful when beginning to work the brain and spinal cord. This protocol will be developed in detail in Chapters 33 and 34.

Phase 0

Phase 0 supports practitioners to initially treat whatever your assessment finds as the dominant lesion in the body: in the CNS or the periphery of the body. Basically in phase 0, you do what you feel you need to do first, at whatever level you need to do it.

Phase 1

Phase 1 comprises techniques that support downregulation and help bring the tissue into an autonomic nervous system neutral state. For example, some tissues in sympathetic hyperactivity need to be downregulated first before being able to touch the body tissue with any kind of efficiency.

Phase 2: nervous system's anatomic and physiologic structures

Once the tissue is downregulated (i.e., once the tissue accepts your touch without any reaction), phase 2 is mainly the work on body structures or any dysfunction that may hold these structures in lesion. Using diagnostic procedures, such as the one described previously, advanced practitioners should be able to assess the CNS and find the dominant lesions and supporting treatment for any of the following structures:

1 Bones: intraosseous and interosseous restrictions.

2 Membranes in all three dimensions.

3 Intracranial fluid: from the surface to the depths:
   a Subarachnoid spaces (SAS) and cisterns
   b CNS parenchyma and lymphatic pathways
   c Ventricular system: fluid, ependymal, and solid approach.

4 Grey matter: nuclei, three-layer cortex, and six-layer cortex.

5 White matter:
   a Commissural fibers
   b Projection fibers
   c Association fibers.

6 Electromagnetic field.

7 Energetic, emotional, mental, and spiritual fields.

Phase 3: brain and spinal cord mobility

Once phase 2 has been completed, the brain and spinal cord can usually come back to their natural seat, to their "throne." We can respectfully help these structures come back where they want to return, where they "belong."

Phase 4 other structures (autonomic nervous system, peripheral nervous system, etc.)

This phase will be addressed in Chapters 34 and 35.

Phase 5

This is a phase to recheck and address compensations and other structures as needed and help the patient integrate the treatment as well as prevent, as much as possible, any treatment reaction.

Further reading

1. Frymann, V.M.: A study of the rhythmic motions of the living cranium. *J. Am. Osteopath. Assoc.* 70 (1971) 928–945.

2. Becker, R.E.: Craniosacral trauma in the adult. *Osteopathic Ann.* 4 (1976) 43–59.

3. Upledger, J.E., Vredevoogd, J.D. 1983. *Craniosacral Therapy.* Seattle: Eastland Press: 7.

4. Lay, E.. 1997. *Cranial field.* In Ward R.C.: (ed) *Foundations for osteopathic medicine.* Baltimore: Williams and Wilkins, 901–913.

5. Magoun, H.I. 1976. *Osteopathy in the cranial field.* 3rd ed. Kirksville: Journal Printing Company: p. 26, 34.

6. Magoun, H.I. 1951. *Osteopathy in the cranial field.* 1st ed. Kirksville: Journal Printing Company: 15f.

7. Lay, E.. 1997. *Cranial field.* In Ward R.C.: (ed) *Foundations for osteopathic medicine.* Baltimore: Williams and Wilkins, 901–913.

8. Magoun, H.I. 1976. *Osteopathy in the cranial field.* 3rd ed. Kirksville: Journal Printing Company: 23.

9. Woods, J.M., Woods, R.H.: A physical finding relating to psychiatric disorders. *J. Am. Osteopath. Assoc.* 60 (1961) 988–993.

10. Frymann, V.M.: A study of the rhythmic motions of the living cranium. *J. Am. Osteopath. Assoc.* 70 (1971) 928–945.

11. Lay, e.M., Cicorda, R.A., Tettambel, M.: Recording of the cranial rhythmic impulse. *JAOA*, 78 (10/1978) 149.

12. Wirth-Pattullo, V., Hayes, K.W.: Inter-rater reliability of craniosacral measurements and their relationship with subjects and examiners heart and respiratory measurements. *Phys. Ther.* 1994 (Oct). 74 (10/1994), 908-16; Discussion 917–20.

13. Becker, A.R. 1996 Personal communication Hawaii

14. Sutherland, W.G. 1939. *The cranial bowl.* USA: Free Press Company, 52.

15. Liem T. 2009. *Cranial Osteopathy - A Practical Textbook,* Eastland Press, Vista.

16. Barral JP 1996. *Manual Thermal Diagnosis.* Vista, CA: Eastland Press.

33

Treating the brain

Bruno Chikly and Torsten Liem

Introduction

Following some of the diagnostic procedures described in Chapter 32, this chapter will present a basic protocol for treating the central nervous system (CNS).

Phase 1

Bruno Chikly

This first phase includes any technique that supports downregulation of the nervous system and helps bring the autonomic nervous system (ANS) into a more "neutral" place. The following subchapters are just a few examples of phase 1 techniques applied to the brain and spinal cord. (See also Chapters 20 and 38)

Tissue trauma or cellular fear

Before being able to physically touch the body, the practitioner needs to be assured that his or her touch and his or her overall information will be accepted by the body. During treatment, the practitioner may not be aware that a specific tissue or region can be in a state of trauma, namely, in hypersympathetic activation or in a hyposympathetic state. But if, for example, the body is in a strong hypersympathetic state, the tissue is most often pushing away any tentative physical treatment, any approach of the hands, and the healing intention of a practitioner. This can possibly lessen the efficiency of a treatment and may create some unwanted post-treatment effects. Accordingly, it is important to address such tissue states at the beginning of a treatment.

Treating tissue hypersympathetic or hyposympathetic dysregulations

There are a few ways to identify areas in hypersympathetic or hyposympathetic dysregulations.

- **Patient's position:** the patient is in prone or supine position.

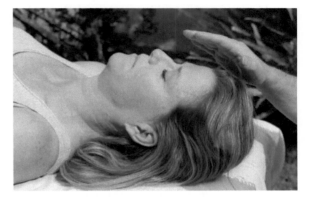

Figure 33.1
Phase 1 Finding the barrier on the cranium or face, and identifying hyper- or hyposympathetic states

- **Practitioner:** the practitioner can approach the patient's body with their hand, in this case, specifically the cranium, face, or neck regions.

- **Method:** feel for clear resistance on the way to touching the skin. This resistance should be felt as a "push away" even before touching the skin. This is not to identify areas with hyperthermia or hyperthermic zones[1]; areas felt as a "pull", with soft, fluidic resistance. There is nothing wrong with these findings, they are just different types of information.

- In this area you may feel a "push," a resistance, like a wall, but respect it; do not pass this "barrier." The body presents a resistance. This reaction occurs most often in the presence of a (known or unknown) trauma. It is as if the tissue is telling the practitioner "you do not have permission to cross this barrier".

- The practitioner should stay at the interface, at the barrier, and initially appreciate the reactions of the patient. These reactions are usually bimodal.
  - Hypersympathetic reaction: the patient becomes aware of a hyperreactivity, fight or flight reaction. Support the patient to exaggerate the movements and amplify its sensations. Hence, the body's inherent self-correcting forces will help rebalance the ANS dysfunction in this area as much as possible. Be aware not to retraumatize the patient by making him or her enter an uncontrollable hypersympathetic state where the patient loses all control and can reenter an overwhelming trauma state.
  - Hyposympathetic arousal: "frozen" state (very little reaction). If the practitioner feels a clear barrier but there are no reactions from the patient, they are probably in a frozen state or hyposympathetic reaction. Let the patient open their eyes, breathe with the mouth, and open and close their hands alternately so they can slowly and safely leave this state in the protected environment you are giving them.

Note that this specific process is not an "off-body" technique. It is just the attempt by the practitioner to contact the skin of the patient and the response of patient's tissue to this manual approach.

- At the end of the treatment, recheck the barrier—to see whether it has vanished. Check also whether previous musculoskeletal lesions have disappeared. The practitioner may appreciate a clear difference in their pre-/post-clinical assessment as many measurements should have regularized - for instance limited passive range of motion, skin discoloration, as well as subjective sensations such as pain, tension, and so forth.

- Recheck if an additional area of the body also presents another ANS barrier that may need to be addressed.

Motility or fluid approach

Any type of motility, as described earlier, can be used in phase 1. For example, synchronizing with a specific tissue rhythm or motility of a patient can be a simple way to start downregulating patients at the beginning of a treatment.

Treating the reticular alarm system

For some patients, especially when cooperation is not possible, such as when in a coma, with babies, patients with stroke, or even when treating animals, the practitioner can have a more specific manual approach on the nuclei of the reticular alarm system (or reticular activation system) to help downregulate ANS.

The reticular formation (RF) is phylogenetically one of the oldest parts of the brain. It is made up of about 100–120 nuclei oriented more or less vertically in the brainstem. These nuclei are located close to midline within the brainstem. At least three main components or "columns" of nuclei have been identified.

1 Midline (or median) column of nuclei also called "nuclei of the raphe." These nuclei are serotonergic and participate in the RF but not the reticular alarm system (RAS). We won't discuss these nuclei here.

2 Medial column nuclei: They contain numerous large reticular RAS neurons and the descending lateral reticulospinal, medial reticulospinal tract, and reticulothalamic tract.

3 Lateral column nuclei and the locus ceruleus (LC): The lateral column nuclei have many small to intermediate RAS neurons. The LC or nucleus pigmentosus located in the floor of the fourth ventricle and higher, near the sulcus limitans, mainly secretes norepinephrine and dopamine neurons. The LC has an orthosympathetic-like effect within the brain. The LC is usually activated during states of heightened vigilance, arousal, pleasure, or, for example, worry and anger.

- **Treating the reticular alarm system:**
  - **Patient's position:** the patient is in prone or supine position.
  - **Hand position:** place your fingers in the brainstem area
  - **Method:**
    - RAS medial nuclei: the practitioner brings all their fingers (except thumbs) midline vertically on the occipital area and separates them about 2–3 mm. The practitioner should be on the RAS medial nuclei or column. He/she can pay attention to whether one of the areas anywhere on

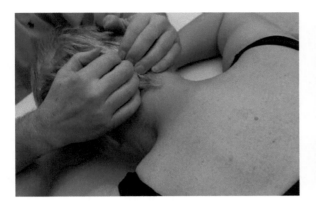

Figure 33.2
Phase 1 RAS - treatment of the median column nuclei

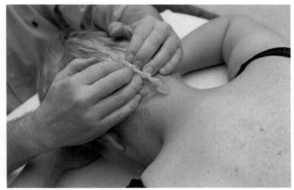

Figure 33.3
Phase 1 RAS treatment of the lateral column nuclei - the fingers are separated approximately 1 to 1.5 cm

these left and right median RAS columns is hyperactive unilaterally or bilaterally, and help downregulate this area. If another structure becomes activated at the same time, the practitioner could also connect this area with this structure of the cerebrum or spinal cord to facilitate downregulation.

- RAS lateral nuclei: when the practitioner has finished with the RAS medial nuclei, he /she can separate their fingers a little more so the space between them is now about 1 cm to synchronize with the RAS lateral column nuclei. Assess if any region, unilaterally or bilaterally, is hyperactive, and pay special attention to the region of the LC (usually just superior to inion, if present). If one nucleus is hyperactive, the patient should immediately feel significant relaxation. It is not rare that patients declare that RAS techniques put them in one of the most relaxing states they have ever been in. After this type of approach, phase two can begin.

Phase 2

Introduction
Bruno Chikly

Once phase one has been completed, the practitioner can feel much more comfortable about making contact with the body. The tissue will accept information from the practitioner much more easily.

In phase two we will describe different cerebral tissue layers and structures that can present osteopathic dysfunctions and may need to be assessed and treated.

Bones: intrarestrictions and interrestrictions
Bruno Chikly

In this phase, the practitioners may need to specifically examine each articulation and intraosseous lesion of the cranium. If an intraosseous lesion is found, or one between sutures, for example, use appropriate approaches to help these lesions. They have been accurately described in many other places.

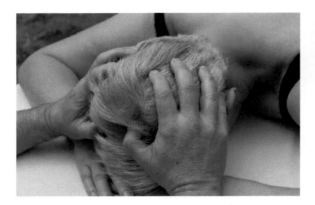

Figure 33.4
Treatment of the posterior membranes and tentorium cerebelli

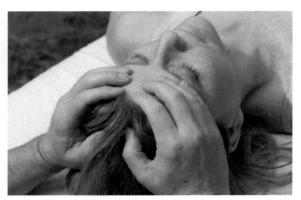

Figure 33.5
Ventricular system - treatment of the lateral ventricles

Membranes
Bruno Chikly

If we delve medially to the calvarium or skullcap, we will find the three different layers of cerebral meninges (dura, arachnoid, and pia mater). They should be checked separately because they have completely different characteristics and can present different dysfunctions.

Periosteal dura is the inner layer of the cranial bone and should be specifically checked around 360 degrees. The bones could be used gently and skillfully as a great handle to release the periosteal dura. Beryl Arbuckle has drawn wonderful maps that could help you prepare for this work[2].

Treatment of all associated dural structures in their respective three dimensions often needs to be completed in order to release dominant osteopathic dysfunctions.

Cerebral fluid compartments
Bruno Chikly

Three levels of fluids can be treated in the cerebrum:

Ventricular system

As we mentioned in the previous chapter, the fluid deep within the cerebral ventricles is a very important location for balancing intracranial fluid dynamics, as well as helping to orient oneself in the brain, and to start to diagnose intracranial grey or white matter lesions. The function of the cerebral ventricles as the main source of cerebrospinal fluid (CSF) production has been strongly contested[4].

Ventricles of fluid hydrodynamics can be disturbed as well as compressed from outside or from within (choroid plexi). A noninvasive diagnosis of all these elements is fundamental for complete CNS assessment.[3,4]

Parenchyma

Cerebral interstitial fluid and glymphatic pathways. The parenchyma does not have either CSF proper (or lymph) but a fluid called the cerebral interstitial fluid (CIF). Considering the new hypothesis for CSF circulation mentioned earlier, manual techniques should be adapted to the flow of CIF described by the new directions in CSF physiology.

One of the interesting aspects of this new description of CSF secretion and reabsorption is the glymphatic system[5]. These passageways are located between the tunica externa (adventitia) of the main intracerebral arteries and veins and the foot of the glial cells called astrocytes. They can be perceived within the brain parenchyma as perivascular spaces that are filled with numerous substances that the brain "drains" out, including amyloid substances. Hence the word glymphatic pathways associated with (lymphatic-like) pathways of cerebral drainage located outside of the main intracerebral vasculature.

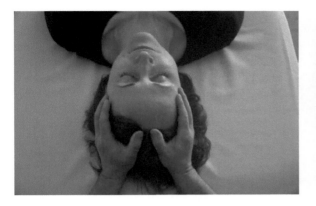

Figure 33.6
Treatment of the brain intraparenchymatous region and the glymphatic system

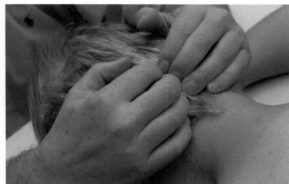

Figure 33.7
Treatment of the cisterna magna

These important glymphatic spaces are often filled with materials including amyloid substances or other toxic substances. Practitioners should be able to identify what type of material is possibly causing pathologic reactions in a specific patient's internal milieu or environment.

Manual therapy should help in any possible way to support "drainage" of these spaces. These substances should be cleared on a regular basis to maintain the CNS in a state of optimum functioning.

Subarachnoid spaces and main cerebral cisterns

Cisterns (and some subarachnoid spaces [SAS]) are the most external CIF palpable. They need to be assessed especially when brain functions may be decreased or damaged, for example, in trauma, cranial surgery, attention deficit disorders, autism, trisomy, and so forth.

The interstitial fluid has the characteristics of a relatively "free" fluid, for example compared to lymph. Lymph is constrained into lymphatic vessels and moves in a specific direction, with a specific rhythm and a specific depth. The little "unbounded" interstitial fluid should have a much greater degree of free-dom within the tissues. The loss of the interstitial fluid freedom of movement in the intracranial cisterns or SAS can be a dominant lesion in the cranium and would need to be addressed.

The interstitial fluid of the following four major subarachnoid cisterns can be considered:

- Ambient cistern (cisterna ambiens)

- Cisterna magna or cerebellomedullary cistern (the largest of the subarachnoid cisterns)

- Cisterna basalis

- Pontine cistern or Hilton's waterbed.

Grey matter: cortex and nuclei

General techniques for phase 2: cerebral grey matter

Balanced tension of the brain and spinal cord:
Torsten Liem

- Go with the tension or tissue pattern of the part of the brain into the position or shape in which the

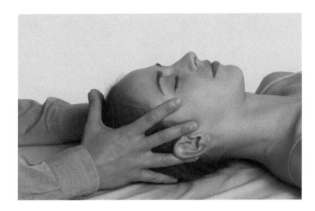

Figure 33.8
General treatment of the regions of the cerebral hemispheres

tension is most evenly balanced (point of balanced tension [PBT]). Perform this in all three spatial dimensions.

- Then "copy" the tension and tissue qualities of the cerebral region by allowing the force of your hand contact to match or mirror them. The more accurate this copying process, the better the resonance in the tissue structures.

- Once you have exactly copied the prevailing tissue qualities, you will sense a PBT becoming established.

- The PBT may also be ushered in by embryologic force vectors. Embryologic force vectors are extremely fine organ motions that would appear to be associated with the embryologic development pathway of the organs. (This is a conceptual model that requires further scientific investigation.) Gentle compression (or more rarely, disengagement) of relationship patterns in the tissues as reflected in embryologic development supports the process of releasing dysfunctional force vectors and relationship patterns. (The inhalation and exhalation phases can be sensed within the compression field.) Tissue reacts to practitioner-induced compression by displaying its original pattern of rotation and allows

a fulcrum or mechanical balance point to emerge for the pattern in question. During gentle compression, the practitioner should sense all the dynamics in the tissue without intervening. In general, you will be able to sense a fulcrum being created between the two regions. Once the fulcrum has been established, you will sense the two structures moving apart.

- Support this process by allowing it to unfold in a gentle compression field (or use minimal counter-pressure to resist disengagement) and go with the disengagement.

- Depending on the tissue, an opposite process may occur in that the structures draw closer together. Support this process of drawing closer by allowing it to unfold in a gentle expansion field (or use minimal counterpressure to resist the process of drawing closer or convergent suction) and thus gently invite and go with the process of drawing closer or convergent suction.

  Dynamic balanced tension (DBT) and balanced fluid tension (BFT) may also be useful when treating the brain and spinal cord (see Chapter 20, pp. 362f.).

Dynamic balanced tension:
Torsten Liem

- Synchronize your hands with the primary respiration of the patient.

- During the inhalation phase, bring about a very slight intensification of the motion or tension that is present in the cerebral tissue but without altering the speed of these motions. Do not confront any tissue restrictions or tissue barriers in the dysfunction.

- During the exhalation phase, simply follow the tissue tensions passively. Repeat this process until, at the end of an inhalation phase, you clearly sense a spontaneous disengagement, *not* one that you have elicited.

  Balanced fluid tension may also be applied (see Chapter 20)

General treatment of the cerebral hemispheres
Torsten Liem

Practitioner: take up a position at the head of the patient.

Hand position: Sutherland cranial vault hold.

Method:

- Palpate the mobility of the cranial bones against the cerebral hemispheres.
- Passively test the cerebral hemispheres: form; symmetry; frequency; force; and ease of "motion," amplitude, end feeling, natural disengagement, natural closeness or retraction, tensions, aberrant movements, density, volume, and so forth.
- Allow resonance with the developmental dynamic force vectors to develop, for example, by delivering gentle compression via the cranial base (as well as the cranial vault) on the cerebral hemispheres.
- Sense the inhalation and exhalation phases within the compression field.
- PBT, DBT or BFT.
- A fulcrum becomes established in the relationship pattern between the mesoectoderm and cerebral hemispheres, for example, between the cranial base and cerebrum.
- After the fulcrum has become established, disengagement usually occurs within the cerebral hemispheres and between them and the surrounding structures. Support the disengagement process by allowing it to unfold in a gentle compression field (or use minimal pressure to counteract the force of disengagement) and so go with the disengagement.
- To begin with, for example, you will usually sense an eccentric force of the head and cerebrum directed superiorly and anteriorly.
- If necessary, you may deliver a fluid drive from the diagonally opposite region of the dysfunctional structure. However, it is not uncommon for a spontaneous fluid drive to be noted during the course of therapeutic interaction.
- At the end of treatment, if necessary, balance the cranial vault and the reciprocal tension membrane.

Each of the cerebral lobes can be tested and treated individually or in conjunction with other tissues. However, it is worth pointing out that in some instances, the boundaries of the lobes cannot be definitively identified.

Treatment of vascular structures
Torsten Liem

Arterial blood supply and venous drainage are naturally also of major importance when treating the brain and spinal cord. The vascular structures involved, for example, the venous sinuses and the internal jugular vein (and facial veins) as well as the arterial supply in the cervical region, should be treated as appropriate (for details on treating the individual cerebral ventricles, see Liem).

On the integration of emotional, mental, and spiritual aspects, see page 371ff. and Chapter 38. (On the treatment of the brain, see Chapters 22 and 31. See also Liem's books *Cranial Osteopathy: a practical textbook* and *Cranial Osteopathy: principles and practice*, which describe fluctuation techniques and the treatment of the individual cerebral ventricles and the intracranial dura.)

Treating the lobes and sulci of the brain
Torsten Liem

See Liem,[3] for a description of fluctuation techniques and of treatment of the individual cerebral ventricles and the intracranial dura.

The frontal lobe:

- **Location:** the frontal lobe lies anterior to the central sulcus; not all its regions can be localized precisely in functional and anatomical terms: the primary motor cortex, premotor cortex, Broca area, medial cortex, and prefrontal cortex.

- **Function:**
  - Involved in virtually all behavioral modalities.
  - Left prefrontal cortex: movement control associated with language.
  - Right prefrontal cortex: movement control not associated with language.
  - Possible lesions associated with dysfunctions of motor activity (fine motor coordination, speed and strength, movement programming, voluntary gaze movement, Broca aphasia), inflexible behavior; and disturbed response suppression (increased risk taking and rule violation, disturbed associative learning), loss of divergent thinking

(behavioral spontaneity, impaired ability to plan, and develop problem-solving strategies), lapses of temporary memory (e.g., inability to estimate frequency), impaired spatial orientation, altered personality or social behavior (pseudo depression with apathy, indifference, loss of sexual interest, lack of emotion), altered sexual behaviors because of lowering of inhibitory threshold (e.g., masturbating in public), and disturbed sense of smell.

Treating the region of the frontal lobe

Hand position:

- Place one hand over the frontal bone and, in front of the vertex, over the anterior part of the parietal bones.

- Position your middle finger on the median line.

- Position your index and ring fingers close to the frontal eminences.

- Position your thumb and little finger in the region of the pterion.

- Place your other caudally directed hand underneath the patient's occiput.

Method:

- Passively test the frontal lobe: form, symmetry, frequency, force and ease of 'motion', amplitude, end feeling, natural disengagement, natural closeness/retraction, tensions, aberrant movements, density, volume etc.

- Go with the frontal bone into flexion and external rotation in order to assess the mobility of the frontal lobe.

- Resonance with the developmental dynamic force vectors: e.g. by gently compressing the frontal lobe.

- Sense the inhalation and exhalation phases within the compression field.

- First treat the side with the less pronounced motion restriction.

- Synchronise with form, density/hardness, tissue elasticity, involuntary rhythms, amplitude, end

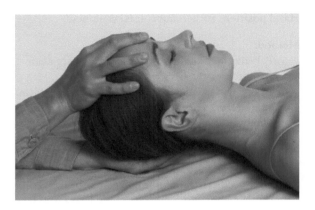

Figure 33.9
Treating the region of the frontal lobe

feel of the particular phase, natural disengagement at the end of the inhalation phase, natural compression/closeness at the end of the exhalation phase, ease of movement, strength/force of movement, fullness/emptiness in the tissue, additional asynchronous chaotic motions during the (sub-)phase(s), tensions.

- Establish a balanced tension BT: a local, regional, global point of balanced tension (PBT), dynamic balanced tension (DBT), balanced fluid tension (BFT), balanced electrodynamic tension (BET) and apply further treatment modalities if needed (Chapters 20 and 38).

- A fulcrum becomes established in the relationship pattern between the mesoectoderm and the frontal lobe, e.g. between the cranial base and frontal lobe, anterior dural band and frontal lobe, frontal lobe and insular cortex, frontal lobe and terminal plate etc.

- After the fulcrum has been established, disengagement usually occurs within the frontal lobe and between the frontal lobe and the surrounding structures. Support the disengagement process by allowing it to unfold in a gentle compression field (or use minimal pressure to counteract the force of disengagement) and so go with the disengagement.

- If necessary, you may deliver a fluid drive from the diagonally opposite region of the occiput. However, it is not uncommon for a spontaneous fluid drive to be noted during the course of therapeutic interaction.

- At the end of treatment, if necessary, balance the frontal bone and the reciprocal tension membrane, or treat the cranial base to open the vessels carrying the blood supply (internal carotid artery, anterior cerebral artery).

The parietal lobe:

- **Location:** the parietal lobe lies beneath the parietal bone and is bounded anteriorly by the central sulcus, inferiorly by the lateral sulcus, and posteriorly by the parietooccipital (PO) sulcus.

- **Function:**
  - Anterior: sensorimotor function (somatic sensation and perception).
  - Posterior: Integration of sensory information from somatic and visual regions (and to a lesser extent also from other sensory regions); possibly also information processing regarding the position and movement of the body in space. The left side tends to be more involved in language processes and the right side in spatial processing.
  - Possible lesions associated with the following: left side – finger agnosia, left–right confusion, impaired ability to write and count; right side – contralateral neglect of visual, auditory, and somatosensory stimuli (e.g., impaired ability to count spots on a dice or to cut paper or to manage the topography of getting dressed).

Treating the region of the parietal lobe

Hand position:

- Position the palms of your hands over the parietal bone on both sides. (Your palms are in contact with the parietal lobe.)

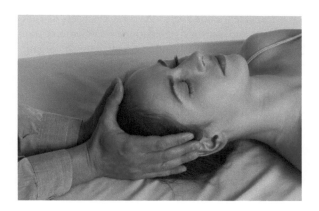

Figure 33.10
Treating the region of the parietal lobe

- Your thumbs should be touching each other to form a fulcrum.

Method:

- As for the frontal lobe.

The temporal lobe:

- **Location:** lying below the lateral sulcus, the temporal region is somewhat arbitrarily defined (the right and left temporal lobes are connected via the corpus callosum and the anterior commissure of the cerebrum).

- **Function:**
  - It does not have a single uniform function but forms part of the primary and secondary auditory cortex, the secondary visual cortex, the tertiary sensory cortex, and the limbic cortex.
  - Three principal functions: auditory and visual perception, long-term storage of sensory information, and affective coloring of afferent sensory information.
  - Left side: linguistic memory, processing of speech sounds.
  - Right side: nonverbal memory, processing of music, and interpretation of facial expressions.

- Possible lesions associated with disorders of auditory and sensory perception, selective attention vis-à-vis auditory and sensory stimuli, organization and categorization of linguistic stimuli, linguistic comprehension, long-term memory (together with the hippocampus), personality changes, affective behavior (anxiety feelings, overemphasis on trivialities, and unimportant aspects of daily living), and sexual behavior (increase in heterosexual and homosexual behaviors).

Treating the region of the temporal lobe

Hand position:

- Position the palms of your hands over the temporal bones on both sides, approximately in the region of the squamoparietal suture (and extending backward beyond the suture).

- Your fingers should be directed caudally.

- Locate your thenar eminences anteriorly and your hypothenar eminences posteriorly on the temporal lobe on each side.

Alternative hand position (Figure 33.11b):

- Position your thumbs on the greater wing of the sphenoid bone on each side, with your metacarpophalangeal joint and thenar eminence approximately over each temporal lobe region.

- Interlace your other fingers beneath the patient's neck.

Method:

- As for the frontal lobe.

The occipital lobe:

- **Location:** this lobe presents a triangular shape. It is localized on the medial surface by the PO sulcus, on the inferior face by a line that connects the preoccipital notch to the beginning of the PO sulcus; and on the lateral surface by an arbitrary line connecting the end of the PO sulcus to the preoccipital notch. The occipital lobe presents Brodmann visual areas 17, 18, and 19.

- **Function:** the occipital lobe mainly constitutes the primary and secondary visual cortex.

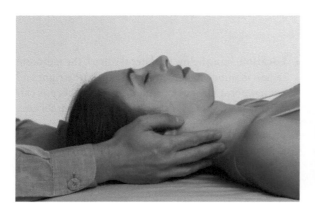

Figure 33.11a
Treating the region of the temporal lobe

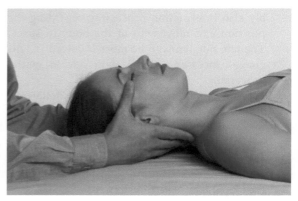

Figure 33.11b
Treating the region of the temporal lobe, alternative hand position

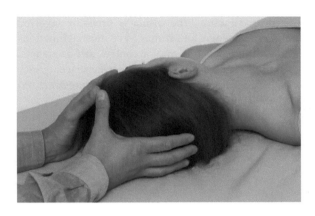

Figure 33.12
Treating the region of the occipital lobe

Treating the region of the occipital lobe

Patient:

- Supine with head turned to one side.

Hand position:

- Position the fingers of one hand, directed caudally, above the superior nuchal line. The distal finger pads are in contact with the occipital lobe.

- Place your other hand over the patient's frontal bone.

- Your thumbs should be touching.

Method:

- As for the frontal lobe.

Primary and secondary motor centres

- The motor cortex which is responsible for voluntary movements includes the primary motor cortex, the adjacent rostral areas, the pre-motor and supplementary motor cortices, and the frontal eye field.

The primary motor cortex

Location

- In the frontal lobe on the pre-central gyrus from the lateral sulcus to the parasagittal cortex and medial side of the hemisphere. In the motor homunculus the pharynx and larynx are situated farthest down. The trunk and legs are situated above.

Function

- Initiating movements, fine controlled voluntary movement of the contralateral side of the body.

Supplementary motor cortex

Location

- Rostrally in the frontal lobe adjacent to M1 on the medial side of the hemisphere.

Function

- Planning of movements.

Pre-motor cortex

Location

- In the frontal lobe, rostrally subsequent to the primary motor cortex.

Function

- Broad movements (e.g. whole arm), planning of movements.

Palpatory approach to the region of the pre-motor and primary motor cortex

Hand position:

- The fingertips of both hands are placed together about 0.5 cm posterior to the coronal suture.

Method:

- The fingers of one hand project into the region of the pre-motor cortex, the fingers of the other hand project into the primary motor cortex.

- **Application:** According to the frontal lobe.

Primary and secondary somatosensory centres

Somatosensory cortex

Overview and location

- The primary somatosensory cortex is the convergence point of the ascending paths carrying sensations from the skin, the muscles, tendons and joints. It is a part of the parietal lobe and is located in the post-central gyrus; the secondary somatosensory cortex adjoins ventrally, the primary motor cortex lies rostrally. The location of the sensory information coming from the body is represented in somatotopic maps of the

Insula (or island) of Reil, insular cortex or insular lobe:
Anatomy: Bruno Chikly

- **Anatomy/structure:** discovered by Johann Christian Reil, it is a layer of cortex medial to the temporal, parietal, and frontal cortex. The insula is located deep within the lateral sulcus. It has different cortex layers (the anterior insula present six cortical layers, whereas the posterior insula has three layers).

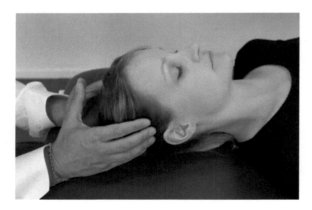

Figure 33.13
Treating the region of the insular cortex

- **Known function:** the insula is probably involved in consciousness and it may have diverse functions including perception, motor control, self-awareness, cognitive functioning, and social experience.
  - Interoceptive awareness (body representation) and emotional experience.
  - Motor control: hand and eye motor movement, swallowing, gastric motility, and speech articulation.
  - Sympathetic and parasympathetic systems regulation.
  - Vestibular sensations processing.
  - Role in addiction.

Treating the region of the insula:
Torsten Liem

Hand position:

Index, middle and ring finger are placed above and below the squamo-parietal suture on each side. Index finger is placed anterior, middle finger is placed medial and ring finger in the posterior area, with thumbs touching each other above the head.

Method:

Your fingers should project deeply toward the insular region.

The index finger tries to palpate the region of the anterior insula, the middle finger palpates the mid insula and ring finger palpates the region of the dorsal posterior insula through skull and lobus temporalis.

In the second step, the dorsal posterior insula can be assessed from rostral to caudal, also the representation fields of the nucleus tractus solitarii, as well as the trigeminal, cervical, thoracic, lumbar and sacral regions can be explored.

In the third step, the ring finger palpates the dorsal posterior insula and the thumb explores the region of the thalamus, both regions can be counterbalanced.

In the fourth step, the middle finger palpates on the mid insula and the thumb goes for the region of the amygdala, both regions can be counterbalanced.

In the fifth step, the index finger palpates the anterior insula and the thumb reaches for the region of the orbito-frontal and posterior-lateral cortex and anterior gyrus cinguli, those regions can be counterbalanced if necessary.

The osteopath palpates the anterior, mid and dorsal posterior insula.

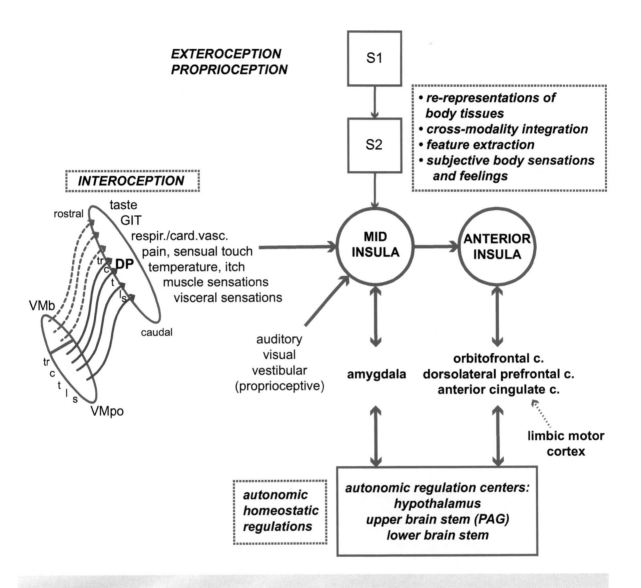

**EXTEROCEPTION
PROPRIOCEPTION**

S1

- *re-representations of body tissues*
- *cross-modality integration*
- *feature extraction*
- *subjective body sensations and feelings*

S2

INTEROCEPTION

rostral

taste
GIT
respir./card.vasc.
pain, sensual touch
temperature, itch
muscle sensations
visceral sensations

tr
c DP
t
l s

VMb

caudal

tr
c
t
l s

VMpo

auditory
visual
vestibular
(proprioceptive)

**MID
INSULA**

**ANTERIOR
INSULA**

amygdala

orbitofrontal c.
dorsolateral prefrontal c.
anterior cingulate c.

limbic motor
cortex

*autonomic
homeostatic
regulations*

*autonomic regulation centers:
hypothalamus
upper brain stem (PAG)
lower brain stem*

Figure 33.14

Integration at the level of the Insular Cortex, from Craig 2006, Jänig 2006, modified by Liem. DP dorsal posterior (insula), S1,S2 somatosensory cortices, VMpo Nucleus ventromedialis posterior thalami, VMb Nucleus ventromedialis basalis thalami, tr trigeminal, c cervical, t thoracic, l lumbar, s sacral, PAG periaqueductal gray matter

- Anterior Insula: re-representations of body tissues, cross-modality integration, feature extraction, subjective body sensations and feelings

- Midinsula receives auditory, visual, vestibular input and has an important connection to the amygdala

- Palpation of the dorsal posterior Insula (Introspection): Nucleus tractus solitarii, trigeminal, cervical, thoracic, lumbar, sacral; from rostral to caudal (taste, GIT, respiration/card,vasc., pain, sensual touch, temperature, itching, muscle sensations, visceral sensations).

Alternative Handhold 1 for treating the region of the insula
Torsten Liem

Hand position: Position your thumbs along the squamoparietal suture on each side. Use your other fingers to cradle the cranial base.

- Your thumbs should project deeply toward the insular region.

Alternative Handhold 2 for treating the insula
Bruno Chikly

Patient: the patient is in supine position.

Practitioner: the practitioner is positioned at the head of the patient.

Method: put your fingers on the frontal cortex with the thumbs touching the lateral area, the region of the temple. Feel the one-layered cortex in the frontal lobe and compared to the sensation on the lateral side, with the insular cortex. You should naturally feel a different sensation between the one-layer and a two-layer cortex. If you feel any change in symmetry, position, quality, rhythm, activity, synchronize precisely with the insula and let the intrinsic self-correcting mechanisms bring back this structure in a balanced/ aligned/ neutral place. Recheck position, rhythm, activity, even energetic or emotional component should be back to homeostasis/allostasis and present no "signaling" at all.

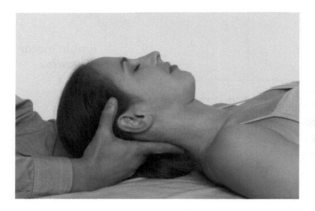

Figure 33.15
Treating the region of the insular cortex

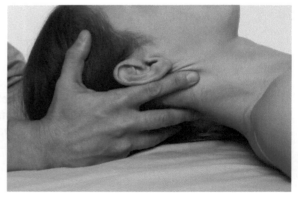

Figure 33.16
Treating the region of the cingulate gyrus

The cingulate lobe and cingulate gyrus:
Torsten Liem

- **Location:** the cingulate gyrus curves round the corpus callosum from above and runs parallel to it; posteriorly and inferiorly, it passes through the narrow isthmus of the cingulate gyrus to become continuous with the parahippocampal gyrus of the temporal lobe.

- **Function:** it regulates autonomic processes, food intake, and psychomotor and locomotor drive.

Treating the region of the cingulate gyrus

Hand position: position your thumbs about 1 cm above and parallel to the squamoparietal suture on both sides. Span the cranial base with your fingers.

Method: your thumbs should project deeply into the region of the cingulate gyrus above the corpus callosum.

Synchronize with the tissue qualities of the region

Balance the tensions of the region

The lateral sulcus (Sylvian fissure):
Torsten Liem

- **Locations:** overlying the region of the insula, the lateral sulcus principally separates the frontal lobe and the temporal lobe; it is surrounded by fields involved with language and hearing. The lateral sulcus follows an inferomedial course, from anterior lateral to posterior medial; it is formed from gestational week 20 onward.

Treating the lateral sulcus

Patient: supine position with head turned to the right.

Practitioner: take up a position at the head of the patient.

Hand position:
- Position your right thumb on the parietal bone, close to the squamoparietal suture. Arrange the other fingers of your right hand caudally so that they form a right angle with your thumb.
- Position your left thumb on the temporal bone below the squamoparietal suture. Arrange the other fingers

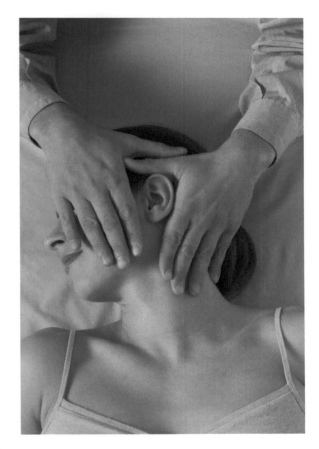

Figure 33.17
Treating the lateral sulcus

of your left hand caudally on the patient's neck so that they form a right angle with your thumb.

Method:
- Go with the temporal bone and parietal bone into external rotation in the inhalation phase.
- Project your thumbs into the course of the lateral sulcus, inferomedially, and from anterior lateral to posterior medial.

- During the next inhalation phase, use your left thumb to go with the temporal lobe in a downward and forward arc while your right thumb goes with the parietal lobe anteriorly.
- Establish a balanced tension BT: a local, regional, global PBT, dynamic balanced tension (DBT), balanced fluid tension, balanced electrodynamic tension (BET).
- A fulcrum becomes established in the relationship pattern between the frontal lobe and temporal lobe.

- **Alternative method:**
  - Allow resonance with the developmental dynamic force vectors to develop, for example, by delivering gentle compression via the cranial vault on to the brain (this copies the embryonic growth resistances in the antibasal and laterodorsal cranial wall, which caused the regions of the expanding brain to fold against each other and the fissures to be formed).
  - Sense the inhalation and exhalation phases.
  - PBT, DBT or BFT.
  - A fulcrum becomes established in the relationship pattern between the mesoectoderm and the cerebral hemispheres, for example, between the cranium and cerebrum and between the frontal lobe and the temporal lobe.

The central sulcus:
Torsten Liem

- **Location:** the central sulcus lies between the frontal lobe and the parietal lobe; it is the site of the primary motor and sensory cortical fields (and is formed from gestational week 24 onward).

Treating the central sulcus

Practitioner: take up a position at the head of the patient.

Hand position:
- Position one hand so that your index and middle fingers are anterior to the central sulcus over the frontal lobe, covering the side of the patient's head anteriorly from the vertex.
- Position the other hand so that your index and middle fingers are posterior to the central sulcus

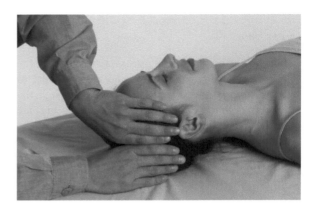

Figure 33.18
Treating the central sulcus

over the parietal lobe, covering the side of the patient's head posteriorly from the vertex.
- Ensure that your thumbs are touching on the other side of the patient's head to act as a fulcrum.

Method: as for the lateral sulcus.

The parieto-occipital sulcus:
Torsten Liem

- **Location:** the PO sulcus lies between the parietal lobe and the occipital lobe.

Treating the parieto-occipital sulcus

Practitioner: take up a position at the head of the patient.

Hand position:
- Position one hand so that your wrist is anterior to the PO sulcus over the parietal lobe (above an imaginary line running about 2 cm above the lambda point). Span the cranium between your thumb and little finger.
- Position the other hand so that your wrist is posterior or inferior to the PO sulcus over the occipital lobe (below an imaginary line running about

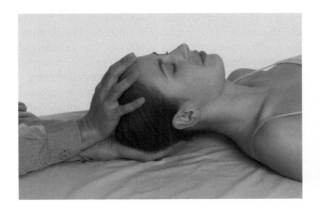

Figure 33.19
Treating the parieto-occipital sulcus

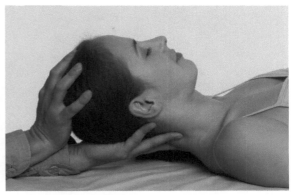

Figure 33.20
Treating the calcarine sulcus

2 cm above the lambda point). Span the cranium between your thumb and little finger.

Method: as for the lateral sulcus.

The calcarine sulcus:
Torsten Liem

- **Location:** the calcarine sulcus runs almost at right angles to the PO sulcus on the medial surface of the occipital lobe and on the under surface of the cuneus. It is the site of the primary visual projection area.

Treating the calcarine sulcus

Hand position:
- Position one hand anterior to the calcarine sulcus over the cuneus. Your wrist should be anterior to the lambda point. Span the cranium between your thumb and little finger.
- Position the other hand so that your wrist is posterior to the calcarine sulcus and posterior to the lambda point. Span the cranium between your thumb and little finger.

Method: as for the lateral sulcus.

Layers of the cerebral cortex
Bruno Chikly

Treating the superficial gyri and superficial sulci

Sulci are depressions in the surface of the brain. They surround specific gyri (or cerebral convolutions) that have been very specifically classified in human brains. The numerous convex folds or ridges of the surface of the brain appear at about 5 months in the embryo and continue to develop at least into the baby's first year.

Lesions can be present within the gyri or sulci of the brain. Be aware that lesions can actually be intragyrus, intergyri, gyrus–sulcus, intrasulcus, intersulci, or a combination of any of these patterns.

The three-layer and six-layer cortex

The brain cortex is divided into two main structures:

- The neocortex or isocortex: The neocortex is only present in mammals. It is like a mantle (pallium) with 1.5–4.5 mm in thickness around the hemispheres.

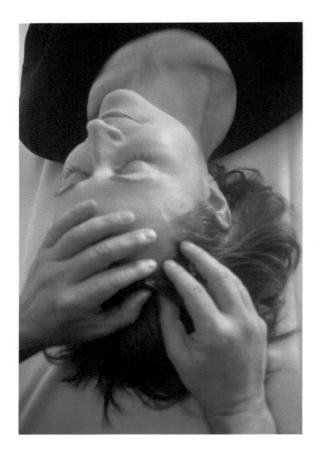

Figure 33.21
Treatment of cerebral sulci and gyri

- The phylogenetically oldest part or allocortex made up of the archicortex and paleocortex:
  - The archicortex comprises the hippocampal formation (including the dentate gyrus).
  - The paleocortex comprises the olfactory cortex (piriform cortex), including the uncus area).
  The cerebellum is also a three-layer cortex.

The regions of the brain with three-layer cortex are usually the areas where we can often find the most important physical or "mechanical" osteopathic

lesions. Hippocampal formation or cerebellar lesions are the place of very common intracerebral lesions. They often create physical problems that can spread anywhere throughout the whole body. For example, a rotated and ascending cerebellum created during a car accident can through its pull on the filum terminal internum or externum easily pull on the spinal cord, reducing lumbar intervertebral disc spaces, and further down the chain create a clinical lesion on the knee or the ipsilateral foot.

General nuclei of the cerebrum

Callosal and supracallosal structures:

- Location: all these structures are located on the roof of the lateral ventricles.

- Main method: first, connect with the motility of the cerebral ventricles and assess a specific structure in relation to the ventricular system when possible.

Corpus callosum: "tough body"
Anatomy and function: Bruno Chikly, Torsten Liem

1 **Anatomy/structure:** the corpus callosum is the largest commissure of the CNS. It comprises 200–300 million myelinated fibers connecting the two cerebral hemispheres. The corpus callosum lies above the third ventricle at the floor of the longitudinal cerebral fissure; a strong myelinated bundle of transverse fibers that connects the two cerebral hemispheres.

2 **Relation to the ventricular system:** the corpus callosum is located in the "roof" of the lateral ventricles.

3 **Known function:** communicates and integrates information across cerebral hemispheres. It may also be involved in maintaining arousal and attention and tactile localization.

Treating the region of corpus callosum
Torsten Liem

Location: The corpus callosum lies above the third ventricle at the floor of the longitudinal cerebral fissure; a strong myelinated bundle of transverse fibers that connects the two cerebral hemispheres.

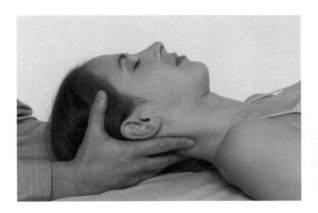

Figure 32.22a
Treating the region of the corpus callosum

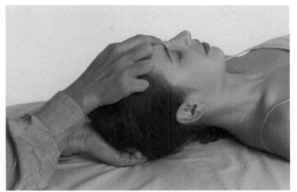

Figure 32.22b
Treating the region of the corpus callosum,
alternative hand position

Hand position:

- Position your thumbs above and parallel to the squamoparietal suture on both sides. Cradle the cranial base with your other fingers.

- Your thumbs should project deeply toward the corpus callosum region.

Alternative hand position:

- Place the index finger of one hand on the glabella, and the index finger of the other hand on the inion.

- Your fingers should project toward the corpus callosum.

Method:

- As for the frontal lobe.

Indusium griseum: "grey tunic"
Bruno Chikly

- **Anatomy/structure**: the indusium griseum is a thin layer of white and grey matter in continuity with the gyrus fasciolaris and the dentate gyrus.

- **Relation to the ventricular system**: the indusium griseum is located just superior to the corpus callosum on the "roof" of the lateral ventricles.

- **Known function**: its function has not been well studied. The indusium griseum is sometimes assumed to be vestigial and nonfunctional in adults. It may help consolidation of memories.

- **Treating the indusium griseum**: palpate the corpus callosum on the roof of the lateral ventricles of the brain. Just superior to it find a thin structure with a slightly different quality, the indusium griseum, connected to the hippocampus.

Medial and Lateral Longitudinal Striae (of Lancisi)
Bruno Chikly

- **Anatomy/structure:** the medial and lateral longitudinal striae are embedded in the indusium griseum. They are bundles of fibers connecting the hippocampal formation with the septal area.

- **Known function:** the functions of these hippocampal related structures are not well understood.

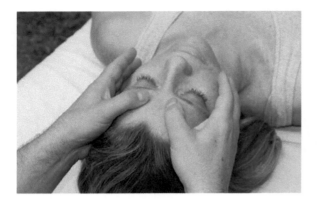

Figure 33.23
Treatment of the anterior part of the corpus callosum and indusium griseum

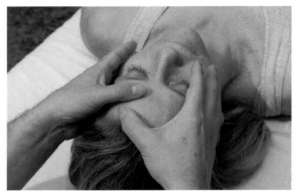

Figure 33.24
Treatment of the left medial longitudinal stria

- **Treating the medial and lateral longitudinal striae (of Lancisi):**

Patient: the patient is in supine position.

Practitioner: the practitioner is positioned at the head of the patient. First, connect with the motility of the lateral ventricles and assess the corpus callosum on the roof of the lateral ventricles of the brain. Just superior to it find longitudinal structures. Two striae are located close to midline and two more laterally.

Method: the practitioner will assess the four striae separately by putting one finger cephalic and one finger caudal to assess the whole length of a stria. It is common to find one of the four striae in lesion in a patient. Synchronize precisely with this structure in lesion and let the intrinsic self-correcting mechanisms bring back this structure in a balanced/aligned/neutral place. Recheck position, rhythm, activity, even energetic or emotional component should be back to homeostasis/allostasis and present no "signaling" at all.

Septum pellucidum (previously called septum lucidum): "transparent separation"
Bruno Chikly

- **Anatomy/structure:** the septum pellucidum is a midline vertical membrane of both white and grey matter present between the frontal horns of the left and right lateral ventricles. The septum pellucidum spreads between the corpus callosum superiorly and the fornix inferiorly. The septum pellucidum is made up of two membrane layers with a virtual cavity in between them sometimes called the "cavum pellucidum."

- **Relation to the ventricular system:** located midline, it is a vertical structure situated between the two ventricles.

Treating the septum pellucidum:

Patient: the patient is in supine position.

Practitioner: the practitioner is positioned at the head of the patient.

Method: first, connect with the motility of the lateral ventricles and assess the structures located just medial to them. If you feel any change in symmetry, position, quality, rhythm, activity, synchronize precisely with this structure and let the intrinsic self-correcting mechanisms bring back this structure to a balanced/aligned/neutral place. Recheck that position, rhythm, activity, even the energetic or emotional component are back to homeostasis/allostasis and present no "signaling" whatsoever. All nuclei will be treated here with this method.

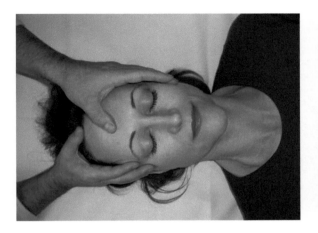

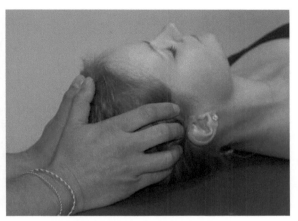

Figure 33.25
Treatment of the septum pellucidum

Figure 33.26
Alternative hand position for treating. Treating the region of the hippocampus and fornix

Fornix: "arched" structure
Anatomy and function: Torsten Liem, Bruno Chikly

- **Anatomy and structure:** the fornix is a C-shaped bundle of fibers placed between the fimbria of the hippocampus and the mammillary bodies (hypothalamus). The fornix is located beneath the corpus callosum and above the third ventricle. It starts as a continuation of the hippocampus, with the two crura of the fornix and the commissure of the fornix, and then unites to become the body of the fornix. Anteriorly, it divides again to form the columns of the fornix, which terminate in the mammillary bodies.

- **Relation to the ventricular system:** the fornix lays at the inferior aspect of the septum pellucidum inferior to the lateral ventricles.

- **Known function:** memory function. Its damage may provoke anterograde amnesia (*memory loss* related to events occurring after a trauma). Efferent conduction from the hippocampus to the septum, amygdaloid body, hypothalamus, and mammillary bodies.

Treating the region of the hippocampus and fornix
Torsten Liem

Hand position

- Index, middle and ring finger are positioned inferior to the temporal/inferior horn of the lateral ventricle.

- The points of contact range from slightly posterior to the lower half of the sphenofrontal suture up to the area superior to asterion.

- The thumbs touch anteriorly and diverge slightly posteriorly about 0.5 cm beside the midline.

- The contact of the thumbs ranges from anterior to the bregma running up to the level of the asterion.

Method:

- Project your fingers towards the region of the hippocampus.

- Project your thumbs toward the region of the fornix, beneath the corpus callosum and above the third ventricle.

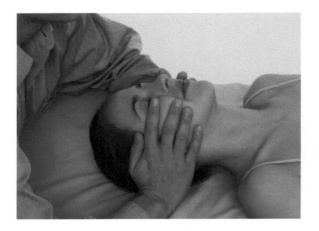

Figure 33.27
Alternative hand position for treating the region of the hippocampus and fornix

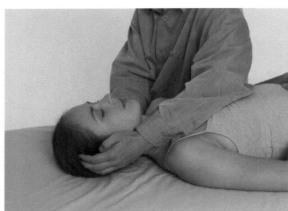

Figure 33.28
Treating the caudate nucleus

- Synchronise with tissue qualities and dynamics

- Synchronise with form, density/hardness, tissue elasticity, involuntary rhythms, amplitude, end feel of the particular phase, natural disengagement at the end of the inhalation phase, natural compression/closeness at the end of the exhalation phase, ease of movement, ,strength/force of movement, fullness/emptiness in the tissue, additional asynchronous chaotic motions during the (sub-) phase(s), tensions.

- Establish a balanced tension BT: a local, regional, global PBT, DBT, BFT, a balanced electrodynamic tension (BET)

- Apply further treatment modalities if needed (Chapters 20 and 38).

Alternative hand position 1 for treating the region of the hippocampus and fornix
Torsten Liem

Hand position
- Position the metacarpophalangeal joint of your index finger approximately midway between the tragus and the squamoparietal suture on each side

- Locate your thumbs immediately below the squamoparietal suture on each side

- Make contact with your thenar eminences Your other fingers should lie passively on either side of the patient's face

Alternative technique 2 for treating the fornix
Bruno Chikly

The caudate nucleus: "tailed nuclei"
Anatomy, function: Bruno Chikly, Torsten Liem

- **Anatomy/structure:** the caudate nucleus is also a C-shaped structure located lateral to the lateral ventricles. It encircles the putamen from above. The wider "head" of the caudate nucleus protrudes inside the lateral ventricles, constituting its lateral wall and floor. The thin "tail" of the caudate nucleus ends up in the amygdaloid body.

- **Relation to the ventricular system:** just lateral to the lateral ventricles . In the upper part of each lateral ventricle, the caudate nucleus together with the thalamus

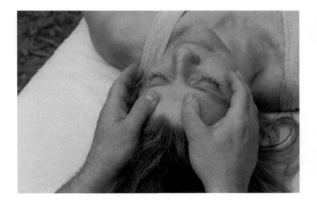

Figure 33.29
Treatment of the caudate nucleus

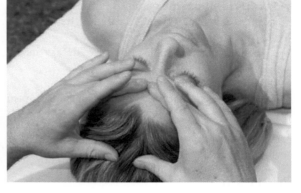

Figure 33.30
Treatment of the fornix

forms the floor of the ventricle, and in the inferior part of each lateral ventricle it forms the roof of the ventricle. Its shape results from the torsion of the cerebral hemispheres during embryological development.

- **Known function:**
  - Regulation of voluntary and involuntary movements (the direct and indirect pathways).
  - Learning and memory (left caudate).
  - Obsessive–compulsive disorder (right caudate).

Treating the caudate nucleus:
Bruno Chikly

Patient: the patient is in supine position.

Practitioner: the practitioner is positioned at the head of the patient.

Method: first, connect with the motility of the lateral ventricles and assess the structures located just lateral to them. If you feel any change in symmetry, position, quality, rhythm, activity, synchronize precisely with this structure and let the intrinsic self-correcting mechanisms bring back this structure in a balanced/aligned/neutral place. Recheck position, rhythm, activity, even energetic or emotional component should be back to homeostasis/allostasis and present no "signaling" at al.

Alternative hand position for treating the region of the caudate nucleus:
Torsten Liem

Practitioner:

- Take up a position to one side level with the patient's shoulder region.

Hand position:

- Position the fingers of each hand in a semi-circle about 1 – 2 cm above the squamoparietal suture on both sides (slightly below the upper boundaries of the lateral ventricles).

Putamen: the "shell"
Anatomy and function: Bruno Chikly, Torsten Liem

- **Anatomy/structure:** the putamen lies lateral to the caudate nucleus. The putamen is shaped like an oval disk. The caudate nucleus and putamen are separated during embryologic development by the ingrowth of the internal capsule.

- **Relation to the ventricular system:** the putamen is not directly connected with the ventricular system. It is located lateral to the caudate nucleus.

- **Known function:** the putamen is connected to the substantia nigra and globus pallidus. Its functions are close to the caudate nucleus.
  - Regulation of voluntary and involuntary movements.
  - Learning: learning reinforcement.
  - "Hate circuit": perception of contempt and disgust.

Treating the putamen:
Torsten Liem

Practitioner:

- Take up a position at the head of the patient.

Hand position:

- Position the second phalanx of your index, middle and ring fingers at the level of the squamoparietal suture on both sides.

- Your thumbs should be touching, to act as a fulcrum.

- Project your index, middle and ring fingers toward the location of the putamen (especially the middle phalanges).

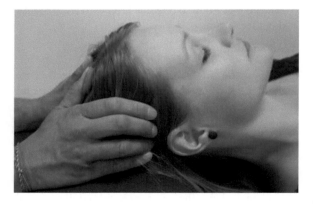

Figure 33.31
Treating the putamen

Globus pallidus: "pale body"
Anatomy and function: Bruno Chikly, Torsten Liem

- **Anatomy/structure:** the globus pallidus is constituted of two parts—the globus pallidus externa (GPe) and the globus pallidus interna (GPi). Both regions communicate with the subthalamic nucleus.

- **Afferents:** corpus striatum, subthalamic nucleus, thalamus.

- **Efferents:** thalamus.

- **Relation to the ventricular system:** the globus pallidus is located medial to the putamen.

- **Known function:** very ancient phylogenetic center for movement. Principally, its function is antagonistic to that of the corpus striatum. Regulation of voluntary and involuntary movements.

Treating the globus pallidus
Torsten Liem

Hand position:

- As for the putamen.

- However, your hands should project further medially.

- Try to differentiate a medial and a lateral segment.

The subthalamic nucleus:
Torsten Liem

- **Anatomy/structure:** the subthalamic nucleus lies ventromedially to the globus pallidus and is derived from the diencephalon.

- **Known function:** inhibit movement-triggering impulses.

Treatment of the region of the subthalamic nuclei

Hand position:

- Position both index fingers approximately 0,5 cm lateral from nasion.

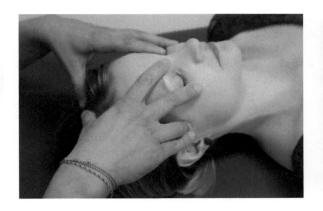

Figure 33.32
Treating the region of the subthalamic nuclei

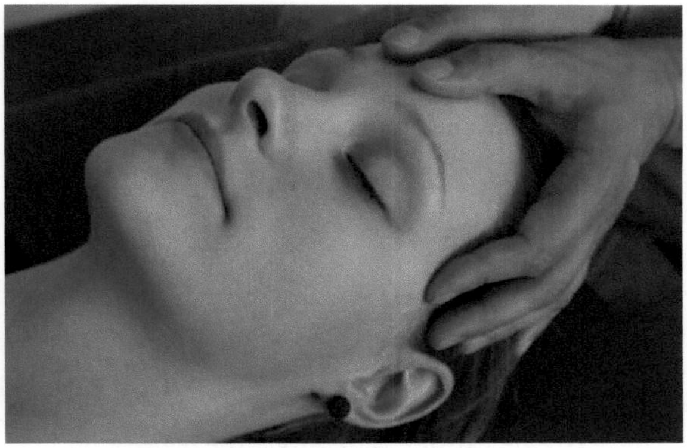

Figure 33.33
Treating the region of the nucleus accumbens

- Position both thumbs approximately 0,5 cm lateral from bregma.

- Position both ringfingers approximately 0,5 cm below pterion.

Method:

- Focus with thumbs, index and middle fingers towards the subthalamic nuclei.

- Balance the structure.

Nucleus accumbens
Torsten Liem

- **Anatomy/structure:** the nucleus accumbens is a small cluster of neurons, which are part of the basal ganglia. It is located in the limbic system in the basal forebrain, between the caudate nucleus and the putamen; it is stimulated by dopaminergic afferents of the ventral tegmental area (VTA)

- **Known function:** It is associated with the experience of pleasure ("wanting", as opposed to the feeling of happiness or "liking" something). It plays an essential role for the reward system and addiction.

Treating the region of the nucleus accumbens

Patient: the patient is in the supine position.

Practitioner: the practitioner is positioned at the head of the patient.

Hand position:

- Each thumb is positioned 1/2 cm lateral of the midline and about ½ to 1 cm superior of the eye.

- The index fingers are located on the side close to pterion.

Method:

- Thumbs and index fingers project towards each other.

- To adress the frontal lobe, e.g. establish a resonance with the dynamics and qualities of that region and let the intrinsic self-correcting dynamics bring back this structure to a balanced state.

- Note: Afterwards connect the nucleus accumbens with the VTA specifically and with respect to the reward system also to the substantia nigra, the locus coeruleus and the prefrontal cortex.

Claustrum: "barrier, fence, and separation"
Bruno Chikly

- **Anatomy/structure:** the claustrum is a vertical sheet of grey matter lateral to the putamen and medial to the insular cortex. The claustrum sets between the white matter tracts of the external (medially) and the extreme capsule (laterally). The claustrum presents some uniformity in the types of its cells. Some researchers believe that the claustrum could be considered a seventh layer of the cortex.

- **Known function:** the claustrum may improve communication and synchronization between the two hemispheres of the brain and may help a uniform quality of conscious experience.

Treating the claustrum:

Patient: the patient is in supine position.

Practitioner: the practitioner is positioned at the head of the patient.

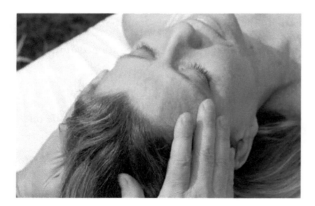

Figure 33.34
Treatment of the insula or claustrum

Method: coming back lateral, by palpation we can isolate first the insula of Reil, then medial to it a thin layer of white matter and further medially the claustrum layer of grey matter. If you feel any change in symmetry, position, quality, rhythm, activity, synchronize precisely with this structure and let the intrinsic self-correcting mechanisms bring back this structure in a balanced/ aligned/ neutral place. Recheck position, rhythm, activity, even energetic or emotional component should be back to homeostasis/allostasis and present no "signaling" at all.

Thalamus: "inner chamber or bridal chamber"
Anatomy and function: Bruno Chikly, Torsten Liem

- **Anatomy/structure:** the thalami of the diencephalon regions are two ovoid masses of grey matter on each side of the third ventricle. They measure approximately 2 cm × 2.5 cm × 5.5 cm, converging anteriorly and diverging posteriorly. The thalami are often separated by an interthalamic adhesion that contains some grey fibers (also called massa intermedia, soft commissure, or grey commissure).

- **Relation to the ventricular system:** the thalami are located medial inside the "C" of the lateral ventricles.

- **Known function:** the "gateway" to consciousness, the thalami have numerous functions:
  - Process all sensory information to (and from) the cortex (except olfactory stimuli).
  - Regulation of consciousness and sleep.

Treating the thalamus:
Bruno Chikly

Patient: the patient is in supine position.

Practitioner: the practitioner is positioned at the head of the patient.

Method:
- Assess all nuclei of thalamus.
- Patient is in supine position; practitioner is positioned at the head of the patient.
- Position the fingers laterally in the temples area, over the area where the temporal horn of the lateral ventricles are located.
- Find the thalamus inside the C of the lateral ventricles.

– Bring thumbs superiorly on the coronal suture. The thalamus is usually positioned just anterior or posterior to the coronal suture. Assess each separate nucleus. You can associate each nucleus in relation to its main cortical projection.

Thalamus nuclei

There is no standard terminology and classification of thalamus nuclei.

1 **Medial group of thalamus nuclei**: All cortex associations of medial group of nuclei are typically with the prefrontal cortex but many other cortical associations are possible.

a **Midline nuclei:** connections with reticular activating system (RAS), hypothalamus.

b **Mediodorsal nuclei (MD):** connections with amygdala, hypothalamus, olfactory cortex, substantia nigra. Anxiety states.

c **Medioventral nuclei (MV):** connections with amygdala and hypothalamus. Related with anxiety.

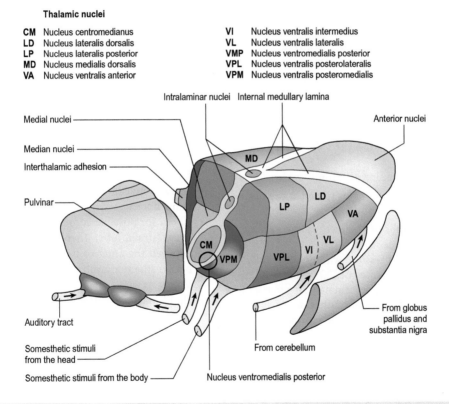

Thalamic nuclei

CM Nucleus centromedianus
LD Nucleus lateralis dorsalis
LP Nucleus lateralis posterior
MD Nucleus medialis dorsalis
VA Nucleus ventralis anterior

VI Nucleus ventralis intermedius
VL Nucleus ventralis lateralis
VMP Nucleus ventromedialis posterior
VPL Nucleus ventralis posterolateralis
VPM Nucleus ventralis posteromedialis

Figure 33.35
The thalamic nuclei

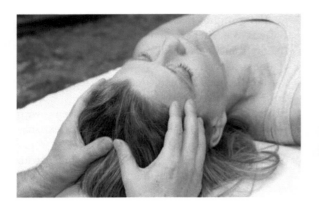

Figure 33.36
Treatment of the medial nuclei of the thalamus

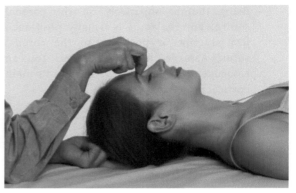

Figure 33.37
Alternative handhold for treating the region of the thalamus

Treating the medial group of thalamus nuclei:

Patient: the patient is in supine position.

Practitioner: the practitioner is positioned at the head of the patient.

Method: put your thumbs at the level of the coronal suture very close to midline.

Try first to get an impression whether the interthalamic adhesion (massa intermedia) is present. In humans, it is only found in approximately 70 percent of adults. If present, the interthalamic adhesion is usually a little bit anterior or posterior to the coronal suture. Go a little lateral and you will first be in relation to the midline nuclei. Then continue a little more laterally, you will find nuclei with a different "quality," the mediodorsal nuclei (MD) which can be also connected with anxiety states. You can possibly connect any of these nuclei with an associated cortex (such as the prefrontal cortex) or any cortical or subcortical structure (such as the amygdaloid bodies or the hypothalamus).

2 **Anterior thalamus nuclei:**
   a Anterior nuclei: learning, memory, and emotions.
   b Classical cortex association: cingulate gyrus.

Treating the anterior group of thalamus nuclei:
   • First, feel the thalamus, as previously described, and go anterior to connect with the anterior thalamic nuclei.
   • Check for possible connection with the cingulate gyrus (limbic lobe). Then feel if a connection exists between the anterior nuclei and the mammillary bodies (the mammillothalamic tract or bundle of Vicq d'Azyr).
   • Hand placement: thumbs on anterior nucleus of thalamus, middle fingers on mammillary body. Stay there if needed until the connection downregulates or balances.

3 **Lateral group of thalamus nuclei:**
   a Lateral dorsal nuclei (LD): memory and vision. Classical cortex association: anterior parietal cortex.
   b Lateral posterior nuclei (LP): vision and complex behaviors. Classical cortex association: posterior parietal cortex.

4 **Ventral group of thalamus nuclei:**
   a Ventral anterior nuclei (VA): motor. Classical cortex association: supplementary motor cortex (area 6).

b Ventral lateral nuclei (VL), anterior division: motor. Classical cortex association: primary motor cortex (area 4).

c Ventral intermediate (VI) and ventral lateral (VL) posterior division nuclei: motor. Classical cortex association: primary motor cortex (area 4); cerebellum.

d Ventral posterior lateral nuclei (VPL): sensory. Classical cortex association: primary somatosensory cortex; lower body.

Ventral posterior medial nuclei (VPM): sensory. Classical cortex association: primary somatosensory cortex, upper body, and face.

5 **Posterior nuclei: pulvinar**

Vision, language, and sensory integration. Lesion in pulvinar may result in attention-deficit problems. Classical cortex association: superior visual cortex.

6 **Intralaminar group of thalamus nuclei**

These nuclei are responsible for many functions including alertness, movement, sensations of pain, and so forth. Coma usually occurs if both sides of intralaminar nuclei are destroyed.

a Centromedian nuclei (associated with RAS)

b Central lateral nuclei (associated with RAS)

c Parafascicular nuclei.

7 **Reticular thalamus nuclei (optional):** connections with cortex and thalamus. The reticular thalamus nuclei inhibits the thalamocortical pathways (gamma-aminobutyric acid - GABA).

8 **Geniculate bodies**:

a Lateral geniculate body: in relation with the visual cortex.

b Medial geniculate body: in relation with the auditory cortex.

Alternative handhold for treating the region of the thalamus
Torsten Liem

Practitioner

- Take up a position at the head of the patient.

Hand position:

- Position the index and middle finger of one hand immediately to the right and left of the region of glabella.

- Position the index and middle finger of your other hand 1 cm above the inion and about 1 cm to the right and left of the median line.

- Align your left and right index fingers and your left and right middle fingers along the longitudinal axes of the two thalami.

Method:

- Project your fingers laterally alongside the third ventricle, approximately at the level of the posterior part of the greater wings of the sphenoid and the superior part of the temporal squama.

- Either assess and treat the two thalamic bodies as a single entity or attempt to differentiate the individual nuclei.

- Then proceed as for PBT, DBT or BFT.

Hippocampal formation: the "seahorse"
Anatomy, function: Torsten Liem, Bruno Chikly

- **Anatomy/structure:** located in the medial aspect of the temporal lobe; the entire hippocampal formation has a length of about 5 cm.

The parahippocampal gyrus, including the entorhinal cortex, lies medial to the hippocampus. It is involved in memory processes and is responsible for relaying sensory information to other parts of the limbic system.

- **Afferents:** rhinencephalon, amygdaloid body, neocortex, thalamus, cingulate gyrus, septum.

- **Efferents:** (via the fornix) septum, amygdaloid body, hypothalamus, mamillary bodies.

- **Relation to the ventricular system:** the hippocampal formation is located inferior and medial to the C of the lateral ventricles.

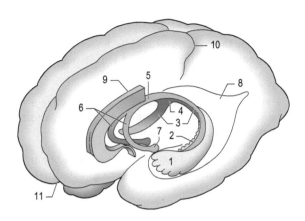

Figure 33.38
Hippocampus and fornix. (1) Hippocampus with the pes hippocampi; (2) dentate gyrus; (3) crura of the fornix; (4) commissure of the fornix; (5) body of the fornix; (6) division into two columns of the fornix that continue to become the mamillary bodies (= 7); (8) posterior horn of the lateral ventricle; (9) corpus callosum.

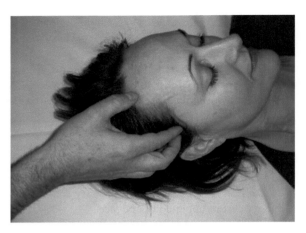

Figure 33.39
Treatment of the hippocampus

- **Known functions:**
  - Memory (especially transfer of content from short-term to long-term memory)
  - Spatial orientation
  - Learning
  - Behavior (involved in development of aggression and affective behaviors).

Treating the hippocampal formation:
Bruno Chikly

- **Patient:** the patient is in supine position.
- **Practitioner:** the practitioner is positioned at the head of the patient.
- **Method:** position the fingers laterally in the temples area, over the area where the temporal horn of the lateral ventricles is located. Find the hippocampal formation inferior to the C of the lateral ventricles. If you feel any change in symmetry, position, quality, rhythm, activity, synchronize precisely with this structure and let the intrinsic

self-correcting mechanisms bring back this structure in a balanced/aligned/neutral place. Recheck position, rhythm, activity, even energetic or emotional component should be back to homeostasis/allostasis and present no "signaling".

(See also page 581 Treating the hippocampus and fornix)

Amygdala (amygdaloid bodies): "almond"
Anatomy, function: Bruno Chikly, Torsten Liem

- **Anatomy/structure:** the amygdaloid body is a small ovoid complex of grey matter consisting of several individual nuclei. It is located in the anterior temporal lobe within the uncus, at the rostral end of the caudate nucleus. The amygdaloid body is usually positioned anterior, superior, and slightly medial to the hippocampus.

- **Known function:** the amygdaloid body has a modulating influence on autonomic centers of the hypothalamus – affective behaviors and affective motor activity (e.g., flight and anxiety reactions). It is also involved in storage of emotionally charged memory content.

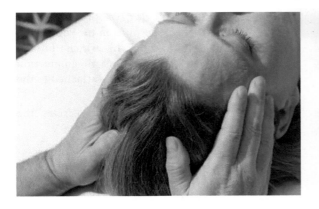

Figure 33.40
Treatment of the amygdala

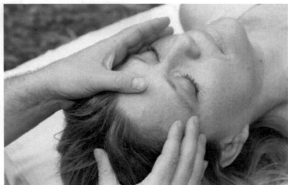

Figure 33.41
Relation amygdala-caudate nucleus

- Older part (centromedial) related to anger, rage, fear, and recognition of threats also smell, feeding, and so forth.
- New part (basolateral) connected to social and sexual behavior, states of bliss, and so forth.

Treating the amygdaloid body:
Bruno Chikly

- **Patient:** the patient is in supine position.
- **Practitioner:** the practitioner is positioned at the head of the patient.
- **Method:** position your middle fingers in an area between the lateral side of the orbit, the projection of the greater wing of the sphenoid and the beginning of the temporal hair if present. The amygdala is very medial within the cranium. Project your middle fingers toward the amygdaloid body. Typically, an amygdala on one side is usually more affected than the other. When one amygdala is in lesion, it will often present a hypersympathetic reaction and be more easily palpable than the other side.

Connect caudate nucleus to amygdala: Place the fingers of one hand on the head of the caudate nucleus (see instruction mentioned earlier) and the other hand on the ipsilateral amygdala. There is an anatomic connection between these two structures; perhaps you could feel a continuity between the hands.

Bridge hippocampus to amygdala: Align the fingers of one hand along the hippocampus and the other hand on the ipsilateral amygdala. This is a physiological connection (hippocampus can regulate amygdala functions in mammals).

Alternative handhold for treating the region of the amygdala:
Torsten Liem

Position your middle fingers posterior to the squamoparietal suture on both sides, approximately on a level with the mid-point of the vertical path of the sphenosquamous suture.

Method:

Project your middle fingers toward the amygdaloid body.

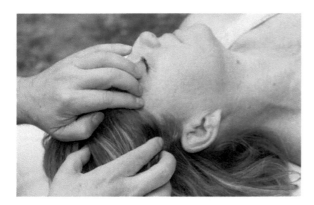

Figure 33.42
Relation hippocampus-amygdala 2

Pituitary (hypophysis)
Anatomy, function: Torsten Liem, Bruno Chikly

- **Anatomy/structure:** located within the sella turcica (hypophyseal fossa) of the sphenoid bone, the pituitary (or hypophysis) is a small structure weighing about 0.5 g (0.018 oz) in humans.

- **Known function:** the pituitary comprises the adenohypophysis (anterior pituitary lobe) and the neurohypophysis (posterior pituitary lobe). The neurohypophysis forms part of the hypothalamus. It is connected with the anterior inferior region of the hypothalamus, the tuber cinereum, via the infundibulum. The pituitary produces numerous hormones but the posterior pituitary only stores the antidiuretic hormone and oxytocin produced in the hypothalamus. Because this region is not characterized by an impervious blood–brain barrier, these hormones are able to enter the blood stream by a process known as "neurosecretion." The adenohypophysis lies below the optic chiasm and it is related on each side to the cavernous sinus. It contains glandular epithelia and, as a glandular secretory organ, it does not form part of the brain

proper. During embryologic development, it arises as an outgrowth of ectoderm from the roof of the pharynx (called Rathke pouch), which initially arches upward and finally loses all connection with the pharynx before becoming attached to the diencephalon.

The pituitary anterior lobe (adeno) secretes the following:

Glandotropic hormones:
thyroid-stimulating hormone (TSH)
follicle-stimulating hormone (FSH) and luteinizing hormone (LH)
adrenocorticotropic hormone (ACTH).

Effector hormones:
growth hormone (GH)
prolactin.

The release of these hormones is regulated by the releasing or release-inhibiting hormones synthesized by the hypothalamus and carried in the hypothalamic pituitary portal system. The intermediate or middle lobe secretes melanin-stimulating hormone (MSH). The pituitary posterior lobe (neuro) stores the following:

Vasopressin or antidiuretic hormone (ADH)

Oxytocin (stimulate uterine contractions; help the initiation of milk secretion; and is described as a "bonding" hormone [impulse to "cuddle" or attachment]).

Treating the pituitary:
Bruno Chikly

Patient: the patient is in supine position.
Practitioner: the practitioner is positioned at the head of the patient.

Gland–infundibulum

Hand position and method: place one finger at the level of the nasion, the other one on the bridge of the nose. Direct your fingers toward the pituitary in the sella turcica (a depression of the sphenoid bone). Assess if there is any lesion between the infundibulum (stalk) of the pituitary and its stem, especially a rotation or torque. If you feel any change in symmetry, position,

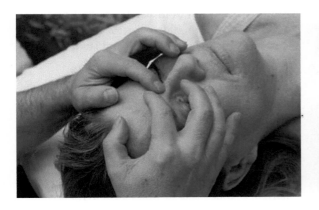

Figure 33.43
Treatment of the pituitary - fingers superior and inferior

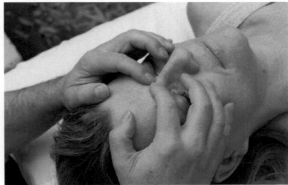

Figure 33.44
Treatment of the pituitary - fingers lateral

quality, rhythm, activity, synchronize precisely with this structure and let the intrinsic self-correcting mechanisms bring back this structure in a balanced/ aligned/ neutral place. Recheck position, rhythm, activity, even energetic or emotional component should be back to homeostasis/allostasis and present no "signaling".

Intraglandular assessment and treatment
Hand position and method: place one finger at the level of the nasion and the other finger next to it. Direct your fingers toward the pituitary in the sella turcica and assess if there is any lesion between or within the pituitary. Treat with the same method as above.

- **Additional notes on treatment:**
Torsten Liem

  – Assess if there is any dominant dysfunctions of the sphenoid bone and the sphenobasilar synchondrosis (SBS).
  – The tension of the cranial dura mater (the diaphragm of the sella turcica, etc.) may need to be normalized during treatment.
  – Treat the third ventricle, where appropriate.
  – Chronic inflammation of the sphenoid sinuses should be assessed.

  – It may be necessary to improve venous drainage because the pituitary is surrounded by the cavernous sinus.
  – The pituitary lies close to the internal carotid artery.

Alternative handhold for treating the region of the pituitary:
Torsten Liem

- Position your index and middle fingers in the upper part of the sphenosquamous suture on both sides.

- Place your thumbs at the level of the bregma point.

- Direct your fingers toward the pituitary in the sella turcica.

Method:

- You may sense developmental dynamic vectors.

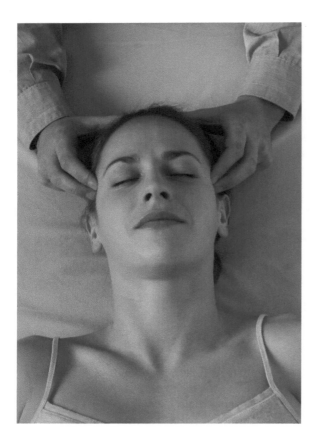

Figure 33.45
Alternative handhold: Treating the pituitary

- These may be ascending from the pharyngeal membrane, descending from the hypothalamus

- Then proceed as for PBT, DBT or BFT.

Hypothalamus
Anatomy, function: Torsten Liem

- **Anatomy/structure:** the hypothalamus is located rostroventrally to the thalamus at the base of the brain, at the floor, and partly at the lateral and anterior wall of the third ventricle. It is bordered anteriorly by the optic chiasm and laterally by the optic tract.

- **Known function:** its principal function is the maintenance and regulation of respiration, circulation, fluid and food intake, body temperature, and reproductive behavior. In the setting of psychoneuroimmunology, the hypothalamus occupies a central position for several reasons: Firstly, because of the anterior lobe pituitary hormones, especially growth hormone, which acts to stimulate T cells. Secondly, because the lymphatic organs are largely subject to sympathetic innervation and modulation; and thirdly, because the hypothalamus is under the control of the limbic system.

Many hormones are secreted by the hypothalamic complex. These include the following:

- Thyrotropin-releasing hormone (TRH), thyrotropin-releasing factor (TRF), or prolactin-releasing hormone (PRH)

- Dopamine (DA) or prolactin-inhibiting hormone (PIH)

- Growth hormone-releasing hormone (GHRH)

- Somatostatin (SS), growth hormone-inhibiting hormone (GHIH), or somatostain release-inhibiting factor (SRIF) in the periventricular nucleus

- Gonadotropin-releasing hormone (GnRH) or luteinizing hormone-releasing hormone (LHRH)

- Corticotropin-releasing hormone (CRH) or corticotropin-releasing factor (CRF)

- Oxytocin

- Vasopressin or antidiuretic hormone (ADH or arginine vasopressin [AVP]).

Many nuclei may secrete the same component. For example, the paraventricular nuclei (PVN) and supraoptic nuclei (SON) can secrete ADH. Some nuclei can secrete different components. For example, the arcuate nucleus secretes DA and GHRH.

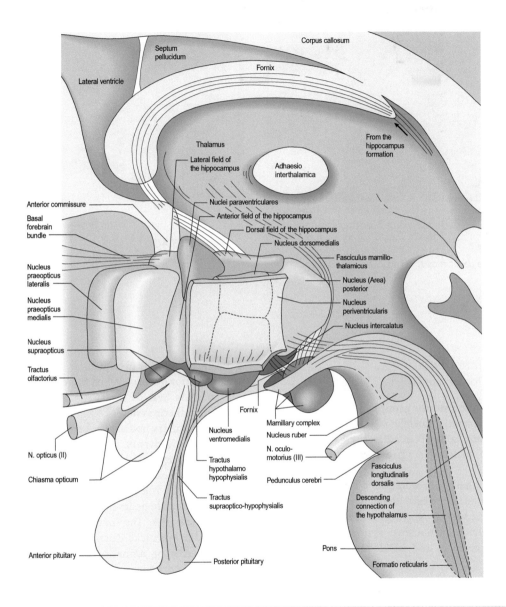

Figure 33.46
The hypothalamus

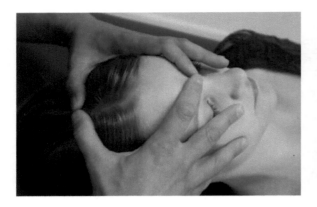

Figure 33.47
Treating the region of the hypothalamus

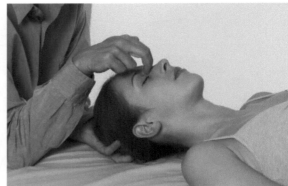

Figure 33.48
Treating the hypothalamus

Hypothalamic nuclei:
Bruno Chikly, Torsten Liem

1 **Hypothalamic anterior group:**
   a Suprachiasmatic nuclei (SCN): master biologic clock. Helps control circadian rhythms.
   b Preoptic nuclei: related to parasympathetic processes
   c SON: synthesis and secretion of ADH
   d Anterior nuclei: release high temperature; diffuses heat in the body by sweating and releasing heat.
   e Paraventricular nucleus: synthesis and secretion of oxytocin and ADH. May helps regulate hunger.

2 **Tuberal nuclear group:**
   a Dorsomedial nucleus: satiety center
   b Ventromedial nucleus: larger satiety center
   c Arcuate nucleus: Regulates release of gonadotrophin. Can stimulate food intake.

3 **Lateral group:**
   a Lateral nuclei: produces "orexins" (hypocretins). Their deficiency can provoke narcolepsy.

4 **Posterior nuclear group:**
   a Posterior nucleus: When there is an excess of cold, increase heat in the tissue. Associated with the sympathetic system.
   b Mammillary bodies: They are located at the rostral end of the fornix. They consist of two groups of nuclei (the medial mammillary nuclei and the lateral mammillary nuclei). They contain histamine and have a role in alertness and memory processing. They are believed to add the element of smell to memories. The mammillary bodies are damaged in Wernicke-Korsakoff syndrome (Korsakoff dementia or amnesic confabulatory syndrome) caused by a lack of thiamine (vitamin B_1), often seen in chronic alcoholism.

Treating the region of the hypothalamus:
Torsten Liem

Practitioner
• Take up a position at the head of the patient.

Hand position:
• Position both index fingers on glabella.
• Position both thumbs on Bregma.

Method:

- Focus with index fingers and thumbs towards the hypothalamus

- Direct your fingers toward the individual hypothalamic nucleus regions.

- Either assess and treat the hypothalamus as a whole entity or attempt to differentiate the individual nucleus groups or nuclei.

- Synchronise with form, density/hardness, activity, tissue elasticity, involuntary dynamics/rhythms, ease of movement, strength/force of movement, fullness/emptiness in the tissue, additional asynchronous chaotic motions during the (sub-) phase(s), tensions and let the intrinsic self-correcting dynamics bring back this structure in a balanced state.

- Proceed as for PBT, DBT or BFT

Alternative handhold: treating the region of the hypothalamus:

- Position the index and middle finger of one hand to the right and left of the median line, above the frontonasal suture.

- Position the index and middle finger of your other hand approximately 0.5 cm above the inion and approximately 1 cm to the right and left of the median line.

Method:

- Direct your fingers toward the individual hypothalamic nucleus regions.

- Either assess and treat the hypothalamus as a whole entity or attempt to differentiate the individual nucleus groups or nuclei.

- Then proceed as for PBT, DBT or BFT.

The pineal gland (or epiphysis)
Anatomy, function: Bruno Chikly, Torsten Liem

- **Anatomy/structure:** the pineal gland lies in the diencephalon, or epithalamus, between the two diverging thalamic bodies in the posterior roof region of the third ventricle. The base of the pineal gland marks the meeting point of the two pineal stalks (habenulae), which form a connection with the thalamus and accommodate, among other things, a relay center for olfactory stimuli.

- **Relation to the ventricular system:** located posterior and midline in relation to the third ventricle.

- **Known functions:**
  - Secretion of melatonin (which is stimulated by darkness).
  - Secretes pinoline (antioxidant), similar to that function of melatonin. It is also connected with higher states of consciousness (e.g., during meditation).

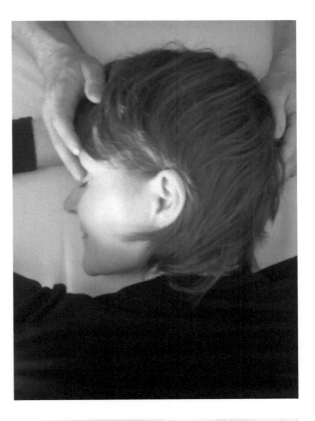

Figure 33.49
Treatment of the pineal-suprachiasmatic nuclei of the hypothalamus

- Action on the immune system: lower levels associated with prostate and breast cancer.

The pineal gland is believed to possess a kind of *zeitgeber* function in mediating circadian rhythm.

Fibers project from the SCN to the paraventricular nuclei (PVN), which relay the circadian signals to the spinal cord and out via the sympathetic system to superior cervical ganglia (SCG), and from there into the pineal gland.

Treating the pineal gland:
Bruno Chikly

Patient: the patient is in prone position.

Practitioner: the practitioner is positioned at the head of the patient.

1 Pineal gland: when patient is in prone position, put your fingers in an area above inion and below the top of bregma on a flat location. Ask the patient to open and close the eyes to help localize more precisely the pineal gland.

2 You can connect the pineal gland with the suprachiasmatic nuclei (SCN) anteriorly. The SCN is a relay for the light information coming from the retina.

Alternative handhold for treating the pineal gland:
Torsten Liem

- Position the tip of the index finger of one hand on the nasion, pointing toward the pineal gland (the roof of the third ventricle).

- Position the index finger of your other hand on the lambda point.

Habenula
Bruno Chikly

- **Anatomy/structure:** this structure is located in the diencephalon, or epithalamus, posterior to the lateral ventricles and lateral to the pineal gland. On each side, we can find two habenulae nuclei (the medial and lateral habenulae). A habenular commissure connects the paired habenular nuclei. The habenulae form part of the dorsal diencephalic conduction system—a system found in all vertebrates.

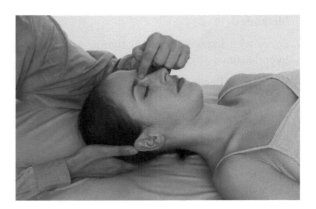

Figure 33.50
Alternative handhold for treating the pineal gland

- **Known function:** the habenulae receive input from the brain via the stria medullaris thalami and outputs to many midbrain areas involved in releasing neuromodulators such as dopamine, norepinephrine, and serotonin. The habenulae seem to inhibit the activity of dopaminergic cells in the ventral midbrain, ventral tegmental area, as well as nucleus accumbens (involved in reward, pleasure, and motivation). The habenulae might also be involved in learning (integration of hippocampal signals) reproductive behavior, sleep, response to noxious stimuli, and among other things, they may be relay centers for olfactory stimuli.

Treating the habenulae:

Patient: the patient is in supine position.

Practitioner: the practitioner is positioned at the head of the patient.

Method: first, connect with the pineal gland and move laterally to find very active structures on the posterior side of the third ventricle. If you feel any change in symmetry, position, quality, rhythm, activity, synchronize precisely with this structure and let the intrinsic self-correcting mechanisms bring back this structure in a balanced/aligned/neutral place. Recheck position, rhythm, activity, even energetic or emotional component should be back to homeostasis/allostasis and present no "signaling".

The midbrain (mesencephalon)
Torsten Liem

Location:
The midbrain (comprising the cerebral peduncles, tegmentum, and tectum including the four rounded elevations known as the colliculi) lies between the pons and diencephalon and surrounds the mesencephalic aqueduct. The midbrain contains the nuclei for cranial nerves III and IV as well as the ascending and descending conduction pathways (pyramidal tract, medial and lateral lemniscus, medial and dorsal longitudinal fascicles, the cerebellothalamic tract, cerebropontine tract, cerebellum-optic thalamus tract) and parts of the reticular formation.

Treating the midbrain

Hand position:
- Position your thenar eminences between the external acoustic meatus and the squamoparietal suture, approximately level with the middle of the eye.

- Project your thenar eminences deeply (toward the midbrain region around the mesencephalic aqueduct).

Method:
As for the frontal lobe, e.g. synchronise with form, density/hardness, tissue elasticity, involuntary dynamics/rhythms, amplitude, end feel of the particular phase, natural disengagement at the end of the inhalation phase, natural compression/ closeness at the end of the exhalation phase, ease of movement, strength/force of movement, fullness/ emptiness in the tissue, additional asynchronous chaotic motions during the (sub-) phase(s), tensions and let the intrinsic self-correcting dynamics bring back this structure in a balanced state.

Note: The individual constituent parts of the midbrain may also be treated in a targeted manner. When adopting this approach, establish a resonance with the the qualities of the particular tissue in question.

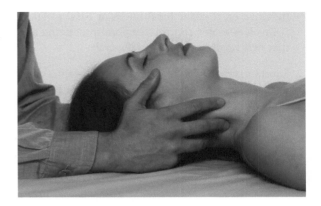

Figure 33.51
Treating the midbrain

Substantia nigra
Anatomy, function: Bruno Chikly, Torsten Liem

- **Anatomy/structure:** the substantia nigra is the largest nucleus of the mesencephalon (midbrain). It is located at the boundary with the cerebral peduncles and with the mesencephalic tegmentum. It consists of three parts: the substantia nigra pars compacta, the pars lateralis, and the substantia nigra pars reticulata.

- **Afferents:** corpus striatum, cortex (especially motor and premotor)

- **Efferents:** corpus striatum (inhibitory action)

- **Known function:** the substantia nigra participates in the control and modulation of motor activity, (movement motivation and movement initiation, in particular), motor planning, eye movement, reward seeking, learning, and addiction. (Clinically important in Parkinson's disease.)

1 Substantia nigra pars compacta and pars lateralis. The substantia nigra pars compacta and pars lateralis is part of an input circuit to the caudate nucleus and

putamen (part of the basal nuclei or basal ganglia). It involves motor control, temporal processing and may help regulate the sleep-wake cycle.

2 Substantia nigra pars reticulata. The substantia nigra pars reticulata is part of an output circuit to many brain structures such as the thalamus and superior colliculus. It resembles anatomically and physiologically the internal part of the globus pallidus.

Treating the substantia nigra:
Bruno Chikly

Patient: the patient is in supine position

Practitioner: the practitioner is positioned at the head of the patient.

Method: an easy way to connect to the substantia nigra is to approach it laterally. Bring your fingers close to the tragus of the ear. Focus your attention medially. The pars lateralis, for example, will often give you a sense of calm and expansiveness. If you feel any change in symmetry, position, quality, rhythm, activity, synchronize precisely with this structure and let the intrinsic self-correcting mechanisms bring back this structure in a balanced/aligned/neutral place. Recheck position; rhythm, activity, even energetic or emotional component - all should be back to homeostasis/allostasis and present no "signaling".

Red nucleus
Bruno Chikly

*   **Anatomy and structure:** the red nucleus is located in the tegmentum of the midbrain, medial to the substantia nigra.

*   **Known function:** the functions of the red nucleus in humans are still subject to debate. It is a subcortical center of the extrapyramidal motor system. It is mainly involved in motor functions and motor coordination such as helping with arm swinging and (in babies) with crawling. The red nucleus receives many inputs from the contralateral cerebellum (deep cerebellar nuclei) and motor cortex (ipsilateral corticorubral tract). Its outputs are mainly to the contralateral spinal (rubrospinal tract) and the ipsilateral inferior olive.

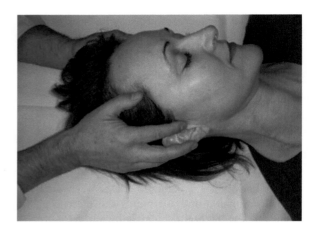

Figure 33.52
Treatment of the substantia nigra-red nucleus or VTA

Treating the red nucleus:

Patient: the patient is in supine position.

Practitioner: the practitioner is positioned at the head of the patient.

Method: repeat the same procedure as for the substantia nigra but focus your attention medially. You can feel a compact nucleus on each side that is much more active and vital than the perception felt in the substantia nigra.

Ventral tegmental area
Bruno Chikly

*   **Anatomy and structure:** the ventral tegmental area (VTA) originally called the ventral tegmentum) is a group of neurons with a heterogeneous cytoarchitecture located in the medial part of the mesencephalon.

*   **Known function:** the VTA is rich in dopaminergic (reward or addiction) and GABAergic (inhibitory) cells and a small percentage of glutamatergic (excitatory) neurons. The VTA is important in cognition; reward or motivation; drug addiction; the emotions of

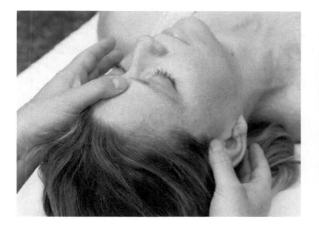

Figure 33.53
Treatment of the nucleus accumbens and VTA

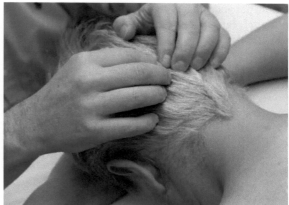

Figure 33.54
Treatment of the brainstem

fear, avoidance, and love. Some neurons of the VTA inhibit the lateral habenula to help promote reward.

Treatment of the nucleus accumbens and VTA

Bruno Chikly

Patient: the patient is in a supine position

Practitioner: the practitioner is positioned at the head of the patient.

Method: In the case of addiction, one nucleus accumbens is usually more active than the other. Identify which one of the left or right nucleus accumbens is more active, place one finger on this nucleus while the finger of the other hand is located on the ipsilateral or contralateral VTA. The VTA is to be found approximately laterally at the level of the attachment of the helix of the ear to the head. Contacting VTA and nucleus accumbens will naturally help downregulate the hyperactivity of the nucleus accumbens. The patient may feel the sense of calm or emptiness replacing the nucleus accumbens hyperactivity. Treating the brainstem, the cranial nerves nuclei, and ganglia

Brainstem:

The brainstem is a very complex and very important structure to treat. It is often implicated in mechanical lesions of the body. The brainstem may be responsible for lesions of the neck, brachial plexus, shoulders, elbow, wrist, lower back, knee, foot, and so forth.

The brainstem has three parts:
- Medulla oblongata (hindbrain): about 3 cm
- Pons: about 2.5 cm
- Midbrain: about 1.5 cm.

Treating the brainstem:

Bruno Chikly

Patient: the patient is in supine position.

Practitioner: the practitioner is positioned at the head of the patient.

Hand position and method: the brainstem is located more or less superior and inferior to inion. Connect with the ventricular system of the brain and follow the intraventricluar cerebrospinal fluid below the third ventricles of the brain to the central canal of the spinal cord inside the brainstem. Where you assessed a brainstem lesion, put your fingers vertically close to midline in the occipital region above and/or below inion. You can treat the brainstem globally for rotation, side bending, and so forth as well as the "columns" and tracts or nuclei of the brainstem locally. The brainstem is organized into vertical columns (e.g., the corticospinal tract, the posterior column-medial lemniscus pathway, etc.). You can treat between two columns, inside a column, and specifically treat a particular nucleus of the brainstem.

The cranial nerves nuclei and ganglia
Bruno Chikly

Nervus terminalis (special sensory nerve)

- **Anatomy and structure:** the nervus terminalis (terminal nerve) lies on the medial side of the olfactory nerve.

- **Known function:** its function in humans is still controversial.

  This nerve projects to the medial and lateral septal nuclei and the preoptic areas; it is probably related to pheromones and associated with the small vomeronasal.

  We will treat it with the olfactory nerve.

Olfactory nucleus (special sensory nerve)
Olfactory nuclei relay olfactory information to the brain.

- **Treating the olfactory bulb and tract:** patient is in the supine position; practitioner is at the head of the table.

- **Assessment:** put each medius or index finger medial to the supraorbital foramen. With the tip of the finger, assess which olfactory bulb and tract may be in lesion.

- **Treatment:**
  Patient: the patient is in supine position.
  Practitioner: the practitioner is positioned at the head of the patient.
  Method: treat unilaterally, with one finger in front of the tip of the bulb and the fingers of the other hand aligned at the level of the sphenoid along the olfactory tract.

Optic nerve pathways (special sensory nerves)

Optic nerve nuclei carry visual information to the brain. The main relays to optic pathways from the ganglion cells of the retina are the lateral geniculate nucleus of the thalamus (visual perception), the superior colliculus of the midbrain (eye movements control), the pretectum of the midbrain (pupillary light reflex), and the suprachiasmatic nucleus of the hypothalamus (circadian rhythms, melatonin changes, etc.).

Oculomotor (motor nerve)

- **Overview:** general somatic motor (efferent) to four extraocular muscles and levator palpebrae superioris.

- Visceral motor: intrinsic muscles of the eye—ciliary muscle and constrictor muscle and sphincter pupillae of the iris (ciliary ganglion).
  - **Oculomotor nuclei:** situated at the level of the superior colliculi. The oculomotor nucleus is made of three subunits: central subnucleus (levator palpebrae superioris), medial subnucleus (superior rectus) and lateral subnucleus combining three units (dorsally in the inferior rectus, ventrally in the medial rectus, and intermediately in the inferior oblique).
  - **Parasympathetic nuclei:** Edinger-Westphal nuclei (parasympathetic and preganglionic) located just posteriorly to motor nuclei of III. Preganglionic fibers may synapse in the ciliary ganglion. Postganglionic fibers, called the short ciliary nerves, innervate the constrictor and ciliary muscles.
  - **Ciliary ganglion:** Located lateral to the optic nerve.

- Afferents: receive mainly three types of nerves:
  - Parasympathetic preganglionic fibers from the Edinger-Westphal nuclei
  - Sympathetic nerves from the "ciliospinal center" (C8–T2) of the spinal cord to the superior cervical ganglion then along the internal carotid artery
  - Sensory fibers from the nasociliary nerve (a branch of V1 [the ophthalmic division of the trigeminal nerve]).

- Efferents: short ciliary nerves.

Trochlear (motor nerve)

- **Overview**: strictly somatic motor for superior oblique.

- **Nucleus of IV**: located just inferior to the inferior colliculi, inferior to the nucleus of III.

- **Treating the ciliary ganglion**:
  Patient: the patient is in supine position.
  Practitioner: the practitioner is positioned at the head of the patient.
  Mothod: the ciliary ganglion is located lateral to the optic globe. Put one finger gently in the region of the greater wing of the sphenoid. To help localize the ganglion specifically, have the patient converge or have him or her imagine going from light to dark.

Trigeminal: "three-twins" nerves (mixed nerve)

- **Overview**: motor for all the muscles of mastication and a few other muscles (motor trigeminal nucleus) and sensory for the cranium, face and neck, sinus, meninges (anterior two-third), and external surface of the tympanic membrane (sensory trigeminal nucleus [mesencephalic, pontine, and principal sensory nuclei])
  The trigeminal is the largest cranial nerve (CN) nuclei and the largest ganglion of the CNS. The sensory ganglion is also called the semilunar or Gasserian ganglion. It is an equivalent to dorsal root ganglia of the spinal cord, containing the cell bodies of incoming sensory fibers. There are three main divisions of the sensory trigeminal nuclei extending throughout the entire brainstem (and the upper part of the spinal cord, as far as C2 to C3).

- **As a simplification** there are three main divisions of the trigeminal nuclei for the sensory functions:
  - **The spinal (inferior or caudal) nucleus:** pain and temperature (protopathic) information for the face. The spinal trigeminal nucleus is made up of three parts, from superior to inferior: pars oralis, pars interpolaris, and pars caudalis.
  - **The pontine (principal or chief) sensory nucleus:** touch (epicritic) and position in space (proprioceptive) sensations.

  - **The mesencephalic nucleus:** proprioception; mechanoreceptors for the jaw and teeth.

- **Treating the trigeminal CN (V) nuclei and ganglia:**
  Patient is in prone position.
  Practitioner is at the head of the table.
  Mothod: Put your fingers laterally on the lateral part of the brainstem. Assess along the line of the trigeminal nuclei, motor or sensory (mesencephalic, pontine, and principal sensory nuclei), if an area is upregulated or downregulated. Treat until balanced.

Abducens (motor nerve)

- **Overview:** strictly motor for the lateral rectus muscle.

- **The abducens nucleus** is located in the fourth ventricle, inferior to the facial colliculus (CN VII), and close to midline in the superior pons (rhomboid fossa).

Facial (mixed nerve)

- **Overview:**
  - Branchial motor for muscles of facial expression and three other muscles (facial motor nucleus)
  - Visceral motor for lacrimal, nasal, and salivatory glands, except the parotid gland (superior salivatory also called lacrimal nucleus, pterygopalatine, and submandibular ganglion)
  - Taste of anterior two-thirds of the tongue (nucleus solitarius cephalic end also called gustatory nucleus or geniculate ganglion).
  - General sensation for a little area of external ear and the external surface of the tympanic membrane (spinal nucleus of the trigeminal nerve)

Superior salivatory (lacrimal) nucleus: This nucleus is located medial to the motor nucleus of the facial nerve; the position of these nuclei in humans is not yet exactly known. It connects to the lacrimal and nasal glands (with a relay in the pterygopalatine ganglion) and submandibular and sublingual glands (with a relay in the submandibular ganglion).

Pterygopalatine ganglion (sometimes called sphenopalatine ganglion): This ganglion is located in the superior area of the pterygopalatine fossa.

Afferents: It receives mainly four types of nerves.

1 Parasympathetic preganglionic fibers: nerve of the pterygoid canal (vidian nerve)

2 Sympathetic nerves along the maxillary artery

3 Sensory fibers from the maxillary nerve (CN V2) they pass through the ganglion

4 Taste fibers for the soft palate.

Efferents: lacrimal and nasal mucosa nerves.

Submandibular ganglion: The submandibular ganglion (and sometime some small sublingual ganglions) are located in the mouth floor.

Afferents: receive mainly two types of nerves.

1 Parasympathetic preganglionic lingual fibers from the superior salivatory nucleus.

2 Sympathetic nerves along the internal carotid artery from the superior cervical ganglion.

Efferents: glandular nerves.

Vestibulocochlear (special sensory nerve)

The vestibular nuclei and ganglion: maintenance of equilibrium

- **Anatomy and function:**
  - Maculae of utricle and saccule respond to gravity, linear acceleration, and deceleration.
  - Ampullae (cristae ampullares) of semicircular ducts (kinetic labyrinth) respond to circular acceleration.

Vestibular nerves pass through the vestibular (Scarpa) ganglion before going to one of the four vestibular nuclei.

The lateral vestibular nucleus (Deiter nucleus) is important for position and motion of head in space. It is connected to the (lateral) vestibulospinal fasciculus (tract), an uncrossed lateral descending pathway.

The three other vestibular nuclei, (the superior, inferior, and medial vestibular nuclei), are connected to the medial longitudinal fasciculus (MLF) or medial vestibulospinal fasciculus, an uncrossed descending pathway as well as the cerebellum (nodule, floccule, uvula,

and fastigial nucleus). The vestibular nuclei can also connect to all nuclei of intraocular muscles and to the thalamus (ventral posterior medial thalamic nucleus) and the cerebral cortex.

- **Treating the vestibular pathways:** a lot of these structures need to be learned within the context of a guided hands-on seminar.
  Patient: the patient is in supine position
  Practitioner: the practitioner is positioned at the head of the patient.
  Method: fingers are vertically aligned mainly below the inion.

1 Connect with the four vestibular nuclei (superior, inferior, medial, and lateral) and assess possible intranuclear and internuclear lesions.

2 Connect any of the four vestibular nuclei to the semicircular canals (utricule or saccule) or vestibular (Scarpa) ganglion.

3 Connect any of the four vestibular nuclei to the flocculonodular lobe of the cerebellum and the fastigial nucleus (slightly inferior to a horizontal line 2–3 mm inferior to the inion). These pathways are usually ipsilateral.

The cochlear nuclei

- **Anatomy and structure:** pathways of audition.

From the cochlea, the CN VIII (mostly myelinated) bifurcates to relay to the anterior (ventral) cochlear nuclei or the posterior (dorsal) cochlear nuclei. The anterior cochlear nuclei pathway ascends to the ipsilateral superior olivary nuclei or continues within the ipsilateral or contralateral lateral lemniscate. The posterior cochlear nuclei pathway normally ascends to the contralateral superior olivary nuclei then to the lateral lemniscate. The lateral lemniscate pathway continues to the inferior colliculus and to the medial geniculate body. These fibers end in the primary auditory cortex (Brodman area 41 and 42).

- **Treating the cochlear nuclei:** a lot of these structures need to be learned within the context of a guided hands-on seminar.
  Patient: the patient is in supine position.

Practitioner: the practitioner is positioned at the head of the patient.

Method:
- Find the anterior and posterior cochlear nuclei.
- Connect them to the cochlea.
- Connect the cochlear nuclei to superior olive, then superior olive to inferior colliculi, and inferior colliculi to medial geniculate body. Finally, connect medial geniculate body to auditory cortex (medial to lateral fissure of the brain).

Glossopharyngeal (mixed nerve)

- **Overview:**
  - Branchial motor: stylopharyngeus muscle (help swallowing [nucleus ambiguous])
  - Visceral motor to parotid gland (inferior salivatory nucleus, otic ganglion)
  - Visceral sensory functions to carotid body and carotid sinus (nucleus of the tractus solitarius, caudal part)
  - Taste of posterior one-third of the tongue (nucleus of the tractus solitarius, superior or rostral part)
  - General sensation for the posterior one-third of the tongue, pharynx (participate in "gag" and vomit reflex), tonsil, small area of the posterior ear, internal surface of the tympanic membrane, eustachian tube, and mastoid cells (**spinal trigeminal nucleus**)

The glossopharyngeal nerve emerges behind the inferior olive and exit through the jugular foramen.

Otic ganglion

- **Nucleus ambiguus:** control of blood vessels in the carotid body.

- **Inferior salivatory nucleus:** parasympathetic fibers to parotid gland.

- **Otic ganglion** is a flat ganglion located on the medial surface of the CN V3, inferior to the foramen ovale.

- **Afferents:** receive mainly three types of nerves.

1 Parasympathetic preganglionic deep petrosal nerve; fibers of the CN IX not only innervating the parotid but also the buccal and labial glands.

2 Sympathetic nerves along the middle meningeal artery, from the superior cervical ganglion.

3 Sensory fibers from the mandibular nerve (CN V3); they pass through the ganglion without stopping and without making a relay.

Efferents: glandular nerves.

Spinal trigeminal nucleus: fibers go through the inferior glossopharyngeal (petrosal or plexiform) ganglion and end in the spinal trigeminal nucleus.

- **Treating the glossopharyngeal (CN IX) ganglia:**
  Patient: the patient is in supine position.
  Practitioner: the practitioner is positioned at the head of the patient.
  Method:
  - Otic ganglion: inferior salivatory nucleus (CN IX; it is a flat ganglion located on the medial surface of the CN V3, inferior to the foramen ovale, and slightly anterior and inferior to the tragus).
  - Glossopharyngeal (CN IX) sensory ganglia: They are usually located straight posterior to the external auditory meatus.
    ◊ Superior (or jugular) ganglion: sensory pathway
    ◊ Inferior ganglion or petrosal or plexiform ganglion (just inferior to the jugular foramen): sensory, taste, and chemoreceptors pathways.

Vagus: "wandering nerve" (mixed nerve)

It is the only cranial nerve to extend beyond head and neck. The vagus nerve is a nerve with about 80 percent sensory (tractus solitarius) and 20 percent motor function.

- **Overview:**
  - Branchial motor to larynx and pharynx (nucleus ambiguus [dorsal division])
  - Visceral motor to the heart, lungs, and abdominal organs as far as the right two-thirds of colon (nucleus ambiguus [parasympathetic motor function of the heart]) and dorsal motor nucleus of the vagus (parasympathetic motor function of pharynx, larynx, and thoracic and abdominal viscera)

- Visceral sensation from larynx, trachea, esophagus, thoracic and abdominal viscera, and from baroreceptors and chemoreceptors in the aortic sinus (nucleus tractus solitarius, caudal or inferior part)
- Taste for the posterior part of the throat (nucleus solitarius, cephalic part)
- General sensation for skin of lower pharynx, larynx, posterior meninges, external auditory meatus, external surface of tympanic membrane, small part of skin of external ear (superior vagus ganglion or jugular ganglion and trigeminal nucleus)

- **Treating the vagus nuclei (CN X) and ganglia:**
  Patient: the patient is in supine position.
  Practitioner: the practitioner is positioned at the head of the patient.
  Method:
  – Nucleus ambiguus (CN IX and X): *stimulation = movement of larynx, swallowing*
    ◊ CN X: dorsal division motor (pharynx, larynx, esophagus, upper trachea); ventrolateral division (heart)
  – Dorsal motor nucleus of CN X: motoricity (preganglionic parasympathetic fibers) for heart, lungs, and abdominal organs as far as right two-thirds of colon
  – Nucleus solitarius caudal end:
    ◊ Stimulation: gently move lungs
    ◊ CN X (inferior nucleus, nodose)
    ◊ Stimulation: sensation in thoracic and abdominal viscera.
  – Nucleus solitarius cephalic end (gustatory nucleus)
    ◊ Stimulation: taste your own saliva
    ◊ CN X: posterior of the throat.
  – Vagus sensory ganglia (CN X)
    ◊ Superior (or rostral) ganglion (just superior to the jugular foramen): (branchial) sensory pathway. It is located posterior to the external auditory meatus.
    ◊ Stimulation: touch concha of ear.
    ◊ Inferior (or nodose) ganglion (just inferior to the jugular foramen): mainly taste pathway. It is located straight inferior to the jugular ganglions.

  Stimulation: taste your own saliva (posterior of the throat).

Accessory (motor nerve)

- **Overview:** strictly motor for SCM and trapezius muscles.

- **Treating the accessory nuclei (CN XI):**
  - **Patient:** the patient is in supine position.
  - **Practitioner:** the practitioner is positioned at the head of the patient.
  - **Brief description:** accessory nucleus (CN XI): SCM and trapezius muscles. Stimulation: Gently shrug shoulder (trapezius, for lower and contralateral part of nucleus).

Hypoglossal (motor nerve)

- **Overview:** strictly motor (intrinsic and extrinsic muscles of the tongue)

- **Treating the hypoglossal nuclei (CN XII):**
  Patient: the patient is in supine position
  Practitioner: the practitioner is positioned at the head of the patient.
  Method: the nucleus of CN XII is located very inferior and medial in the floor of the fourth ventricle (hypoglossal triangle). It contains magnocellular cells and is the most medial nuclei in the brainstem. The hypoglossal nerve exits between the inferior olive and the pyramid of the brainstem. It exits the cranium through the hypoglossal foramen (anterior condylar foramen).

- Stimulation: move tongue inside the mouth.

Treating the cranial nerves

Torsten Liem

The cranial nerves (CNs) are part of the peripheral nervous system (PNS), with maybe the exception of CN I (olfactory nerve) that makes it synapse within the CNS and CN II (optic nerve), which is a tract of the brain synapsing in the retina.

Olfactory nerve (cranial nerve I) and olfactory placode

Mobility Testing CN I:
Flexion and contralateral side bending in the upper cervical area are introduced. For testing, additional move-

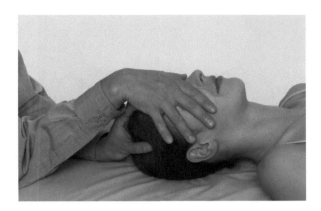

Figure 33.55
Treating the olfactory nerve and olfactory placode

- PBT, DBT or BFT.
- Sense the resultant tissue dynamics but without reacting to them. A fulcrum usually becomes established among the regions of the eyes, brain, and nose (original metabolic field in the development of the olfactory placode).
- Once the fulcrum has been established, disengagement may occur between the original nasal region and the surrounding structures. Support the process of disengagement by allowing it to unfold in a gentle compression field (or resist the force of disengagement using minimal counter-pressure) and so go with the process of disengagement.
- Then your hand on the cranial vault projects toward the region of the corpus striatum (on each side at the floor of the lateral ventricles) and the cerebrum.
- It may sometimes become necessary also to apply gentle disengagement caudally in the nasal region, approximately along the longitudinal axis of the olfactory nerve fibers.
- During or at the end of treatment, the osseous e.g. the ethmoid bone and dural region around the olfactory nerve can be balanced.

Optic Nerve (Cranial Nerve II) and Optic Nerve Tract

Mobility Testing CN II:
Flexion and contralateral side bending in the upper cervical area are introduced. Resilience and mobility in all planes of movement is tested on the bulbus. Additional movements can be performed on the Os sphenoidale and the orbita.

Treatment of CN II:
Practitioner: take up a position at the head of the patient.

Hand position:
- Cup the fingers of one hand around the eyeball.
- Position your other hand on the opposite side beneath the occiput (occipital lobe), above the superior nuchal line.

ments can be performed on the os ethmoidalis in the region of the lamina cribrosa, the nasal septum and the conchae. Motion restrictions or occurrence of symptoms are assessed.

Treatment of CN I:
Practitioner: take up a position at the head of the patient.

Hand position:
- Position the middle and index fingers of one hand over the zygomatic process of the maxillary and covering the orbit; locate the metacarpophalangeal joint of your index finger on the root of the nose.
- Position your other hand anteriorly to cover the cranial vault (frontal bone and parietal bone).

Method:
- With the middle and index fingers of one hand and with your other hand covering the cranial vault, deliver gentle convergent pressure on the orbits, cerebral hemispheres, and corpus striatum toward the nasal region to establish a resonance with the developmental dynamic force vectors.

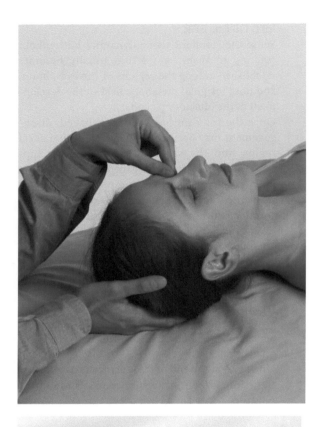

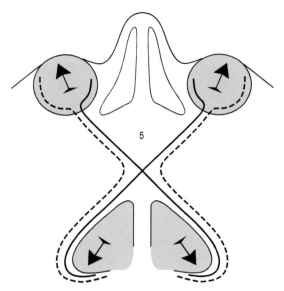

Figure 33.57
Diagram showing growth directions of the optic nerve fibers (5=optic chiasm)

Figure 33.56
Treating the optic nerve and optic nerve tract

Method:
- Flexion and contralateral side bending in the upper cervical area can be introduced.
- Deliver gentle compression (or gentle disengagement) between the eyeball and the occiput (occipital lobe) on the opposite side and the diencephalon (at the level of the third ventricle) to establish a resonance with the developmental dynamic force vectors.
- PBT, DBT or BFT.

- Sense the resultant tissue dynamics but without reacting to them. A fulcrum usually becomes established between the regions.
- Once the fulcrum has been established, disengagement may occur between the eyeball on the one hand and the diencephalon or occipital lobe on the other. Support the process of disengagement by allowing it to unfold in a gentle compression field (or resist the force of disengagement using minimal counterpressure) and so go with the process of disengagement.
- During or at the end of treatment, the osseous and dural region around the optic nerve can be balanced.

Oculomotor Nerve (Cranial Nerve III), Trochlear Nerve (Cranial Nerve IV) and Abducens Nerve (Cranial Nerve VI)

Palpation CN III:
It is possible that small rami are palpable infraorbital on the orbita. These can be sensitive to stretch and pressure.

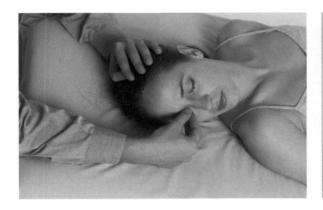

Figure 33.58A
Treating the trochlear nerve

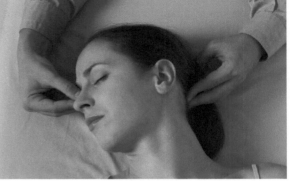

Figure 33.58B
Treating the abducens nerve

Mobility Testing CN III:
Flexion and contralateral side bending in the upper cervical area are introduced. The bulbus is moved towards cranial (lateral). Additional movements can be performed on the Os sphenoidale and the orbita.

Mobility Testing CN IV:
Flexion and contralateral side bending in the upper cervical area are introduced. The bulbus is moved towards caudal (lateral). Additional movements can be performed on the Os sphenoidale and the orbita.

Palpation CN VI:
Probably some fibres can be palpated on the orbital edge.

Mobility Testing CN VI:
Flexion and contralateral side bending in the upper cervical area are introduced. The bulbus is moved towards medial. Additional movements can be performed at the Os sphenoidale and the orbita.

Treatment of CN III, IV, VI:
Practitioner: take up a position at the head of the patient.

Hand position:
- Cup the fingers of one hand around the eyeball.
- For CNs III and IV: Position the palm of your other hand over the posterior third of the parietal bone - for CN IV on the opposite side - (approximately parallel to the cerebral peduncles in the region around the aqueduct), with the fingers pointing anteriorly (Figure 34.46A).
- For CN VI: Direct the fingers of your other hand caudally, placing them beneath the superior nuchal line on the occiput (in the region of the pons, cerebellum, and fourth ventricle; Figure 34.46B).

Method:
- Flexion and contralateral side bending in the upper cervical area can be introduced.
- Deliver a gentle pull on the eyeball: for CN III superior (lateral), for CN IV caudal (lateral) and for CN VI medial and follow the dynamics of the nerve until the tensions got balanced and the neurodynamics improved. Direct your attention to the ocular muscles.

- PBT, DBT or BFT.
- Sense the resultant tissue dynamics but without reacting to them. A fulcrum usually becomes established between the regions.
- Once the fulcrum has been established, you may sense that the nerves are being attracted by the ocular muscles. Support this process by allowing it to unfold in a gentle expansion field (or resist the force of approximation or attraction using minimal counterpressure) and so go with the process of drawing closer.
- It may also be necessary to deliver a gentle disengagement among the region of the cerebral peduncles, tectum, and tegmentum on the one hand and the eyeball on the other (CN III and IV) or a corresponding disengagement in the region of the pons and cerebellum (CN VI).
- During or at the end of treatment, the the Os phenoidale and other bones of the orbit and the dural region around the oculomotor, trochlear, and abducens nerves can be balanced.

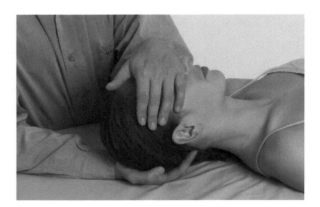

Figure 33.59A
Treating the ophthalmic nerve

Trigeminal nerve (cranial nerve V)

Palpation CN V:

- Palpation CN V/1: at the Foramen ophthalmicum

- Palpation CN V/2: at the Foramen infraorbitale; branches of the N. zygomaticus at the Proc. frontalis ossis zygomaticus

- Palpation CN V/3 - N. alveolaris inferior: at the Foramen mentale

- V/3 - N. auriculotemporalis is best palpable between Tragus and Caput mandibulae with an open mouth.

- V/3 - N. lingualis: mediodorsal, is palpable on the mandibula, approx 1cm caudal of the Caput mandibulae, in the superior region of the M. pterygoideus medialis.

Mobility Testing CN V:
- Flexion and contralateral side bending in the upper cervical area are introduced for all branches.

- V/1-N. frontalis: additional movement of the bulbus towards caudal. Additional movements can be performed on the Os frontale and Os temporale.

- V/1-N. lacrimalis: additional movement of the bulbus towards medial. Additional movements can be performed on the maxilla, Os zygomaticum, Os lacrimale, Os ethmoidale, Os nasale and Os temporale.

- V/1-N. nasociliaris: additional movement of the bulbus towards lateral. Additional movements can be performed on the Os sphenoidale, Os lacrimale and Os temporale.

- V/2: additional movement of the bulbus towards cranial (medial). Additional movements can be performed on the maxilla for infraorbital branches, a cranial pull on the Os zygomaticum for zygomaticofascial branches and a cranial pull on the Os palatinum for palatine branches.

- V/3: for N. mentalis and N. lingualis a caudal pull on the mandibula (>2 cm) and a contralateral laterotrusion can be performed. For N. auriculotemporalis and N. buccalis a caudal pull on the mandibula (>2 cm) and latero- or mediotrusion movements can be performed. Additional movements can be performed on the Os sphenoidale and Os temporale.

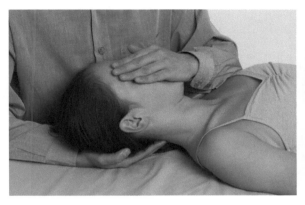

Figure 33.59B
Treating the maxillary nerve

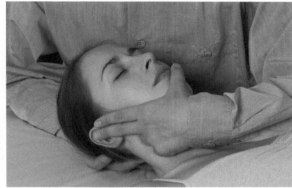

Figure 33.59C
Treating the mandibular nerve

Treatment of CN V:
Practitioner: take up a position to one side of the patient's head.

Hand position:
- Use your cranial hand to cradle the patient's occiput (contact with the cerebellum, pons, and [for CN V1], the midbrain).
- Caudal hand:
  – For CN V1: The palm of your caudal hand covers the contralateral eye (Figure 33.59A).
  – For CN V2: Position your index, middle, and ring fingers so as to cover the contralateral eye, with your wrist spanning the oral region.
  – For CN V3 (unilateral): With your thumb spanning the oral region, position your index and middle fingers on the tragus and external acoustic meatus (in contact with the tympanum; Figure 33.59C).

Method:
  – Flexion and contralateral side bending in the upper cervical area can be introduced.
  – To induce a slight stretch, the parameters as described in the mobility testing can be included

while following the (inherent) dynamics of the nerve, until the tensions got balanced and the neurodynamics improved.
- For CN V1: Deliver or sense gentle disengagement at the eye longitudinally to the nerve.
- For CN V2: Deliver or sense gentle disengagement between the oral region and the eye.
- For CN V3: Deliver or sense gentle disengagement (less commonly, compression) between the oral region and tympanum.
- PBT, DBT or BFT.
- Sense the resultant tissue dynamics but without reacting to them. A fulcrum usually becomes established between the regions.
- Once the fulcrum has been established, you may sense a kind of suction of the nerve toward the organ. Support this process by allowing it to unfold in a gentle expansion field (or resist the force of approximation or suction using minimal counterpressure) and so go with the process of drawing closer.
- During or at the end of treatment, the osseous (see above) and dural region around the trigeminal nerve and its branches can be balanced, as well as the spinal nucleus at the level of C1–C3.

Facial Nerve (Cranial Nerve VII)

Palpation CN VII:
- The ramus auricularis posterior can be palpated on the ventral Pars petrosa from caudal to cranial (it can also be explored on the Os occipitale).

- The temporal branch can be palpated laterally from the eyebrow (superiorlateral of the M. orbicularis oris).

- The buccal branch can be palpated underneath Os zygomaticum (it passes M. buccalis).

- The mandibular branch can be localised when biting, along the chin line in the frontal region of M. masseter, ventral from the salivary glands.

Mobility Testing CN VII:

Flexion, contralateral side bending and ipsilateral rotation in the upper cervical area are introduced. Whilst the patient engages the ipsilateral mimic musculature, additional movements can be performed at the Os temporale.

For the other areas and branches of CN VII, flexion and contralateral sidebending in the upper cervical area are introduced.

For the areas of the inner auditory canal, the canalis facialis and the Foramen styloideum, additional movements can be performed at the Os temporale, e.g. on the mastoid/pars petrosa.

For the ramus buccalis and ramus mandibularis, additional movements can be performed at the Os temporale, and the mandibula can be moved towards caudal and can be contralaterally laterotrusionised. At the same time, the patient engages his ipsilateral mimic musculature.

For branches of CN VII in the region of the hyoid, additional movements at the Os temporale can be performed and the hyoid can be moved towards caudal.

Treatment of CN VII:
Practitioner: take up a position at the head of the patient.

Hand position:
- Place one hand so as to cover one-half of the patient's face.
- Position your other hand in the neck region and on the inferior part of the occiput (at the level of the medulla oblongata, olivary bodies, and fourth ventricle).

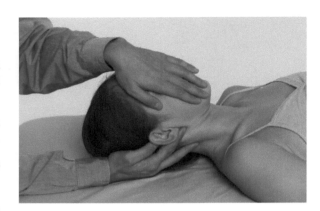

Figure 33.60
Treating the facial nerve

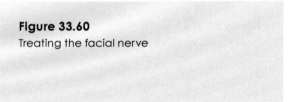

- Locate your index finger anteriorly and your middle finger posteriorly to the mastoid process close to the facial nerve at the stylomastoid foramen and try to palpate it.

Method:
- Flexion, contralateral side bending and ipsilateral rotation in the upper cervical can be introduced.
- Use your hand covering the patient's face to exert a gentle divergent force on the facial musculature.
- PBT, DBT or BFT.
- Slightly stretch the nerve with your index finger and follow the dynamics of the nerve until the tensions got balanced and the neurodynamics improved.
- Sense the resultant tissue dynamics but without reacting to them. A fulcrum usually becomes established between the regions.
- Once the fulcrum has been established, you may sense that the nerve is being attracted by the facial musculature. Support this process by allowing it to unfold in a gentle expansion field (or resist the force of approximation or attraction using minimal counterpressure) and so go with the process of drawing closer.

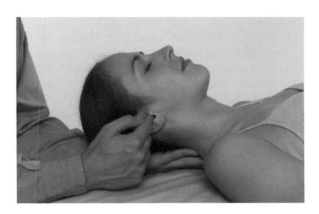

Figure 33.61
Treating the vestibulocochlear nerve

- It may also be necessary to deliver a gentle disengagement between the region of the medulla oblongata and olivary bodies on the one hand and the face on the other.
- During or at the end of treatment, the Os temporale and its parts and the dural region around the facial nerve can be balanced.

Vestibulocochlear Nerve (Cranial Nerve VIII)

Mobility Testing CN VIII:

Flexion and contralateral side bending in the upper cervical area are introduced. Additional movements at the Os temporale, in particular at the Mastoid/Pars petrosa, Os occipitale and Os sphenoidale are performed.

Treatment of CN VIII:

Practitioner: take up a position at the head of the patient.

Hand position:

- Insert the index finger of one hand into the external acoustic meatus.
- Position your other hand in the neck region and on the inferior part of the occiput (at the level of the medulla oblongata, olivary bodies, and fourth ventricle).

Method:

- Flexion and contralateral side bending in the upper cervical area can be introduced.
- Use your hands to exert a gentle disengagement between the region of the medulla oblongata and olivary bodies on the one hand and the inner ear on the other.
- PBT, DBT or BFT.
- Sense the resultant tissue dynamics but without reacting to them. A fulcrum usually becomes established between the regions.
- Once the fulcrum has been established, you may sense a kind of suction of the nerve toward the inner ear. Support this process by allowing it to unfold in a gentle expansion field (or resist the force of approximation or suction using minimal counterpressure) and so go with the process of drawing closer.
- During or at the end of treatment, the Os temporale, in particular at the Mastoid/Pars petrosa, Os occipitale and Os sphenoidale and the dural region around the vestibulocochlear nerve can be balanced.

Glossopharyngeal Nerve (Cranial Nerve IX)

Function: The glossopharyngeal nerve contains motor, general sensory, special sensory, and secretory fibers. It is located primarily in the region of the tongue and pharynx; it also innervates the tympanic cavity and parotid gland and regulates blood pressure.

Palpation CN IX:

Can probably be palpated anteriorly of the styloid process. The palpation is easier if initially a homolateral sidebending of the head is performed in order to relax the tissues in the region of the nerve.

Mobility Testing CN IX:

Flexion and contralateral side bending in the upper cervical area are introduced. Additional movements are performed at the Os temporale and Os occipitale in the region of the foramen jugulare.

- For the motoric rami, the Os temporale (styloid process) is medially moved.

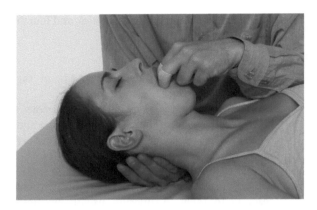

Figure 33.62
Treating the glossopharyngeal nerve

- For the sensoric parts, a movement of the Os sphenoidale is performed.

- For the parts of the tongue, the patient is performing a tongue protrusion.

- For extracranial branches, a contralateral laterotrusion and protrusion of the mandibula is performed.

Treatment of CN IX:

Practitioner: Take up a position to one side of the patient's head.

Hand position:
- Position your cranial hand transversely under the patient's neck and under the inferior part of the occiput (at the level of the medulla oblongata, olivary bodies, and fourth ventricle).
- With the thumb, index, and middle fingers of your caudal hand, take hold of the patient's tongue.
- Alternatively, position your caudal hand over the parotid gland.

Method:
- Flexion and contralateral side bending in the upper cervical area can be introduced.
- To induce a slight stretch, the parameters as described in the mobility testing can be included while following the (inherent) dynamics of the nerve, until the tensions got balanced and the neurodynamics improved.
- Use your hands to exert a gentle disengagement between the region of the medulla oblongata and olivary bodies on the one hand and the lingual and pharyngeal region on the other.
- PBT, DBT or BFT.
- Sense the resultant tissue dynamics but without reacting to them. A fulcrum usually becomes established between the region of the medulla oblongata and olivary bodies on the one hand and the region of the tongue and pharynx on the other.
- Once the fulcrum has been established, you may sense a converging force between the nerve and the tongue or pharynx or parotid. Support this process by allowing it to unfold in a gentle expansion field (or resist the force of approximation or suction using minimal counterpressure) and so go with the process of drawing closer.
- During or at the end of treatment, the Os temporale and Os occipitale and the dural region around the glossopharyngeal nerve can be balanced.

Vagus Nerve (Cranial Nerve X)

Palpation CN X:
In the Vagina carotica, medially from M. sternocleidomastoideus; auricular branches are palpable on the mastoid process.

Mobility Testing CN X:
Flexion and contralateral side bending in the upper cervical area are introduced. Middle and lower cervical extension is introduced for assessment of the lateral branches that are connecting to the hyoid. Additional movements are performed at the Os temporale and Os occipitale in the region of the Foramen jugulare.

- For the assessment of the pharyngeal branches, the hyoid is moved laterally.

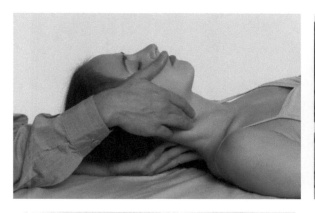

Figure 33.63
Treating the vagus nerve

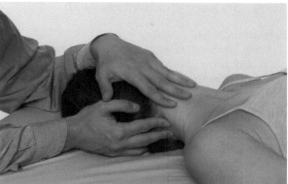

Figure 33.64
Treating the accessory nerve

- For bronchialmotoric branches, a contralateral lateral and caudal movement at the cricohyoid is performed.

- For visceral sensoric and general sensoric branches, the cricohyoid is moved caudally.

- For cardial and pulmonar plexus, the sternum/thorax is mobilised.

Treatment of CN X:
Practitioner: Take up a position at the head of the patient.

Hand position:
- Position one hand in the patient's neck region covering the inferior part of the occiput (at the level of the medulla oblongata, olivary bodies, and fourth ventricle).
- Place your other hand on the vagus nerve above the common carotid artery within the carotid sheath. Palpate the nerve by using your fingers to seek out the nerve strands of CN X, first, medially and then posteriorly to the carotid artery.

- In addition, locate your fingers medially to the sternocleidomastoid muscle on the esophagus.

Method:
- Flexion and contralateral side bending in the upper cervical area can be introduced.
- To induce a slight stretch, the parameters as described in the mobility testing can be included while following the (inherent) dynamics of the nerve, until the tensions got balanced and the neurodynamics improved.
- Use both hands to exert a gentle disengagement between the region of the medulla oblongata and olivary bodies on the one hand and the esophagus on the other.
- For further details, see above.
- During or at the end of treatment, the Os temporale and Os occipitale and the dural region around the vagus nerve can be balanced.
- Note: Alternatively, you can also palpate the superior laryngeal nerve (a branch of CN X), which is located in the thyrohyoid membrane between the thyroid cartilage and the hyoid bone.

Accessory nerve (cranial nerve XI)

Palpation CN XI:
Can be localised at the posterior triangle of the neck, anteriorly from and parallel to the M. trapezius. Approximately five thumb widths superiorly of the clavicula, CN XI passes underneath the M. trapezius.

Mobility Testing CN XI:
Flexion and contralateral side bending in the upper cervical area and extension in the infracervical area are introduced. At the same time, the shoulder is moved towards caudal and posteriorly. Additional movements are performed at the Os temporale and Os occipitale in the region of the Foramen jugulare.

Treatment of CN XI:
Patient: head turned toward opposite side.

Practitioner: take up a position at the head of the patient.

Hand position:
- Position one hand in the patient's neck region over the inferior part of the occiput (at the level of the medulla oblongata, olivary bodies, and fourth ventricle).
- Position your other hand so that your middle finger is on the accessory nerve (this travels across the levator scapulae, which lies between the SCM and trapezius muscles). At the same time, locate your index finger on the SCM and your ring finger on the trapezius.

Method:
- Using your hand located on the SCM and trapezius, exert a gentle divergent force on these muscles.
- Then proceed further as described for the facial nerve (CN VII).
- To induce a slight stretch, the parameters as described in the mobility testing can be included while following the (inherent) dynamics of the nerve, until the tensions are balanced.

Hypoglossal nerve (cranial nerve XII)

Palpation CN XII:
Function: this purely somatomotor nerve, (in phylogenetic terms) which as a spinal nerve has been taken into the cranium, is responsible for innervating the tongue.

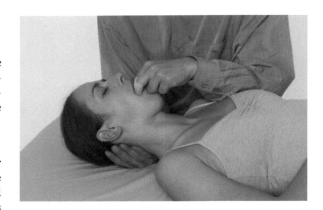

Figure 33.65
Treating the hypoglossal nerve

Localize underneath the mandibula, above the hyoid, anteriorly from the carotid artery externa/communis and anteriorly from the glandula submandibularis, CN XII. One finger of the other hand can support the palpation intraorally, by palpating through the soft tissues and serving the outer finger as a counterfort.

Mobility Testing CN XII:
Flexion and contralateral side bending in the upper cervical area are introduced. The hyoid is moved caudally and contralaterally whilst the patient moves his tongue towards the front and lateral. Additional movements are performed at the Os occipitale.

Treatment of CN XI:
Practitioner: take up a position to one side of the patient's head.

Hand position:
- Use the thumb, index, and middle finger of your caudal hand to take hold of the patient's tongue.
- Position your cranial hand transversely under the patient's neck and under the inferior part of the occiput (at the level of the medulla oblongata, olivary bodies, and fourth ventricle).

- (An approach to this nerve is also possible in the cervical region between the mylohyoid and hyoglossus muscles.)

Method:
- Exert a gentle divergent force on the muscles of the tongue.
- To induce a slight stretch, the nerve can be palpated and the parameters as described in the mobility testing can be included while following the (inherent) dynamics of the nerve, until the tensions are balanced.
- For further details, proceed as described above.
- **Note:** Via the tongue, it is possible to achieve morphodynamic integration of the pharyngeal arch nerves (the precursors of CNs V3, VII, IX, and X and, as such, involved in the formation of the tongue). The brain (and with it the head) arches upward and forward in the antibasal region. The weak endodermal oropharyngeal tube adapts to these growth dynamics, arching convexly upward and widening transversely. The epithelial anlage of the tongue develops on the basal side of the oropharyngeal tube, which is more arched than the upper side. The musculature follows this pattern and develops in the stroma of the tongue anlage in all three principal dimensions, (i.e. longitudinal, transverse, and vertical). Because the tongue is a large organ near the brain, it displays particularly generous cranial nerve innervation.

White Matter of the Cerebrum
Bruno Chikly, Torsten Liem

Anatomy: Bruno Chikly

There are three types of white (myelinated) fibers in the cerebrum:

- Commissural fibers: They connect the corresponding regions of two cerebral hemispheres.

- Projection fibers: They connect various cortical regions within the same cerebral hemisphere.

- Association fibers connect the cerebral cortex with the lower part of the brain or brainstem and the spinal cord. Association fibers can be corticofugal (efferent) fibers or corticopetal (afferent) fibers.

Commissural fibers
The cerebrum contains many commissural fibers:

- The corpus callosum (neocortical) is the largest commissure in human.

- The fornix (archicortical) or hippocampal commissure, previously called psalterium or David's lyre.

- The interthalamic adhesion (soft or grey commissure).

- The habenular commissure.

These four commissures have been previously dealt with.

- The *posterior commissure* (or epithalamic commissure), previously called the dorsal white commissure, is located in the superior end of the cerebral aqueduct or posterior third ventricle. It connects the pretectal nuclei and is important in the bilateral pupillary light reflex.

- The *anterior commissure* (paleocortical), previously called the ventral white commissure, is the first commissure to appear in the human embryo. It is located within the upper portion of the lamina terminalis and runs across the midline just in front of the fornix. The anterior commissure connects the middle and inferior temporal gyri of the two hemispheres, the olfactory tracts, amygdala, and most likely the orbitofrontal cortex. The anterior commissure is also part of the neospinothalamic tract for nociception and pain sensation.

Treating the anterior commissure:
Bruno Chikly

Patient: the patient is in supine position.
Practitioner: the practitioner is positioned at the head of the patient.
Hand Position: the practitioner put both hands midline on the frontal area, just above the supraorbital ridges.
Method: first distinguish the correct layer of brain parenchyma by doing a layered palpation. Assessing the anterior commissure can be done with ease or by testing the barrier.
- With ease: testing the barrier necessitates an extremely gentle approach so as not to lesion

the brain. Contact the two frontal lobes and perceive if there is a local pull deep between the two lobes at the level of the anterior commissure (and not a pull between the two lobes in relation to the whole width of the frontal lobe).

◊ Treat by following the ease within the anterior commissure. Recheck that both lobes are completely free.

– Direct test: Very softly and gradually, try to separate the two frontal lobes and assess if there is a small band of matter preventing this separation at the level of the anterior commissure (and not a global barrier between both cerebral lobes).

Treat by following the ease within the anterior commissure. Recheck that both lobes are completely free.

Projection fibers: internal, external, and extreme capsules

I. The internal capsule and the Corona Radiata

The internal capsule is a layer of white matter lying vertically approximately between the thalamus or caudate nucleus medially and the lentiform nucleus laterally. The internal capsule continues as the widening corona radiata toward the cerebral cortex. Internal capsule and corona radiata contain both ascending and descending fibers and are the foremost connection among the cerebral cortex, the brainstem, and the spinal cord.

The *anterior limb* of the internal capsule contains the following:

1 The frontopontine (corticofugal) fibers project from frontal cortex to pons.

2 The thalamocortical fibers (part of the thalamocortical radiations) connect the medial and anterior nuclei of the thalamus to the frontal lobes.

• The *genu* contains the corticobulbar fibers, which run between the cortex and the brainstem.

• The *posterior limb* of the internal capsule contains corticospinal fibers, sensory fibers (including the medial lemniscus and the anterolateral system) from the body, and a few corticobulbar fibers.

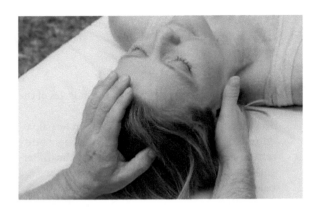

Figure 33.66
Treatment of the corona radiata and internal capsule

• The *retrolenticular part* contains fibers from the optic system coming from the lateral geniculate nucleus of the thalamus. More posteriorly, this becomes the optic radiation. Some fibers from the medial geniculate nucleus (which carry auditory information) also pass in the retrolenticular internal capsule but most are in the sublenticular part.

• The *sublenticular part* contains fibers connecting with the temporal lobe. These include the auditory radiations and temporopontine fibers.

Treating the internal capsule and the corona radiata:
Bruno Chikly

Patient: the patient is in supine position.

Practitioner: the practitioner is positioned at the head of the patient.

Hand position: the practitioner brings one hand posterior to the coronal suture (motor area 4 and 6 of Broadmann's cytoarchitectonic regions).

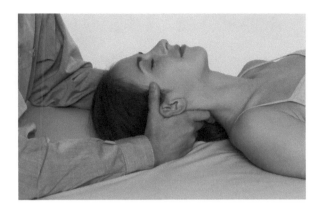

Figure 33.67
Alternative hand position, internal capsule

Later on, this hand can be adjusted and also placed more anteriorly to assess another area such as the sensorimotor area 3–1–2 of Brodmann.

Place your other hand as close as you can to the foramen magnum. With this second hand, you will have the inferior end of the internal capsule, at the most inferior part of the brainstem, after the pyramidal decussation. Adjust both hands so you can feel the place of maximum tension between the two hands.

Method: Find the position for both hands with the maximum barrier and synchronize with it with ease until it naturally lets go. Recheck to make sure all barriers have disappeared.

Alternative hand position for treating the region of the internal capsule
Torsten Liem

• Position your thumbs below the squamoparietal suture on both sides. Cradle the cranial base with your other fingers.

• Your thumbs should project deeply toward the center of the cranium, toward the region of the internal capsule

between the lentiform nucleus and thalamus medially and the caudate nucleus laterally.

• The palpation resonates with the density and other tissue qualities of the fan-like mass of myelinated projection fibers of the cerebral peduncle from the frontal, parietal and occipital lobes.

• Further functional relationships could be acknowledged by palpating with one hand the region of the corticospinal tract, pyramidal tract or cranial nerves VII, XII or II (see below) as supranuclear tracts are related to cranial nerves VII and XII and the optic tract. All these tracts are present together in an extremely confined space.

• Establish a balanced tension BT between the region of the internal capsule and the other region: a local, regional, global point of balanced tension (PBT), dynamic balanced tension (DBT), balanced fluid tension, (BFT) balanced electrodynamic tension (BET) and apply further treatment modalities if needed.

II. The external capsule

The external capsule is a thin white sheet of white matter that runs between the lateral part of the lentiform nucleus and the claustrum.

III. The extreme capsule

The extreme capsule is another thin sheet of white matter that runs between the lateral part of the lentiform nucleus and the insula of Reil. The extreme capsule has bidirectional connection between the Broca and Wernicke speech areas and it could play a role in language.

Association fibers

Association fibers connect regions of the cerebral cortex within one hemisphere. There are two categories of association fibers:

• The short association fibers or "U-fibers" connect neighboring cerebral gyri

• The long association fibers connect distant gyri usually among different lobes.

The main long association fibers are:

- The superior longitudinal fasciculus. It connects parts of the frontal lobe with the occipital and temporal cortices.

- The inferior longitudinal fasciculus. It connects the temporal and occipital cortices.

- The occipitofrontal fasciculus. It extends posteriorly from the frontal lobe, radiating into the temporal and occipital lobes.

Numerous association fibers can be distinguished by the following:

- The superior longitudinal fasciculus originates from the parietal and frontal lobe and terminates in the occipital lobe.

- The fronto-occipital fasciculus originates from the occipitoparietal region and terminates in the occipital lobe.

- The middle longitudinal fasciculus originates from the anterior portion of the temporal lobe and terminates in the parietal lobe.

- The inferior longitudinal fasciculus originates from the occipitotemporal region and terminates in the temporal lobe.

- The cingulum bundle originates from the cingulate gyrus and terminates in the entorhinal cortex.

- The uncinate fasciculus originates from the frontal lobe and terminates in the temporal lobe.

- The arcuate fasciculus originates from the frontal lobe and terminates in the temporal lobe. (Schmahmann J, Pandya D, Wang R, et al. Association fibre pathways of the brain: Parallel observations from diffusion spectrum imaging and autoradiography. *Brain*. 2007; 130:630–653.)

Treatment of the association fibers : occipi-to-frontal - white matter fasciculus:

Patient: the patient is in supine position.

Practitioner: the practitioner is positioned at the head of the patient.

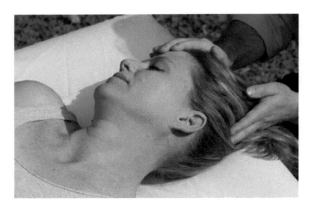

Figure 33.68
Treatment of the association fibers - occipito-frontal -white matter fasciculus

Method: One flat hand of the practitioner is located on one occipital area lay the other hand gently on the ipsilateral frontal area.

Focus your attention on the fibers between the two hands with the minimum pressure and use any of the fascia approaches necessary to release these white fibers indirectly, until there is no fascia pull or "draw" .

The Cerebellum
Anatomy and function: Torsten Liem, Bruno Chikly

Cortex, Nuclei, and White Matter

- **Anatomy and structure:** the *cerebellum* is a major structure of the metencephalon located posterior to the cerebrum, inferior to the occipital cortex. It occupies about 10% of the cranial cavity but it contains more than 50% of the total number of cerebral neurons. The cerebellum is made up of a three-layer cortex with six types of cells. The small granular cells in the cerebellum cortex are the most numerous neurons in the brain. The cerebellar (deep) nuclei are the sole output pathways of the cerebellum.

- **Known function:**
  - Motor control: maintenance of balance and posture

The cerebellum modulates commands to motor neurons and coordinates the timing and force of the different muscle groups to produce flowing body movements:

- Coordination of walking: anterior lobe.
- Maintenance of postural tone and modulation of motor activities: posterior lobe.
- Maintenance of balance: flocculonodular lobe.
  - Motor learning: The cerebellum plays a major role in adapting and fine tuning motor programs to make accurate movements through a trial-and-error process.
    - Fine control of motor activity: most of its afferents run from the cerebral cortex via nuclei from the pontine region to motor and premotor cortices.
    - Coordination of planned and actual activities: The intermediate zone of the cerebellum receives information about the extremities principally via the cortex (via the pons) and spinal cord (spinocerebellar tract).
    - Posture: The vermis receives information about the axial musculature and body position via the vestibular nucleus, the spinal cord, and the fastigial nucleus.
    - Control of eye movement: flocculonodular lobe via the vestibular nucleus; each of the deep cerebellar nuclei has connections with the brainstem. Other important relay stations are the red nucleus and the RF.
  - Cognitive functions: The cerebellum seems to play a role in language and memory.
    - Compensation of frontal lobe function.
    - Further interconnections with the hypothalamus, parts of the autonomic nervous system, the prefrontal cortex (evidence of higher cognitive functions), other regions of the cerebral cortex, and the limbic and mesolimbic system.
  - Sensory functions: The cerebellum also has sensory functions.
- **Cerebellar pathology:**
  - Cerebellar disorders are possibly involved in:

- Attention-deficit hyperactive disorder (ADHD; children with ADHD have a smaller posterior, inferior vermis)
- Cognitive and emotional functions·
- Epilepsy
- Depression
- Psychoses
- Schizophrenia
- Bipolar disorders[14]
- Dyslexia.

Treatment of the Cerebellum
Bruno Chikly

- **Treating the Global Cerebellum**
  Practitioner: take up a position at the head of the patient.
  Patient: in supine position. Prone position is suggested for beginners in order to avoid having the full weight of the cranium on the sensitive parts of the hand.

- **Treating cerebellum–cerebrum restrictions**

Hand position:
  - Position one hand on the cerebellum inferior to the tentorium cerebelli.
  - Position the other hand on the cerebrum superior to the tentorium cerebelli.

Method: assess if there is any somatic dysfunction between cerebellum–cerebrum and release with ease if needed.

- **Treating intercerebellar restrictions**

Hand position:
  - Position one hand on the left lobe and one hand on the right lobe of the cerebellum. Both hands are inferior to the tentorium cerebellum.

Method: assess if there is any somatic dysfunction between the two lobes of the cerebellum. Release with ease if needed.

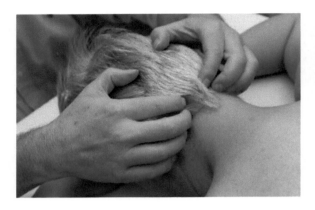

Figure 33.69
Treatment of cerebello-cerebral dysfunctions

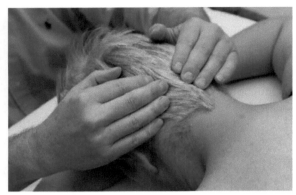

Figure 33.70
Treatment of intercerebellar dysfunctions

- **Treating intracerebellar restrictions**

Hand position:
- Position both hands on the cerebellum, inferior to the tentorium cerebellum.

Method: Assess if there is any somatic dysfunction within the cerebellum. You can more specifically assess white matter, cortex layers, fissures, and nuclei. Release with ease if needed.

- **Treating the cerebellum nuclei: fastigial, globose, emboliform, and dentate**

The cerebellar nuclei are usually located on a horizontal line below the level of the inion.

Hand position:
- Position each hand symmetrically on each side of midline.

Method: Start with the most medial position within the vermis (fastigial nuclei) where the fingers of each hand are about 1–2 mm apart; and move each hand more and more lateral each time by about 2–3 mm to assess respectively the globose, emboliform, and dentate nuclei. A cerebellar nuclei in dysfunction usu-

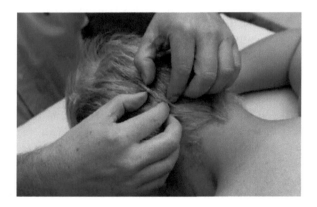

Figure 33.71
Treatment of intracerebellar dysfunctions

ally present a very intense vibration or heat under the practitioner's finger. Synchronize very specifically with the deep cerebellar nucleus that needs help and release with ease.

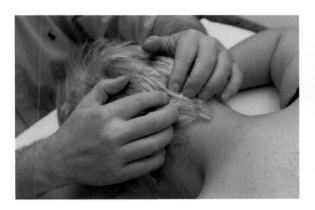

Figure 33.72
Treatment of the cerebellar nuclei - fastigial nuclei

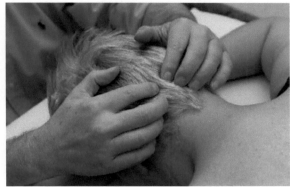

Figure 33.73
Treatment of the cerebellar nuclei - globose nuclei

The cerebellar peduncles

Cerebellar peduncles are myelinated axons. The practitioner can globally assess the superior, middle, and inferior cerebellar peduncles by feeling the deep peduncular "pull". Assessment is bilateral; treatment of cerebellar peduncles is usually unilateral.

1 Treating the superior cerebellar peduncles (SCP): contralateral. The SCP contain fibers from the globose, emboliform, and dentate nuclei. These fibers decussate to the contralateral red nucleus, or the thalamic ventrolateral or ventroanterior nuclei.

Practitioner: Take up a position at the head of the patient.

Patient: in prone (or supine) position.

Hand position:
  • Position one hand on the middle of the cerebellum inferior to inion; and position the other hand on the controlateral red nucleus or thalamic nuclei.

Method: Assess if there is any somatic dysfunction within the SCP or within the practitioner's two hands and release with ease if needed. Recheck that the somatic dysfunction has disappeared.

2 Treating the middle cerebellar peduncles (MCP). The middle cerebellar peduncles (MCP) contain fibers going from the nuclei of the pons to contralateral cerebellum (pontocerebellar fibers).

Practitioner: Take up a position at the head of the patient.

Patient: in prone (or supine) position.

Hand position:
  • Position one hand on the middle of the inferior cerebellum; and position the other hand on the most lateral part of the ipsilateral cerebellum, close to the posterior ear.

Method: Assess if there is any somatic dysfunction within the MCP or within the practitioner's two hands and release with ease if needed. Recheck that the somatic dysfunction has disappeared.

3 Treating the inferior cerebellar peduncles (ICP). The inferior cerebellar peduncles receive mainly olivocerebellar fibers from contralateral inferior olive (also anterior and posterior spinocerebellar fibers, vestibular nuclei, and lateral reticular). Efferent fibers go from fastigial to ipsilateral vestibular nuclei and the reticular formation.

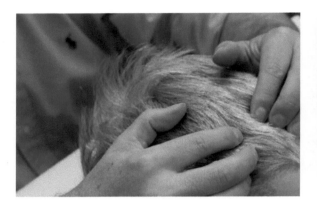

Figure 33.74
Treatment of the cerebellar nuclei - emboliform nuclei

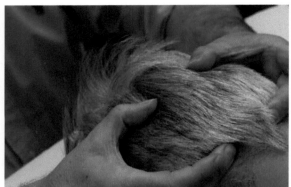

Figure 33.75
Treatment of the cerebellar nuclei - dentate nuclei

Practitioner: Take up a position at the head of the patient.

Patient: in prone (or supine) position.

Hand position:
- Position one hand on the middle of the cerebellum inferior to inion, and position the other hand on the contralateral inferior olive or on the ipsilateral spinal cord.

Method: Assess if there is a pull between the two hands, indicating a somatic dysfunction within the ICP. Release with ease if needed. Recheck that the somatic dysfunction disappeared.

Treating the Cerebellum (according to Plothe)
Torsten Liem

Patient is in supine position;

Practitioner is at the head of the table.

Hand position:
- Cradle the patient's cranium in both your hands.

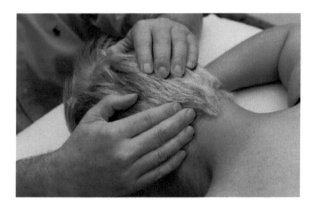

Figure 33.76
Treatment of the superior cerebellar peduncle

- Locate your index, middle, ring, and little fingers beneath the nuchal line on both sides to sense the cerebellar hemispheres (Figure 33. 79A).

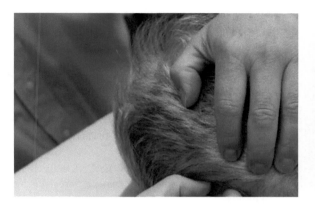

Figure 33.77
Treatment of the middle cerebellar peduncle

Figure 33.78
Treatment of the inferior cerebellar peduncle

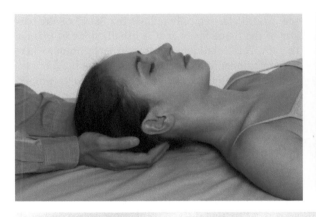
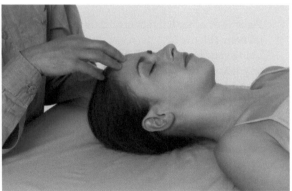

Figure 33.79A, B
Treating the cerebellum

Method:
- By gently guiding the occiput toward flexion at the SBS, you can gain a good impression of the mobility of the cerebellar hemispheres.

- Treat the side with the less pronounced movement restriction first.
- On the side of the hemisphere to be treated, keep your hand under the patient's occiput. This serves simultaneously to stabilize the cranium.

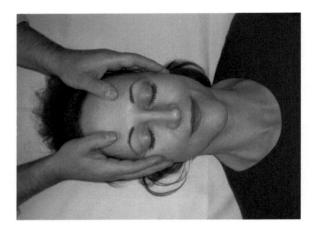

Figure 33.80
Phase 3 - brain mobility treatment

- Place your other hand contralaterally on the frontal bone (Figure 32.27b).
- Using your hand under the occiput, gently go with or guide the bone into flexion so as to ensure maximum freedom for the underlying brain structure and, hence, to open the associated blood vessels, that is, the territories supplied by the superior cerebellar artery (branch of the basilar artery), inferior anterior cerebellar artery (branch of the basilar artery), and inferior posterior cerebellar artery (branch of the vertebral artery).
- Simultaneously, using light pressure from your hand on the frontal bone, deliver a fluid drive diagonally toward the hemisphere to be treated and wait for the sensory feedback from the stabilizing hand.
- Once release has been successfully achieved, change to the side where there is greater movement restriction and repeat the procedure.
- **Note:** According to work published in the 1990s by Nicolson and Fawcett, impairment of cerebellar function results in increased frontal lobe activity as a compensatory phenomenon.

It is therefore advisable also to treat the frontal lobe. To do this, use your posterior hand during the inhalation phase to send a fluid drive to the diagonally opposite frontal lobe. Here too, you should start with the side with the less pronounced movement restriction.
- Conclude by balancing the dural system.

Electromagnetic Field of the Brain and Spinal Cord

The electromagnetic (EM) field of the CNS activity in general creates an EM field that can be perceived by human hands[9].

Energetic, emotional, mental, and spiritual fields will not be addressed here; see Chapters 18, 20, 25, 32, 38

Phase 3: Brain Mobility
Bruno Chikly

The technique of phase three is not an approach where the practitioner typically follows the "ease" or the barrier of the tissue fibers as it is usually done in manual therapy. This technique is a *parenchyma* technique where the practitioner follows the movement (not the motility) of the brain parenchyma trying to go back to its (proper) place, to its "throne." In this approach, the practitioner does not initially need to pay much attention to the ease or the resistance of the surrounding fibers.

When the practitioner brings awareness to the brain (or spinal cord) parenchyma, and perfectly synchronizes with it, the organ will have the tendency to come back to its appropriate place, which we sometimes call the "seat of the brain" or its throne.

From a functional standpoint, most brains do not sit properly in their optimum position within the cranium. Over time, countless traumas accumulate within the body system, such as: birth trauma; physical injuries; car accidents; or possibly chemical, nutritional, and environmental toxicity; allergy to specific food or dyes. Something as benign as repainting the room of the child or changing cleaning products could potentially affect the brain's location.

Numerous types of injuries can create minute inflammation in the brain that can eventually lead to some degree of fibrosis and asymmetrical position of the brain and spinal cord. The accumulation of a whole life of unrecognized, unreleased, CNS trauma can set the brain in a wrong functional location.

Many patients may need to have their CNS checked and eventually respectfully set free.

In clinical practice, patients are often found to have a brain in a relative flexed position. This can create numerous problems because, for example, the eyes and vestibular system do their best to maintain gaze in a horizontal orientation. A life of unreleased accumulated brain traumas can clinically create a collection of chronic symptoms such as poor memory or focus, mental sluggishness, difficulty to find words, dyslexia, faulty space or time orientation, mental fatigue, and so forth.

To use this approach, the practitioner needs to use the correct pressure, the precise depth needed to engage someone's particular brain (or spinal cord) tissue. During treatment, these brains in lesion will often naturally extend, coming back posteriorly.

It is of utmost importance to exactly follow the cerebral tissue and stop when it stops to avoid possible side effects. In this approach, the cerebral tissue is in complete command. It is not the time to "impose" a specific rhythm, direction, and pressure on the brain parenchyma.

In some pathologies, unknown aneurysms are present and it is of the utmost importance to have a clear diagnosis and strictly follow the lead of the brain in order to avoid severe potential problems. In other pathologies, such as Arnold-Chiari malformation, for example, the brain parenchyma will direct itself during treatment in flexion rather than extension so it is not the occasion for insisting on "therapist agenda" and imposing any mental picture on the brain. Every tissue will respond very specifically to your touch.

This approach may need, in some cases, a certain pressure to completely synchronize with the "need" of the tissue. So be aware of any contraindications applied to the CNS—any pressure more than a few grams that could be contraindicated for your patient, including, but not limited to bleeding, possible hidden fracture, fever, and so forth. Practitioners need to develop specific skills for this technique that need to be learned properly within the context of a supervised hands-on seminar.

Phase 4: Autonomic nervous system, peripheral nervous system, etc.

This phase will be addressed in Chapters 34 and 35.

Phase 5: completion

Bruno Chikly, Torsten Liem

This phase provides for rechecking and addressing compensations and other structures as needed, and for helping the patient integrate the treatment as well as, so far as possible, prevent any treatment reaction.

Also a sacro-occipital balancing can be done, synchronising occiput and sacrum with deep in- and exhalation of the patient (see also Liem *Cranial Osteopathy: A Practical Textbook*) .

Further reading

1. Barral JP, Manual Thermal Evaluation, Eastland Press, 2003.

2. Arbuckle BE, *The selected writings of Beryl E. Arbuckle, D.O., F.A.C.O.P.* National Osteopathic Institute and Cerebral Palsy Foundation; 1977.

3. Chikly B, Quaghebeur J. Reassessing cerebrospinal fluid (CSF) hydrodynamics: A literature review presenting a novel hypothesis for CSF physiology. *J Bodyw Mov Ther.* 2013;17(3):344–354.

4. Igarashia H, Tsujitaa M, Kwee IL, Nakada T, Water influx into cerebrospinal fluid is primarily controlled by aquaporin-4, not by aquaporin-1: 17O JJVCPE MRI study in knockout mice, *Neuroreport,* 2014;25(1):39–43.

5. Iliif J, Wang M, Liao Y, et al. A paravascular pathway facilitates CSF flow through the brain parenchyma and the clearance of interstitial solutes, including amyloid β. *Sci Transl Med.* 2012;4(147):147ra111.

6. Gaskell W. H., The Electrical changes in the Quiescent Cardiac Muscle which accompany Stimulation of the Vagus Nerve, J Physiol November 1886; 7; (5-6) 451-452.

7. Herrick C.J., The Cranial and First Spinal Nerves of Menidia. A Contribution Upon the Nerve Components of the Bony Fishes, J. Compl Neurol,.1913, 23: 635-675.

8. Schmahmann J, Pandya D, Wang R, et al. Association fibre pathways of the brain: Parallel observations from diffusion spectrum imaging and autoradiography, *Brain*, 2007; 130:630–653.

9. Oschman J., *Energy Medicine: The Scientific Basis*. London, UK: Harcourt Publishers; 2000.

10. Jealous J. *Automatic Shifting*. 1989.

11. Haines DE, Dietrichs E, Mihailoff GA, McDonald EF. The cerebellar-hypothalamic axis: Basic circuits and clinical observations. *Int Rev Neurobiol*. 1997;41:83–107.

12. Dempsey CW, Tootle DM, Fontana CJ, Fitzjarrell AT, Garey RE, Heath RG. Stimulation of the paleocerebellar cortex of the cat: Increased rate of synthesis and release of catecholamines at limbic sites. *Biol Psychiatry*. 1983;18:127–132.

13. Castellanos FX, Giedd JN, Berquin PC, et al. Quantitative brain magnetic resonance imaging in girls with attention-deficit hyperactivity disorder. *Arch Gen Psychiatry*. 2001;58:289–295.

14. Castellanos FX, Giedd JN, Marsh WL, et al. Quantitative brain magnetic resonance imaging in attention-deficit hyperactivity disorder. *Arch Gen Psychiatry*. 1996;53(7):607–616.

15. Mostofsky SH, Mazzocco MM, Aakalu G, Warsofsky IS, Denckla MB, Reiss AL. Decreased cerebellar posterior vermis size in fragile X syndrome: Correlation with neurocognitive performance. *Neurology*. 1998;50(1):121–130.

16. Schmahmann JD. An emerging concept. The cerebellar contribution to higher function. *Arch Neurol*. 1991;48(11):1178–1187.

17. Schmahmann JD. Cerebellum – the true thinking machine. In: Zigmond M, Bloom F, Landis S, Roberts J, Squire L, eds. *Fundamental Neuroscience*. San Diego, CA: Academic Press; 1998:985.

18. Loeber RT, Sherwood AR, Renshaw PF, Cohen BM, Yurgelun-Todd DA. Differences in cerebellar blood volume in schizophrenia and bipolar disorder. *Schizophr Res*. 1999;37:81–89.

19. Jacobsen LK, Giedd JN, Berquin PC, et al. Quantitative morphology of the cerebellum and fourth ventricle in childhood-onset schizophrenia. *Am J Psychiatry*. 1997;154:1663–1669.

20. Lauterbach EC. Bipolar disorders dystonia and compulsion after dysfunction of the cerebellum dentatorubrothalamic tract and substantia nigra. *Biol Psychiatry*. 1996;40:726–730.

21. Nicolson RI, Fawcett AJ. Automaticity: A new framework for dyslexia research? *Cognition*. 1990;35:159–182.

22. Nicolson RI, Fawcett AJ. Performance of dyslexic children on cerebellar and cognitive tests. *J Mot Behav*. 1999;31(1):68–78.

23. Blechschmidt E. *Humanembryologie Prinzipien und Grundbegriffe*. Stuttgart: Hippokrates; 1974:57.

24. Blechschmidt E. *Humanembryologie Prinzipien und Grundbegriffe*. Stuttgart: Hippokrates; 1974:65.

25. Teilhard de Chardin P. *Das Herz der Materie*. Düsseldorf: Patmos; 2002:120.

26. Liem T. *Kraniosakrale Osteopathie*. Stuttgart: Hippokrates; 2005.

27. Jealous J. Course Notes on Automatic Shifting. 1989.

28. Liem T. Cranial Osteopathy: A Practical Textbook. Seattle, WA: Eastland Press; 2009.

29. Blechschmidt E, Gasser RF. Biokinetics and Biodynamics of Human Differentiation. Springfield, IL: Charles C. Thomas; 1978:132.

30. Haines DE, Dietrichs E, Mihailoff GA, McDonald EF. The cerebellar-hypothalamic axis: basic circuits and clinical observations. Int Rev Neurobiol. 1997;41:83–107.

31. Dempsey CW, Tootle DM, Fontana CJ, Fitzjarrell AT, Garey RE, Heath RG. Stimulation of the palaeocerebellar cortex of the cat: Increased rate of synthesis and release of catecholamines at limbic sites. Biol Psychiatr. 1983;18:127–132.

32. Castellanos FX, Giedd JN, Berquin PC, et al. Quantitative brain magnetic resonance imaging in girls with attention-deficit hyperactivity disorder. Arch Gen Psychiatr. 2001;58:289–295.

33. Castellanos FX, Giedd JN, March WL, et al. Quantitative brain magnetic resonance imaging in attention-deficit hyperactivity disorder. Arch Gen Psychiatr. 1996;53:607–616.

34. Mostofsky SH, Mazzocco MM, Aakalu G, Warsofsky IS, Denckla MB, Reiss AL. Decreased cerebellar posterior vermis size in fragile X syndrome: Correlation with neurocognitive performance. Neurology. 1998;50:121–130.

35. Schmahmann JD. An emerging concept. The cerebellar contribution to higher function. Arch Neurol. 1991;48:1178–1187.

36. Schmahmann JD. Cerebellum – the true thinking machine. In: Zigmond M, Bloom F, Landis S, Roberts J, Squire L, eds. Fundamental Neuroscience. San Diego, CA: Academic Press; 1998:985.

37. Cooper IS, Upton AR. Therapeutic implications of modulation of metabolism and functional activity of cerebral cortex by chronic stimulation of cerebellum and thalamus. Biol Psychiatry. 1985;20:811–813.

38. Beauregard M, Leroux JM, Bergman S, et al. The functional neuroanatomy of major depression: An fMRI study using an emotional activation paradigm. Neuroreport. 1998;9:3253–3258.

39. Heath RG. Modulation of emotion with a brain pacemaker. Treatment for intractable psychiatric illness. J Nerv Ment Dis. 1977;165:300–317.

40. Loeber RT, Sherwood AR, Renshaw PF, Cohen BM, Yurgelun-Todd DA. Differences in cerebellar blood volume in schizophrenia and bipolar disorder. Schizophr Res. 1999;37:81–89.

41. Jacobsen LK, Giedd JN, Berquin PC, et al. Quantitative morphology of the cerebellum and fourth ventricle in childhood-onset schizophrenia. Am J Psychiatr. 1997;154:1663–1669.

42. Lauterbach EC. Bipolar disorders, dystonia and compulsion after dysfunction of the cerebellum dentatorubrothalamic tract and substantia nigra. Biol Psychiatr. 1996;40:726–730.

43. Plothe C. Die osteopathische behandlung des zerebellums bei legasthenie. In: Liem T, Schleupen A, Altmeyer P, Zweedijk R, eds. Osteopathische Behandlung von Kindern. Stuttgart: Hippokrates; 2010:688–691.

44. Nicolson RI, Fawcett AJ. Automaticity: A new framework for dyslexia research? Cognition. 1990;35:159–182.

45. Fawcett AJ, Nicolson RI. Performance of dyslexic children on cerebellar and cognitive tests. J Mot Behav. 1999;31:68–78.

46. Schmahmann J, Pandya D, Wang R, et al. Association fibre pathways of the brain: Parallel observations from diffusion spectrum imaging and autoradiography. Brain. 2007; 130:630–653. 66

34

Treating the spinal cord

Bruno Chikly and Torsten Liem

Introduction
Bruno Chikly

In treating the spinal cord we can use any phase approach, for example, down regulation with tissue trauma, or cellular fear technique, or different motilities including Sutherland motility, asynchronous motility, or any other spinal cord motilities (see Chapter 33).

Phase 1: developmental dynamic treatment of the spinal cord
Torsten Liem

- Practitioner: take up a seated position to one side of the patient.

- Hand position:
  - From the side, locate your cranial hand underneath the patient's occiput.
  - From the side, locate your caudal hand underneath the patient's sacrum.

- Method:
  - Deliver gentle compression between the occiput and sacrum to produce a resonance with the developmental dynamic force vectors of the spinal cord.
  - Point of balance (PBT), dynamic balance tension (DBT), or balance fluid tension (BFT).
  - Sense the resultant tissue dynamics but without reacting to them. A fulcrum usually becomes established between the regions.
  - Once the fulcrum has been established, disengagement may occur in the spinal cord. Support the process of disengagement by allowing it to unfold in a gentle compression field (or use minimal pressure to counteract the force of disengagement) and go with the process of disengagement. Sense the primary respiration.
  - The inhalation and exhalation phases can be sensed within the compression field.

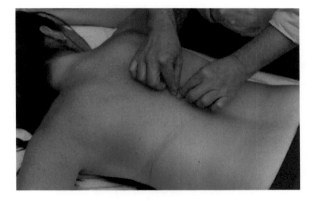

Figure 34.1
Spinal cord assessment

- At the end of treatment, the osseous and dural region around the spinal cord can be brought into balance.

Phase 2: spinal cord white (projection) fibers and grey matter
Bruno Chikly

As we did for the brain during phase 2 (see Chapter 33), we can assess the white fibers and grey matter of the spinal cord.

Assessment and treatment of spinal cord dysfunction

- Patient's position: the patient is in a prone or supine position.

- Practitioner: place your hands on the caudal part and thoracic most cephalic part of the spinal cord.

- Method: the practitioner may find the location of the main spinal cord restriction by slightly pulling on each end of the spinal cord to find which area is most involved/restricted. Find a tension or restriction and follow its path. Determine if it is the following:

1 Located on the left or right side of the spinal cord.

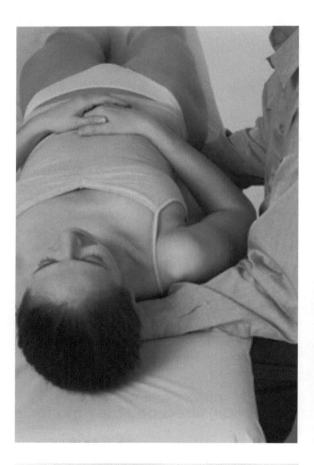

Figure 34.2
Developmental dynamic treatment of the spinal cord.

2 Whether it is grey or white matter: (i) if it is grey, assess the 10 layers of Rexed laminae and possibly check if it is a neuron, interneuron, or synapse(s). Synapse problems are often seen in scoliosis and if released can create an immediate change in the physical spine and associated ribs. (ii) If it is white, assess if it is an ascending, descending, or bidirectional pathway first, then, as usual, synchronize locally, regionally, or with the whole white matter path and release it with ease. You may want to have one hand in relation to the beginning or the end of a fasciculus. For example, have one hand on the white descending rubrospinal fasciculus and the other hand on the contralateral red nucleus.

The main fasciculi of the spinal cord are the following:

1 Descending pathways (fasciculus or tract):
   a Lateral (or crossed) corticospinal (pyramidal) fasciculus: voluntary movement (inferior to the face)
   b Rubrospinal fasciculus: from contralateral red nucleus
   c Lateral (medullary) reticulospinal fasciculus: posture and gait-related movements
   d Medial (pontine) reticulospinal fasciculus: posture and gait-related movements
   e Vestibulospinal fasciculus: from lateral vestibular nucleus (nucleus of Deiters)

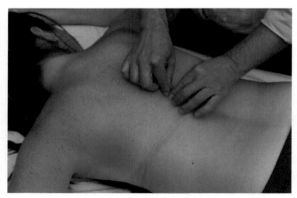

Figure 34.3
Inside the spinal cord - white or grey matter?

f Tectospinal fasciculus: from contralateral superior colliculus

g Anterior (ventral or uncrossed) corticospinal fasciculus: mainly voluntary movement of the trunk

h Hypothalamospinal fasciculus: from paraventricular nucleus of hypothalamus

i Interfascicular fasciculus and septomarginal fasciculus.

2 Ascending pathways (fasciculus or tract):

a Fasciculus gracilis

b Fasciculus cuneatus

c Posterior (dorsal) spinocerebellar fasciculus: unconscious proprioception and

d stereognosis

e Anterior (ventral) spinocerebellar fasciculus: originates at L3

f Spino-olivary fasciculus: to the inferior olivary nucleus of the medulla

g Spinothalamic fasciculus: pain (nociception), temperature, and coarse touch (protopathic sensitivity)

h Spinoreticular fasciculus

i Spinotectal (spinomesencephalic) fasciculus: ascends to the superior colliculus.

3 Bidirectional pathways:

a Medial longitudinal fasciculus: contains the medial vestibulospinal fasciculus (from medial, superior, and inferior vestibular nucleus)

b Fasciculus proprius (long and short propriospinal or spinospinalis neurons): interneurons; intersegmental reflexes

c Dorsolateral fasciculus of Lissauer.

Phase 3: spinal cord motility and spinal cord attachments

Bruno Chikly

Once the grey and white matter have been checked, it may be important to release all compensations and tensions in the spinal cord, and depending on the order of priority given by your assessment.[1]

Phase 3: assess dura, arachnoid, and pia (DAP) in the spinal cord

Same technique as for the brain (see Chapter 33) and applied to the spinal cord.

• Patient's position: the patient is in a prone or supine position.

• Practitioner: place your hands over one of the meninges covering the spinal cord.

• Method: find an area of tension in the spinal cord for one segment. Do a systematic layer palpation and discriminate if the tension is more predominant in the dura, arachnoid, or pia. Release the associated spinal root (or rootlet) if needed. Do mobility treatment to the spinal cord (same technique as the brain; see Chapter 33) with awareness of the most restricted area. Re-check as the spinal cord should be without any tension at all.

Spinal cord attachments

To complete the spinal cord the osteopath often needs to assess each dural ending (cervical and/or sacral) and check spinal cord attachments.

Assessing the main dural attachments of the spinal cord

• Patient's position: the patient is in a prone or supine position.

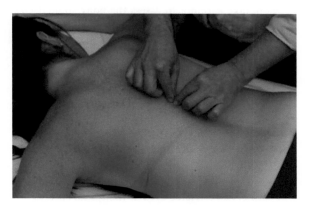

Figure 34.4
Spinal Cord - is it dura, arachnoid or pia?

- Practitioner: is positioned at the head of the patient.

- Method: to assess each dural ending (cervical and/or sacral ending), stabilize a segment of the spinal cord (take care not to assess the bony spine itself) and check which of the two ends has the most tension. You can hold the spinal cord and notice if it pulls more toward the sacrum or the upper cervical region. If the main pull is cephalic, then do the next treatment on the inferior attachments, especially the filum terminale. If the main pull is caudal, treat the cervical attachments.

Treating the filum terminale internum, terminal filament, or central ligament

If the main pull is cephalic, connect an area of the spinal cord to the filum terminale internum at its sacral attachments at S2.

- Patient's position: the patient is in prone or supine position.

- Practitioner: is positioned at the head of the patient.

- Hands position and method: put the fingers of one hand on a (restricted) area of the spinal cord (and again, take care not to assess the bony spine itself). Put the fingers of the other hand approximately on S2 (S1–S3). Assess if there is any tension between the two hands pulling the spinal cord caudally. Let the tissue release by following it until no tension is left between the two hands. Re-check the spinal cord tension. If there is no tension left, proceed to the next maneuver.

Filum terminale externum (terminal filament or central ligament) or coccygeal ligament

This maneuver is similar, but this time the practitioner will connect a restricted area of the spinal cord to the coccygeal ligament (sacrococcygeal junction).

- Patient's position: the patient is in a prone or supine position.

- Practitioner: is positioned at the head of the patient.

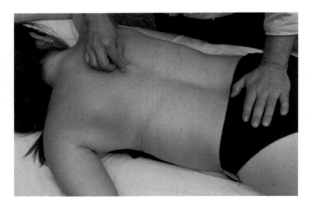

Figure 34.5
Filum terminale - spinal cord to S2

- Hands position and method: put the fingers of one hand on an (restricted) area of the spinal cord. Put the fingers of the other hand approximately on the coccygeal ligament (sacrococcygeal junction). Assess the left–middle–right sides of the sacrococcygeal junction. Assess if there is any tension between the superior hand and the left, middle, or right side of the sacrococcygeal junction, pulling the spinal cord caudally. If a tension is present in any of these three locations, let the tissue release by following it until no tension is left between the two hands. Recheck the spinal cord tension. If there is no tension left, proceed to the next maneuver.

Connect filum terminale internum (S2) to the end of the coccygeal ligament (coccyx)

S2–coccyx 1–coccyx 2: assess left–middle–right sides. This time, the practitioner will connect the area around S2 (filum terminale internum) to the coccygeal ligament (filum terminale externum).

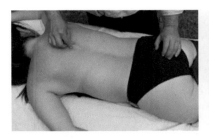

Figure 34.6
Filum terminale - spinal cord to middle of sacro-coccygeal junction

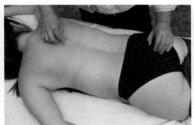

Figure 34.7
Filum terminale - spinal cord to left attachment of sacro-coccygeal junction

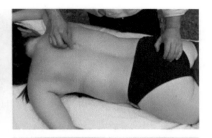

Figure 34.8
Filum terminale - spinal cord to right attachment of sacro-coccygeal junction

- Patient's position: the patient is in a prone or supine position.

- Practitioner: is positioned at the head of the patient.

- Hands position and method: put the fingers of one hand on the area around S2 (filum terminale internum) and the other hand on the coccygeal ligament where your previous assessment found the maximum tension (assess left, middle, or right side of the sacrococcygeal junction). Assess whether there is any tension between the superior hand and the left, middle, or right side of the sacrococcygeal junction. If a tension is present in any of these three locations, let the tissue release by following it until no tension is left between the two hands. Recheck the spinal cord tension if there is any tension left.

Superior attachments of the spinal cord: C0–C1–C3 and other cervical levels

You can assess the cervical region if your initial assessment found that the spinal cord was pulling you in a cephalic direction or if you have completed the caudal treatment.

- Patient's position: the patient is in a prone or supine position.

- Practitioner: is positioned at the head of the patient.

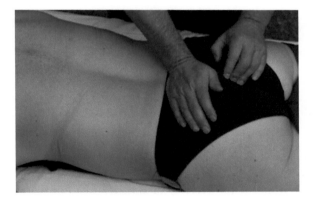

Figure 34.9
Filum terminale - S2 to sacro-coccygeal junction

- Hands position and method: put the fingers of one hand on a (restricted) area of the spinal cord. Put the fingers of the other hand on the cervical region (C0, C1, or C2). Assess the area of maximum tension between the two hands. Let the tissue release by following it until no tension is left between the two

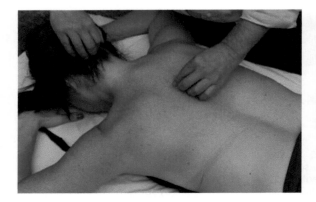

Figure 34.10
Spinal cord to C0 1

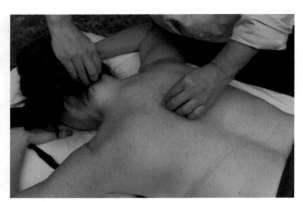

Figure 34.11
Spinal cord to C1

hands. Re-check the spinal cord tension.[2]

Other spinal cord attachments

There are few weaker spinal cord attachments along the spinal cord:

- Anterior attachments: anterior meningo-vertebral ligament (of Trolard) or anterior sacro-vertebral ligament.

- Lateral attachments: ligament of Hoffman (dorsolateral ligaments) and opercules of Forestier (vertebral foramen attachments).

- Posterior attachments and fibers of Soulié.[2]

Caudal traction on the filum terminale (terminal filament) according to Paul Chauffour and Eric Prat
Torsten Liem

- Practitioner: take up a seated position to one side of the patient at the level of the sacrum.

- Hand position: hook your index finger on to the terminal filament in the sacral hiatus (approximately at the level of the third or fourth sacral vertebra).

- Method:
  - Deliver gentle caudal traction on the terminal filament. This releases tensions in the spinal cord
  - Various methods may be used such as PBT, DBT, and BFT.

Note

- Phase 4: Electromagnetic (EM) field: see Chapters 20 and 32.

- Phase 5: Energetic, emotional, mental, and spiritual fields will not be addressed.

- Phase 5/compensations: see Chapter 32.

References

1. Osteopathische Behandlung der Dura mater spinalis in der hochzervikalen region. Torsten Liem - Osteopathische Medizin, 15. Jahrg., Heft 2/2014, S. 4-11

2. Osteopathic treatment of the dura. In: Liem, Tozzi, Chila: Fascia in the Osteopathic Field. (Handspring 2017)

For more details see also Liem T. Anatomy of dura mater cranialis. In: Liem, Tozzi, Chila: Fascia in the Osteopathic Field. (Handspring 2017)

35

Treating the autonomic and peripheral nervous systems

Bruno Chikly and Torsten Liem

Treating the autonomic nervous system: arteries, veins, peripheral fascia, viscera, articulations, and sense organs

Bruno Chikly, Torsten Liem

The autonomic nervous system (ANS) allows the body to respond involuntarily, subconsciously, and automatically to the body's demands for daily adjustments and maintenance of homeostasis/allostasis.

The ANS has two mainly involuntary actions to maintain the internal environment:

- Contraction of smooth muscles (viscera, eyes, blood vessels, etc.) and cardiac muscles.
- Glandular secretion (adrenal, lacrimal, salivary, digestive, cutaneous, etc.).

Two divisions have been conventionally associated with the ANS: the parasympathetic and sympathetic nervous systems. They harmonize and counteract each other. Under normal conditions, these two main branches of the ANS are usually in balance. A third division, the enteric nervous system, which deals with the diffuse visceral (especially enteric) sensory input, has more recently been isolated.[1–4]

The ANS is comprised of at least two neurons outside of the central nervous system that synapse together (preganglionic and postganglionic neurons). An added interneuron gives the ANS its autonomy and capacity to control local "decisions."

ANS neurological "control groups"
Bruno Chikly

We can anatomically distinguish five types of ANS neurological "control groups" that can influence the state of the local tissue:

1 When the ANS is active, the most cephalic control group can be located in the cortical and subcortical regions.

2 Another possible ANS control group could be located in the intermediolateral segments of the spinal cord: from T1 to L2 or L3.

3 A third group can be in the sympathetic chain (paravertebral): cervical, thoracic, lumbar, and sacral ganglia, and one midline impar (coccygeal) ganglion.

4 The fourth control group can be part of the prevertebral (preaortic) ganglia:

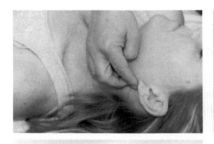

Figure 35.1
Superior cervical ganglion

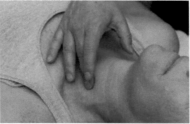

Figure 35.2
Middle cervical ganglion

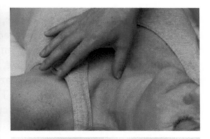

Figure 35.3
Inferior cervical ganglion

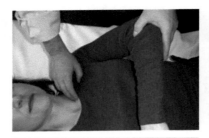

Figure 35.4
ANS technique - left stellate ganglion to release elbow joint

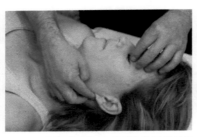

Figure 35.5
ANS Technique - superior cervical ganglion to release eye

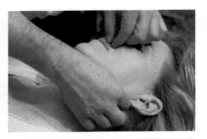

Figure 35.6
ANS Technique - superior cervical ganglion to release tooth

a The celiac ganglion or semilunar ganglion ("solar plexus," epigastric plexus) is the largest ganglion in the body. It is anterior to the aorta and the crura of the diaphragm
b The superior mesenteric ganglion
c The inferior mesenteric ganglion
d The aorticorenal ganglion
e As well as the adrenal medulla, sometimes compared to a modified sympathetic ganglia (postganglionic neurons) because there are only preganglionic fibers (T8–L1) stimulating them and no postganglionic fibers.

5 The last group encompasses other ANS control centers that can be located in variable, anatomically unconventional locations. They can be, for example, close to known groups of lymph nodes or near arteries or ANS plexus. Numerous anatomic variations can exist for the ANS.

Principles of treatment for the autonomic nervous system

Bruno Chikly

When working with arteries, veins, fascia, viscera, articulations, or sense organs, the practitioner will try to help release the ANS "control" on the tissue. The practitioner will try to help regularize, for example, the vasoconstriction or dilation of vascular structures of all sizes or the release of fascia tension. The same general principles can be used on most structures presenting somatic dysfunction.

• Patient's position: the patient is lying in a supine or prone position.

• Practitioner's position: the practitioner finds a somatic dysfunction and goes slightly and gradually in the direction of the lesion. The practitioner maintains, in this manner, a very small tension on the tissue "against the barrier."

• Hand position: one hand is on the tissue dysfunction and the other hand on the related ANS ganglion.

• Method:
  ◦ One hand keeps a small tension on the somatic dysfunction ("against the barrier") while the other hand finds the ANS control group that reacts while this small tension is maintained.
  ◦ The practitioner readjusts the small tension on the somatic dysfunction's hand and "gets rid of the slack", until the whole barrier releases completely.
  ◦ The practitioner waits until the tension in both hands is released. The somatic dysfunction can be re-checked and if the technique has been properly applied it should be completely released.

Inhibition of the superior cervical ganglion

Torsten Liem

Therapist: Take up a position at the head of the patient.

Hand position: On one side of the patient's head, place an index finger anterior of the transverse process of the second and third cervical vertebra and of the Musculus longus capitis, posterior of the internal carotid artery.

On each side, place your middle fingers on the posterior margin of the transverse process of the second cervical

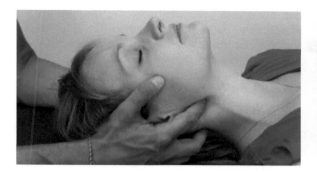

Figure 35.7
Inhibition of the superior cervical ganglion

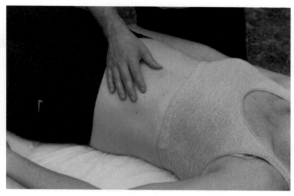

Figure 35.8
Celiac ganglion

vertebrae and your ring fingers on the posterior margin of the transverse process of the third cervical vertebrae.

Method:

Place the patient's head in slight extension.

With your middle and ring fingers, apply gentle pressure in an anterior direction on to the vertebrae. Hold this pressure for 90 s.

At the same time synchronize your index finger with the tissue tension and tissue dynamics and follow in the direction of ease until the tension is released.

Alternatively the other hand can be placed at the area of the preganglionic area (T1-T2) or at the symptomatic region of the body.

According to the description treat the other cervical ganglia:

the medial cervical ganglion at the level of C6

the inferior cervical ganglion at the level above of the pleural dome and between the transverse process of the seventh cervical vertebrae and the collum of the first rib

or the cervicothoracic ganglion posterior to the pleural dome and superior to the head of the first rib.

Treating the autonomic nervous system: additional information

Bruno Chikly

Any tension against the barrier could possibly create even a small hypersympathetic reaction in the body. This reaction can be felt, with training, in a specific ANS control center (as described earlier). These "cent-

ers" are clinically very often located in the inferior or superior cervical ganglia or the celiac ganglia.

Maintaining the tension also helps "monitor" whether the technique works, e.g. if the tension is released. If possible, it is best to have the clients feel the tension in the ANS control center, and actively exaggerate or amplify the agitation of this center. It may feel unusual for new clients but they'll get used to it and they will really like the results. You can easily work multiple hands with this technique or use the help of the client.

Robert Fulford technique for treating the solar plexus

Torsten Liem

Any emotion that we experience leaves traces behind somewhere in the life blueprint of every individual. Every emotionally tinged experience can also have repercussions on the organism as a whole via a network of neuro–endocrine–immunologic connections. According to Robert C. Fulford,[5] D.O. (1905–1997) emotional centers exert their governing influence via the energy reserves in the body that are located in the nerve centers (ganglia, plexuses, and brain). One of the largest of these centers is the solar plexus.[5]

Fulford believed that at some original point in our phylogenetic history, the emotions fulfilled a protec-

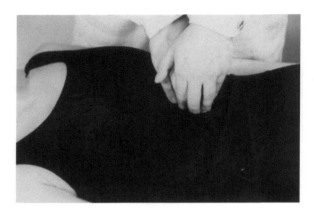

Figure 35.9
Fulford's technique for treating the solar plexus.

tive function; however, the body's energy reserves can still be used to activate emotions. All that is necessary is for the activity patterns to be transcended from lower emotions ("fight or flight" reactions in conjunction with instinctive responses) to higher emotions that are linked with the spiritual aspect. This allows creative activity to take the place of destructive activity. The healing process results when the creative energy that was held captive in fight or flight patterns is able to flow into those areas that require repair, work, and healing. In this way, emotions can act as a spiritual force that impinges on physical and mental resistance in the subconscious to activate and reshape old behavioral patterns.

According to Fulford, all biologic impulses can be traced back to the fundamental functions of expansion and contraction. The parasympathetic nervous system is associated with expansion, broadening, hyperemia, and bringing fullness and joy, whereas the sympathetic nervous system is associated with contraction, central blood pooling, pallor, anxiety, pain, and a concentration of biologic energy. The autonomic center of this biologic energy is located in the abdomen. The life process, especially breathing, can be understood as a constant state of pulsation in which the organism alternates back-and-forth between parasympathetic

expansion and sympathetic contraction. A disturbance of this pulsation – either from the center to the periphery or from the periphery to the center – leads in the long term to a disturbance of biological equilibrium in the organism.[3]

Fulford also believed that chronic fixed anxiety combined with a fear of expansion lies at the center of an agitated sympathetic state. This is associated with respiratory impairment because of abdominal tension. In anxiety, there is a tendency to hold the breath. When this happens, breathing out is incomplete, superficial, and associated with fixation of the diaphragm. This, in turn, disturbs the celiac ganglion and the flow of energy in the body. It results in physiological (hypertension, stomach ulcers, etc.), emotional, behavioral (e.g., neuroses, psychoses), and structural changes (hyperlordosis, excessive kyphosis, pelvic imbalance, etc.).

- Indications for use of Fulford technique for treating the solar plexus: release of tension in the celiac ganglion or solar plexus, therapy blockage, emotional trauma, diaphragm dysfunction, and pulmonary respiratory disturbance.

- Practitioner's position: take up a position to one side of the patient on a level with the solar plexus.

- Hand position: place one or both your hands on the patient's solar plexus.

- Method:
  - Apply gentle downward pressure, that is, in a posterior direction.
  - Administer gentle vibrations or go with the tissue tension until you sense a marked softening of the tissue.
  - The celiac, superior mesenteric and inferior mesenteric ganglia may be treated simultaneously by placing the fingers of both hands in a line from T12 down to L4. Posterior pressure is then applied.
  - Fossum suggests treating each ganglion individually and in relation to the sympathetic trunk. For the celiac ganglion this entails placing one hand posteriorly in the paravertebral area along the line of T6-T9. The superior mesenteric ganglion (at the level of L1) is treated by placing the hand in the posterior paravertebral area at the level of T10-T11. Likewise, the inferior mesenteric gangli-

on (level of L3/L4) is treated by placing the hand in the posterior paravertebral region of T12-L2. These areas are inhibited through light thenar and finger pressure on both sides of the region.

- Contraindication or precaution: if the technique is applied quite heavily, cautiously monitor the celiac plexus and proximity of the abdominal aorta.

Note

According to Robert Fulford, the solar plexus is the emotional memory of the body. Emotional traumas are "stored" in the solar plexus in the ANC. For treatment to be successful, it is imperative to release tension at the level of the solar plexus. In doing so, this technique has far-reaching effects similar to those of CV4.

References

1. Chambers JD, Thomas EA, Bornstein JC, Mathematical modelling of enteric neural motor patterns, Clin Exp Pharmacol Physiol. 2014 Mar;41(3s):155-64. doi: 10.1111/1440-1681.1220.

2. Yarandi SS, Srinivasan S, Diabetic gastrointestinal motility disorders and the role of enteric nervous system: Current status and future directions, Neurogastroenterol Motil. 2014 Mar 24. doi: 10.1111/nmo.12330.

3. Cheeseman BL, Zhang D, Binder BJ, Newgreen DF, Landman KA, Cell lineage tracing in the developing enteric nervous system: superstars revealed by experiment and simulation, J R Soc Interface. 2014 Feb 5;11(93):20130815. doi: 10.1098/rsif.2013.0815.

4. Gershon M, Columbia University, The Second Brain, 1998.

5. Fulford RC. From Center to Periphery. AAO Convocation: 1980.

36

Developmental patterns and influence upon body organization

Patrick van den Heede and Torsten Liem

Developmental patterns related to ectodermal differentiation

Embryological considerations

According to Blechschmidt, the structural development of an organ is inherently bound up with the development of its form (morphogenesis) and this in turn is part of its positional development (topogenesis).[1-6] The development of a new structure requires firstly a spatial opportunity and secondly a developmental dynamic occasion, i.e. in space and time. The future function of the organ in question is already foreshadowed during embryonic development. No organ at any time in its development is without function. As a metabolic field, each cell aggregation and each organ at least has a formative function in the shaping processes of the body as a whole and is always part of a spatial and kinetic entirety.

From Blechschmidt's perspective, the spinal cord and brain develop according to identical principles. Modifications arise as a result of respective differences in local topogenesis and morphogenesis.

During Blechschmidt's time, it was impossible to sufficiently recognize the importance of molecular biological, biochemical as well as biophysical findings in embryological design processes. Despite that, Blechschmidt's descriptions of growth dynamics did not lose their meaning; his statements are only relativized by often underlying biomolecular processes.

The descriptions in the following chapter are supported by biomolecular findings, with such molecular processes being discussed as far as they are important from the osteopathic perspective of embryonic and fetal development.

Cephalization and space modifying processes during the embryonic period

The development of the head and the neck begins early in embryonic life and continues until cessation of postnatal growth in the late teens.

Cephalization starts with the rapid expansion of the rostral end of the neural plate.

Almost immediately the ectodermal plate at the rostral end of chorda becomes the dominant component in the further differentiation of the entocyst disc. Later on during embryogenesis a subtle interaction between the ectoderm of the rostral part and the adjacent and surrounding mesenchyme (prechordal and parachordal mesoderm) will induce the differentiation of the cranio-facial region as also further morphogenesis of the brain.

The early cranio-facial region consists of a massive neural tube with underneath the bottom of the notochord, a ventrally situated pro-enteron surrounded by a series of aortic arches, an ectodermal covering, segregation of neuronal cells forming the neural crest and a mesodermally derived mesenchyme filling and surrounding the remaining spaces.

Early cellular migration and tissue displacements in the cranio-facial region qualify the intensive metabolic needs of the rostral ectoderm and the subsequent structure/function differentiation that progressively develops. Brain development and structuration are already a function as underlined Blechschmidt.[7]

- The neural crest cells are one of the first components that exhibit massive migratory behavior. These populations of cells become confluent during their migration through and towards the pharyngeal arches. They exhibit a morphogenetic pattern by behaving as wandering mesenchymal cell and differentiated neuronal cells at once. They inform function and structure at the same time.

They relate the prechordal and parachordal differentiation of nerve and brain centers to an anterior confluens that mainly consists of a glandular (thyroid, parathyroid, thymic and parafollicular cell mass) and rhythmic, electrical component (heart, fibronective system and epicardial, subhyoidal muscles) in the pharyngeal arch region.

In the viscero-cranium they relate the hindbrain to the neurosensorial areas (otic and optic placodes). In a certain sense they transport the cellular message of the ventral and dorsal midline towards an integrated structure/function relationship situated in a ventral confluens. This ventral confluens displays different functions ranging from Ca² control (parathormone-calcitonine), hematopoïetic function, rhythmic zone and immune cell maturation. This could be considered as an anterior midline function.

- The cranial mesoderm consists mainly of para-axial and prechordal mesenchymal cells. They form the connective tissue and the skeletal elements of most of the neck and the cranium in combination with the migrated neural crest cells.

Somitomere derived myogenic cells undergo extensive migration to form the bulk of the muscles of the cranial region. The morphogenetic control appears to reside within the connective tissue elements of the muscles rather than in the myogenic cells.

- The prechordal mesoderm is a transient mass of cells located in the midline rostral to the tip of the notochord. Myoblasts contributing to the extra-ocular muscles take their origin in this part that belongs to the first occipital somites.

The basic structure of the cranio-facial segment is established between the 4th and the 8th week. Changes in proportionality of the various regions continue until well after birth. In particular the midface remains underdeveloped during embryogenesis and even in early postnatal life.

The development of the neural plate is the first stage in the formation of the neural tube. Shaping of the neural plate is accomplished by region specific changes in shape of neuro-epithelial cells. Neurulation is started by a lateral folding of the neural plate resulting in an elevation of each side of the neural plate along a midline neural groove. The ventral midline of the neural plate appears to act like an anchoring point, the median hinge point. Closure of the neural groove and separation of the neural crest cells can be considered as the endpoint of this differentiation.

Organization and structure of the developing nervous system

The embryonic nervous system (after Blechschmidt)

Topogenesis and morphogenesis

- Flexion of the neural tube: As a result of the increasing longitudinal growth of the neural tube coupled simultaneously with the relative growth lag (restraining function) of the accompanying neural tube vessels, the brain is bridled. It displays ventral, concave bending over the heart swelling, leading to the formation of flexion folds ventrally in the endoderm and ectoderm.

- Development of the peripheral nervous system: The second month of embryonic development is characterized by surface ectoderm expansion dorsally (due to the rapid eccentric growth of the brain and spinal cord) and ventrally (due to the growth of the heart and liver). Between the dorsal and ventral regions the surface growth of the body wall is hindered, causing the surface ectoderm in this zone to thicken and the underlying stroma to become dense. It is in this field that the locomotor apparatus and the early embryonic peripheral nervous system make their first appearance.

- Whereas the spinal cord is anchored in the trunk by numerous spinal nerves, only a few cranial nerves course from the brain to the face, which is still relatively small.

- The brain is enclosed in tissue that will form the wall of the cranial cavity, and it is therefore hindered in its longitudinal growth. Consequently, the brain bends upon itself as it grows. At its frontal end the anlagen of the cerebral hemispheres and optic cups appear as blind-sac expansions on each side. A definite kink develops at the junction with the spinal cord and there is lateral expansion in the temporal region (Figure 36.1).

- Dorsally the embryonic brain encounters only low resistance to growth from the neighboring body wall. The body wall in this area therefore becomes easily expanded over the growing brain. As a result of this, the mesenchyme adjacent to the vertex of the embryonic brain becomes so extremely flattened during the second month that it shows almost no further growth. Ultimately, this retarded growth of the flattened tissue causes the cerebral and cerebellar hemispheres to remain close together.

- The cerebral hemispheres grow dorsally relative to the frontal brain region. They achieve this by bending convexly upward above the eye and laterally over the outer aspect of the brainstem.

From a functional viewpoint, subdivision of the cerebrum into lobes is arbitrary and is useful only to a very limited extent because it is not possible to assign memory, language, spatial behavior, emotion or movement precisely to any one brain region. As a general pattern in processing, it seems that sensory information is divided into a spatial and a formal component, analyzed in the parietal and temporal lobes, and transmitted to the frontal and medial temporal lobes, where the information is then re-integrated. When assessing findings it must also be remembered that disorders of the association cortex are commonly characterized by partial right-left overlap of symptoms.

- These conditions mean that the mesenchyme later becomes flattened and compressed between the two cerebral hemispheres and between the cerebrum and cerebellum to form the falx cerebri and the tentorium cerebelli.

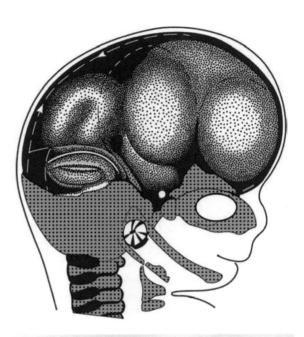

Figure 36.1

Head region of a 29 mm embryo at the end of the eighth week. The dural bands are shown as arching interrupted lines, the chondrocranium as sparse stipple, and the arachnoid occupies the solid dark areas.[8]

- The size of the cerebral hemispheres is one of the key prerequisites for the functional development of the organism as a whole.

Structural development

At the beginning of the second month, following the differentiation of the brain and spinal cord, the neural tube clearly exhibits three distinct zones (Table 36.1):

- The innermost layer of the neural tube close to the lumen or ventricle initially remains undifferentiated, compared with the higher differentiation exhibited by the outer layer.

- The outer zone is near the source of nourishment and is considered by Blechschmidt to be an assimilation field (photographically light).

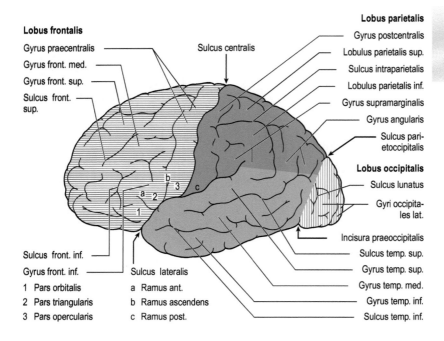

Lobus frontalis

Gyrus praecentralis

Gyrus front. med.

Gyrus front. sup.

Sulcus front. sup.

Sulcus centralis

Lobus parietalis

Gyrus postcentralis

Lobulus parietalis sup.

Sulcus intraparietalis

Lobulus parietalis inf.

Gyrus supramarginalis

Gyrus angularis

Sulcus parietoccipitalis

Lobus occipitalis

Sulcus lunatus

Gyri occipitales lat.

Incisura praeoccipitalis

Sulcus temp. sup.

Gyrus temp. sup.

Gyrus temp. med.

Gyrus temp. inf.

Sulcus temp. inf.

Sulcus front. inf.

Gyrus front. inf.

1 Pars orbitalis

2 Pars triangularis

3 Pars opercularis

Sulcus lateralis

a Ramus ant.

b Ramus ascendens

c Ramus post.

Figure 36.2
Lateral view of cerebrum: subdivision into lobes.

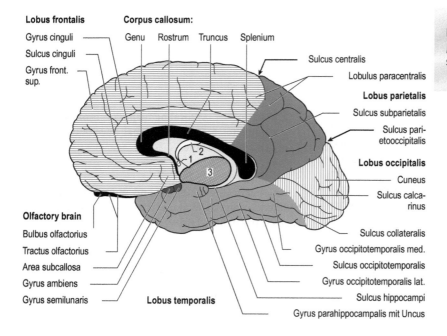

Lobus frontalis

Gyrus cinguli

Sulcus cinguli

Gyrus front. sup.

Corpus callosum:

Genu   Rostrum   Truncus   Splenium

Sulcus centralis

Lobulus paracentralis

Lobus parietalis

Sulcus subparietalis

Sulcus parietoccipitalis

Lobus occipitalis

Cuneus

Sulcus calcarinus

Sulcus collateralis

Gyrus occipitotemporalis med.

Sulcus occipitotemporalis

Gyrus occipitotemporalis lat.

Sulcus hippocampi

Gyrus parahippocampalis mit Uncus

Olfactory brain

Bulbus olfactorius

Tractus olfactorius

Area subcallosa

Gyrus ambiens

Gyrus semilunaris

Lobus temporalis

Figure 36.3
Medial view of cerebrum: subdivision into lobes.

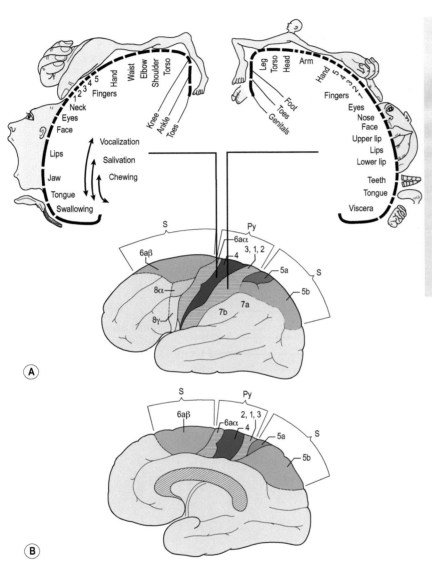

Figure 36.4a and b

Sensorimotor systems at the central sulcus; cortical fields of the pyramidal system (Py) and associated supplementary regions (S) that are counted as belonging to the non-pyramidal or para-pyramidal system. The diagram shows the primary motor cortical fields in the frontal lobe and the primary sensory cortical fields in the parietal lobe. The two regions are separated by the central sulcus. A) Lateral view; B) medial view (adapted from Rohen).[9]

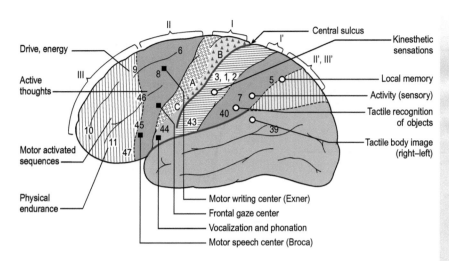

Figure 36.5
The higher (secondary and tertiary) cortical fields of the sensorimotor system, according to Rohen. The Arabic numerals denote Brodmann's areas.
The subdivisions of the frontal and parietal lobes incorporate the labels proposed by Kleist. I, I', II, II', III and III' denote the primary, secondary and tertiary cortical fields of the frontal and parietal lobes respectively.

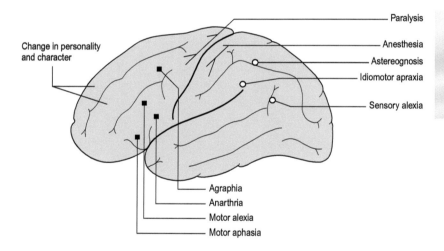

Figure 36.6
Clinical deficits manifested in response to lesions of the cerebral lobes (after DeJong).[10]

- The innermost zone (photographically dark) is considered to be a dissimilation field.

- Between the two there exists an intermediate zone characterized by cell nuclei superimposed at central-peripheral positions to each other and by juxtaposed cytoplasm. The rate of growth of the embryonic anlage of the nervous system is variable and is related to local position:

- Dorsally, the body wall is thin (with plate-like mesenchymal cells), and there is minimal resistance to neural tube growth: high mitotic rate, appositional growth of the nervous system.

- Ventrally, in the region of the floor plate, there is marked resistance to growth: minimal growth.

These unequal growth movements are one of the factors contributing to the kyphotic bending of the embryo and are responsible for the differing development of the mesenchyme of the neural tube (dura). As early as week 4, by the time the somites first appear, the dura ventrally already envelopes the neural tube relatively tightly and

Innermost layer close to the ventricle	Intermediate layer	Outermost layer
Dissimilation zone	Transitional zone	Assimilation zone
Contains large amount of liquid, with high internal mobility, and numerous mitoses occur	Long spindle-shaped cell bodies, cell nuclei superimposed at central-peripheral positions, and juxtaposed cytoplasm	Almost free of cell bodies and nuclei, with very narrow cell processes aligned perpendicularly to the primitive pia
Initially undifferentiated		Higher degree of differentiation
Black	Gray	White

TABLE 36.1: Organization of the brain and spinal cord into three zones.

in the course of its further development it becomes thickened ventrally far more than dorsally – due to the dorsal appositional growth of the neural tube.

Ventrally, the dura becomes so extremely stretched that it becomes highly resistant to tension and thus acts as a restraining apparatus. As a result of its tangential growth pull it initiates the formation of the large sensory ganglia and of the dorsal nerve roots that are located dorsally on each side of the neural tube (Figure 36.3, left). The dura is supported in this forming function in the trunk region by the dorsal branches of the aorta because these vessels remain short and are anchored in the pia mater, and in the head region by the pharyngeal arch vessels. The early embryonic gray matter of the dorsal neural tube and the ganglia that form as slips dorsolaterally from the neural tube therefore reflect the net cooperative action of the tensile strength of the dura, of the restraining function of the dorsal branches of the aorta, and of the dorsal growth of the neural tube (Figure 36.8).

After they have grown to a certain size in any tissue, all blood vessels have a restraining function. The longitudinal growth of the larger vessels is retarded when compared with the total length of their numerous branches. In this way blood vessels have the capacity to cause growth resistance that is directed against the organs they supply. Consequently, according to Blechschmidt, the restraining function of the embryonic dorsal aorta is responsible for the increased bending of the embryo (Figure 36.7).

- Formation of the ventral median fissure: The primitive dura restrains the ventral part of the neural tube so severely that the ventral median fissure forms there when the growth of the floor plate of the neural tube becomes retarded (Figure 36.9).

- Formation of the cisterns: The ventral part of the primitive dura becomes so strong that the arachnoid fluid pressed out of the neural tube becomes con-

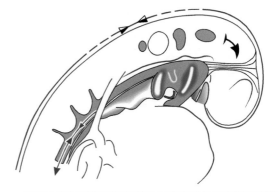

Figure 36.7
Restraining function of the dorsal aorta (convergent arrows) in a 2.57 mm embryo.[11]

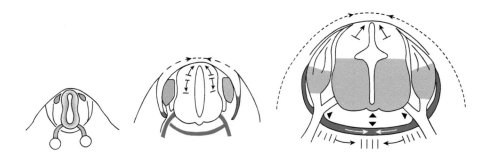

Figure 36.8
Cross-sectional diagrams showing the developmental movements of the dura and spinal ganglia in embryos approximately 3 mm, 7 mm and 8 mm.[12]

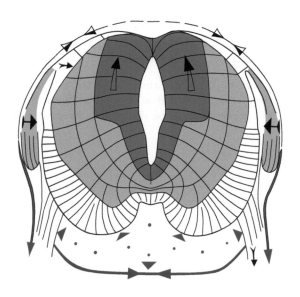

Figure 36.9
Cross-sectional diagram of the spinal cord of a 19 mm embryo showing the developmental movements and alignment of the cell limiting membranes. Arrowheads represent fluid pressure in the arachnoid; tailed arrows show karyofugal flow movements.[13]

gested between the dura and the pia mater, and the first cisterns are formed, i.e. on the ventral aspect of the spinal cord, on the basal aspect of the brain, and beneath the mesencephalon.

- Nerves as structures that are subject to pull: From the biomechanical and metabolic mechanical viewpoint, nerve fibers are structures that are subject to pull. For example, the distance between the origin and insertion of the optic nerve becomes clearly greater as the brain expands, with the result that the optic nerve lengthens in response to pull and develops high tensile strength.

- Guiding structure of the dorsal branches: The dorsal branches of the paired aortas supply the early embryonic pia. They originate even before the spinal nerves and act as a guiding structure for the latter along the cisterna spinalis toward the body wall. Subsequently, cartilage and finally bone are formed around these vessels and nerves.

The development of the central nervous system

The brain

According to Blechschmidt, the embryonic brain is characterized by outer and inner limiting layers that are separated by an intermediate zone. The basal dura becomes flattened due to the increasing growth of the brain. This results in a basal dura that is stretched and

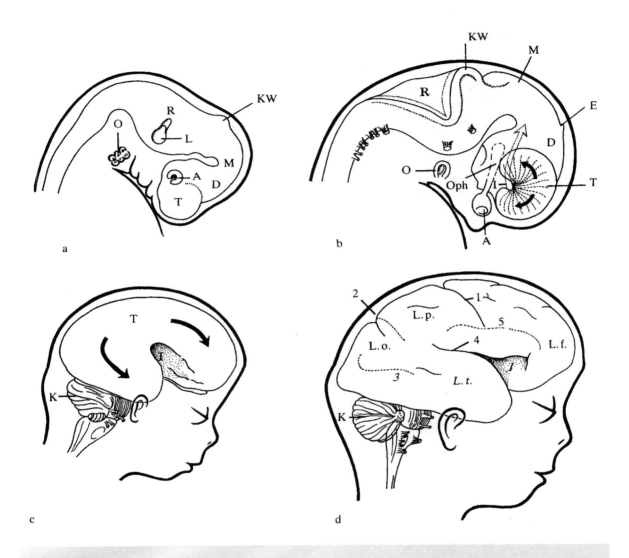

Figure 36.10

Coronal section through the forebrain showing growth development and alignment of cell limiting membranes in a 27.2 mm embryo at the end of the eighth week. Black convergent arrows at the base of the brain represent the restraining function of the ectomeninx (anlage of the dura); tailed arrows show the formation of cerebrospinal fluid; stippled outer layers represent the gray matter.[14]

thus strong and resistant to tension; this structure exerts a certain restraining function vis-à-vis the brain.

The brain enlarges eccentrically in the area of least resistance, primarily in the antibasal region (where the dura has not yet become resistant to tension). The brain (and the head too) grows convexly upward and forward in the antibasal region Figure 36.10).

- *Growth direction of the cerebral hemispheres and development of the insular cortex.* Because the cerebral hemispheres are firmly attached medially to the diencephalon, they too are capable of expansion only in an anterior and posteroinferior direction. Originating from a center of relatively minor growth on the lateral surface of the hemispheres, the insula, the hemispheres grow around the insula. The temporal lobe grows downward and forward in an arching movement and partially encompasses the insula. The hemispheres also grow laterally – the exception to this process being the insula itself, which thus becomes increasingly covered by the temporal, parietal and frontal lobes. As a result, the insular cortex comes to be situated deep in the lateral fissure where the cerebral hemispheres meet with the diencephalon.

- *Fissures.* The increasing eccentric growth of the brain causes growth resistances in the antibasal and laterodorsal cranial wall also to increase gradually to such an extent that regions of the expanding brain fold against each other. This leads to the formation of

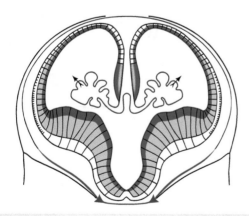

Figure 36.11
Restraining function of stretched mesenchyme in the vicinity of the olfactory placode (4) in a 3.4 mm embryo at approximately 27 days.[15]

fissures in which the falx cerebri and the tentorium cerebelli become stretched.

- *Dural band system.* Because of the strengthening of the dura between the differently thickening parts of the brain, surface expansion of the brain is possible only in the 'windows' between the dural bands or girdles. Surface growth then occurs primarily in the forebrain region as it expands forward.

- *Fontanelles.* The brain is bridled or restrained basally to such an extent that it bulges in the windows between the dural bands. The spaces in the antibasal regions between the dural bands develop into the fontanelles.

- *Basal ganglia formation.* At the base of the brain the surface growth of the cerebrum is retarded. Cells grow toward the brain ventricle, i.e. in the direction of least resistance. The result is a local thickening of the brain wall (basal ganglia formation).

- *Development of gray matter.* In the antibasal region, in contrast, the wall of the cerebrum is encouraged in its surface growth and offers sufficient room to cells close to the pia mater. As a result, nucleus-rich cells migrate – opposite to the situation in the spinal cord – outward into the cerebral cortex and form the gray matter (Figure 36.11).

- *Choroid plexuses.* At the medial wall of the cerebrum the highly vascular embryonic pia mater causes the ventricle wall to expand with each pulsation. The thin, weak wall (choroid fissure) protrudes inward toward the ventricles and with heavily proliferating vascular networks forms the initially very large choroid plexuses, which release fluid into the ventricles (Figure 36.11).

- *Olfactory (nasal) placode.* The stroma compressed between the optic vesicle and the embryonic forebrain becomes stretched (Figure 36.12). As it stretches, its rate of growth becomes less intense. The stroma connects to a very small area of ectoderm (anlage of cutis) and in this area it functions as a restraining apparatus. The ectoderm in the locally restrained area is thereby hindered in its surface growth, which

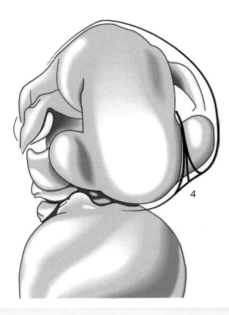

Figure 36.12
Restraining function of stretched mesenchyme in the vicinity of the olfactory placode (4) in a 3.4 mm embryo at approximately 27 days.[16]

causes it to thicken.* This initiates the formation of the olfactory (nasal) placode.

On a molecular level, early manifestations are characterized by cell migrations and differentiation organized around a central line represented in this case by the apex of the notochord. The whole complex of three-dimensional structuration of the brain and its connecting pathways depends upon genetic-molecular interactions. The physical component that permits this *intrinsic* information pattern to manifest itself is however dependent upon the 'mechanical' surrounding that constitutes the *extrinsic* patterning. Fluid pressure in the ependyme canal and the brain vesicles together

---

* The varying thickness of limiting tissue reflects differences in rates of growth. Minimal spatial growth resistances coupled with high developmental dynamics occasioned by the kinetic circumstances result in a relatively thin tissue layer. Hindrances to surface growth cause the limiting tissue to be relatively thick.

with the restraining function of the surrounding primitive meninx will organize the 3-dimensional pattern of the brain and the spinal cord.

The sequence of structure/function differentiation will follow a general pattern of centralization around the midline, ascension against the bony environment of the vertebral column and coiling movements of the developing brain.

- *Ascension of spinal cord and brain with dorsal appositional growth of the early neural structures.*

  There exists increasing evidence that the seemingly featureless cerebral cortex is a matrix of discrete columnar radial units, which consist of radial glial cell and neuroblasts that migrate along them. The development of the spinal cord displays an identical pattern.

  One can say that during neurulation the general pattern of differentiation is the same for the immature brain vesicles and for the closing neural tube. I.e. they both show a dorsal appositional outgrowing and differentiation, which increase height and volume of the cord and the brain. This volume change makes that the spinal cord will ascend in the vertebral canal against a fluid cushion that is created by compression of the arachnoid layer of the primitive meninx at the ventral side of the spinal cord. Blechschmidt defined it as an ascensus cerebri against a descensus viscerum.

- *Myelencephalon.* The major part of the medulla oblongata serves as a conduit for tracts that link the spinal cord to the brain and vice versa. It contains centers for the regulation of the vital functions of the body (heart rhythm, respiratory rhythm).

  The arrangement of the alar and basal plates is almost the same as in the spinal cord but there is a pronounced expansion of the roof plate to form the characteristic thin roof overlying the expanded central canal. Mechanical components like the appearance of the cervical flexure and the pontine flexure will support the differentiation process of the 4th ventricle.

  The dorsal lying afferent columns of nuclei migrate downwards and concentrate on the ventral site. They accommodate structures derived from the branchial arches.

Here again we have a clear example of synergism between mechanical factors (as bending of the tube) and neurotrophism dependent upon local secretion of vital organs, nuclei or cellmasses. Local, topographically determined, differentiation is capable of secreting a neurotrophic factor (NGF) that facilitates the further differentiation of the function/structure relationship.

- *Metencephalon (Pons-cerebellum).* Its fundamental organization remains like that of the myelencephalon with three sets of afferent nuclei and three sets of efferent nuclei. The future site of the cerebellum is first represented by the rhombic lips, which represent the mechanical landmarks of cell differentiation and outgrowth. They first grow medially, partly into the ventricle. Later growth is directed outwards. These 2 movements support respectively a crowding of developing cells and a bulging of fully differentiated tissues: vermis, flocculus and cerebellar hemispheres.

The cerebellum is formed as a bilaterally symmetrical anlage from the dorsolateral part of the alar plates of the mesencephalon; on each side the alar plates thicken to form the rhombic lips and the primordium of the cerebellum. In this process an intraventricular part and an extraventricular part develop around the fourth ventricle. By the end of the third month the cerebellar plate has formed outside the ventricle to bridge its rostral part.

The lateral anlagen in this region grow more rapidly than the medial section, giving rise to the development of two lateral portions, the cerebellar hemispheres, and a smaller midline portion, the vermis. From that point onward fissures (the posterolateral, primary, secondary and pre-pyramidal fissures) also start to develop on the surface of the cerebellum. All the important fissures have normally appeared by the end of the fourth month. The cerebellum then continues to enlarge in a dorsal direction.

- *Mesencephalon.* In the region of the alar plate neuroblasts migrate towards the roof (tectum) forming 2 prominent bulges: the corpora quadrigemina.
  - The inferior nuclei are related to the auditory system.
  - The superior nuclei are related to the visual system.

- The basal plate develops the tegmentum (somatic efferent nuclei of III and IV cranial nerves, nucleus ruber and niger).
- The crus cerebri, the passageways for the ascending and descending pathways to and from the brain, are situated more basically.

The mesencephalic and submesencephalic nuclei are the place of secretion and diffusion of most of the chemicals of the reticular integrating system. Noradrenaline is particularly associated with the locus ceruleus (pons), dopamine with the substantia nigra (midbrain), serotonin with the raphe nuclei (center of the brainstem), acetylcholine with nuclei in the pons, histamine in the hypothalamus and released by the thalamus.[17] By this means the mesencephalon together with the submesencephalon represents a molecular and mechanical force plate between the cortex and the brainstem. The neurological substrate is the reticular formation that is not only activating or inhibiting but an integrative centrum. It represents a molecular, neurological and mechanical hinge point (pontine flexure).

- *Diencephalon.* The forebrain structures (diencephalon and telencephalon) are highly modified derivatives of the alar plates without significant representation of the basal plates.

The early diencephalon is characterized by the development of 2 pairs of lateral swellings on the walls of the third ventricle (thalamic nuclei). The hypothalamus serves as the major interface between neural integration of sensory information and the humoral environment of the body. The epithalamus develops dorsal to the thalamus and displays interference with masticator and swallowing functions.

The thalamus, epithalamus, metathalamus and hypothalamus form another articulating force plate. This time between the higher and lower brain centers. This articulation can be considered as an ionic-molecular articulation. It controls cell to cell transmitters and cellular homeostasis.

In summary, the third, respectively the fourth ventricle and their nucleic surroundings can be considered as the center of two different primary respiratory rhythms. Cell respiration and its homeostasis versus whole body homeostasis respectively. The primary respiratory mechanism is probably 'supervised' by a primary inner cell respiratory mechanism. The first (PRM) is governing the chemical metabolic environment of the body, the cell respiratory mechanism (CRM) is governing the ionic-electron balance of the cell.

- *Telencephalon.* Its development is characterized by a tremendous expansion of the bilateral telencephalic vesicles. They surround the expanded lateral ventricles, outpocketings from the midline third ventricle. Growth dynamics cause them to approach to the midline over the roofs of the diencephalon and mesencephalon. They never meet because they are separated by a thin septum of connective tissue. Later on one of the most massive folding involves the large temporal lobes which protrude laterally and rostral. Starting from the 4th to 9th month the expanding temporal, frontal and parietal lobes will completely cover the insula. Fissures and sulci start to appear around the 6th month and some take definitive shape at the 8th month already: sulcus centralis, sylvian fissure and sulcus temporalis superior for instance.

The base of each telencephalic vesicle thickens to form a comma-shaped corpus striatum located dorsal from the thalamus. They develop into the n. lentiformis and n. caudatus (control of muscle tone and complex body movements). At the rostral part of the early telencephalon we find the lamina terminalis.

- *Ventricles, meninges and LCS.* As certain parts of the brain take shape the central canal expands into well-defined ventricles. The ventricles are lined by ependymal epithelium and filled with clear LCS. They probably play an important role in regulating the trophic environment of the differentiating neurons. They also serve as a guiding structure along which glial cell and neurons expose their migration trajectories. Once production, fluctuation and exchange of LCS starts the ventricles could assume a more mechanical function in cooperation with the enveloping meninges.

Two layers of mesenchyme appear around the brain and the spinal cord. One is a thick outer layer of mesodermal origin, which will constitute the dura, and the membranes of the bones of the calvarium. The other is a thin inner layer that is from neural crest origin and represents the pia mater and the arachnoidea.

The spinal cord

In the first 3 months the spinal cord extends the entire length of the embryonic body. The spinal nerves pass through the intervertebral spaces directly opposite to their site of origin.

Through growth of the body the vertebral column grows faster than the spinal cord. This creates a regressing of the caudal portion of the cord. It ends up at level L3 at birth. In the adult it ends at level L2. So the spinal cord is 'pressed' towards the foramen magnum by fluid pressure and at the same time it is retained downwards by the insertion of the filum terminale at the coccyx and the sacral insertion at the level of the 2nd sacral vertebra.

According to Blechschmidt, the growth pull of the ventral roots causes the neural tube to assume a rhomboid shape in transverse section. As a result of this growth pull the internal structure of the floor plate becomes characterized by an increase in cell numbers and by the formation of progressively larger cells (ventral horn cells → motor centers of the spinal cord). First the pathways are formed and then the centers.

The dorsal appositional growth of the neural tube causes the embryo to rapidly increase in its longitudinal and transverse diameters. As this occurs, the emerging anlagen of the dorsal ganglia are anchored ventrally in place by the strong, dense primitive dura, causing the distance to increase between the ganglia anlagen and the dorsal zone of the neural tube as early as week 4 (Figure 36.9).

In accordance with this positional development, the spinal ganglia send processes called 'neurites' to the spinal cord; in the neural tube these neurites follow the principal ascending growth direction of the spinal cord and form the first ascending central pathways (anlage for the future longitudinal sensory bundles) (Figure 36.9). This example of the development of afferent and efferent pathways clearly illustrates how future function already has its beginnings in morphogenesis, i.e. in the development of the position, shape and structure of the nervous system.

The spinal cord grows intensely in length in the relatively narrow vertebral canal and becomes slender whereas the brain develops over a broader area. The spinal cord lengthens with its nerve anlagen remaining anchored in the body wall. The white matter located in the sliding zone of the spinal cord organizes itself in a longitudinal manner in line with the growth direction of the spinal cord (the nerve pathways are established before their corresponding centers develop).

Trajectorial structure and formation of the white commissure

The cell-limiting membranes in the developing spinal cord cross perpendicularly to one another because the diameter growth of the spinal cord is also associated with circular alignment of the nerve fibers. The more central layers slide in a dorsal direction against the more peripherally situated layers. The ventral nerves appear as U-shaped fiber paths and their apex in the floor plate of the central canal forms the white anterior commissure (Figure 36.9).

During the first trimester of pregnancy the ectodermal neural tube and its surrounding mesodermal structures (meninges and osseous vertebral elements) are relatively identical in length and exhibit synchronous development. During the second trimester the vertebral column—which is sensitive to growth hormone—develops more rapidly than the nerve tissue. As a result the lumbar nerve roots increase in length and begin to assume the shape of the cauda equina.[18] In this process the tension of medullary traction increases gradually and, in normal circumstances, a number of physiological compensatory mechanisms develop to offset these forces. The result is the development of the physiological curvatures of the vertebral column.

Ultimately this development means that the medullary cone in 94% of adults is situated at the level of L1. However, this situation may also result in an abnormal increase in the tension of medullary traction. The lower the location of the medullary cone, the greater the medullary traction force (MTF).

According to investigations conducted by Royo-Salvador,[19-21] it could be hypothesized that tension between the cranium and sacrum is transmitted not via the spinal dura mater but via the spinal cord. In patients suffering from syringomyelia and idiopathic scoliosis he recorded a markedly abnormal tension increase in medullary traction and he regards this phenomenon

as the cause of the medical conditions in question. Eighty percent of patients with idiopathic syringomyelia are characterized by a marked increase in MTF. The deformities associated with idiopathic syringomyelia are believed to be provoked by MTF – which is transmitted from the sacrum via the filum terminale and spinal cord to the brain. This produces changes in the interior of the spinal cord. The MTF is transmitted via the spinal dura mater to the cranium and the intracranial dura system and also results in changes involving the bony attachments of the dura. Surgery to release tension at the filum terminale leads to a marked improvement in symptoms.

According to Royo-Salvador, abnormal MTF produced the following changes at the cranial level: caudal pull on the brain stem and increased tension in the dural meninges surrounding the brain stem and in the periosteal attachment of the meninges (e.g. the tentorium cerebelli). The cerebellar tonsils are drawn downward and compressed, leading to deformation of the fourth ventricle, an increase in the basal cranial angle, clivus deformation, and approximation of the petrous portion of the temporal bone and the sacrum. The cerebellar hemispheres are pressed into the posterior cranial fossa, and this in turn leads to deformation of the foramen magnum.

At the cervical level, the caudal pull at C1/C2 is associated with an anteroposterior force and thus with a posterior rocking motion of the dens. In the cervical region it is the nerve tissue that is most severely affected, with subsequent compression, ischemia and necrosis.

In the thoracic region increased MTF provides one explanation for the development of idiopathic scoliosis. The vertebral column attempts to reduce the tension caused by the spinal cord. The development of thoracic curvature minimizes the effect of medullary traction. In the thoracic region, in particular, abnormal traction on the spinal cord leads to the development of scoliosis. This arises as a result of compression that develops increasingly during the growth phase in particular. Increased pressure on the growth zone of the vertebra (the epiphyseal plate) retards the growth of this vertebral component compared with the other components, leading to deformation of the vertebral arch. The increase in pressure produces greater density and more trabeculae in the vertebra.

In the lumbosacral region increased MTF causes an abnormally low position of the medullary cone and increased tension at the filum terminale. Increased tension at the filum terminale in turn has the capacity to produce detrimental repercussions for the dural sac. In extreme cases the filum terminale may even perforate. According to the results of studies by Royo-Salvador, force is transmitted from the sacrum to the cranial interior via the spinal cord.

Under physiological conditions, MTF measurements oscillate between maximum and minimum values. Symptoms are found to worsen during flexion/ extension of the vertebral column, during Valsalva's maneuver, defecation, and other movements involving the vertebral column.

Filum terminale

The filum terminale varies between 1.5 mm and 3 mm in thickness. Tension at the level of the filum terminale is increased in syringomyelia and in scoliosis.

The development of the peripheral nervous system

Neural crest development and its functional significance

The future neural crest cells are located along the lateral borders of the neural plate where it interfaces with the general cutaneous ectoderm. They break away from the neural plate and change their shape and properties from neuro-epithelial cells to mesenchymal cells. These cells break through the basal lamina before neural tube closure and then start their migration. They lose their cell to cell adhesives (CAM) after migration when definitive location CAM adhesion is again expressed.

In the head region they leave the neural tube before closure (day 24-26). In the trunk region they leave after neural tube closure. Migration of the neural crest cells is determined by their intrinsic properties and by external environmental factors. Permissive factors are substrate containing fibronectin, laminin, and collagen of type IV. They do not penetrate the posterior, dorsal region of the somites (sclerotomes).

Pre-migratory neural crest cells are programmed to ultimately migrate to a specific environment where they are determined to reside. There is also a correlation between the time of migration and the intrinsic developmental potential. Most experiments suggest that early neural crest cells segregate into intermediate lineages preserving the option of differentiation in several but not all types of phenotypes.

A number of neural crest cells are bipotential and depend upon signals from their local environment. For example the sympatho-adrenal lineage cells can form adrenal medullar cells when exposed to adrenal glucocorticoids. If they are exposed to FGF or NGF they convert to postmitotic cholinergic phenotypes.

The trunk neural crest cells follow three different pathways:

- a dorsolateral pathway where they differentiate into melanocytes,

- a ventromedial pathway belonging to the sympatho-adrenal lineage, already mentioned above,

- a ventrolateral pathway where they differentiate in segmental sensory ganglia. They contain no level-specific instructions.

The cranial neural crest represents the major morphological substrate for the morphogenetic transformation of the vertebrate head. There are overlapping migratory territories for the major neural crest cells contributing to the sensorial and motor pathways of most of the cranial nerves. They migrate in diffuse streams throughout the cranial mesenchyme to reach their final destination.

Interactions between the neural crest cells and surface ectoderm of the pharyngeal arches may specify transformation of the tissue levels belonging to these arches. The circumpharyngeal crest for example passes behind the 6th pharyngeal arch ventral to the pharynx; it sweeps in cranial direction providing the pathway through which the XII cranial nerve passes. All the muscles innervated by this n. XII and the hypopharyngeal muscles together with their connective tissue substrate find their origin in the same neural crest origin.

The cranial neural crest, in contrast with the trunk neural crest, contains level-specific instruction. The occipital neural crest for example migrates towards the cardiac neural crest and informs the septal differentiation and the outflow tract.

Nerve fiber growth

Conduction pathways are guided in situ by previously formed mesenchymal structures. Later these pathways act as restraining structures. Existing canalization zones to enable nerves to find their way are referred to by Blechschmidt as 'fluxion zones'.[22]

Just as in the vascular system, a metabolic gradient is necessary to determine the direction of nerve growth. However, whereas extracellular flowing movements are thought to occur in the canalization zones of the vascular system, Blechschmidt suspects the development of intracellular fluxion in the nerve canalization zones.

Example: Trigeminal nerve

During the formation of the trigeminal nerve the inner tissue (mesenchyme) in the facial region is not of uniform thickness. Rather like the skin over a flexed knuckle, the mesenchymal tissue stretched over the brain protrusions is thin and pale: tissue with this appearance is found over the embryonic cerebellum, mesencephalon and cerebrum. It is also present lateral to the optic vesicle, lateral to the mouth and at the embryonic eardrum. In the areas between these thin fields of mesenchyme, the inner tissue is thick in the form of relatively large bands that serve as guiding structures for the three main divisions of the trigeminal nerve:

- Guiding structure for the establishment of the ophthalmic division (CN V/1): inner tissue band between the optic vesicle and mesencephalon

- Guiding structure for the establishment of the maxillary division (CN V/2): inner tissue band between the optic vesicle and mouth

- Guiding structure for the establishment of the mandibular division (CN V/3): inner tissue band between the mouth and eardrum anlage in the middle ear.

The spatial and the kinetic/biodynamic occasion for the establishment of the three trigeminal nerve divisions must come from those body parts that are capable of being innervated.

Sensory and motor pathways

According to Blechschmidt, the dynamics in the development of sensory and motor pathways display polar growth gestures. Sensory pathways draw themselves toward a substance source by using outside molecules to construct their growing membrane.

By contrast, motor pathways grow toward the embryonic anlagen of the growth-stretched muscle fiber. The motor neurite tips are drawn by the suction spaces of the growth-stretched muscle fibers and, according to Blechschmidt, are thought to release substances into the muscle cell (growth innervation). He suspects that electrophysiological innervation processes unfold between neurite tips and muscle fiber that contribute to the development of the muscle fiber. In the light of the processes described, muscle fibers that are lengthening at a rapid pace would develop extensive innervation while slowly lengthening muscle fibers would receive a less extensive innervation.

	Developmental tendency	Morphological structure	Dominant function	Psychophysical aspect
Head, CNS	Concentration	Nuclei	Integration (afferents from the sensory systems)	Capacity for conscious experience
Spinal cord	Segmentation	Metameric arrangement	Reflexive processes (relative equilibrium between afferent and efferent neurons)	Partly unconscious (reflexes), but sometimes also subject to conscious influence
Peripheral autonomic nervous system	Decentralization	Ganglia and plexuses	Visceral regulation (efferents)	Unconscious processes

TABLE 36.2: Morphological divisions of the nervous system, modified from Rohen.[23]

Primary embryonic brain vesicle	Secondary embryonic brain vesicle	Brain region	Cortical regions and nuclei	Ventricle	Cranial nerves
Prosencephalon	Telencephalon	Endbrain	Cerebral cortex, caudate nucleus, corpus striatum, putamen	Lateral ventricle (paired)	I (olfactory nerve)
	Diencephalon	Inter-brain	Globus pallidus, thalamus, hypo- and metathalamus, organ of sight, epithalamus (pineal gland and habenulae)	Third ventricle	II (optic nerve)
(Mesencephalon)	(Mesencephalon)	Midbrain	Tectum (superior and inferior colliculi), tegmentum, cerebral peduncle	Cerebral aqueduct	III (oculomotor nerve) IV (trochlear nerve)
Rhombencephalon	Metencephalon	Cranial slope of hindbrain	Cerebellum, pons	Fourth ventricle	V (trigeminal nerve) VI (abducens nerve) VII (facial nerve) VIII (vestibulocochlear nerve) IX (glossopharyngeal nerve) X (vagus nerve) XI (accessory nerve) XII (hypoglossal nerve)
	Myelencephalon	Caudal slope of hindbrain	Medulla oblongata, olives		

TABLE 36.3: Development and organization of the nervous system (according to Rohen).[25]

Cranial nerves[24]

The nuclei of cranial nerves III and IV are located in the midbrain region. Cranial nerve III exits from the ventral aspect of the midbrain, while cranial nerve IV is unique in that it exits from the midbrain dorsally.

The nuclei of cranial nerves V to XII are located in the rhombencephalon. These are comparable with the spinal nerves. Rohen identifies two novel structural principles in these cranial nerves:

- The principle of individuation: the nuclear material of the basal plate is divided into individual nuclei so that the anterior and posterior roots remain separate.

- The principle of specialization: each cranial nerve possesses one or more special functions and, in contrast to the spinal nerves, does not possess all four qualities simultaneously (somatic afferent, somatic efferent, visceral afferent, and visceral efferent).

The motor cranial nerves (CN III, IV, VI and XII) that are comparable to the anterior roots of the spinal cord exit dorsally from the brain stem.

The sensory cranial nerves (CN V and VIII) that are comparable to the posterior roots of the spinal cord exit from the lateral aspect of the brain stem.

The pharyngeal arch nerves, which were originally associated with autonomic functions, have modified their function and are comparable to the lateral horn of the spinal cord (visceral afferents and efferents):

- First pharyngeal arch nerve: CN V/3

- Second pharyngeal arch nerve: CN VII

- Third pharyngeal arch nerve: CN IX

- Fourth pharyngeal arch nerve: CN X

The optic nerve (CN II) and olfactory nerve (CN I) are not cranial nerves in the true sense. CN II originates as an outpouching from the embryonic diencephalon, and CN I is associated with the telencephalon.

Brain growth and development.

Methods for evaluating brain growth and development

Different indicators and components of brain growth have been studied in scientific literature to discover the patterning of brain development, the rate of growth, the direction of growth, the mechanical support and the time of brain growth and maturation.

The most representative components are:

- Myelination of cortical lobes and brain centers.

- Glial cell distribution during cortical development.

- Mechanical events, both intrinsic and extrinsic.

- Gyration.

Myelination

Myelination can be used as a reliable indicator of brain maturation during the fetal and postnatal period. Myelination first occurs in the globus pallidus, the pallido-thalamic fibers of the posterior internal capsule and the thalamus at 25 weeks post conception. The striatum and the precentral and postcentral gyri start their myelination at 35 weeks.[26]

Gyration and myelination studied in 50 children between 30-240 weeks postconceptional age (PCA) progressed in an occipito-rostral direction. Myelin appeared in the telencephalon between 55-65 weeks (3-6 months postnatal). It was clear in this study that the morphological differentiation of the brain surface preceded biochemical by an average of 12 months.[27]

One may remark that there is a tendency for myelination from the center to the periphery. In fact the periventricular structures display a first myelination pattern. In this process the thalamus can be considered as a central structure. Myelination of this nucleus indicates the importance of the cortico-thalamic and thalamo-cortical pathways in installing cortical integrative function.

The second remarkable fact is that myelination displays a postero-anterior, occipito-rostral progression. This coincides with the general organization of the base of the skull and progression of its ossification.

Glial cells

Glial cells are commonly known as the structures that radiate from the ventricle to the periphery of the future brain cortex and nuclei. They play the role of mechanical structuring bridges between the peri-ependymal germ layer and the outer cortical layers. Microglial cell localization (especially ramified cells) in the brain structure and their morphological forms correlate precisely with the appropriate stages of brain development.[28]

Nerve cells seem to be in constant movement, so that they pass through their eventual permanent sites and then return to them. The ventricular germinal zone gradually becomes thinner whilst the cortical zone progressively gets thicker.

Glial cells migrate with the neurons to their permanent location. Phylogenetically older parts of the brain tend to arise earlier in ontogeny.[29]

Mechanical events

The mechanical events that are important for definitive brain formation and growth are based upon both

Brain growth and development.

661

intrinsic and extrinsic mechanisms. The intrinsic mechanism is based upon neuronal cell crowding by which form and structure change during late embryonic and fetal life. Overproduction of neuronal cells is followed by sometimes massive cell-death till late in teenage life.

Another intrinsic factor is the myelination process that starts much later in fetal life (7th-8th month). It is responsible for huge brain growth in the postnatal period (2-fold the brain size during the first year of life, 3-fold during the first 10 years of life). The myelination pattern is a good indicator for brain maturation.

The extrinsic factors are dependent upon the interaction between the brain and the developing skull. Cortical folding is largely dependent upon intra-cortical mechanical forces but the regular distribution of the sulci, together with the orderly spatio-temporal pattern of growth point to the conclusion that this process may be controlled by extra-cortical signals.[30]

Gyration

Gyration appears later on the left than on the right sides of the brain and can be considered as an indicator for brain asymmetry. Gyration and myelination can also be considered as reliable indicators for brain maturation. Brain maturation starts in the central area and proceeds towards the parieto-occipital cortex. The frontal cortex develops last.[31]

In summary, brain development displays an occipito-rostral way of developing and maturation. It also shows a central to lateral pattern of neuronal migration and maturation. The architectural older parts also indicate the phylogenetically older structures of the brain. They form the base for an eccentrically directed growth movement.

When we consider that brain maturation is also dependent upon mechanical events in which the interaction between the meninges, skull and brain play an important role then a global parieto-occipito-frontal curve or pathway can be described. (cfr. Ruoss. K. et al.).

In general, the morphological differentiation of the brain surface precedes the biochemical maturation (myelination) by an average of 12 months.

Conclusions:

- the mechanical events are particularly important for bulging of the gyri and the formation of sulci,

- genetic components are important for the direction and emplacement of gyri,

- extra-cortical signaling plays an important role,

- biochemical maturation is preceded by morphological differentiation.

Biodynamical considerations concerning brain growth and its spatial organization

The brain and the spinal cord both grow eccentrically, later on they develop by means of the successive flexures around the brain vesicles and the relative ascension of the spinal cord. Eventually the brain 'sits down' at the base of the skull near the occipital bone, directing the developing cerebellum into the deepest of its squame (fossa cerebellaris o. occipitalis).

An important part of brain expansion and development will be controlled by mechanical parameters.

The surrounding mesenchyme, i.e. the later endo- and ectomeninx, and the inner fluid pressure in the ependymal canal and the ventricles, will restrain, guide and orientate brain development.

The anti-basal part of the cranial wall yields to the growing brain by intensive surface enlargement. In contrast growth of the mesenchyme surrounding the growing brain is hindered at the future skull base. The mesenchyme of the basal aspect of the brain becomes very strong and resistant to tension. It obliges the brain and also the cord to grow in the direction of least resistance.

This means that the dorsal part of the CNS and the spinal cord grow appositional, which creates:

- a kyphotic bending of the embryo,

- a stretched mesenchyme at the basal part that starts to function as a restraining apparatus (Halteapparat),

- a fluid (LCS) compressed between the dura mater and the pial sleeve especially at the mesencephalic part of the brain.

At the level of the mesencephalon this fluid acts as a biomechanical expansion force and supports the brain folding at this site.

In the area of cortical abutment the ectomeninx (dural sleeve) becomes stronger and starts to form restraining bands or dural girdles. Only the surface between the dural girdles grows intensively. This means that there are two sequences in brain and medullar development; an extrinsic processing and an intrinsic processing.

The extrinsic processing.

The ascensus cerebri is supported by compressive forces created by interaction between the developing somites and dura at one level and the spinal cord, surrounded by its leptomeninx at the other. As a final result of compression an increase in fluid secretion by the retiform tissue of the arachnoideal layer can be remarked.

This fluid does not only stabilize the spinal cord and the future brain but these are also 'pressed' upward by fluid pressure. It seems as if this 'ascension' is the first original flexion movement ever made by the cortex and the medulla.

An important quantity of fluid is concentrated at the base of the brain. The brain builds its own fluid 'cushions' which will be later be individualized as the cisternae of the brain. They function as mechanical 'fulcrums' by which the brain is stabilized against its bony environment and guided during its expansion movements.

They also favor the intrinsic mechanical episodes of brain development.

Intrinsic processing.

The fluid pressure at the base of the skull, between the meninges and the brain, organizes an external ascending appositional growth of the brain by means of neuronal crowding and migration around a more or less expanded ependymal canal.

At the upper side of the future skull the expanding brain will also be compressed by the ectomeninx. This fact obliges the two hemispheres of the future brain to grow toward the median level.

Neuronal crowding will first create cellular 'condensations' at the base of the brain recognized in the thalamic nuclei and the striatum. Later on the metathalamus and epithalamus are constructed in a cranial dorsal direction. The phrenulum habenulae and the pineal gland are the final witnesses of the intrinsic mechanical organization of the brain around the primitive brain ventricles.

During the further development of the roof plate of the different ventricles neurons are progressively crowded along their surface forming the basal nuclei of the primitive brain. Not only neurons are concentrated

but also blood vessels located in the pial layer become concentrated around the roof and will later bulge into the cavity of the ventricle. In this way the choroid plexuses of the different brain ventricles are formed.

The ventricles and the ependymal canal finally accomplish two functions at the same time:

- The fluid pressure inside functions as a potency that permits the ventricle and the canal to function as dynamical axle for structure proliferation and orientation.

- The outer peri-ependymal layer functions as a geographical field across which cell proliferate, differentiate and mature.

The final establishment of the central nuclei of the brain already displays a geographic and chronological ordering that can be studied as a landmark of progression in hierarchy in function of the different nuclei. But it also displays the geometrical pattern by which nuclei are 'laid down' from the center to the periphery of the brain and also how they 'unwind' from posterior to anterior and then from anterior to superior and to lateral. The pattern they demonstrate coincides with the curling pattern described in cranial osteopathy.

Increasing differentiation of structure and function in the primitive brain creates an increasing need for metabolic exchange. That means that the ventricles and their membranes not only function as mechanical support for further brain development but that they also organize the metabolic field of the expanding brain.

The 4th *ventricle* for instance regulates the metabolic field of the nuclei that are concerned with the survival strategy of the whole body. Metabolism of cells and nuclei is dependent upon mechanisms that by chemical and hydroelectrical exchange support maturation and that later by the same mechanism will support their function. One could propose that almost each function was a local metabolic field at first.

The functions of the periventricular nuclei and the intrinsic physiology of the ventricle itself are intimately linked. One can suggest that the 4th ventricle is related to the basic physiological survival techniques of the body (regulation of heart-pulse, heart rhythm, breathing rhythm, acid-base balance of the body and so on). It concentrates a totally different part of the archipallium around its cavity than the 3rd ventricle and consequently represents a complete different part of physiology.

It surveys basic homeostasis of the body and can do so by activating or inhibiting the basal nuclei and the vegetative part of some cranial nuclei. The method of activation or inhibition is certainly governed by interneuronal connections but the intrinsic physiology of the ventricle might play a more important role than ever suspected.

The hydrodynamic properties of the flux of cerebrospinal fluid in the floor of the 4th ventricle are such that it is organized in two different flux patterns:

- A central flux pattern is orientated to the foramen of Magendie and represents a rapid and powerful interference between fluid and the floor.

- A peripheral pattern is orientated to the foramina of Monro and is a slow flowing pattern.

The pressure and the velocity of the flow patterns of the cerebrospinal fluid are in one way or another sensed by the nuclei in the floor and possibly modifiy basal physiology (cardio-motor, vasopressure, and respiratory function…). Other nuclei in the pons and medulla oblongata are probably also influenced by the mechanical properties of the fluctuating LCS because of the changes in pressure it induces (n. tractus solitarius, dorsal motor nuclei, nucleus lacrymalis, and nucleus salivatorii…).

As one can see, an important part of the autonomous function of the body and of the vegetative tonus are not only dependent upon the electrical properties of these structures but are possibly modified by the mechanical properties of fluids.

Through the physiology of the 4th ventricle the brain is relieved of taking care of the body's basic needs for survival. It serves as a first step towards 'ascension' of the brain by which it is able to construct central nuclei around a second hydraulic cushion that controls the biochemistry and electrical exchange of the brain itself. All these periventricular nuclei serve in one way or another as a relay between the brain cortex and the basal physiology at the base of the brain.

When we study the content of the 3rd ventricle we observe the presence of cytokines, sugars, hormones, proteins in this cavity. Apparently the refined biochemistry of the fluid content in the ventricle is important for part of the function of the surrounding nuclei. Certain substances can cross the blood-brain barrier by which they can be 'sensed' by these nuclei. In particular the hypothalamic nuclei are sensitive to base/acid changes and cytokines through which the basic vegetative and motor tonus of the whole body can be changed (ergotrophic/trophotrophic nuclei, increase in body temperature).

It is clear that at this level the ionic/molecular and endocrine level of the brain and the body are equilibrated. The physiological environment of the 3rd ventricle serves the subtle biochemistry of the body as of the higher brain centers as well. Simultaneously it displays a very dynamic pattern of contraction and relaxation being constantly squeezed by the thalamic nuclei. These nuclei function as mechanical tools transmitting the heart pulse of the aa. thalamici to the walls of the ventricle.

The mechanical pattern not only activates expulsion and resorption of LCS but also probably is necessary for generating the electrical pulse of the cortex. One has to remember that most of the basic nuclei are central and that from here the brain displays an eccentric growth pattern towards the peripheral cortex. It is evident that the wiring of the brain that coordinates the electrical transmission is conceived in the same pattern as the migratory circuit of the neurons.

Looking at the flow pattern of the LCS one can observe two different progressions of cerebrospinal fluid. The 4th ventricle displays an 'organized' pattern consisting of a central and two lateral flow directions, coinciding with the biophysical laws of pressure and velocity of flow. It behaves almost like the macro shear-force observed in the flow patterns inside the arteries.

By contrast the 3rd ventricle shows a rather 'turbulent' pattern of compression/decompression by which constant intrinsic power is generated.

This guarantees a more or less constant volume of LCS present in the cavity because only small amounts of fluid progress towards the aqueductus Sylvii. Because of the rhythm of the arterial surrounding which exceeds a rapid adaptation of the ventricle walls, turbulence rather than well-organized flow occurs.

A progressive/regressive mode has been established in the flow pattern of the LCS from the 3rd ventricle towards, and inside the aqueductus of Sylvii. This proves the presence of turbulence in the ventricle as in the ductus as well.

That means that besides a chemical/electrical exponent in the efficacy of the fluid, it also provides a relatively constant volume in the ventricle by means of turbulence. By this means it creates a more or less stable center around which the coiling and uncoiling of the lateral hemispheres of the brain are organized.

The brain hemispheres can, generally speaking, open up laterally and downwards anteriorly, following the pattern earlier described in the chapter on brain development and patterning. That means that they follow a general pattern of the coiling 'like a ramhorn', as described by Magoun.[32] They pivot around the foramina of Monro in a frontal, parietal, occipital and temporal direction and succession. Sutherland described this coiling as the property of a bird flying away by opening its wings.

When the bird opens its wings it pushes slightly downwards and in a frontal direction to find a support, then the bird tilts up. In the same way the movement of the hemispheres tilts the brain up and it is lifted around the fluid pivot of the 3rd ventricle and the foramina of Monro. The increase in fluid pressure at this level creates a second hydrostatic pivot at the level of the aqueductus of Sylvii. This stabilizes the 3rd ventricle.

The axle of the aqueductus serves in two ways:

- by permitting a more or less lateralizing pattern of the two hemispheres, a little bit like a torsion pattern around a central axle,

- by generating a fluid pressure column in direction of the 4th ventricle which will be used to influence the vital nuclei in the floor of the ventricle by generating to patterns of flow.

A major part of the fluid will be expelled in the cisternae, which in their way will stabilize the brain in its bony and fascial environment.

In summary we can conclude that the two centralized ventricles exhibit a distinct physiology:

- First they display a different pattern of LCS flux. The 3rd ventricle displays a chaotic pattern guaranteeing an almost constant volume supported by turbulence of the LCS-flux. The squeezing of the ventricle by the thalamic nuclei, organized by the arterial rhythm and pulse of the thalamic arteries, is probably one of the main components in creating this turbulence pattern. The turbulence continues in a to and fro movement in the aqueduct of Sylvius although the general pattern is one of constant progression of the fluid towards the 4th ventricle.

The 4th ventricle at his turn 'canalizes' the fluid forces of the LCS in two distinct 'main-ways':
  - a central pathway that displays a fast flux pattern,
  - a lateral pathway that displays a slow flux pattern.

- Second, the 3rd ventricle is more involved in the 'balancing' of the ionic-endocrine milieu of the cell-environment of the brain itself. The final result is transmitted to the periphery of the body determining the basic physiology of the whole body or from specific body domains (redox system, pH and electron poising are basic events determining cell tonus). The 'mechanical' interference of the thalamic nuclei with the 3rd ventricle could be an excellent tool in transmitting the physical property of the periphery, retained in the arterial mechanics' towards the center of the brain and afterwards to the cortex.

The 4th ventricle transforms the 'power' of the LCS stream into a more or less compressive energy and activates with that the vital nuclei led down in its floor. These nuclei are essentially involved with supporting the basic body physiology and homeostasis. Both ventricles express a different kind of physiological involvement and we think that it is justified to define two distinct physiological mechanics for the two ventricles.

The 3rd ventricle seems to be involved with the cell-respiratory mechanism of the brain and in contrast, the 4th ventricle seems to be involved in the primary respiratory mechanism of the peripheral mechanism, included all deep and superficial compartments of fasciae (thus also the lepto- and pachymeninges).

Self-evident the primary mechanism is distinct from the secondary respiratory mechanism.

Summarizing, one can distinguish:

- a cranial respiratory mechanism (CRM),

- a primary respiratory mechanism (PRM),

- a secondary respiratory mechanism (SRM).
  - Third, the peri-ependymal gray matter is a transit structure containing the switching on and of network to and from the cortex. It acts as a

modulating circuit that integrates local metabolic and mechanical components of the ventricles into the modulating activity of the electrical circuit of neurons. The constant turbulence in the fluid axles of the brain and the squeezing activity of the thalamic nuclei proves that there must exist continuity between the intrinsic electrical activity of the brain and its central nuclei with the integrated physiology of the body periphery.

This interaction should function in two directions by means of which the cortex should not only be able to change electrical patterns but also to facilitate secretory activity of the periventricular and intra-ventricular organs (glandular physiology or choroid secretion).

Palpation of cranial stages of flexion

Hand positioning

Modified positioning at the roof of the skull according to Sutherland - fingers are placed in a line above the suture parietosquamosa. The thumbs touch each other at the roof of the skull and serve as a fulcrum. Likewise, the practitioner's forearms that are placed on the treatment table serve as a fulcrum.

Flexura submesencephalica

The submesencephalic suture forms in the area of the mesencephalon, on day 29 (Carnegie stage 10) with an angle of 150°. Within approximately four days, this area of the apex of the notochord (day 33, Carnegie Stage 14) decreases to 105° and finally to an angle of 50°. The flexure submesencephalica is organized around the apex of the notochord. At the same time, the heart anlage is carried along with this dynamic system, rotating at around 180°. Simultaneously, with the erection of the organs, the flexure submesencephalica verticalizes.

This flexure develops in two phases:

- The first phase runs towards the Pre-sphenoid (1a)

- The second phase of the flexure is directed towards the Tentorium cerebelli (1b)

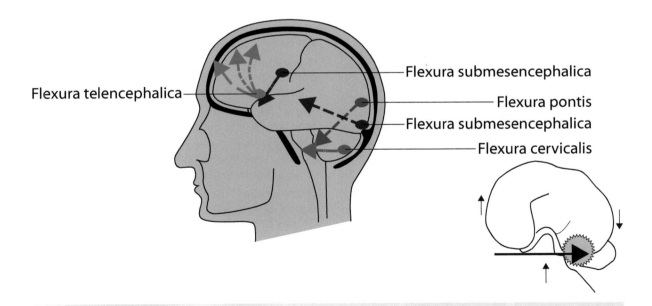

Figure 36.13
Palpatory vectors providing information about different cranial stages of flexion.

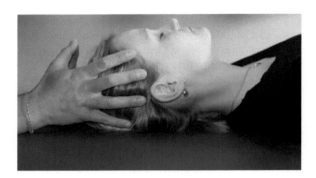

Figure 36.14
Hand position: modified positioning at the roof of the skull according to Sutherland.

Palpatory approach

- Index and middle finger introduce a gentle induction inferiorly to the Pre-sphenoid, directed towards the angle of the mandibula

- Subsequently, gentle induction of ring and little finger anteriorly towards the Glabella

Flexura cervicalis

The cervical flexure develops shortly after (Carnegie stage 13) in the hindbrain. The development of the cervical flexure takes place around the area of the apex of the dens and the Supra-occiput (Somites 1 and 2).

Palpatory approach: little fingers perform a gentle induction anteriorly towards the Nasion. Induction at the brain can be introduced gently and anteriorly.

Flexura pontis

With increased bending, the flexure pontis dorsally arises between Metencephalon and Myelencephalon in the area of the later Basiocciput (Carnegie stage 14-15), in the form of an opponent curvature of the neural tube.

Palpatory approach: middle and ring finger perform an induction anteriorly into the direction of the mandibular angle, carefully balancing the cerebellum at this stage.

Telencephalon

Finally, as part of the Telencephalisation, which continues after birth, the Flexura telencephalica arises around the Pre-sphenoid.

Palpatory approach: index and middle finger are located in the region of the insula, performing a gentle induction towards cephalad and posterior.

References

[1]Blechschmidt E. Humanembryologie: Prinzipien und Grundbegriffe. Stuttgart: Hippokrates; 1974.

[2]Blechschmidt E, Gasser RF. Biokinetics and Biodynamics of Human Differentiation. Springfield, Illinois: Charles C. Thomas; 1978.

[3]Blechschmidt E. The Ontogenetic Basis of Human Anatomy. Berkeley, California: North Atlantic Books; 2004.

[4]Blechschmidt E. Die pränatalen Organsysteme des Menschen. Stuttgart: Hippokrates; 1973.

[5]Blechschmidt E. Sein und Werden. Stuttgart: Urachhaus; 1982.

[6]Blechschmidt E. Wie beginnt das menschliche Leben. 6th edn. Stein am Rhein: Christiana; 1989.

[7]E. Blechschmidt. The stages of human development before birth. S. Karger, NY., 1961.

[8]Blechschmidt E, Gasser RF. Biokinetics and Biodynamics of Human Differentiation. Springfield, Illinois: Charles C. Thomas; 1978:89.

[9]Rohen JW. Funktionelle Anatomie des Nervensystems. 5th edition. Stuttgart: Schattauer: 1994:105.

[10]Campbell WW, DeJong RN, Haerer AF. DeJong's The Neurologic Examination. Philadelphia: Lippincott Williams & Wilkins; 2005.

[11]Blechschmidt E, Gasser RF. Biokinetics and Biodynamics of Human Differentiation. Springfield, Illinois: Charles C. Thomas; 1978:83.

[12]Blechschmidt E, Gasser RF. Biokinetics and Biodynamics of Human Differentiation. Springfield, Illinois: Charles C. Thomas; 1978:95.

[13]Blechschmidt E, Gasser RF. Biokinetics and Biodynamics of Human Differentiation. Springfield, Illinois: Charles C. Thomas; 1978:107.

[14]Rohen JW. Funktionelle Anatomie des Nervensystems. 5th edition. Stuttgart: Schattauer: 1994:38.

[15]Blechschmidt E, Gasser RF. Biokinetics and Bio-dynamics of Human Differentiation. Springfield, Illinois: Charles C. Thomas; 1978:108.

[16]Blechschmidt E, Gasser RF. Biokinetics and Bio-dynamics of Human Differentiation. Springfield, Illinois: Charles C. Thomas; 1978:127.

[17]A. Zeman. Consciousness a users guide. Yale Press.,Yale University Press, 2002.

[18]Ruiz de Azua A: La force de la traction médullaire. Apostill 2002; 11/12:7-14.

[19]Ruiz de Azua A. La force de la traction médullaire. Apostill 2002; 11/12:7-14.

[20]Royo-Salvador MB. Aportación a la etiología de la siringomielia idiopática. Doctoral thesis. Barcelona; 1992.

[21]Royo-Salvador MB. Siringomielia, escoliosis y malformaciónes de Arnold-Chiari idiopáticas: Etiología commún. Rev Neurol 1996;24:937-959.

[22]Blechschmidt E, Gasser RF. Biokinetics and Biodynamics of Human Differentiation. Springfield, Illinois: Charles C. Thomas; 1978:112.

[23]Rohen JW. Funktionelle Anatomie des Nervensy-stems. 5th edition. Stuttgart: Schattauer: 1994:59.

[24]Rohen JW. Funktionelle Anatomie des Nervensystems. 5th edition. Stuttgart: Schattauer: 1994:21.

[25]Rohen JW. Funktionelle Anatomie des Nervensystems. 5th edition. Stuttgart: Schattauer: 1994:54.

[26]M. Hasegava et al., Brain Dev. 14(1), 1-6, 1992.

[27]E. Martin et al., J Comput Assist Tomogr. 12(6), 917-22, 1988.

[28]D. Malinska et al., Folio Neuropathol. 36(3), 145-51, 1998.

[29]N. Geschwind et A.M. Galaburda., Cerebral lateralization. Bradford book, 1987.

[30]I. Ferrez et al., J Anat. 160, 89-100, 1988.

[31]K. Ruoss et al., Neuropediatrics. 32(2), 69-74, 2001.

[32]H.I. Magoun., osteopathy in the cranial field. The journal printing company, Kirksville, 1976.

37

Polyvagal theory: an introduction

Stephen W. Porges

The basis for the Polyvagal Theory: The role of the vagus in the bidirectional communication between the brain and the body

During the phylogenetic transition from ancient reptiles to mammals, the autonomic nervous system changed. In the ancient reptiles, the autonomic nervous system regulated bodily organs via two subsystems: the sympathetic nervous system and the parasympathetic nervous system. Modern reptiles share these global features. The sympathetic nervous system provides the neural pathways for visceral changes that support fight and flight behaviors. The sympathetic nervous system functions to support mobilization by increasing heart rate and suppressing digestion.

Complementing the sympathetic nervous system, the reptilian parasympathetic nervous system serves two functions. First, it supports processes of health, growth and restoration. Second, when recruited as a defense system, the parasympathetic nervous system reduces metabolic activity by dampening heart rate and respiration, enabling immobilized reptiles to appear inanimate to potential predators. When not under threat the two components of the autonomic nervous system in reptiles function antagonistically and simultaneously innervate several of the body organs to support bodily functions.

Most of the neural pathways of the parasympathetic nervous system travel through the vagus. The vagus is a large cranial nerve that originates in the brainstem and connects visceral organs with the brain. In contrast to the nerves that emerge from the spinal cord, the vagus connects the brain directly to bodily organs. The vagus contains both motor fibers to change the function of visceral organs and sensory fibers to provide the brain with continuous information about the status of these organs. The flow of information between body and brain informs specific brain circuits that regulate target organs. Bidirectional communication provides a neural basis for a mind–body science, or brain–body

medicine, by providing plausible portals of intervention to correct brain dysfunction via peripheral vagal stimulation (for example, vagal nerve stimulation for epilepsy) and plausible explanations for exacerbation of clinical symptoms by psychological stressors, such as stress-related episodes of irritable bowel syndrome. In addition, bidirectional communication between the brain and specific visceral organs provides an anatomical basis for historical concepts within physiology and medicine, such as Walter Cannon's homeostasis[1] and Claude Bernard's internal milieu[2].

Polyvagal theory: Overview

Polyvagal theory is a reconceptualization of how autonomic state and behavior interface. The theory emphasizes a hierarchical relation among components of the autonomic nervous system that evolved to support adaptive behaviors in response to the particular environmental features of safety, danger, and life threat[3]. The theory is named "polyvagal" to emphasize that there are two vagal circuits: an ancient vagal circuit associated with defense and a phylogenetically newer circuit related to feeling safe and spontaneous social behavior[4]. The theory articulates two defense systems: (a) the commonly known fight-or-flight system that is associated with activation or the sympathetic nervous system (fight or flight) and (b) a less-known system of immobilization and dissociation that is associated with activation of a phylogenetically more ancient vagal pathway.

The Polyvagal Theory describes the neural mechanisms through which physiological states communicate the experience of safety and contribute to an individual's ability either to feel safe and spontaneously engage with others, or to feel threatened and recruit defensive strategies. The theory articulates how each of three phylogenetic stages in the development of the vertebrate autonomic nervous system is associated with a distinct and measurable autonomic subsystem, each of which remains active and is expressed in humans under certain conditions[5]. These three involuntary autonomic subsystems are phylogenetically ordered and behaviorally linked to three global adaptive domains of behavior: (a) social communication (e.g., facial expression, vocalization, listening), (b) defensive strategies associated with mobilization (e.g., fight-or-flight behaviors), and (c) defensive immobilization (e.g., feigning death, vasovagal syncope, behavioral shutdown, and dissociation). Based on their phylogenetic emergence during the evolution of the vertebrate autonomic nervous system, these neuroanatomically based subsystems form a response hierarchy.

The polyvagal theory emphasizes the distinct roles of two distinct vagal motor pathways identified in the mammalian autonomic nervous system. The vagus is a cranial nerve that exits the brainstem and provides bidirectional communication between brain and several visceral organs. The vagus conveys (and monitors) the primary parasympathetic influence to the viscera. Most of the neural fibers in the vagus are sensory (i.e., approximately 80%). However, most interest has been directed to the motor fibers that regulate the visceral organs, including the heart and the gut. Of these motor fibers, only approximately 15% are myelinated. Myelin, a fatty coating over the neural fiber, is associated with faster and more tightly regulated neural control circuits. Humans and other mammals have two functionally distinct vagal circuits. One vagal circuit is phylogenetically older and unmyelinated. It originates in a brainstem area called the dorsal motor nucleus of the vagus. The other vagal circuit is uniquely mammalian and myelinated. The myelinated vagal circuit originates in a brainstem area called the nucleus ambiguus. The phylogenetically older unmyelinated vagal motor pathways are shared with most vertebrates and, in mammals when not recruited as a defense system, function to support health, growth, and restoration via neurally regulation of subdiaphragmatic organs (i.e., internal organs below the diaphragm). The "newer" myelinated vagal motor pathways, which are observed only in mammals, regulate the supradiaphragmatic organs (e.g., heart and lungs). This newer vagal circuit slows heart rate and supports states of calmness

The Face–Heart Connection: The Emergence of the Social Engagement System

When the individual feels safe, two important features are expressed. First, bodily state is regulated in an efficient manner to promote growth and restoration (e.g., visceral homeostasis). Functionally, this is accomplished through an increase in the influence of myelinated vagal motor pathways on the cardiac pacemaker to slow heart rate, inhibit the fight-or-flight mechanisms of the sympathetic nervous system, dampen the stress response system of the hypothalamic–pituitary- adrenal axis (e.g., cortisol), and reduce inflammation by modulating immune reactions (e.g., cytokines). Second, through the process of evolution, the brainstem nuclei that regulate the myelinated vagus became integrated with the nuclei that regulate the muscles of the face and head. These emergent changes in neuroanatomy provide a face–heart connection in which there are mutual interactions between the vagal influences to the heart and the neural regulation of the striated muscles of the face and head. The phylogenetically novel face–heart connection provided mammals with an ability to convey physiological state via facial expression and prosody (intonation of voice), enabling facial expression and voice to calm physiological state[3,4,6,7].

The integration of neuroanatomical structures in the brainstem provides the neural pathways for a functional social engagement system characterized by a bidirectional coupling between bodily states and the spontaneous social engagement behaviors expressed in facial expressions and prosodic vocalizations. As illustrated in Figure 37.1, the behavioral manifestation of this integrated social engagement system observed in mammals emerged specifically as a consequence of the neural pathways regulating visceral states (via the myelinated vagus), becoming neuroanatomically and neurophysiologically linked with the neural pathways regulating the muscles (via special visceral efferent pathways) controlling gaze, facial expression, head gesture, listening, and prosody[8,9,5].

The face–heart connection enabled mammals to detect whether a conspecific was in a calm physiological state and 'safe' to approach, or in a highly mobilized and reactive physiological state during which engagement would be dangerous. The face–heart connection concurrently enables an individual to signal 'safety' through patterns of facial expression and vocal intonation, and potentially calm an agitated conspecific to form a social relationship. When the newer mammalian vagus is optimally functioning in social interactions (i.e., inhibiting the sympathetic excitation that

The basis for the Polyvagal Theory: The role of the vagus in the bidirectional communication between the brain and the body

671

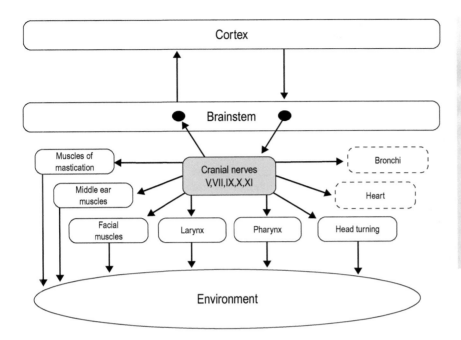

Figure 37.1

The Social Engagement System. The Social Engagement System consists of a somatomotor compnent (i.e., special visceral effernt pathways that regulate the striated muscles of the face and head) and a visceromotor component (i.e., the myelinated vagus that regulates the heart and bronchi). Solid blocks indicate the somatomotor component. Dashed blocks indicate the visceromotor component.

promotes fight-or-flight behaviors), emotions are well regulated, vocal prosody is rich, and the autonomic state supports calm spontaneous social engagement behaviors. The face–heart system is bidirectional with the newer myelinated vagal circuit influencing social interactions and positive social interactions influencing vagal function to optimize health, dampen stress-related physiological states, and support growth and restoration. Social communication and the ability to co-regulate another, via reciprocal social engagement systems, leads to a sense of connectedness, which is a defining feature of the human experience.

The Polyvagal Theory proposes that physiological state is a fundamental part, and not a correlate, of emotion and mood. The theory emphasizes a bidirectional link between brain and viscera, which would explain both how thoughts can change our physiology, and how physiological state influences our thoughts. As individuals change their facial expressions, the intonation of their voices, the pattern in which they are breathing, and their posture, they are also changing their physiology primarily through manipulating function of the myelinated vagus to the heart.

Dissolution

The three circuits defined by the Polyvagal Theory are organized and respond to challenges in a phylogenetically determined hierarchy consistent with the Jacksonian principle of dissolution. Jackson proposed that in the brain, higher (i.e., phylogenetically newer) neural circuits inhibit lower (i.e., phylogenetically older) neural circuits and "when the higher are suddenly rendered functionless, the lower rise in activity"[10]. Although Jackson proposed dissolution to explain changes in brain function due to damage and illness, polyvagal theory proposes a similar phylogenetically ordered hierarchical model to describe the sequence of autonomic response strategies to challenges.

The human nervous system, similar to that of other mammals, evolved not solely to survive in safe environments but also to promote survival in dangerous and life-threatening contexts. To accomplish this adaptive flexibility, the mammalian autonomic nervous system, in addition to the myelinated vagal pathway that is integrated into the Social Engagement System, retained two more primitive neural circuits to regulate defensive strategies (i.e., fight–flight and death-feigning behaviors). It is important to note that social behavior, social communication, and visceral homeostasis are incompatible with the neurophysiological states that support defense. Thus, via evolution, the human nervous system retains three neural circuits, consistent with the Jacksonian principle of dissolution, that are in a phylogenetically organized hierarchy. In this hierarchy of adaptive responses, the newest circuit is used first; if that circuit fails to provide safety, the older circuits are recruited sequentially.

Neuroception

To effectively switch from defensive to social engagement strategies, the mammalian nervous system needs to perform two important adaptive tasks: (1) assess risk, and (2) if the environment is safe, inhibit the more primitive limbic structures involved in fight, flight, or immobilization (e.g., death feigning) behaviors. Any stimulus that has the potential for signaling cues of safety has the potential to recruit an evolutionarily more advanced neural circuit that promotes calm behavioral states and supports the prosocial behaviors of the social engagement system.

The nervous system, through the processing of sensory information from the environment and from the viscera, continuously evaluates risk. Polyvagal Theory proposes that the neural evaluation of risk does not require conscious awareness and functions through neural circuits that are shared with our phylogenetic vertebrate ancestors. Thus, the term neuroception[11] was introduced to emphasize a neural process, distinct from perception, which is capable of distinguishing environmental (and visceral) features that are safe, dangerous, or life-threatening. In safe environments, autonomic state is adaptively regulated to dampen sympathetic activation and to protect the oxygen-dependent central nervous system, especially the cortex, from the metabolically conservative reactions of the dorsal vagal complex (e.g., vasovagal syncope).

Neuroception is proposed as a plausible mechanism mediating both the expression and the disruption of positive social behavior, emotion regulation, and visceral homeostasis[9,11]. Neuroception might be triggered by feature detectors involving areas of temporal cortex that communicate with the central nucleus of the amygdala and the periaqueductal gray, since limbic reactivity is modulated by temporal cortex responses to biological movements including voices, faces, and hand movements. Embedded in the construct of neuroception is the capacity of the nervous system to react to the 'intention' of these movements. Neuroception functionally decodes and interprets the assumed goal of movements and sounds of inanimate and living objects. This process occurs without awareness. Although we are often unaware of the stimuli that trigger different neuroceptive responses, we are aware of our body's reactions. Thus, the neuroception of familiar individuals and individuals with appropriately prosodic voices and warm, expressive faces translates into a positive social interaction promoting a sense of safety.

The features of risk in the external environment do not solely drive neuroception. Afferent feedback from the viscera provides a major mediator of the accessibility of prosocial circuits associated with social engagement behaviors. For example, the polyvagal theory predicts that states of mobilization would compromise our ability to detect positive social cues. Functionally, visceral states color our perception of objects and others. Thus, the same features of one person engaging another may result in a range of outcomes, depending on the physiological state of the target individual. If the person being engaged is in a state in which the social engagement system is easily accessible, the reciprocal prosocial interactions are likely to occur. However, if the individual is in a state of mobilization, the same engaging response might be responded to with the asocial features of withdrawal or aggression. In such a state, it might be very difficult to dampen the mobilization circuit and enable the social engagement system to come back on line. The insula may be involved in the mediation of neuroception, since it has been proposed as a brain structure involved in conveying the diffuse feedback from the viscera into cognitive awareness. Functional imaging experiments have demonstrated that the insula plays an important role in the experience of pain and the experience of several emotions, including anger, fear, disgust, happiness, and sadness. Critchley proposes that internal body states are represented in the insula and contribute to states of subjective feeling, and he has demonstrated that activity in the insula correlates with interoceptive accuracy[12].

In most individuals (i.e., those without a psychiatric disorder or neuropathology), the nervous system evaluates risk and matches neurophysiological state with the actual risk of the environment. When the environment is appraised as being safe, the defensive limbic structures are inhibited, enabling social engagement and calm visceral states to emerge. In contrast, some individuals experience a mismatch and the nervous system appraises the environment as being dangerous even when it is safe. This mismatch results in physiological states that support fight, flight, or freeze behaviors, but not social engagement behaviors. According to the theory, social communication can be expressed efficiently through the social engagement system only when these defensive circuits are inhibited. The autonomic nervous system will shift state to support defense, when triggered by a physical event, a mental thought, or the body's reaction to illness (e.g., fever). The shift in physiological state is frequently a reflexive reaction to events and signals that do not require awareness to process. Thus, for manipulative therapeutic practices to be functional and to have positive outcomes, they must be implemented during a physiological state in which the autonomic nervous system is not supporting defense and in context that does not elicit a neuroception of danger or life threat.

References

[1]Cannon, WB (1932) Wisdom of the body. New York: WW Norton

[2]Bernard, C (1872) De la physiologie générale. Paris: Librairie Hachette

[3]Porges, SW (2011) The Polyvagal Theory: Neurophysiological foundations of emotions, attachment, communication, and self-regulation. New York: WW Norton

[4]Porges, SW (2012) What therapists need to know about the polyvagal theory. Presentation at Leading Edge Seminars, Toronto, Ontario, Canada

[5]Porges, SW (2009) The polyvagal theory: New insights into adaptive reactions of the autonomic nervous system. Cleveland Clinic Journal of Medicine, 76, S86–90

[6]Porges, SW & Lewis, G F (2009) The polyvagal hypothesis: Common mechanisms mediating autonomic regulation, vocalizations, and listening. In S. M. Brudzynski (Ed) Handbook of mammalian vocalizations: An integrative neuroscience approach (pp 255–264). Amsterdam: Academic Press.

[7]Stewart, AM, Lewis, GF, Heilman, KJ, Davila, MI, Coleman, DD, Aylward, SA, & Porges, S W (2013) The covariation of acoustic features of infant cries and autonomic state. Physiology and Behavior, 120, 203– 210

[8]Porges, SW (2001) The Polyvagal Theory: Phylogenetic substrates of a social nervous system. International Journal of Psychophysiology, 42, 123–146

[9]Porges, SW (2007) The polyvagal perspective. BiologicalPsychology, 74, 116–143

[10]Jackson, JH (1958) Evolution and dissolution of the nervous system. In J Taylor (Ed) Selected writings of John Hughlings Jackson (pp 45–118). London: Staples Press.

[11]Porges, SW (2004) Neuroception: A subconscious system for detecting threat and safety. Zero to Three: Bulletin of the National Center for Clinical Infant Programs, 24(5), 19– 24

[12]Critchley HD (2005) Neural mechanisms of autonomic,affective, and cognitive integration. Journal of Comparative Neurology, 493, 154–166

38

An osteopathic approach to the treatment of trauma and emotional integration

Torsten Liem

I slept and dreamed that life was joy. I awoke and saw that life was service. I acted, and behold, service was joy.

R. Tagore[1]

Traumatic experiences may lead to unwanted reactions such as hyperarousal and states of dissociation that persist long after a trauma has occurred. Over time, these originally lifesaving response patterns evolve to be a heavy burden to bear. The integration of traumatic experiences allows a change of these stressful reaction patterns.

Osteopathic treatments leading to emotional integration may be based on different strategies including polyvagal theory[1]a (see also Chapter 37), osteopathic tissue palpations and approaches of resource work, positive psychology, Eye Movement Desensitization and Reprocessing (EMDR), Neuro-Linguistic Programming (NLP), neurogenic tremors, somatic experiencing, and meditative practices. In this chapter, aspects of the therapeutic relationship between osteopath and patient are discussed, and specific techniques for emotional integration as part of the osteopathic treatment approach, both in the stabilization and confrontation phases, are introduced.

Osteopathic implications of the Polyvagal theory

The Polyvagal theory is of great significance for osteopathic treatment in general, especially in relation to the treatment of trauma. The severity of traumatic experiences manifests in hyper-sympathetic arousal or immobilization linked to activation of the unmyelinated subdiaphragmatic vagus. Osteopaths can help patients to perceive and integrate reflex triggered physical reaction patterns. They can educate their patients to experience feelings of security and safety that are conveyed through the body.

The aim of treatment is to activate resources of the myelinated supradiaphragmatic vagus in conjunction with mindfulness during the stabilization phase (see below), in order to safely meet and integrate traumatic experiences in the confrontation phase. This may be achieved by recruiting the myelinated supradiaphragmatic vagus, which will promote relaxed behaviors and dampen active sympathetic arousal and the entire HPA axis.

Due to the presence of the myelinated vagal state, and with support of osteopathic treatment techniques, past traumatic experiences are increasingly associated with a relaxed body feedback during trauma confrontation. This may be reflected in slow breathing with a focus on exhalation (i.e., vagal efferent actions on the heart's pacemaker are optimized during exhalation), a slow heart rate, relaxed facial and neck muscles, and support of the development of an explicit mnemonic or interpretational frame in relation to trauma.

In a resource-rich myelinated vagal state it is possible to be aware of covariation between one's own biography, life circumstances, inner experience and behavior on the one hand and the related disturbed inner peace and disorders on the other hand. For this, the active involvement of the patient in the healing process is necessary, as well as the development of methodologies and skills in order to acknowledge and integrate inner components of awareness in patients into the treatment. This can be achieved for example by a palpation practice that supports the patient in experiencing and understanding important correlations between state of health disorders, dysfunction and internal as well as external contexts of their life. In addition, the treatment could assist patients to acquire competencies that increasingly enable them to gain access to a myelinated vagus excitation state in daily life.

Role of amygdala and hippocampus

In early traumatic childhood experiences, emotional components are not stored in the declarative memory, since the hippocampus is not sufficiently mature. In the amygdala, incoming sensory stimuli are coupled to affective qualities by activation of phylogenetically older neural structures and networks[1].

A substantial factor in this process is the question of how sustainably the experience has been stored. The amygdala is responsible for activating the emotional memory content in certain situations. Since it receives afferents from sensory brain regions, feelings of, for example, panic and palpitations can be triggered in seemingly harmless situations, if certain triggers cause the amygdala to evoke past emotional experiences. The hippocampus, however stores emotional experiences as facts only.

In order to integrate traumatic experiences, the therapeutic encounter consists of the inhibition of amygdala activity, by means of the hippocampus that combines implicit memory contents with explicit declarative memory and learning. The polyvagal theory complements these functions through the process of neuroception, which may inhibit limbic circuits and down-regulate defensive reactions. For all these processes, promoting reactions of the myelinated vagus is essential. In the case of trigger stimuli that evoke regressive memory, instead of responding by escape/fight or flight reactions, patients are brought into a relaxed state, enabling them in conjunction with their available resources to observe their internal states and communicate current feelings and needs.

Touch rather than language as a form of communication may enable easier access to the anti-episodic memory of early childhood experiences, since the sense of touch developed long before language and represents the most developed of the senses in newborns. Perhaps this is why during palpation of somatic dysfunction patterns regressive inner memories can be evoked in patients. Here it is important that these regressions are not forced in any way. On the contrary, attention is first given to the establishment of resources and eyewitness awareness that is anchored in the present, and a visceral state that support a feeling of safety so that re-traumatisation is avoided. Only on this basis can a secure encounter with stressful experience content occur.

---

[1] Two ways are described: a fast connection as a protective reaction - from the thalamus to the amygdala, and a slower connection from the thalamus via the cortex to the amygdala, essential in fear conditioning.

Physical feedback

Experience of fear requires four components: the working memory in order to place experiences in relation to each other, the amygdala (see above), the nucleus basalis to perceive fear as a physical arousal, and feedback of fear-specific physical reactions in the region of the solar plexus and by tensioning of facial muscles. For example, an experimental study has demonstrated that changing the feedback signal of participants' own heartbeat influenced their feeling of fear[2]. When feedback to the participant presented the heartbeats as slower than the heart was really beating, the subjects reported perceiving less fear.[13]

In another study by Ekman[3], subjects were instructed to move certain facial muscles. The participants did not know that these muscles were those that are innervated with expression of specific emotions. Participants rated their mood much more positive if those muscles were activated that are characteristic of a positive emotion, in contrast to the activation of those muscles that would express negative emotions. In the treatment setting, these findings have to be considered, for example by asking the patient during the confrontation with stress triggering memories to gently breathe into the belly and the body, and especially to relax the face. Through this physical feedback - in addition to an intuitive sensitive palpation by the practitioner - a myelinated vagal excitation state is stimulated, in which a deconditioning of traumatising experiences can occur. The neuroanatomy supports this speculation, since the afferent pathways from the facial nerve and trigeminal nerve provide major inputs into the source nucleus of myelinated vagus (i.e., nucleus ambiguus).

The confrontation with fear-provoking triggers is important, in order to ensure that the competence of their inhibition can be learned by the patient. A resolution of these activity patterns in the amygdala does not seem to be possible, but rather their integration or cortical inhibition of other fear reactions. Le Doux[4,5] suggested that the fear response stored in the amygdala is not erased, but the wider effects are inhibited via the prefrontal cortex. This has been hypothesized in a study where patients with arachnophobia were successfully treated[6]. After behavioral therapy, in confrontation with spiders there were no fear reactions, neither in behavior nor subjective emotions or autonomic reactions (skin conductance and heart rate).

However, the brain activity measured by an electroencephalogram (EEG) still differed from subjects without arachnophobia. The authors suggested that the amygdala remains activatable by an appropriate stimulus, but a possible inhibition of another chain of reactions, and thus the fear reaction in the body, may take place in the orbitofrontal cortex. Van der Kolk[7] could show in patients with post-traumatic stress disorder an increased metabolic activity in the prefrontal cortex after treatment with eye movement desensitization and reprocessing (EMDR), and decreased activity in the limbic system[18]. Inhibition of fear responses mainly occurs in the left prefrontal cortex, particularly in its medial part[8,9]. The left prefrontal area probably also inhibits the right prefrontal lobe (seat of negative emotions, such as fear)[10].

Emotional integration and treatment of trauma in osteopathy

In addition to the following proposed method, it is important that patients increasingly learn to anchor their attention in the present, to perceive and respect boundaries, to enter into beneficial relationships with themselves and others, and to develop perseverance and courage in order to stand up for goals that give meaning to their lives.

A calming practice environment is essential, together with pleasant practice facilities, empathic communication skills of the practitioner (see below), a calm and relaxed palpation by the osteopath, and a treatment session offering plenty of time. In this way, the patient most likely will feel sufficiently protected and guarded.

Regression-promoting therapies stimulate the occurrence of early memories. For traumatised patients, these memories are, however, hardly bearable and to be rated as negative, as usually these patients are already suffering, as they are unable to separate the present from the experience of the past. Most importantly, the patient needs to understand that what has happened in the past is now over, and to develop and activate resources and distancing techniques (see page 682). On this basis, it is possible to work with stressful memories and images and to integrate them. It is important not to provoke regressive experiences.

The following procedures described below should not be used without prior training on the topic. The structure of the treatment is divided into four phases:

1 Therapeutic relationship

2 Stabilization Phase

3 Confrontation Phase

4 Integration into everyday life, stress management and a new beginning

The therapeutic relationship – a working unit between patient and osteopath

Firstly, the aims and objectives of the therapeutic interaction need to be developed; patients should be informed about the therapeutic approach (including the requirement for its acceptance by patients), and the development of a stable therapeutic relationship.

The adult 'parts' of a patient must be strengthened[ii] so that they can take care of the traumatised parts. The patient's need for control and coping strategies has to be acknowledged.

Trauma patients often exhibit conflicting subpersonalities. Through parts therapy (Box 38.1) these may be heard, identified and differentiated. The vulnerable portions, often the traumatized childlike parts, for example, could be afraid of a therapeutic encounter.

Childlike behavior – behavior that does not match normal adult behavior – can be communicated. It leads to the question of how old patients are, resulting in them feeling and behaving in that particular way. Working with childlike parts means giving patients security and comfort in the stabilization phase. Patients learn to take care of their own childlike parts. In the confrontation stage, the painful experiences are looked at.

Offender-introjection, by contrast, can be strongly directed against the therapeutic process, trying to thwart it[iii]

[ii] No regression is to be admitted in the relationship between practitioner and patient.

[iii] Offender-introjections are - by border violation of the offender - internalized complex mental parts that are loyal towards the offender, which operate mostly in secret.

Box 38.1

Parts therapy

Parts therapy generally refers to the therapeutic management of various proportions of a human personality. These proportions are in contact with each other by more or less permeable boundaries. In the case of condensed boundaries, strong resistances between individual proportions are created, potentially leading to high loads accompanied by complete detachment of personality aspects. These are expressed not only mentally, but also neuro-autonomic, neuro-hormonal, and neuro-immunological. The aim of parts therapy is to stimulate processes of becoming aware of (diverging) personality traits/proportions and integrate them.

Forms of treatment within parts therapy are based on the concept of multiplicity and relate to internal models of the variety of different parts. Examples are Transactional Analysis by Berne[16,17], Ego-state therapy[18], systemic therapy[19], Voice Dialogue[20], and growth-oriented family therapy[21].

Parts therapy includes the integration of detached emotional contents/proportions and body regions

- The practitioner works exclusively in the here and now with an aspect of fear, a memory or a body region

- Assessment of load intensity with respect to the affected body region, or the image of the memory (scale 0-10)

- Careful palpation of the associated body part and perception of the related field

- Very slow bilateral stimulation (slow motion 2–3 x)

- Neurogenic tremors if necessary

- Slow and relaxed breathing, repeat if necessary

- Not more than 15–30 minutes in highly traumatized and dissociative patients –they decide when it is enough for today's treatment session

It is important to perceive these conflicting proportions, and parts therapy may be helpful in addressing this issue.

Empathy

Empathy arises when we:

- Take others seriously and are sensitive to their needs

- Show presence and pay full attention to patients in the here and now, and perceive their circumstances, feelings and needs, with us being aware of our own circumstances, feelings and needs. Experience of our own depths is a prerequisite to be able to consciously resonate with these levels in a patient when we touch. If there is a projection onto the practitioner, i.e. reacting with strong emotions to the patient, abdominal breathing and becoming aware of as well as integrating one's own inner concerns may be helpful

- Make time for each other, so that patients can fully express their concerns without feeling rushed, and keep attention going until a relief is felt

- Choose words to confirm the connection

- Interrupt to return the patient to the here and now

In order to better understand an empathic contact, it is helpful to identify behaviors that are different from empathy. Empathy is not:

- To instruct ('This can be turned into a very positive experience, if you just ....')

- To reinforce ('This is nothing, listen to what happened to me...')

- To give advice ('It would be good if you ...')

- To comfort ('This was not your fault, you have done the best you could...')

- To sympathise ('I am also familiar with this ...')

- To pity ('Oh dear, it must be really hard for you...')

- To interrogate ('When did it start? Did your mother have a difficult childhood?')

- To explain ('Oh, I would have called if ...')

- To argue ('It was not like that. You cannot put it that way.')

- Telling stories: ('This reminds me, when I ...')

- To encourage/improve ('Come on, cheer up, it's not that bad. Look! The sun is shining...')

- To cut someone short ('Now you're exaggerating....')

The more the osteopath is able to maintain empathic contact in experiencing the patient without judging or condemning, the more he can serve as the fulcrum in the treatment process.

Case history

In the process of case history taking, clinical pictures, qualities and possible causalities, the burden of the complaints/assessment of load (scale of 0-10: 0-1 = no load, 10 = maximum load), the family environment and contraindications will be explored. From the outset, the focus will be to direct attention to what patients enjoy, and what makes them happy. Furthermore, external and internal resources can be explored and developed, and stability can be tested. These resources also provide the basis of an attempt to confront and integrate burdensome unprocessed experiences. The practitioner uses the communication with the patient to establish a relationship, which is characterised by empathy.

Indications:

- Stressful experiences, memories or significant parts thereof arise during an osteopathic treatment or palpation

- For the assessment of biographical backgrounds in somatic dysfunctions

- Current triggers that restrict everyday life

- Allergies

- Irrational negative cognitions

- Traumatisation

Contraindications:

- Current psychotic syndromes

- Organic brain disorders

- Reduced strength of own ego (relative contraindication: Borderline patients)

- Secondary gain of illness

- Low motivation for therapy

- Low physical strength

- Commonly a trauma affects the body in such a way that changes in the ANS may be expected. Therefore precise diagnostic findings are most important. Assess what the patient's facial expression is like; does the patient engage in eye contact? The patient might appear restless and distant or be exhibiting signs of a startle response. What about the heartbeat qualities? What is the skin like - cold or warm - and what about the color? Assess breathing; are the lungs fully expanding and does the abdomen move with inhalation and exhalation? How is the muscle tone, hyper- or hypotonic? How are the joints working? Also, it is possible to assess the ANS by looking at heart rate variability.

Palpation

Through palpation, the therapist approaches the patient in his physicality, in the sense of 'wait and see', and (initially) refuses to assign meaning or importance to any of his findings.

From personal experience, emotional stress and emotional factors are often apparent in tensions around the area of the solar plexus, and in dysfunctions of the vertebral junctions (C0/C1/C2, C7/Th1, Th12/L1, L5/S1). Other areas affected could be the visceral organs in general, the pelvic floor, diaphragm, heart area, shoulders, throat, mandible, lips, tongue, soft palate, and eyes . The heat or activity of the left and right prefrontal area can be assessed. These areas should be specifically assessed in cases of emotional imbalance and trauma.

Stabilisation phase

Stabilization exercises serve to strengthen patients '-own egos and are an important prerequisite for subsequent confrontational approaches with stressful content. Approaches for stress reduction are exclusively adopted. These include the recognition of coping strategies, providing knowledge about the consequences of trauma, learning of imagination exercises for stress reduction, affect differentiation, and regulation, and the development of security/safety (internally and externally).

Stabilization can be achieved through resource work. Transmission distortions are addressed and a differentiated and loving body awareness is promoted, as well as the development of controlled handling of traumatic material or painful feelings, in order for patients to experience and learn how to give themselves comfort. In distancing techniques, patients acquire the competence to deliberately repress painful memories (eg the 'bank vault exercise'). This is also essential if new traumata appear at the surface during the course of the confrontation phase.

Stabilisation-resource-distancing exercises

The detection, acknowledgement and promotion of resources is to be put at one level with the promotion of properties of a myelinated vagal excitation state. Especially in the stabilization phase, dealing with resources is important. Resources form the basis of 'being', and enable us to experience stability, protection and space. This creates appetite for life and a positive fundamental feeling, due to a nourishing relationship with nature, with oneself and others. By promoting appreciation and recognition (e.g. of our needs) through others and ourselves, self-respect develops, meaning that we are allowed to be as we are. By fulfilling tasks in professional or private life, a sense of meaning forms.

- 'Count Your Blessings' according to Martin Seligman[11,12] with bilateral stimulation.[iv]

Patients spend five minutes listing what is going well in their lives and things for which they are most grateful. At the end of this exercise, what has been achieved can be anchored by bilateral stimulation through the butterfly hug.[v]

Ideal for giving patients as a home exercise: 'At the end of a given day, think about three things that have happened during the day, and for which you are most grateful. Also, why do you think these were happening?' This exercise can be carried out over a period of six weeks, 2–3 times a week.

- Imagination of the inner helper: this can be a figure or person, who holds all the power and wisdom and is protective. For children this could be elves, wizards, stuffed animals, grandmother or godfather/godmother. In adults, this might be heroes of Greek mythology (Sisyphus or Odysseus)

- Imagination of the inner healer: In contrast to the inner helper, the inner healer is not personified

- Tree exercise: 'Imagine with all your senses a tree and its nourishing roots going downwards, and feel it opening up – how sunlight can be taken up and converted'[13]

- Body Scan: patients perform a scan of their entire body, which is perceived from toes to the hair ends (e.g. the position of the joints, permeability, temperature, touch, tingling, etc). Patients are also encouraged to breathe into the different body areas. Through this approach, patients localize regions of strength and wellbeing.[vi]

These resources are anchored by bilateral stimulation through the butterfly hug.

- Emergency kit: 10 things, activities, contact details of third persons etc., that convey safety/security, which are available at all times and are executable by patients themselves, which create distance and

---

[iv] Bilateral stimulation can be defined as visual, auditory or tactile stimuli in a rhythmic left-right pattern.

[v] Patients are asked to cross their arms across their chest, as if they were holding themselves. As they experience anxiety or fear, they may tap alternately left and right at a comfortable speed. After tapping for a while, patients are advised to take a deep breath and become aware of how they are feeling. If levels of anxiety or fear do not change, they should continue to tap (please note this exercise may not work for everyone). The butterfly hug can be applied as often as is necessary for patients in order to settle them.

help bridge the time when suddenly overwhelming feelings emerge. These things should be trigger-free in any case. Patients orientate themselves according to which of those things have helped so far, and which promote the ability to act. This list or symbol should always be easily accessible (wallet, smartphone, computer)

- Exercises to get into the here and now, for example the 5-4-3-2-1 exercise by Y. Dolan[14]: patients are asked to rest their eyes on a point in space that is pleasant to look at, and then start to name five things that they see here and now, then five things that they hear and finally five haptic perceptions. The sequence of each modality is then repeated four times, three times, twice, and eventually only once. 'I can see, I can hear, I can feel...' The same perceptions can be mentioned in the following rounds and, if other sensory perceptions also come along, can be changed e.g. from seeing to hearing. The practitioner can encourage the answers through a short 'yes' or 'hmmm'. When used as crisis intervention, for example when patients lose themselves in flashbacks, the exercise can also be performed in a more directive way, and the practitioner can offer patients some perceptions for verification: 'look at the white curtain' etc. If patients do not react at least non-verbally, it can be preceded more directly: 'You see the green bottle of water, right? What else do you see?' The aim is to draw attention - away from a focus of emotionally stressful thoughts - to the outside environment, to anchor it in the present and re-establish a verifiable contact with patients through a 'yes-attitude'.

- Bank vault exercise: this is a distancing exercise, where thoughts or experiences that are burdening are stored for later, until patients are able and want to deal with them. Unpleasant images and memories are deposited and can later - if necessary - be brought up again in a more protected situation. Also, stressful thoughts/experiences that come out at the end of a treatment session may be held until the next meeting, and it may sometimes not be permanently possible

to store things in a vault. In this case, the exercise should be repeated.

- Inner Observer: strengthening and training of an inner observer or witness, who is working closely with the neutral current self. Within the trauma confrontation process, both are to be situated in a safe place, in order to meet the trauma from a safe distance. All experiencing parts remain in security/safety and the practitioner always ensures that this is the case.

- Inner safe place: patients are supported to develop an inward image of a place where they feel absolutely safe, comfortable and secure. This is envisioned with as many senses as possible (*VAKOG - visual, auditory, kinesthetic, olfactory, gustatory*) and can additionally be bilaterally anchored through the butterfly hug. The *perception of security/safety* is checked on a measuring scale of 0-7 (0 = not at all safe, 7 = perfectly safe).

Confrontation phase

A clearly defined setting is to be used where the trauma situation can be worked on. In the confrontation phase it is important on the part of the practitioner that patients maintain and keep contact with their resources.

Implementation

1 A stop signal is agreed with patients, in case the intensity of the activation supersedes the tolerance range, or in case patients do not want to continue for other reasons. The patient's right to a clear stop signal also supports their self-determination and control over the situation.

2 To establish the inner safe place

3 Synchronization with silence (Box 38.2)

4 There are several ways to begin treatment with associated content experience:

- The osteopath asks the patient for content experience, images, sensations, feelings, memories, etc., that correlate with the palpation of dysfunctional tissue regions, or the patient spontaneously and unprompted reports stressful content experience during palpation.

[vi] If nowhere feels at all comfortable, patients are asked to feel where it is most uncomfortable and where it feels less unpleasant. The difference is to be worked on, comparing subjective feelings before and after treatment.

Box 38.2

Synchronization with silence

For an osteopath, to touch means to listen, to be there, to wait with gentle attention for the moment, until the tissues speak, and to learn to understand its own story. The ability of the practitioner to assume a state of silence and to be receptive to the stillness is essential in this process. The more practitioners have learned to integrate their own downsides, and consciously allow polar personality traits some space, the more they will be able to synchronize with silence. The extent of the ability to be able to experience silence is in direct relation to the conscious differentiation, relativization and integration of one's own sensory, mental, and psycho-emotional conditioning or restrictive patterns of perception. Thus, it is an expression of one's own development of consciousness. Maturation, inner balance, being centered in the presence, in silence and in "being", the ability to open up to life (instead of trying to control and manipulate it), to be able to give oneself up, the access to one's own vulnerability and self-awareness will have a direct impact on the therapeutic interaction and on a process of palpation which is free of judgment. The conditioned perceptions and attitudes of the practitioner cannot be arbitrarily changed overnight, but may significantly influence the extent and quality of the silence to which the practitioner can get into contact. The prerequisite for a genuine synchronization with deeper levels of being in others assumes the practitioner's own authentic awareness of these levels, where each aspect of life is enclosed (relationships and perspectives of the body, partner, children, friends, "enemies", sex, food, holidays, money, power, etc.). Thus, a more mature consciousness opens up gradually, not only by being awake but also in deep sleep, and an openness towards silence without expectations.

- The patient performs a scan of the entire body and anchors these by bilateral stimulation. Subsequently, the patient identifies regions of discomfort and the osteopath contacts these regions through palpation.

- Alternatively, the patient identifies a stressful content experience and mentions body regions that are particularly associated with these, as a starting point for the palpatory approach of the osteopath.

5 If the patient responds by sympathetic or immobility signs: *assessment of load* (scale of 0-10: 0-1 = no load, 10 = maximum load)

- Clarify whether sufficient competence on the part of the practitioner and resources from the patient are available in order to continue.

6 Contact with the palpated tissue region: the practitioner follows with his eyes the field of the region around the palpated tissue. Patients are supported, in that they experience their interoception/proprioception and VAKOG during osteopathic palpation:

- *VAKOG* of the palpated somatic dysfunction
  - Body sensation: size, strength / softness, vibration, tension, permeability, pain, elasticity, etc.
  - Associated visual impressions: images, landscapes, figures, people, light / dark, black / white or colour, what colour, etc.
  - Associated noises
  - Associated odor
  - Associated taste

- Are there (emotionally stressful) memories or thoughts occurring during the palpation of somatic dysfunction

- The patient may give the somatic dysfunction and specific body parts a voice: what does it want to tell me? What do you want to tell me? (Box 38.1 - parts therapy)

7 **Assessment of load** (scale of 0-10: 0-1 = no load, 10 = maximum load)/ the intensity level of inner experience: Imagine your worst moment. What did you think during that moment? Checking the sense of safety/security

- Which positive thought is strengthening in this situation? *Validity of Cognition*: How confidently is this felt on a scale of 1-7 (1 = totally unbelievable, 7 = totally believable)

- Now, when you're thinking about it, how distressing is the burdensome experience / the picture now for you? *Subjective units of disturbance*: 0 = no disturbance, 10 = worst disturbance the patient can imagine

8 Patient follows the personal experience *(VAKOG)*, while the osteopath palpates the tissue dynamics and follows the body region with his eyes.

9 Anchoring in the state of myelinated vagus: contacting stressful traumatic conditions can trigger a slight sympathetic arousal. The osteopath, however, ensures that the patient does not descend into an overly strong sympathetic state of excitement or vagal unmyelinated rigid immobility, in order to avoid re-traumatization. To prevent the first of these, patients may be asked to keep quiet and breathe slowly. In the second, patients can gently and carefully deepen their breathing. Patients breathe gently into their stomach and try to relax their face. Should the state of excitement increase to that extent that patients, in spite of these approaches, struggle to find themselves in the here and now, the practitioner will use dissociation stop techniques (Box 38.3) in order to break the contact with the trauma experience. In this event, the patient's resources and tolerance range are not yet sufficiently developed to be able to cope with this trauma. In this case, treatment should initially focus on stability and resource work.

10 *Assessment of load* (scale of 0-10: 0-1 = no load, 10 = maximum load):The patient identifies the emotion

Box 38.3
Dissociation stop techniques

Should patients be at risk of slipping into re-traumatisation, i.e. because their resources are insufficient to deal with stressful memories in a myelinated vagal state, the contact to the trauma experience should be interrupted by Dissociation stop techniques.

Examples of these specific techniques are:

- Making eye contact

- Specifically address the adult proportion of the patient

- Change of posture (upright sitting or standing, neck straightened)

- Moving around in the treatment room

- Interruption of patterns of any kind, i.e. open the window, sip some water

- The 5-4-3-2-1 exercise

- Cognitive re-orientation (place, date, time)

- Giving tasks that may seem absurd in the context of the treatment, such as riddles; reverse calculation; patient has to smell sharp/pungent odours (i.e. camphor); sharp, sour or bitter substances are placed into the mouth of the patient (i.e. ascorbic acid, pepper, chilli); cold, hot, or hard tactile experiences (i.e. spikey ball, cold water, brush massage); or targeted use of loud, shrill dissonant sounds and the stressful experience and describes it as precisely as possible (*VAKOG*).

11 Palpation of tissue dynamics of somatic dysfunction and associated inner experience of the patient: during palpation of somatic dysfunction, patients are assisted to remain within the inner experience in the hope of completing the burdensome emotion/situation (*VAKOG*).

12 The sense of safety, related body representation, and the myelinated vagal state are assessed and supported if necessary.

13 The palpation of tissue dynamics continues.

14 At the same time, a bilateral stimulation via lateral eye movement takes place (kinesthetics or sounds are also possible); initially a short period of 5-20 seconds.

15 Re-checking the sense of security/safety and the associated body representation; if this state is well established, then bilateral stimulation can be carefully extended, accompanied by simultaneous palpation of tissue dynamics

16 Neurogenic tremors according to Berceli[15]: at the same time, the process can be supported by neurogenic tremors: the soles of the feet are placed together; the knees are flexed and fall outwards. The pelvis is lifted up for a few minutes, while the knees stay relaxed and open. Then the pelvis is brought back to the treatment table and the knees still remain open for about a minute. Here, an involuntary trembling or shaking may occur in the legs. Then the knees will be moved towards each other for about five centimetres and remain in this position for a few minutes. There may be reinforcement of the trembling or shaking in the legs. Again, the knees can be moved further towards each other for five centimetres. The tremors and shaking may also spread over the entire legs and pelvis, and even the back. Repeat the process and continue as long as the feeling is not unpleasant for the patient. However, perform for no longer than 15 minutes, as otherwise the body can get tired.

17 Re-checking the sense of security/safety and possible support

18 Assessment of load (scale of 0-10: 0-1 = no load, 10 = maximum load)

19 If the load has decreased, but not yet reached 0-1, the process can be continued.

20 Palpation of tissue dynamics in the areas of somatic dysfunction, bilateral stimulation, neurogenic tremors as necessary

21 Re-orientation in the here and now

22 Repetition of these steps

23 At the end of the process a resource situation is retrieved, and what has been achieved is anchored; if the load intensity has not reached 0-1, if required, the bank vault exercise can be carried out (see above)

Integration in everyday life, stress management and a new beginning

a A positive reassessment of the situation can be performed: 'How am I doing compared to last year and towards other people?'

b Patients practice active problem-oriented action and learn how to realistically evaluate the control of a given situation (only valid if the situation is controllable anyway)

c Patients learn to accept irreversibility

References

[1] Tagore, R. Sadhana: The Realization of Life. London, UK: Macmillan; 1915:188.

[1a] Porges, SW. (2011). The Polyvagal Theory: Neurophysiological Foundations of Emotions, Attachment, Communication, and Self-regulation. New York: WW Norton.

[2] Valins, S. Cognitive effects of false heart-rate feedback. J. Personal. Soc. Psychol. 4: p 400-408, 1966.

[3] Ekman, P. (1993). Facial expression and emotion. American Psychologist, 48, 384-392.

[4] LeDoux, J. E. (2001). Das Netz der Gefühle. München: Deutscher Taschenbuch Verlag.

[5] LeDoux, J. E. (2002). Synaptic Self: How our brains become who we are. New York: Viking Penguin.

[6] Gutberlet, I. & Miltner, W. H. (1999). Therapeutic effects on differential electrocortical processing of

phobic objects in spider and snake phobics. Internat. J. of Psychophysiology, 33, 180.

[7]Van der Kolk BA, *Psychological Trauma*. Washington DC, American Psychiatric Press, 1987.

[8]Fast, K., Markowitsch, H. J. (2004). Neuropsychologie des posttraumatischen Stresssyndroms. In S. Lautenbacher & S. Gauggel (Hrsg.), Neuropsychologie psychischer Störungen (S. 223-248). Berlin: Springer.

[9]Morgan, M. A., LeDoux, J. E. (1995). Differential contribution of dorsal and ventral medial prefrontal cortex to the acquisition and extinction of conditioned fear in rats. Behavioral Neuroscience, 109(4), 681-688.

[10]Morschitzky, H. Angst als biologisches Geschehen - Neurobiologische Modelle der Angstentstehung in: http://www.panikattacken.at/angst-biologie/angst-biologie.htm. Access 20th Oct 2015.

[11]Seligman, Martin E. P. (2005) Der Glücks-Faktor. Warum Optimisten länger leben. Bastei Lübbe.

[12]Seligman, Martin E. P. (2012) Flourish - Wie Menschen aufblühen. Kösel-Verlag, München.

[13]Reddemann, L. (2010) Imagination als heilsame Kraft. Zur Behandlung von Traumafolgen mit ressourcenorientierten Verfahren. Cotta'sche Buchhandlung, Stuttgard.

[14]Dolan, Y. (1991): Resolving Sexual Abuse: Solution-Focused Therapy and Ericksonian Hypnosis for Adult Survivors. Norton & Company.

[15]Berceli, D. (2010) Neurogenes Zittern. Eine körperorientierte Behandlungsmethode für Traumata in großen Bevölkerungsgruppen. Trauma & Gewalt 2010; 4: 148-156.

[16]Berne, E. (1977). Intuition and Ego States, San Francisco: TA Press.

[17]Berne, E. (2001). Die Transaktionsanalyse in der Psychotherapie. Paderborn: Junfermann.

[18]Watkins, J.G. & Watkins, H.H. (2003). Ego-States. Theorie und Therapie. Heidelberg: Cari-AuerSysteme.

[19]Schmidt, G. (2005). Einführung in die hypnosystemische Therapie und Beratung. Heidelberg: CariAuer-Systeme

[20]Stone, H. & S. (1994) Du bist viele. Heyne Verlag, München.

[21]Satir, V. (1978). Your Many Faces. Berkeley, California: Celestial Arts.

Note: Page number followed by f and t indicates figure and table only.

D